AF273050

Drug pocket plus

Contributing Authors:
Albrecht, Carter, Casper, Cheung, Daley, D'Souza, Endres, Freytes, Gilkeson, Jazieh, Kaliszky, Krystal, Levine, Lien, Mukherjee, Pritchard, Russ, Smolinske, Tyor, Ur, Walker, Walsh, Woodson
Cover Illustration: Jaqueline Heumueller, Dipl.-Ing. Verlagsherstellung (FH)
Printer: Koesel GmbH & Co. KG., Am Buchweg 1, 87452 Altusried-Krugzell, Germany
Publisher: Börm Bruckmeier Publishing LLC, www.media4u.com

IMPORTANT NOTICE - PLEASE READ!
This book is based on information from sources believed to be reliable, and every effort has been made to make the book as complete and accurate as possible and to describe generally accepted practices based on information available as of the printing date, but its accuracy and completeness cannot be guaranteed. Despite the best efforts of author and publisher, the book may contain errors, and the reader should use the book only as a general guide and not as the ultimate source of information about the subject matter.
This book is not intended to reprint all of the information available to the author or publisher on the subject, but rather to simplify, complement and supplement other available sources. The reader is encouraged to read all available material and to consult the package insert and other references to learn as much as possible about the subject.
This book is sold without warranties of any kind, expressed or implied, and the publisher and author disclaim any liability, loss or damage caused by the content of this book.
IF YOU DO NOT WISH TO BE BOUND BY THE FOREGOING CAUTIONS AND CONDITIONS , YOU MAY RETURN THIS BOOK TO THE PUBLISHER FOR A FULL REFUND.

Printed in Germany
ISBN 1-59103-217-2
Koesel GmbH & CO. KG

Preface to the First Edition

In clinical drug therapy, there are, at bottom, two major problems.

On the one hand, a known diagnosis brings with it the question of which drug or drug combination can be used in this particular case. The physician wants help in the form of concrete therapy schemes. For this problem, our **Drug Therapy pocket** offers well-structured overviews for all common diagnoses.

The second major problem concerns the drug itself. To avoid medication errors, specific information on dosage instructions, dosage forms, common brand names, etc. is necessary. You will find the answers in our **Drug pocket**.

In this book, we have attempted to combine the information that addresses both of these problems. **Drug pocket plus** incorporates the complete contents of both **Druq pocket** and **Drug Therapy pocket**. In addition, we have included a comprehensive system of cross-references. This kind of networking creates bridges between the information on drug therapy for a given disease and the information on a particular drug.

We hope that the concept of the **Drug pocket plus** will make your work with patients easier. Since any new concept can always be improved upon, we would be very happy to hear your comments, positive or negative. Please e-mail us at info@media4u.com.

The authors and the publisher   August 2004

Contributing Authors

Drugs

Andreas Russ, MD
(all subjects)

Department of Internal Medicine,
Clinic of Rosenheim, Germany

Therapies

Helmut Albrecht, MD
(Infections)

Assistant Professor, Division of Infectious Diseases,
Emory University, Atlanta, GA

Timothy D. Carter, MD
(Neurology)

Associate Professor, Department of Neurology
Medical University of South Carolina, Charleston, SC

Daniel S. Casper, MD
(Ophthalmology)

Assistant Clinical Professor,
Department of Ophthalmology, College of Physicians
& Surgeons, Columbia University, New York, NY

Pamela Cheung, MD
(Ophthalmology)

Assistant Professor, Department of Ophthalmology,
University of Tennessee Health Science Center,
Memphis, TN

Charles L. Daley, MD
(Respiratory System)

Associate Professor, Division of Pulmonary and Critical
Care Medicine, San Francisco General Hospital,
University of California San Francisco, CA

D. Cyril D'Souza, MD
(Psychiatry)

Associate Professor, Department of Psychiatry, School
of Medicine, Yale University School of Medicine,
New Haven, CT

Stefan Endres, MD
(Gastroenterology)

Professor, Chief, Division of Clinical Pharmacology,
University of Munich, Munich, Germany

Cesar O. Freytes, MD
(Hematology)

Associate Professor, FACP,
Director, Adult Bone Marrow Transplant Program,
University of Texas Health Science Center at San
Antonio, TX

Gary Gilkeson, MD
(Rheumatology)

Professor, Division of Rheumatology and Immunology,
Department of Medicine, Medical University of South
Carolina, Charleston, SC

Abdul-Rahman Jazieh, MD
(Oncology)
Associate Professor, M.P.H.,
Co-director, Thoracic Oncology, Barrett Cancer Center
Department of Internal Medicine, University of
Cincinnati, Cincinnati, OH

Zoltan Kaliszky, MD
(Neurology)
Department of Neurology
Medical University of South Carolina, Charleston, SC

John H. Krystal, MD
(Psychiatry)
Professor, Department of Psychiatry,
Yale University School of Medicine,
New Haven, CT

Norman Levine, MD
(Dermatology)
Professor, Chief, Dermatology Section,
Department of Medicine, Arizona Health Sciences
Center, University of Arizona, Tucson, AZ

Y. Howard Lien, MD
(Fluids, Electrolytes,
Urology, Nephrology)
Professor, Chief, Section of Nephrology,
Department of Medicine, College of Medicine,
University of Arizona, Tucson, AZ

Debabrata Mukherjee, MD
(Cardiovascular System)
Assistant Professor, Department of Internal Medicine,
UMHS Cardiovascular Center, University of Michigan,
Ann Arbor, MI

Paul B. Pritchard, III, MD
(Neurology)
Professor, Department of Neurology
Medical University of South Carolina, Charleston, SC

Susan Smolinske, Ph.D.
(Toxicology)
Managing Director, Regional Poison Control Center,
Children's Hospital of Michigan, Wayne State
University, Detroit, MI

William R. Tyor, MD
(Neurology)
Professor, Department of Neurology
Medical University of South Carolina, Charleston, SC

Ehud Ur, MB, FRCP
(Metabolic, Endocrine)
Head, Division of Endocrinology & Metabolism
Dalhousie University, Halifax, Nova Scotia, Canada

Aljoeson Walker, MD
(Neurology)
Assistant Professor, Department of Neurology
Medical University of South Carolina, Charleston, SC

Tracey Walsh, Pharm.D.
(Hematology)
Pharm.D., BCOP,
Adult Bone Marrow Transplant Program, University of
Texas Health Science Center at San Antonio, TX

Gayle Ellen Woodson, MD
(ENT)
Professor, FACS, FRCS (C),
Department of Otolaryngology
University of Florida, Gainesville, FL

Additional titles in this series:

Anatomy pocket
Canadian Drug pocket
Differential Diagnosis pocket
Drug pocket
Drug Therapy pocket
ECG pocket
EMS pocket
Homeopathy pocket
Medical Abbreviations pocket
Medical Spanish pocket
Medical Spanish Dictionary pocket
Medical Spanish pocket plus
Normal Values pocket
Respiratory pocket

Contents

14.   Ophthalmology   377

14 A. Ophthalmology – Drugs   377

14 B. Ophthalmology – Therapies   386

15.   ENT   408

15 A. ENT – Drugs   408

15 B. ENT – Therapies   416

19.   Toxicology   470

19 A. Toxicology – Drugs   470

19 B. Toxicology – Therapies   472

20.   Index   485

1 A. Emergency - Drugs

Adenosine	→38
Adenocard *Inj 3mg/ml* **Adenoscan** *Inj 3mg/ml*	**SVT** (not AF) →61: 6mg rapidly IV, if no response, in 1-2min 12mg IV, then 12-18mg IV prn; **CH** ini 50µg/kg IV, incr to 100µg/kg, then to 200µg/kg
Albuterol	→95
Ventolin *MDI 100µg/puff*	**Asthma** →101: 1-2puffs q4-6h prn
Atropine	→38
Atropine Sulfate *Inj 0.04, 0.1, 0.3, 0.4, 0.5, 0.6, 0.8, 1mg/ml*	**Bradycardia** →63/**CPR:** 0.5mg IV/ET, rep prn in 1min, max 2mg; **CH** (CPR): 0.02mg/kg/dose, total dose ≥ 0.1mg; **organophosphate intoxication** →483: 0.05mg/kg IV
Biperiden	→294
Akineton *Inj 5mg/ml*	**Drug-induced extrapyramidal DO** →344: 2mg IM/IV q30min prn, max 8mg/24h; **CH** 0.04mg/kg/dose or 1.2mg/square meter/dose IM, rep prn q30min, max 4 doses/d
Bretylium	→37
Bretylol *Inj 50mg/ml*	**VF, VT** →62, →20: 5mg/kg IV, prn rep 10mg/kg IV in 10min
Cimetidine	→117
Tagamet *Inj 300mg/2ml, 300mg/50ml*	**Allergy/anaphylaxis:** 300mg IV/IM or 5mg/kg IV/IM
Dextrose	→155
Dextrose *Inj 50% Dextrose/ 50ml vial*	**Hypoglycemia** →167: 25g (50ml of D50W) IV; **CH** >6mo: 0.5-1g/kg (D25W 2-4ml/kg/dose) slowly IV, max 25g/dose, <6mo: 0.2-0.4g/kg (D10W 2-4ml/kg) slowly IV
Diazepam	→287, →330
Diastat *Gel (rectal) 2.5mg, 5mg, 10mg, 15mg, 20mg* **Valium** *Inj 5mg/ml* **Generics** *Inj 5mg/ml*	**Seizures** →312, **status epilepticus** →311: 5-10mg IV, max rate 1mg/min, rep prn q5min, max 30mg, or 10mg PR, rep prn; **CH** 1 mo-5 y: 0.2-0.5mg/kg slowly IV, rep prn q5min, max 5mg, or 0.5mg/kg PR, rep prn in 4-12h, >5 y: 1mg IV, rep prn q5min, max 10mg or 0.3mg/kg PR, rep prn in 4-12h; **sedation** →338: 2-10mg IV/IM, rep prn in 4h; **muscle spasm** →304: 5-10mg IV/IM, rep prn in 4h
Digoxin	→40
Lanoxin *Tab 0.0625mg, 0.125mg, 0.25mg, 0.5mg Inj 0.1mg/ml, 0.25mg/ml*	**AF** →60, **Af with tachyarrhythmia** →60: ini 0.5mg IV, rep in 4h, 0.25mg PO in 8h + 12h
Diltiazem	→29
Cardizem *Inj 5mg/ml*	**AF** (rapid) →60: 20mg (0.25mg/kg) IV x 2min, rep in 15min prn 30mg (35mg/kg) IV, then prn inf at 5-15mg/h

Diphenhydramine →331, →409
Benadryl *Inj 10mg/ml, 50mg/ml* | **Anaphylaxis** →21: 1mg/kg IV/IM, max 50mg single dose, rep prn q2-3h, max 400mg/d; **CH** 1.25mg/kg IV/IM qid, max 300mg/d

Dobutamine →22
Dobutrex *Inj 250mg/20ml* | **Low-output-failure:** 1mg/ml (250mg in 250ml D5W) at 2.5-15µg/kg/min, max 40µg/kg/min; →54

Dopamine →22
Intropine *Inj 40mg/ml, 80mg/ml, 160mg/ml* | **Acute hypotension** →49: 400mg in 250ml D5W (1600µg/ml) at 2-20µg/kg/min IV, ini 2-5µg/kg/min, incr by 1-4µg/kg/min q10-30min, max 50µg/kg/min; →54

Epinephrine →22
Adrenalin/Epinephrine *Inj 0.01mg/ml (1:100,000), 0.1mg/ml (1:10,000), 1mg/ml (1:1,000)* | **Cardiac arrest** →20: 1mg (sol 1:10,000) IV/ET q3-5min prn; **CH** ini 0.01mg/kg IV, then prn 0.1mg/kg IV, max 0.2mg/kg IV (sol 1:10,000); **anaphylaxis** →21: 0.3-0.5mg/kg IV/IM/SC, rep q10-15min prn

Esmolol →24
Brevibloc *Inj 10mg/ml, 250mg/ml* | **SVT** →60: ini 500µg/kg IV x 1min, then 50µg/kg/min IV x 4min, if response, do not change rate >25µg/kg/min; if no response, rep 500µg/kg IV x 1min, then 100µg/kg/min x 4min, prn rep 500µg/kg IV x 1min, then incr inf by 50µg/kg/min q4min, max 200µg/kg/min

Etomidate →283
Amidate *Inj 2mg/ml* | **Anesthesia, induction:** 0.3mg/kg IV x 15-60sec, maint 0.01-0.02mg/kg/min; **CH** >10 y: 0.3mg/kg IV x 15-60sec

Fentanyl →270, →282
Sublimaze *Inj 50µg/ml* | **Anaesthesia:** 50-100µg IV/IM; →302

Flumazenil →471
Romazicon *Inj 0.1mg/ml* | **Benzodiazepine overdose** →475: 0.2-0.5mg IV x 30sec, rep q60sec, max 3mg

Furosemide →33
Lasix *Inj 10mg/ml* | **Edema** →163: 20-40mg IV/IM, rep prn in 2h, then incr prn by 20mg > q2h until response; **CH** 1mg/kg/dose, prn incr by 0.25-0.5mg/dose q4-12h, max 10mg/kg/24h; **acute pulmonary edema** →49: ini 40mg slowly IV, prn incr in 1h by 40mg

Haloperidol →329
Haldol *Inj (IM) 5mg/ml* | **Agitation** →338: 2-5mg IM, rep prn q1-8h

Heparin →70
Heparin Sodium *1,000 U/ml, 2,000 U/ml, 5,000 U/ml, 10,000 U/ml, 20,000 U/ml, 40,000 U/ml* | **DVT** →67/**pulmonary embolism** →112: ini 80U/kg IV, then 18 U/kg/h, adjust by PTT testing; **CH** ini 50U/kg IV, then 10-25 U/kg/h

Hyoscyamine →127, →423

Levsin, Generics *Tab 0.125mg, Tab (SL) 0.125mg, Inj 0.5mg/ml* | **GI hypermotility/urinary spasm** →436: 0.25-0.5mg IV/IM/SC prn q4h, max 4 doses/d; **CH** 2-12y. 0.0625mg-0.125mg/dose PO/SL, prn q4h, max 0.75mg/24h, >12y: 0.125-0.25mg/dose PO/SL, prn q4h, max 1.5mg/24h

Ketamine →283

Ketalar *Inj 10mg/ml, 50mg/ml, 100mg/ml* | **Sedation + analgesia:** 2-4mg/kg IM or 0.2-0.75mg/kg IV x 2-3min, then inf of 5-20 µg/kg/min; **CH** 2-10mg/kg IM or 0.2-1mg/kg IV x 2-3min, then inf of 5-20 µg/kg/min, 50% dose reduction in hypovolemia

Lidocaine →39, →285

Xylocaine *Inj 0.5% (5mg/ml), 1% (10mg/ml), 2% (20mg/ml), 4% (40mg/ml)* | **VT/VF** →62: ini 1mg/kg IV, then prn 0.5mg/kg IV q5-10min, max 3mg/kg, maint 1-4mg/min; **CH** 1mg/kg/dose IV q5-10min, max 5 mg/kg, maint 10-50 µg/kg/min; **local anesthesia:** 0.5-1% for infiltration, max 300mg

Lorazepam →289

Ativan *Inj 2mg/ml, 4mg/ml* | **Status epilepticus** →311: 4mg slowly IV, may rep after 10-15min, max 8mg; **CH** 0.1mg/kg IV, max 4mg/dose

Magnesium Sulfate →141

Generics *Inj 100mg/ml (10%), 500mg/ml (50%)* | **Ventricular arrhythmia** →62: 1-6g IV x 15min, then 3-20mg/min; **eclampsia:** ini 1-4g IV x 2-4min as 10-20% sol, maint 2-3g/h IV inf or 4-5g IM as 50% sol, rep prn q4h

Mepivacaine →285

Carbocaine *1% (10mg/ml), 1.5% (15mg/ml), 2% (20mg/ml)* | **Brachial nerve block:** 50-400mg (1-2% sol.); **epidural nerve block:** 150-300mg (1-2% sol.); **local infiltration:** up to 400mg (0.5-1% sol.)

Methylprednisolone →149

Solu-Medrol *Inj 0.04, 0.125, 0.5g, 1, 2g/vial* | **Status asthmaticus:** 1-2mg/kg IV; →102 **anaphylaxis:** 125mg IV/IM or 2mg/kg IV/IM

Methohexital →282

Brevital *Inj 0.5g, 2.5g, 5g* | **Induction of anesthesia:** 1-1.5mg/kg IV (10mg/ml sol)

Metoclopramide →125

Reglan *Inj 5mg/ml* | **Nausea** →453: 10mg IV q2-4h; **CH** 0.1-0.2mg/kg q6-8h

Morphine →270

Morphine Sulfate *Inj 0.5, 1, 2, 3, 4, 5, 8, 10, 15, 20, 25, 50mg/ml* | **Pulmonary edema** →49: 2-8mg IV; **pain** →302: 2-10mg IV, max 20mg prn q2-6h or 1-10mg/h IV inf, max 80mg/h or 5-20mg IM/SC; **CH** 0.1-0.2mg/kg IV/IM/SC q2-4h, max 15mg/dose or 0.025-2.6mg/kg/h IV inf

Naloxone →272

Narcan *Inj 0.02mg/ml, 0.4mg/ml, 1mg/ml* | **Opioid reversal (after anesthesia):** 0.1-0.2mg IV q2-3min prn; **CH** 0.01mg/kg IV, rep q2-3min; **opioid overdose** →483: 0.4-2mg IV, rep q2-3min, max 10mg; **CH** <20kg: 0.1mg/kg IV/IM/ET q2-3min, >20kg: 2mg IV, rep q2-3min

Nitroglycerin →36

Nitroglycerin *Inj 5mg/ml, 10mg/ml, 25mg in 250ml D5W, 50mg in 250ml D5W, 100mg in 250ml D5W*
Nitrolingual
Spray 0.4mg/spray
Nitrostat *Tab (SL) 0.3mg, 0.4mg, 0.6mg*

Acute angina pectoris →50: 1-2 sprays SL, rep prn q5min, max 3 sprays or 0.4mg Tab SL, rep prn q5min, max 3 doses; **acute MI** →52/**angina pectoris** →50: ini 5µg/min IV as inf of 50mg in 250ml D5W (200µg/ml), incr prn by 5µg/min q3-5min to 20µg/min, then incr prn by 10µg/min

Norepinephrine →22

Levophed *Inj 1mg/ml*

Acute hypotension →49: ini 8-12µg/min IV (4mg in 500ml D5W), maint inf at 2-4µg/min

Oxytocin →449

Pitocin, Syntocinon *Inj 10U/ml*

Postpartum hemorrhage: 3-10U IM or 10U IV in 1L NS at 100-200ml/h

Pancuronium →284

Pavulon *Inj 1mg/ml, 2mg/ml*

Paralysis (anesthesia): 0.04-0.1mg/kg IV

Phenobarbital →289

Luminal, Generics *Inj 65mg/ml, 130mg/ml*

Status epilepticus →311: 10-20mg/kg IV, max rate 60mg/min, max 20mg/kg

Phenylephrine →23

Neo-Synephrine *Inj 2mg/ml*

Acute hypotension →49 (mild-mod.): 200µg IV, ini max 500µg IV, rep prn q10-15min; **acute hypotension** (severe): inf 10mg in 500ml D5W, ini at 100-180µg/min, prn decr to 40-60µg/min

Phenytoin →289

Dilantin *Inj 50mg/ml*

Status epilepticus →311: ini 15-18mg/kg IV, max rate 0.5 mg/kg/min, max 30mg/kg, rep 100mg PO/IV q6-8h; **CH** 15-20mg/kg IV, max rate 1-3mg/kg/min

Procainamide →40

Pronestyl *Inj 100mg/ml, 500mg/ml*

VF (refractory)/ paroxysmal SVT with wide QRS →53: 20-30mg/min or 100mg IV q5min, until max 17mg/kg, BP ↓ , dysrhythmia suppressed or QRS/PR widens >50%, maint inf of 2g in 250ml D5W at 2-6 mg/min

Propranolol →24

Inderal *Inj 1mg/ml*

SVT/AF/Af →60: 1-3mg IV, max 1mg/min, rep prn in 2min, rep third dose in >4h; **CH** 0.01-0.15mg/kg IV x 10min, rep prn q6-8h, max 1mg

Rocuronium →284

Zemuron *Inj 10mg/ml*

Paralysis (anesthesia): 0.6-1.2mg/kg IV

Sodium Bicarbonate

Sodium bicarbonate 8.4% *Inj 1mEq/ml (84mg/ml)*

Metabolic acidosis →167: 1mEq/kg IV, rep prn 0.5mEq/kg IV q10min; **CH** 1mEq/kg IV, then 0.5mEq/kg prn q10min

Sodium Nitroprusside →31

Nipride *Inj 50mg/5ml*
Nitropress *Inj 50mg/2ml*

HTN (malignant) →48: 0.3-10µg/kg/min IV; max 70mg/kg within 14d;
CH 0.3-10µg/kg IV

Terbutaline →95, →448

Bricanyl *Inj 1mg/ml*

Asthma →102: 0.25mg SC q20min, max 3 doses;
preterm labor: 0.25-0.5mg SC q2h

Theophylline →97

Generics *Inj 200mg/50ml,*
200mg/100ml, 400mg/100ml,
400mg/250ml, 400mg/500ml,
400mg/1,000ml, 800mg/250mg

Acute bronchospasm: ini 4.6mg/kg IV x 6min, then inf at 0.5mg/kg/h;
→102, →105

Thiopental →282

Pentothal *Inj 250mg/vial,*
400mg/vial, 500mg/vial, 1g/vial,
5g/vial

Anesthesia induction: 3-5mg/kg IV;
convulsions: 75-125mg IV (3-5ml of a 2.5% sol)

Verapamil →29

Calan *Inj 2.5mg/ml*

SVT/AF/Af →59: 5-10mg IV x 2min, rep prn 10mg IV in 30min;
CH >2 y or >15kg (paroxysmal SVT): ini 0.1-0.3mg/kg IV x 2min,
max 5mg/dose, rep prn in 30min, max 10mg

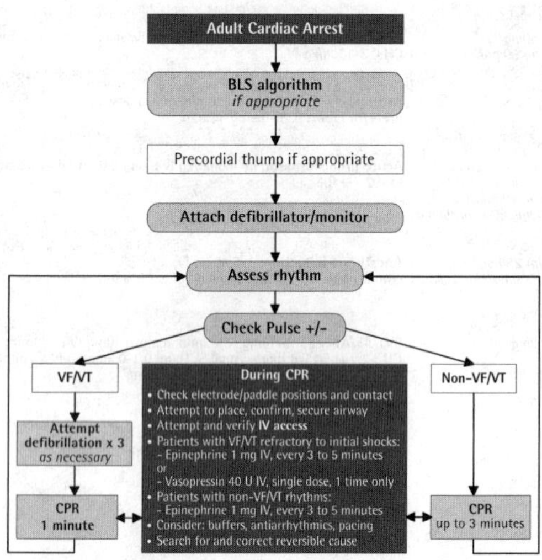

Reference: American Heart Association; Circulation. 2000; 102 (suppl I): I-143

Drug pocket 2005 for PDA (460 kb, US $ 16.95)
Drug Therapy pocket for PDA (840 kb, US $ 16.95)
Homeopathy pocket for PDA (2040 kb, US $ 16.95)
ICD-9-CM 2004 pocket for PDA
(5323 kb, US $ 24.95)
Medical Abbreviations pocket for PDA
(1279 kb, US $ 16.95)
Medical Spanish pocket for PDA
(670 kb, US $ 16.95)
Medical Spanish Dictionary pocket for PDA
(2343 kb, US $ 16.95)
Medical Spanish pocket plus
(2487 kb, US $ 24.95)
Differential Diagnosis pocket
(867 kb, US $ 24.95)
ECG pocket (670 kb, US $ 24.95)
coming soon: Normal Values pocket
(5323 kb, US $ 16.95)

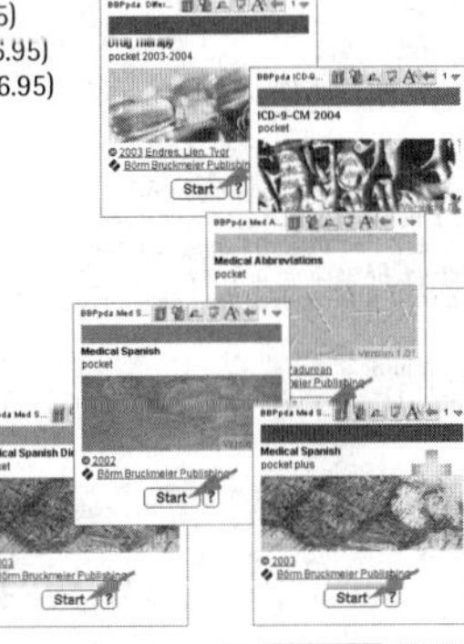

Online-Shop, PDA demo files, FAQs...   http://pda. media4u .com

2 A. Cardiovascular – Drugs

2 A.1 Vasopressors

MA/EF (dobutamine): primarily β-rec. agon., pos. inotropic, no vasoconstriction; **MA/EF** (dopamine): dose-dependent dopamine-, β-/α-rec. agon, renal vasodilation, cardiac output ↓, vasoconstr.;
MA/EF (epinephrine): primarily β-rec. agon., pos. inotropic, chronotropic + bathmotropic effect, syst. BP ↑, diast. BP ↓, bronchodilation; **MA/EF** (norepinephrine): primarily α-rec. agonist ⇒ syst./diast. BP ↑;
MA/EF (midodrine): α-adren. agonism on arteriolar + venous rec. ⇒ vascular tone ↑, venous pooling ↓, BP ↑; **MA/EF** (metaraminol) release of norepinephrine + direct α-(β1) rec. agon. ⇒ vasoconstr., BP ↑;
MA/EF (methoxamine): α1 sel. rec. agon. ⇒ periph. resistance ↑, BP ↑ ⇒ sinus bradycardia
AE: hyperglycemia, arrhythmia, angina, hypertensive reactions, headache
CI: thyrotoxicosis, pheochromocytoma, glaucoma, micturition disturbances, high-frequency continuous arrhythmia, combination with systemic β$_2$-sympathomimetics
CI (methoxamine): hypersensitivity to methoxamine, severe HTN, local anesthetics

Dobutamine	EHL 2min, Dur (1x dose) 10min, PRC B, Lact ?
Dobutrex *Inj 12.5mg/ml* **Generics** *Inj 12.5mg/ml, 50mg/100ml, 100mg/100ml, 200mg/100ml, 400mg/100ml, 1.25g/100ml*	**Cardiac decompensation** →54: ini 0.5–1µg/kg/min IV, incr to 2–20µg/kg/min, max 40µg/kg/min

Dopamine	EHL 2min, Dur 10min, PRC C, Lact ?
Intropin *Inj 40mg/ml, 80mg/ml, 160mg/ml* **Generics** *Inj 1.6mg/ml, 40mg/ml, 80mg/ml, 160mg/ml, 80mg/100ml, 160mg/100ml, 320mg/100ml, 640mg/100ml*	**Hypotension** →49, **heart failure** →56: ini 1–5µg/kg/min IV, incr prn by 5–10µg/kg/min increments, max 50µg/kg/min; →54

Ephedrine sulfate	EHL 3h, PRC C, Lact ?
Generics *Inj 50mg/ml*	**Acute hypotension** →49: 25–50mg SC/IM; **CH:** 750µg/kg IV/SC

Epinephrine	Dur 2min, PRC C, Lact ?
Epipen Jr. *Inj (IM) 0.15mg/delivery* **Epi E Z Pen Jr.** *Inj (IM) 0.15mg/delivery* **Epipen E Z Pen** *Inj (IM) 0.3mg/delivery* **Epipen** *Inj (IM) 0.3mg/delivery* **Sus–phrine Sulfite–free** *Inj 1.5mg/amp, 5mg/ml*	**Cardiac arrest** →20: 0.5–1mg IV/ET, rep prn q3–5min; anaphylaxis: 0.3–0.5 mg SC/IM, rep prn q10–15min; **CH :** 0.01mg/kg IV; 0.1mg/kg ET rep prn with 0.1mg/kg IV/ET q3–5min; **anaphylaxis** →21: 0.01mg/kg SC/IM (use 1: 1000 Sol), then 0.1mg/kg IV prn (IV: use 1:10.000)

Metaraminol	Dur 20–60min, PRC C, Lact ?
Aramine *Inj 10mg/ml* **Generics** *Inj 10mg/ml*	**Acute hypotension (in surgery, spinal anesthesia):** 0.5–5mg IV, then inf of 15–100mg in 500ml; 2–10mg SC; DARF: not req

Methoxamine	Dur 10–15min, PRC C, Lact ?
Vasoxyl *Inj 20mg/ml*	**Acute hypotension in spinal anesthesia:** 3–5mg IV; 10–15mg IM; **termination of SVT** →59: 10mg IV over 3–5min

Midodrine	EHL 0.5h, PRC C, Lact ?		
ProAmatine *Tab 2.5mg, 5mg*	**Orthostatic hypotension** →49: ini 10mg PO tid, incr prn to max 40mg/d; DARF: ini 2.5mg tid		
Norepinephrine	Dur 1-2min, PRC C, Lact ?		
Levophed *Inj 1mg/ml*	**Acute hypotensive states** →49: ini 8-12 µg/min IV, maint 2-4 µg/min		
Phenylephrine	PRC C, Lact ?		
Neo-Synephrine *Inj 10mg/ml* **Generics** *Inj 10mg/ml*	**Acute hypotension** →49: 2-5mg SC/IM, max ini 5mg IV, rep prn q1-2h; 0.2-0.5mg slowly IV, max ini 0.5mg IV		

Systemic Beta Adrenergic Agonists →95, α-β-Adrenergic Agonists →96

2 A.2   Beta Blockers

MA: competitive blockage of β-receptors
EF: neg. inotropic + chronotropic ⇒ cardiac output ↓, myocardial O_2 consumption ↓, renin secretion ↓, high-dose nonspecific membrane-stabilizing effect (quinidine-like);
AE: fatigue, dizziness, N/V, sexual ability ↓, AV block, bradycardia, hypotension, heart failure ↑, peripheral vasoconstriction, bronchospasm, insulin secretion ↓, glycogenolysis ↓
CI: congestive heart failure, bradycardia, AV block II°-III°, SA block, sick sinus syndrome, cardiac shock, hypotension, asthma, hypothyroidism

Acebutolol	EHL 3-4h, PRC B, Lact ?	β_1	ISA
Sectral *Cap 200mg, 400mg* **Generics** *Cap 200mg, 400mg*	**HTN** →47: ini 400mg PO qd or 200mg PO bid, maint 400-800mg/d, max 1200mg/d; **ventricular arrhythmia** →63: ini 200mg PO bid, maint 0.6-1.2g/d; DARF: GFR (ml/min) 25-50: 50%; <25: 25%	+	+
Atenolol	EHL 6-7h, PRC D, Lact ?	+	−
Tenormin *Tab 25mg, 50mg, 100mg, Inj 0.5mg/ml* **Generics** *Tab 25mg, 50mg, 100mg*	**Acute MI** →52: 5mg IV over 5min, rep in 10min, follow with 50-100mg PO qd or div bid; **HTN** →47: ini 50mg PO qd, maint 50-100mg/d; **angina** →50: 50-200mg PO qd; DARF: GFR (ml/min) 15-35: max 50mg/d PO/IV; <15: max 25mg/d PO or 50mg/d IV		
Betaxolol	EHL 12-22h, PRC C, Lact ?	+	−
Kerlone *Tab 10, 20mg* **Generics** *Tab 10, 20mg*	**HTN** →47: ini 10mg PO qd, max 20mg/d; DARF: ini 5mg PO, incr by 5mg q14d, max 20mg/d		
Bisoprolol	EHL 10-12.1h, PRC C, Lact ?	+	−
Zebeta *Tab 5mg, 10mg* **Generics** *Tab 5mg, 10mg*	**HTN** →47: 2.5-5mg PO qd, max 20mg/d; DARF: ini 2.5mg PO qd, incr prn		
Carvedilol	EHL 6-10h, PRC C, Lact ?	−	−
Coreg *Tab 3.125mg, 6.25mg, 12.5mg, 25mg*	**Heart failure** →56: ini 3.125mg PO bid incr dose q2 wk as tolerated to max 25mg bid (<85 kg) or 50mg bid (>85 kg); **HTN** →47: ini 6.25mg PO bid, incr prn, max 50mg/d; DARF: not req		

		β_1	ISA
Esmolol	EHL 9min, PRC C, Lact ?		
Brevibloc *Inj 10mg/ml, 250mg/ml*	**SV tachyarrhythmia** →60: 500µg/kg IV over 1min, then 50µg/kg/min IV over 4min; DARF: not req	+	-
Labetalol	EHL 5-8h, PRC C, Lact +	-	(+)
Normodyne *Tab 100mg, 200mg, 300mg, Inj 5mg/ml* **Trandate** *Tab 100mg, 200mg, 300mg, Inj 5mg/ml* **Generics** *Tab 100mg, 200mg, 300mg, Inj 5mg/ml*	**Hypertensive emergency** →48: 20mg slow IV, then 40-80mg IV q10min prn, max 300mg total; **HTN** →47: ini 100mg PO bid, maint 200-400mg bid, max 2400mg/d; DARF: not req		
Metoprolol	EHL 3-7h, PRC C, Lact ?	+	-
Lopressor *Tab 50mg, 100mg, Inj 1mg/ml* **Toprol-xl** *Tab ext.rel 50mg, 100mg, 200mg* **Generics** *Tab 50mg, 100mg, Inj 1mg/ml*	**HTN** →47, **angina** →50: ini 50mg PO bid or 50-100mg PO qd (ext.rel), incr prn max 400mg/d; **acute MI** →52: ini 5mg IV q2min up to 15mg, if tolerated give 50mg PO q6h for 48h, then 100mg PO bid; **heart failure** →56: ini 6.25-12.5mg PO bid, incr q2 wk as tolerated max 200mg/d; DARF: not req		
Nadolol	EHL 20-24h, PRC C, Lact ?	-	-
Corgard *Tab 20mg, 40mg, 60mg,80mg,120mg,160mg* **Generics** *Tab 20mg, 40mg, 80mg, 120mg, 160mg*	**HTN** →47: ini 40mg PO qd, maint 40-80mg/d, max 320mg/d; **angina** →50: ini 40mg PO qd, maint 40-80mg/d, max 240mg/d; DARF: GFR (ml/min): >50: q24h, 31-50: q24-36h, 10-30: q24-48h, <10: q40-60h		
Penbutolol	EHL 17-26h, PRC C, Lact ?	-	+
Levatol *Tab 20mg*	**Angina pectoris** →50: 10-40mg PO qd; **HTN** →47: 20mg PO qd; DARF: not req		
Pindolol	EHL 3-4h, PRC B, Lact ?	-	+
Visken *Tab 5mg, 10mg* **Generics** *Tab 5mg, 10mg*	**Angina pectoris** →50: ini 2.5-5mg/d PO, maint 10-40mg/d div tid; **HTN** →47: ini 5mg PO bid, maint 10-40mg/d, max 60mg/d; DARF: not req		
Propranolol	EHL 3-4h, PRC C, Lact ?	-	-
Inderal *Tab 10mg, 20mg, 40mg, 60mg, 80mg, Inj 1mg/ml* **Inderal LA** *Cap ext.rel 60mg, 80mg, 120mg, 160mg* **Generics** *Tab 10mg, 20mg, 40mg, 60mg, 80mg, 90mg, Sol (oral) 20mg/5ml, 40mg/5ml, Inj 1mg/ml*	**HTN** →47: ini 40mg PO bid, maint 120-240mg/d, max 640mg/d; ext.rel: ini 60-80mg PO qd, maint 120-160mg/d, max 640mg/d; **angina** →50: ini 10-20mg PO tid-qid, maint 160-240mg/d; **arrhythmias** →59: 1-3mg IV, rep after 2min prn; 10-30mg PO tid-qid; **MI** →52: 180-240mg/d PO div bid-qid; **migraine** →307: ini 80mg/d PO, maint 160-240mg/d; **essential tremor**: ini 40mg PO bid, maint 120mg/d; **pheochromocytoma** →180: preop. 60mg/d PO in div doses bid-tid in combination with an alpha blocking agent; **hypertrophic subaortic stenosis**: 20-40mg PO bid-tid; CH 2-4mg/kg/d PO div bid; DARF: not req		

Timolol	EHL 2-4h, PRC C, Lact ?	β_1	ISA
Blocadren *Tab 5mg, 10mg, 20mg* **Generics** *Tab 5mg, 10mg, 20mg*	**HTN** →47: ini 10mg PO bid, maint 20-40mg/d, max 60mg/d; **MI** →52: 10mg PO bid; **migraine** →306: ini 10mg PO bid, maint 20mg/d qd; DARF: not req	-	-

β_1: selective blockage of β_1-receptors;
ISA: intrinsic sympathomimetic activity = partial agonistic and antagonist activity

2 A.3   ACE Inhibitors

2 A.3.1   ACE Inhibitors – Single Ingredient Drugs

MA: competitive blockage of angiotensin converting enzyme $\Rightarrow$ angiotensin II $\downarrow$, bradykinin $\uparrow$
EF: vasodilation $\Rightarrow$ BP $\downarrow$, renal blood flow $\uparrow$, aldosterone $\downarrow$, catecholamines $\downarrow$, reversal of myocardial and blood vessel wall hypertrophy, protective in diabetic nephropathy
AE: acute RF, rash, dry cough, hair loss, angioneurotic edema, headache, hyperkalemia, hyponatremia, complete blood count changes, urticaria, hypotension
CI: aortic stenosis, primary hyperaldosteronism, creatinine clearance <30ml/min; bilateral renal artery stenosis; angioedema

Benazepril	EHL 0.6 h, PRC C(1), D(2nd, 3rd trim.), Lact +
Lotensin *Tab 5mg, 10mg, 20mg, 40mg*	**HTN** →47: ini 10mg PO qd, maint 20-40mg PO qd or div bid, max 80mg/d; DARF: GFR (ml/min) >50: 100%; 10-50: 50-75%; <10: 25-50%

Captopril	EHL 1.9h, PRC C(1), D(2nd, 3rd trim.), Lact +
Capoten *Tab 12.5mg, 25mg, 50mg, 100mg* **Generics** *Tab 12.5mg, 25mg, 50mg, 100mg*	**HTN** →47: ini 25mg PO bid-tid, maint 25-150mg PO bid tid, max 150mg/d; **heart failure** →56: ini 12.5-25mg PO tid, incr to 150-300mg/d div tid, max 450mg/d; DARF: GFR (ml/min) >50: 100% q8h; 10-50: 50-75% q12-18h; <10: 25-50% q24h

Enalapril	EHL 1.3h, PRC C(1st), D(2nd, 3rd trim.), Lact +
Lexxel *Tab ext.rel 2.5mg, 5mg* **Vasotec** *Tab 2.5mg, 5mg, 10mg, 20mg* **Generics** *Tab 2.5mg, 5mg, 10mg, 20mg*	**HTN** →47: ini 5mg PO qd, maint 10-40mg PO qd or div bid, max 40mg/d; 1.25mg IV q6h, max 5mg IV q6h; **heart failure** →56: ini 2.5 mg PO bid, incr to 10-20mg PO bid, max 40mg/d; **CH heart failure**: 0.1-0.5mg/kg/d PO qd or div bid; DARF: GFR (ml/min) <30: ini 2.5mg PO qd, titrate prn, max 40mg/d

Fosinopril	EHL 11.5h, PRC C(1st), D(2nd, 3rd trim.), Lact +
Monopril *Tab 10mg, 20mg, 40mg*	**HTN** →47: ini 10mg PO qd, maint 10-40mg PO qd, max 80mg/d; **heart failure** →56: ini 5-10mg PO qd, maint 20-40mg PO qd, max 40mg/d; DARF: not req

Lisinopril	EHL 12h, PRC C(1st), D(2nd, 3rd trim.), Lact +
Zestril *Tab 2.5mg, 5mg, 10mg, 20mg, 30mg, 40mg* **Prinivil** *Tab 2.5mg, 5mg, 10mg, 20mg, 40mg*	**HTN** →47: ini 10mg PO qd, maint 20-40mg PO qd, max 80mg/d; **heart failure** →56: ini 2.5-5mg PO qd, maint 5-40mg PO qd, max 80mg/d; DARF: GFR (ml/min) 10-30: ini 5mg PO, <10: ini 2.5mg PO, titrate dosage prn, max 40mg/d
Moexipril	EHL 1 h, PRC C(1st), D(2nd, 3rd trim.), Lact +
Univasc *Tab 7.5, 15mg*	**HTN** →47: ini 7.5mg PO qd, maint 7.5-30mg PO qd, max 60mg/d; DARF: GFR (ml/min) <40: 3.75mg PO qd
Perindopril	EHL 0.9 h, PRC C(1st), D(2nd, 3rd trim.), Lact +
Aceon *Tab 2mg, 4mg, 8mg*	**HTN** →47: ini 4mg PO qd, maint 4-8mg PO qd, max 16mg/d; **heart failure** →56: 4mg PO qd; DARF: GFR (ml/min) <30: ini 2mg PO qd, max 8mg/d
Quinapril	EHL 0.8h, PRC C(1st), D(2nd, 3rd trim.), Lact +
Accupril *Tab 5mg, 10mg, 20mg, 40mg*	**HTN** →47: ini 10mg PO qd, maint 20-80mg PO qd or div bid, max 80mg/d; **heart failure** →56: ini 5 mg PO qd-bid, maint 20-40mg/d div bid; DARF: GFR (ml/min) >60: ini 10mg PO; 30-60: ini 5mg PO; 10-30: ini 2.5mg PO, then titrate to the optimal response
Ramipril	EHL 1-5h, PRC C(1st), D(2nd, 3rd trim.), Lact +
Altace *Cap 1.25mg, 2.5mg, 5mg, 10mg*	**HTN** →47: ini 2.5mg PO qd, maint 2.5-20mg PO qd or div bid, max 20mg/d; **heart failure**: →56 ini 1.25-2.5mg PO bid, maint 2.5-5mg bid, max 10mg/d; DARF: GFR (ml/min) <40: 25%
Trandolapril	EHL 0.6-1.3h, PRC C(1), D(2nd,3rd trim), Lact +
Mavik *Tab 1mg, 2mg, 4mg*	**HTN** →47, **heart failure** →56: ini 1mg PO qd, maint 2-4mg PO qd, max 8mg/d; DARF: GFR (ml/min) <30: ini 0.5mg, titrate to optimal response

2 A.3.2   ACE Inhibitors - Combinations

Benazepril + Hydrochlorothiazide (HCTZ)	PRC C(1st trim.), D(2nd, 3rd trim.), Lact -
Lotensin HCT *Tab 10 + 12.5mg, 20 + 12.5mg, 20 + 25mg, 5 + 6.25mg*	**HTN** →47: 5+6.25 - 20+25mg PO qd; DARF: GFR (ml/min) >30: 100%, <30: not rec
Captopril + HCTZ	PRC C(1st trim.), D(2nd, 3rd trim.), Lact -
Capozide *Tab 25 + 15mg, 25 + 25mg, 50 + 15mg, 50 + 25mg* **Generics** *Tab 25 + 15mg, 25 + 25mg, 50 + 15mg, Tab 50 + 25mg*	**HTN** →47: 25+15 - 50+25mg PO qd-bid; DARF: GFR (ml/min) >30: 100%, <30: not rec
Enalapril + HCTZ	PRC C(1st trim.), D(2nd, 3rd trim.), Lact -
Vaseretic *Tab 5 + 12.5mg* *Tab 10 + 25mg*	**HTN** →47: 5+12.5 - 10+25mg PO qd, max 20+50mg PO qd or div bid; DARF: GFR (ml/min) >30: 100%, <30: not rec

Lisinopril + HCTZ	PRC C(1st trim.), D(2nd, 3rd trim.), Lact -
Prinzide *Tab 10 + 12.5mg, 20 + 12.5mg, 20 + 25mg* **Zestoretic** *Tab 10 + 12.5mg, 20 + 12.5mg, 20 + 25mg*	**HTN** →47: 10+12.5 - 20+25mg PO qd; DARF: GFR (ml/min) >30: 100%, <30: not rec
Moexipril + HCTZ	PRC C(1st trim.), D(2nd, 3rd trim.), Lact -
Uniretic *Tab 7.5 + 12.5mg; 15 + 25mg;*	**HTN** →47: 7.5+12.5 - 15+25mg PO qd, max 30+50mg PO; GFR (ml/min) >40: 100%, <40: not rec
Quinapril + HCTZ	PRC C(1st trim.), D(2nd, 3rd trim.), Lact -
Accuretic *Tab 10 + 12.5mg, 20 + 12.5mg, 20 + 25mg*	**HTN** →47: 10+12.5 - 20+25mg PO, max 40+25mg PO qd; DARF: GFR (ml/min) >30: 100%, <30: not rec

2 A.4   Angiotensin II Receptor Blockers
2 A.4.1   Angiotensin II Receptor Blockers – Single Ingredient Drugs

MA (ARBs): inhibition of type 1 angiotensin II receptor
EF: selective blockage of angiotensin II-effects without action on bradykinin breakdown
AE: headache, dizziness, nausea, abdominal pain; **CI:** renal artery stenosis following renal transplantation, primary hyperaldosteronism, biliary cirrhosis, severe hepatic damage

Candesartan	PRC C(1st), D(2nd, 3rd trim.), Lact ?
Atacand *Tab 4mg, 8mg, 16mg, 32mg*	**HTN** →47: ini 16mg PO qd, max 32mg/d
Eprosartan	EHL 6h, PRC C(1st), D(2nd, 3rd trim.), Lact -
Teveten *Tab 300mg, 400mg, 600mg*	**HTN** →47: ini 600mg PO qd, max 800mg qd
Irbesartan	EHL 11-15h, PRC C(1), D(2nd, 3rd trim.), Lact ?
Avapro *Tab 75mg, 150mg, 300mg*	**HTN** →47: ini 150mg PO qd, max 300mg/d; DARF: not req
Losartan	EHL 1.5-2h, PRC C(1.), D(2nd, 3rd trim.), Lact ?
Cozaar *Tab 25mg, 50mg*	**HTN** →47: ini 50mg PO qd, max 100mg qd or div bid; **heart failure** →56: ini 12.5mg PO qd, incr in 7-d intervals to 25-50mg/d; DARF: not req
Olmesartan	EHL 13h, PRC C(1st), D(2nd, 3rd trim.), Lact ?
Benicar *Tab 5mg, 20mg, 40mg*	**HTN** →47: ini 20mg PO qd, incr prn to 40mg qd
Telmisartan	EHL 24h, PRC C(1st), D(2nd, 3rd trim.), Lact ?
Micardis *Tab 20mg, 40mg, 80mg*	**HTN** →47: ini 40mg PO qd, max 80mg/d
Valsartan	EHL 6-9h, PRC C(1st), D(2nd, 3rd trim.), Lact ?
Diovan *Cap 80mg, 160mg*	**HTN** →47: ini 80mg PO qd, max 320mg/d; DARF: GFR (ml/min) >10: not req

2 A.4.2   Angiotensin II Receptor Blockers – Combinations

Irbesartan + HCTZ	PRC C(1st trim.), D(2nd, 3rd trim.), Lact -
Avalide *Tab 150 + 12.5mg, 300 + 12.5mg*	**HTN** →47: 150+12.5 - 300+25mg PO qd; DARF: GFR (ml/min) >30: 100%, <30: not rec

Losartan + HCTZ	PRC C(1st trim.), D(2nd, 3rd trim.), Lact –
Hyzaar *Tab 50 + 12.5mg, 100 + 25mg*	**HTN** →47: 50+12.5 - 100+25mg PO qd; DARF: GFR (ml/min) >30: 100%, <30: not rec
Eprosartan + HCTZ	EHL 6h, PRC C(1st), D(2nd, 3rd trim.), Lact –
Teveten HCT *Tab 600 + 12.5mg, 600 + 25mg*	**HTN** →47: 600+12.5-25mg PO qd; DARF: GFR (ml/min) >30: 100%, <30: not rec
Valsartan + HCTZ	PRC C(1st trim.), D(2nd, 3rd trim.), Lact –
Diovan HCT *Tab 80 + 12.5mg, 160 + 12.5mg*	**HTN** →47: 80+12.5 - 160+25mg PO qd; DARF: GFR (ml/min) >30: 100%, <30: not rec

2 A.5   Aldosterone Receptor Blockers

MA: blocks binding of aldosterone to the mineralcorticoid receptor
AE: hyperkalemia, headache, dizziness, diarrhea, abdominal pain; **CI:** hyperkalemia > 5.5mEq/l, type 2 diabetes with microalbuminuria, GFR <50ml/min, combination with strong CYP3A-inhibitors (ketoconazole, itraconazole), potassium-sparing diuretics

Eplerenone	EHL 4-6 h, PRC B, Lact ?
Inspra *Tab 25mg, 50mg, 100mg*	**HTN** →47: ini 50mg PO qd, incr prn after 4wk to 50mg bid; DARF: GFR (ml/min) <50: contraind.

2 A.6   Calcium Channel Blockers
2 A.6.1   CCBs – Dihydropyridines

MA: blockage of inflow of calcium ions ⇒ neg. inotropic effect, myocardial O_2 consumption ↓, predominantly arterial vasodilation ⇒ afterload ↓, preload unchanged!
AE: hypotension, flush, reflex tachycardia, ankle edema, headache, complete blood count changes, gingival hyperplasia
CI: shock, hypotension, significant aortic stenosis; heart failure (NYHA III-IV)

Amlodipine	EHL 35-50h, PRC C, Lact ?
Norvasc *Tab 2.5mg, 5mg, 10mg*	**HTN** →47: ini 2.5-5mg PO qd, max 10mg qd; **chron. stable AP** →50: 5-10mg PO qd; DARF: not req
Felodipine	EHL 10-16h, PRC C, Lact ?
Plendil *Tab ext.rel 10mg, 2.5mg, 5mg*	**HTN** →47: ini 5mg PO qd, maint 5-10mg/d; DARF: not req
Isradipine	EHL 5-10.7h, PRC C, Lact ?
Dynacirc *Cap 2.5mg, 5mg* **Dynacirc CR** *Tab ext.rel 5mg, 10mg*	**HTN** →47: ini 2.5mg PO bid, maint 5-10mg/d div bid, max 20mg/d; ext.rel: 5-20mg PO qd
Nicardipine	EHL 8.6h, PRC C, Lact ?
Cardene *Cap 20mg, 30mg* *Inj 2.5mg/ml* **Cardene SR** *Cap ext.rel 30mg, 45mg, 60mg* **Generics** *Cap 20mg, 30mg*	**HTN crisis** →48: ini 5mg/h IV incr prn by 2.5mg/h q5-15min, max 15mg/h; **HTN** →47: ini 20mg PO tid, maint 20-40mg tid; ext.rel.: ini 30mg PO bid, maint 30-60mg PO bid, max 120mg/d; **chronic stable AP** →50: ini 20mg PO tid, maint 20-40mg tid; DARF: not req

Nifedipine — EHL no data, PRC C, Lact +

Adalat *Cap 10mg, 20mg*
Adalat CC *Tab ext.rel 30mg, 60mg, 90mg*
Procardia *Cap 10mg, 20mg*
Procardia XL *Tab ext.rel 30mg, 60mg, 90mg*
Generics *Tab ext.rel 30mg, 60mg, Cap 10mg, 20mg*

HTN →47: ext.rel: ini 30-60mg PO qd, max 120mg/d; **angina pectoris** →50: ini 10mg PO tid, maint 10-20mg tid; ext.rel: ini 30-60mg PO qd, max 120mg/d; DARF: not req

Nisoldipine — EHL 7-12h, PRC C, Lact ?

Sular *Tab ext.rel 10mg, 20mg, 30mg, 40mg*

HTN →47: ini 20mg PO qd, maint 20-40mg qd, max 60mg/d; DARF: not req

2 A.6.2 CCBs–Non–Dihydropyridines

MA: blockage of inflow of calcium ions
EF: neg. inotropic and chronotropic effect, myocardial O_2 consumption ↓, vasodilation (afterload ↓, preload unchanged!), AV conduction time ↑, AV refractory period ↑
AE: AV block, bradycardia, cardiac arrest, hypotension, ankle edema
CI: AV block II°-III°, SA block, bradycardia, sick sinus syndrome, combination with betablockers

Diltiazem — EHL 3-6.6h, PRC C, Lact -

Cardizem *Tab 30mg, 60mg, 90mg, 120mg, Inj 25mg/vial, 100mg/vial, 5mg/ml*
Cardizem CD *Cap ext.rel 180mg, 240mg, 300mg*
Cardizem SR *Cap ext.rel 60mg, 90mg, 120mg*
Cartia XT *Cap ext.rel 120mg, 180mg, 240mg, 300mg*
Tiamate *Tab ext.rel 120mg, 180mg, 240mg*
Tiazac *Cap ext.rel 120mg, 180mg, 240mg, 300mg, 360mg, 420mg*
Generics *Tab 30mg, 60mg, 90mg, 120mg, Tab ext.rel 120mg, 180mg, 240mg, Cap ext.rel 60mg, 90mg, 120mg, 180mg, 240mg, 300mg, Inj 5mg/ml*

Chronic stable and vasospastic AP →50: ini 30mg PO qid, max 360mg/d; ext.rel: 120-480mg qd, max 540mg/d;
HTN →47: ini 60-120mg PO bid, maint 120-180mg bid, max 360mg/d; ext.rel: 240-360mg PO qd;
AF →60: ini 0.25mg/kg IV over 2min, rep prn after 15min with 0.35mg/kg; continuos inf: 5-15mg/h; DARF: not req

Verapamil — EHL 4-12h, PRC C, Lact +

Calan *Tab 40mg, 80mg, 120mg*
Covera–HS *Tab ext.rel 180mg, 240mg*
Isoptin *Tab 40mg, 80mg, 120mg, Inj 2.5mg/ml*
Isoptin SR *Tab ext.rel 120mg, 180mg, 240mg*
Verelan *Cap ext.rel 120mg, 180mg, 240mg, 360mg*
Verelan PM *Cap ext.rel 100mg, 200mg, 300mg*
Generics *Tab ext.rel 120mg, 180mg, 240mg, Tab 40mg, 80mg, 120mg, Cap ext.rel 120mg, 180mg, 240mg, Inj 2.5mg/ml*

HTN →47: ext.rel: 120-240mg PO qd-bid; **chronic stable AP** →50: ext.rel: 180-360mg PO qd, max 480mg/d; **SVT** →60: 5-10mg IV over 2min, rep after 15-30min prn; continuous inf: 5mg/h IV;
AF →60: 240-480mg/d PO div tid-qid;
CH 1-15 y: **arrhythmias**: 0.1-0.3mg/kg IV; DARF: not req

2 A.7 Adrenergic Inhibitors
2 A.7.1 Central Acting Alpha Agonists

MA (clonidine, guanabenz, methyldopa): stimulation of central α_2-receptors (presynaptic effect ⇒ release of noradrenaline ↓, postsynaptic effect ⇒ peripheral sympathetic tone ↓, release of renin ↓, (⇒ inhibition of renin-angiotensin-aldosterone-system); additional agonistic effect on imidazole-receptor; **EF** (clonidine, guanabenz, methyldopa): BP ↓ due to reduction of peripheral resistance, stroke volume and cardiac output
AE (clonidine, guanabenz): AV block, bradycardia, drowsiness, oral dryness
CI (clonidine, guanabenz): bradycardia

Clonidine	EHL 12–16h, PRC C, Lact ?
Catapres *Tab 0.1mg, 0.2mg, 0.3mg,* *Film (ext.rel, TD) 0.1mg/24h, 0.2mg/24h, 0.3mg/24h* **Duraclon** *Inj 0.1mg/ml* **Generics** *Tab 0.1mg, 0.2mg, 0.3mg*	**HTN** →44: ini 0.1 mg PO bid, maint 0.2-0.6mg/d div bid, max 2.4mg/d; TTS: ini 0.1mg/24h patch, max 0.6mg/24h **CH HTN**: ini 5-10µg/kg/d PO div bid-tid, max 0.9mg/d; DARF: not req; →48
Guanabenz	EHL 6h, PRC C, Lact ?
Wytensin *Tab 4mg, 8mg* **Generics** *Tab 4mg*	**HTN** →44: ini 4mg PO bid, incr by 4-8mg/d at 1-2 wk intervals, max 96mg/d
Methyldopa	EHL 1.7h, PRC B, Lact +
Aldomet *Tab 125mg, 250mg, 500mg,* *Susp 250mg/5ml , Inj 50mg/ml* **Generics** *Tab 125mg, 250mg, 500mg, Inj 50mg/ml*	**HTN** →44: ini 250mg PO bid-tid, maint 500-2000mg/d div bid-qid; 250-500mg IV q6h; **CH HTN**: 10mg/kg/d PO div bid-qid, max 65 mg/kg/d; 20-40mg/kg/d IV div qid; DARF: GFR (ml/min) >50: q8h; 10-50: q8-12h; <10: q12-24h

2 A.7.2 Alpha Adrenergic Blockers

MA: reversible blockage of α_1-receptor; **MA** (phenoxybenzamine): irreversible blockage of α_1/α_2-receptor; **EF**: vasodilation, pre- and afterload ↓
AE: reflex tachycardia (not prazosin), arrhythmia, postural hypotension, fatigue, nausea, dyspepsia, diarrhea; "adverse epinephrine effect": epinephrine → vasodilation and BP ↓ when α receptors are blocked due to β-mimetic effect; **AE** (Prazosin): "first-dose phenomenon": postural hypotension after first dose ⇒ slow increase in dosage!; **CI**: aortic and mitral stenosis, pericardial effusion, pulmonary embolism, left ventricular failure, children < 12

Doxazosin	EHL 8.8-22h, PRC C, Lact ?
Cardura *Tab 1mg, 2mg, 4mg, 8mg* **Generics** *Tab 1mg, 2mg, 4mg, 8mg*	**HTN** (not first line) →48: ini 1mg PO qd, max 16mg/d
Phenoxybenzamine	EHL 24h, PRC C, Lact ?
Dibenzyline *Cap 10mg*	**Pheochromocytoma** →49: ini 10mg PO bid, incr slowly qod prn up to 20-40mg bid-tid, max 120mg/d
Phentolamine	EHL 19min, PRC C, Lact ?
Regitine *Inj 5mg/vial* **Rogitine** *Inj 5mg/vial* **Generics** *Inj 5mg/vial*	**Pheochromocytoma surgery** →49: 5mg IV/IM 1-2h prior to surgery, 5mg IV during surgery prn; **CH pheochromocytoma surgery**: 1mg IV/IM 1-2h prior to surgery, 1mg IV during surgery prn

Prazosin	EHL 2-4h, PRC C, Lact ?
Minipress *Cap 1mg, 2mg, 5mg* **Minipress XL** *Tab ext.rcl 2.5mg, 5mg* **Generics** *Cap 1mg, 2mg, 5mg*	**HTN** →48: ini 1mg PO qd, maint 6-15mg/d div bid, max 20mg/d; **CH HTN**: ini 5µg/kg PO as 1x dose; maint 25-150µg/kg/d div q6h, max 0.4 mg/kg/d, DARF: not req
Terazosin	EHL 9-12h, PRC C, Lact ?
Hytrin *Cap 1mg, 2mg, 5mg, 10mg, Tab 1mg, 2mg, 5mg, 10mg* **Generics** *Cap 1mg, 2mg, 5mg, 10mg, Tab 1mg, 2mg, 5mg, 10mg*	**HTN** →48: ini 1mg PO hs, maint 1-5mg PO qd or div bid, max 20mg/d; DARF: not req
Tolazoline	EHL 3-10h, PRC C, Lact ?
Priscoline *Inj 25mg/ml*	**Persistent pulmonary HTN in newborns**: ini 1-2mg/kg IV over 10min, then 1-2mg/kg/h

2 A.7.3 Peripheral Acting Adrenergic Blockers

MA: inhibition of vesicular storage of catecholamines
EF: peripheral resistance ↓ (afterload) ⇒ BP ↓, HR ↓, cardiac output ↓
AE: depression, gut motility↑, bradycardia, postural hypotension, stuffy nose
CI: congestive heart failure, asthma, bronchitis, ulcer disease, depression

Reserpine	EHL 50-100h, PRC C, Lact -
Serpalan *Tab 0.1mg, 0.25mg* **Generics** *Tab 0.1mg, 0.25mg*	**HTN** →44: ini 0.5mg/d PO for 1-2 wk, then reduce to 0.1-0.25mg/d PO qd; DARF: GFR (ml/min) >10: 100%; <10: not rated; →318

2 A.8 Direct Vasodilators

MA/EF: direct effect on the smooth muscles of the small arteries and arterioles ⇒ peripheral resistance ↓ (afterload) ⇒ BP ↓
MA (fenoldopam): selective postsynaptic dopamine-1 (DA-1) receptor agonist
MA (nesiritide): recombinant human B-type natriuretic peptide ⇒ arterial and venous vasodilatation ⇒ PCWP ↓, BP ↓
AE (direct vasodilators): hypotension, Na^+, H_2O retention, tachycardia, dizziness, headache; **AE** (diazoxide): hyperglycemia; **AE** (hydralazine): LE; **AE** (nitroprusside): cyanide poisoning; **AE** (minoxidil): hypertrichosis, pericardial effusion, changes in T-wave;
AE (nesiritide): hypotension, ventricular tachykardia, angina pectoris, bradycardia, headache, abdominal pain, insomnia, dizziness, anxiety, nausea, vomiting
CI (diazoxide): thiazide allergy; **CI** (nesiritide): cardiogenic shock, BP < 90mm Hg
CI (nitroprusside): aortic coarctation, hypothyroidism, metabolic acidosis

Diazoxide	EHL 20-36h, PRC C, Lact ?
Hyperstat *Inj 15mg/ml* **Proglycem** *Cap 50mg, Susp 50mg/ml*	**Malignant HTN** →49: 1-3mg/kg, max 150mg IV q5-15min prn; **(pre-)eclampsia**: 30mg IV q1-2min until diastolic BP <90 mmHg
Epoprostenol	EHL 0-5min, PRC B, Lact ?
Flolan *Inj 0.5mg/vial, 1.5mg/vial*	**Primary pulmonary HTN** →113: 2ng/kg/min IV, incr by 2ng/kg/min q15min

Fenoldopam	EHL 5–10min, PRC B, Lact ?
Corlopam Inj 10mg/ml	**Malignant HTN** →48: ini 0.1 µg/kg/min IV, incr q15–20min by increments of 0.05–0.1µg/kg/min prn to 1.6µg/kg/min
Hydralazine	EHL 3–5h, PRC C, Lact +
Apresoline Tab 10mg 25mg, 50mg, 100mg, **Generics** Tab 10mg, 25mg, 50mg, 100mg, Inj 20mg/ml	**HTN emergencies** →48: 10–20mg IV, 20–40mg IM, rep prn; **HTN** →44: ini 10mg PO qid for 2–4d, incr to 25mg qid, then 50mg qid, max 400mg/d; **CH HTN emergency**: 0.1–0.5mg/kg IM/IV ; **CH HTN**: 0.75–1mg/kg/d PO div q4–6h
Minoxidil	EHL 2.3–28.9h, PRC C, Lact +
Loniten Tab 2.5mg, 10mg **Generics** Tab 2.5mg, 10mg	**Severe HTN** →48: ini 5mg PO qd, incr to 10–40mg/d div bid; **CH** <12 y: ini 0.2mg/kg PO qd, incr q3d up to 0.25–1mg/kg/d qd or div bid, max 50mg/d
Nesiritide	EHL 18min, PRC C , Lact ?
Natrecor Inj 1.5mg/vial	**Acutely decompensated heart failure** →54: ini 2µg/kg IV over 1min, then 0.01µg/kg/min
Nitroprusside Sodium	EHL 3–4min
Nitropress Inj 25mg/ml, 50mg/vial **Generics** Inj 25mg/ml, 50mg/vial	**HTN emergencies** →49: ini 0.3µg/kg/min IV, incr slowly to 10µg/kg/min; DARF: not req
Treprostinil	EHL 2–4h, PRC B, Lact ?
Remodulin Inj 1mg/ml, 2.5mg/ml, 5mg/ml, 10mg/ml	**Pulmonary arterial HTN** →113: ini 1.25ng/kg/min SC, incr. by 1.25ng/kg/min per wk for the first 4 wk, then incr. by max. 2.5ng/kg/min; max 40ng/kg/min

2 A.9   Endothelin Receptor Antagonists

MA/EF (bosentan): specific and competitive antagonist at endothelin receptor types ETΛ and ETB ⇒ inhibition of endothelin-1 effects ⇒ pulmonary artery pressure ↓
AE (bosentan): headache, nasopharyngitis, hypotension, flushing, edema, liver injury
CI (bosentan): pregnancy, coadmin. with cyclosporine A, glyburide; known hypersensitivity

Bosentan	EHL 5h, PRC X, Lact –
Tracleer Tab 62.5mg, 125mg	**Pulmonary arterial HTN** (WHO III–IV) →113: ini 62.5mg PO bid for 4wk, then 125mg bid; DARF: not req

2 A.10 Diuretics
2 A.10.1 Thiazide Diuretics

MA: inhibition of the reabsorption of Na^+, Cl^- and H_2O in the distal convoluted tubule, secretion of K^+ ↑
EF: elimination of Na^+, Cl^-, H_2O and K^+ ↑, excretion of Ca^{2+} and PO_4^{3-} ↓
AE: hypokalemia, hypercalcemia, hyperuricemia, thrombosis, anemia, hyperglycemia
CI: hypokalemia, hypovolemia, renal insuff., sulphonamide hypersensitivity, hepatic coma

Chlorothiazide	EHL 45-120min, PRC C, Lact +
Diuril *Tab 250mg, 500mg, Sol (oral) 50mg/ml, Inj 500mg/vial*	**Edema** →163, **HTN** →47: 0.5-1g/d PO/IV qd or div bid; **CH** 6 mo-2 y: 10-20mg/kg/d PO qd or div bid, max 375mg/d; **CH** 2-12 y: 1g/d PO qd; DARF: GFR (ml/min) 10-50: ineffective, <10: not rec
Chlorthalidone	EHL 40-89h, PRC B, Lact ?
Hygroton *Tab 25mg, 50mg* **Thalitone** *Tab 15mg, 25mg* **Generics** *Tab 25mg, 50mg*	**HTN** →47: 12.5-25mg PO qd, maint 12.5-50mg/d; **edema** →163: ini 30-60mg PO qd or 60mg qod, incr prn to 90-120mg/d
Hydrochlorothiazide	EHL 10-12h, PRC B, Lact +
Esidrix *Tab 25mg, 50mg, 100mg* **Hydrodiuril** *Tab 25mg, 50mg, 100mg* **Microzide** *Cap 12.5mg* **Oretic** *Tab 25mg, 50mg* **Generics** *Tab 12.5mg, 25mg, 50mg, 100mg, Sol (oral) 50mg/5ml*	**Edema** →163: 25-100mg PO qd or qod; **HTN** →47: ini 12.5-25mg PO qd, maint 12.5-50mg/d; **CH** 1-2mg/kg/d PO qd or div bid
Indapamide	EHL 14-15h, PRC B, Lact ?
Lozol *Tab 1.25mg, 2.5mg* **Generics** *Tab 1.25mg, 2.5mg*	**HTN** →47: ini 1.25mg PO qd, incr prn, max 5mg/d; **edema** →163: 2.5-5mg PO qd
Metolazone	EHL 8-14h, PRC B, Lact +
Mykrox *Tab 0.5mg* **Zaroxolyn** *Tab 2.5mg, 5mg, 10mg*	**Edema** →163: 5-10mg PO qd, max 20mg/d; **HTN** →47: ini 2.5-5mg PO qd, maint 5-20mg/d (Zar.); 0.5-1mg PO qd (Mykrox)

2 A.10.2 Loop Diuretics

MA/EF: inhibition of the reabsorption of Na^+, Cl^-, K^+ and H_2O, primarily in the ascending limb of the loop of Henle ⇒ increased elimination of Na^+, Cl^-, K^+, H_2O, Ca^{2+} and Mg^{2+}
AE: hypokalemia, hypocalcemia, hypotension, hyperuricemia, thrombosis, reversible hearing loss;
CI: serious hypokalemia, hypovolemia, anuria, hepatic coma

Bumetanide	EHL 1-1.5h, PRC C, Lact ?
Bumex *Tab 0.5mg, 1mg, 2mg, Inj 0.25mg/ml* **Generics** *Tab 0.5mg, 1mg, 2mg, Inj 0.25mg/ml*	**Edema** →163: 0.5-2mg PO qd, rep prn doses at 4-5h intervals, max 10mg/d; 0.5-1mg IV/IM, rep prn at 2-3h intervals, max 10mg/d; DARF: not req
Ethacrynic Acid	EHL 1-4h, PRC B, Lact -
Edecrin *Tab 25mg, 50mg, Inj 50mg/vial*	**Edema** →163: 50-200mg/d PO; 0.5-1mg/kg IV, max 100mg/d; **CH** ini 25mg PO, incr prn q2-3d by 25mg, max 2-3mg/kg/d

Furosemide	EHL 30-120min, PRC C, Lact ?
Lasix *Tab 20mg, 40mg, 80mg, Sol (oral) 10mg/ml, Inj 10mg/ml* **Generics** *Tab 20mg, 40mg, 80mg, Sol (oral) 10mg/ml, 40mg/5ml, Inj 10mg/ml*	**Edema** →163: ini 20-80mg PO or 20-40mg IV, incr by 20-40mg q6-8h prn, max 600mg/d; **HTN** →47: ini 20-40mg PO bid, incr prn; **CH** ini 2mg/kg IV/IM/PO, incr by 1-2mg q6-8h until desired effect is achieved, max 6mg/kg/dose
Torsemide	EHL 3-6h, PRC B, Lact ?
Demadex *Tab 5mg, 10mg, 20mg, 100mg, Inj 10mg/ml*	**Edema** →163: ini 10-20mg IV/PO qd, incr prn by doubling the dose, max 200mg qd; **HTN** →47: 5-10mg PO qd

2 A.10.3 Potassium-Sparing Diuretics

MA (amiloride, triamterene): inhibition of the reabsorption of Na^+, Cl^- and H_2O as well as inhibition of the K^+-secretion in the distal convoluted tubule
MA (spironolactone): competitive blockage of aldosterone receptor in late-distal tubule
EF: elimination of Na^+, Cl^- and H_2O ↑, K^+ elimination ↓
AE (amiloride, triamterene): hyperkalemia, metabolic acidosis, megaloblastic anemia
AE (spironolactone): hyperkalemia, gynecomastia, impotence, amenorrhea, hirsutism, voice DO, skin DO
CI (amiloride, triamterene): hyperkalemia, renal insufficiency
CI (spironolactone): renal insufficiency, hyperkalemia

Amiloride	EHL 6-9h, PRC B, Lact ?
Midamor *Tab 5mg* **Generics** *Tab 5mg*	**Edema** →163/**HTN** →47: ini 5mg PO qd in combination with another diuretic, max 20mg/d
Spironolactone	EHL 1.3-1.4h, PRC D, Lact +
Aldactone *Tab 25mg, 50mg, 100mg* **Generics** *Tab 25mg, 50mg, 100mg*	**Edema with heart failure, cirrhosis, nephrotic syndrome** →163: ini 100mg PO qd or div bid, incr prn until diuretic effect is achieved, max 200mg/d; **HTN** →47: 50-100mg PO qd or div bid; **CH** 1-3mg/kg/d PO
Triamterene	EHL 1.5-2.5h, PRC D, Lact -
Dyrenium *Cap 50mg, 100mg*	**Edema with cirrhosis, nephrotic syndrome, heart failure** →163: 50-100mg PO bid, max 300mg/d

2 A.10.4 Potassium-Sparing Diuretics – Combinations

HCTZ + Amiloride	PRC B, Lact -
Hydro-ride *Tab 50 + 5mg* **Moduretic** *Tab 50 + 5mg* **Generics** *Tab 50 + 5mg*	**HTN** →47, **edema** →163: 50+5 - 100+10mg PO qd
HCTZ + Spironolactone	PRC C, Lact ?
Aldactazide *Tab 25 + 25mg, 50 + 50mg* **Generics** *Tab 25 + 25mg*	**Edema** →163: 25+25 - 200+200mg PO qd or div bid; **HTN** →47: 50+50 - 100+100mg PO qd or div bid

HCTZ + Triamterene	PRC D, Lact -
Dyazide *Cap 25 + 37.5mg* **Maxzide** *Tab 25 + 37.5mg, 50 + 75mg* **Generics** *Cap 25 + 37.5mg, 25 + 50mg, 50 + 75mg*	**HTN** →47, **edema** →163: 25+37.5 - 50+75mg PO qd or div bid

2 A.10.5 Diuretics – Carbonic Anhydrase Inhibitors

MA/EF: noncompetitive inhibition of the enzyme carbonic anhydrase ⇒ urine volume ↑, urinary excretion of bicarbonate and sodium ↑ ⇒ metabolic acidosis
AE: taste disturbances, paresthesia, metabolic acidosis, tinnitus
CI: hypersensitivity to acetazolamide, sulfonamides or thiazides, hyponatremia, hypokalemia, severe liver or renal impairment, hyperchloremic acidosis

Acetazolamide	EHL 4-8h, PRC C, Lact ?
Diamox *Tab 125mg, 250mg, Cap ext.rel 500mg, Inj 500mg/vial* **Generics** *Tab 125mg, 250mg, Inj 500mg/vial*	**Acute glaucoma** →405: 250mg IV q4h; 250mg PO qd-qid; **heart failure** →56: 250-375mg PO qod; mountain sickness: 0.5-1g PO div bid-tid, ini 24-48h before ascent, continue for 48h at high altitudes

2 A.11 Antihypertensive Combinations

Amlodipine + Benazepril	PRC D, Lact ?
Lotrel *Cap 2.5 + 10mg, 5 + 10mg, 5 + 20mg*	**HTN** →48: 2.5+10 - 5+20mg PO qd; DARF: GFR (ml/min) >30: 100%, <30: not rec
Atenolol + Chlorthalidone	PRC D, Lact -
Tenoretic *Tab 50 + 25mg, 100 + 25mg* **Generics** *Tab 50 + 25mg, 100 + 25mg*	**HTN** →48: 50+25 - 100+25mg PO qd; DARF: GFR (ml/min) 15-35: 50mg qd, <15: 50mg qod
Bisoprolol + HCTZ	PRC C, Lact ?
Ziac *Tab 2.5 + 6.25mg, 5 + 6.25mg, 10 + 6.25mg* **Generics** *Tab 2.5 + 6.25mg, 5 + 6.25mg, 10 + 6.25mg*	**HTN** →48: 2.5+6.25 - 20+12.5mg PO qd
Clonidine + Chlorthalidone	PRC C, Lact ?
Combipres *Tab 0.1 + 15mg, 0.2 + 15mg* **Clorpres** *Tab 0.1 + 15mg, 0.2 + 15mg, 0.3 + 15mg* **Generics** *Tab 0.1 + 15mg, 0.2 + 15mg, 0.3 + 15mg*	**HTN** →48: 0.1+15 - 0.6+30mg PO qd or div bid
Enalapril + Felodipine	PRC D, Lact ?
Lexxel *Tab 5 + 2.5mg, 5 + 5mg*	**HTN** →48: 5+2.5 - 20+10mg PO qd
Hydralazine + HCTZ	PRC C, Lact ?
Apresazide *Cap 25 + 25mg, 50 + 50mg* **Hydra-Zide** *Cap 25 + 25mg, 50 + 50mg, 100 + 50mg* **Generics** *Cap 50 + 50mg*	**HTN** →48: 25+25 - 100+50mg PO qd
Metoprolol + HCTZ	PRC C, Lact +
Lopressor HCT *Tab 50 + 25mg, 100 + 25mg, 100 + 50mg*	**HTN** →48: 50+25 - 100+50mg PO qd

Nadolol + Bendroflumethiazide	PRC C, Lact -
Corzide *Tab 40 + 5mg, 80 + 5mg*	**HTN** →48: 40+5 - 80+5mg PO qd; DARF: GFR (ml/min) >50: q24h, 31-50: q24-36h, 10-30: q28-48h, <10: q40-60h
Prazosin + Polythiazide	PRC C, Lact -
Minizide *Cap 1 + 0.5mg, 2 + 0.5mg, 5 + 0.5mg*	**HTN** →48: 2+1 - 15+1.5mg PO div bid-tid
Propranolol + HCTZ	PRC C, Lact ?
Inderide LA *Cap ext.rel 40 + 25mg, 80 + 25mg, 80 + 50mg, 120 + 50mg, 160 + 50mg* **Generics** *Tab 40 + 25mg, Tab 80 + 25mg*	**HTN** →48: 40+25 - 160+50mg PO qd or div bid; ext.rel: 80+50 -160+50mg PO qd
Timolol + HCTZ	PRC C, Lact -
Timolide 10-25 *Tab 10 + 25mg*	**HTN** →48: 20+50mg PO qd or div bid
Trandolapril + Verapamil	PRC D, Lact -
Tarka *Tab ext.rel 1 + 240mg, 2 + 180mg, 2 + 240mg, 4 + 240mg*	**HTN** →48: 1+180 - 4+480mg PO qd or div bid

2 A.12 Nitrates

MA: NO relaxes smooth musculature of blood vessels
EF: preload ↓ through venous pooling, coronary spasmolysis; afterload ↓
AE: BP ↓, tachycardia, headache, tachyphylaxis (not molsidomine)
CI: hypotension, shock, HOCM

Isosorbide Dinitrate	EHL 4h, PRC C, Lact ?
Dilatrate-SR *Cap ext.rel 40mg* **Isordil** *Cap ext.rel 40mg, Tab 10mg, 20mg, 30mg, 40mg, 50mg, Tab (SL) 2.5mg, 5mg, 10mg* **Sorbitrate** *Tab 5mg, 10mg, 20mg, 40mg, Tab (chew) 5mg, 10mg* **Generics** *Tab 5mg, 10mg, 20mg, 30mg, Tab (SL) 2.5mg, 5mg, Tab ext.rel 40mg*	**AP Tx** →50: 2.5-10mg PO/SL, rep prn q5-10min up to 3 doses in 30min; **angina PRO** →50: ini 5-20mg PO bid-tid, maint 10-40mg bid-tid; ext.rel: ini 40mg PO bid, max 80mg PO bid; a daily dose-free interval of 10-14h is advisable to avoid nitrate tolerance; DARF: not req
Isosorbide Mononitrate	EHL 6.2 and 6.6h, PRC C, Lact ?
Imdur *Tab ext.rel 30mg, 60mg, 120mg* **ISMO** *Tab 20mg* **Monoket** *Tab 10mg, 20mg* **Generics** *Tab 10mg, 20mg, Tab ext.rel 30mg, 60mg, 120mg*	**AP** →50: 20mg PO bid (8 am and 3 pm); ext.rel: ini 30mg PO qd, incr prn to 120mg/d, max 240mg/d
Nitroglycerin IV	EHL 19-33min, PRC C, Lact ?
Nitro-Bid *Inj 5mg/ml* **Tridil** *Inj 0.5mg/ml* **Generics** *Inj 0.1mg/ml, 5mg/ml, 10mg/100ml, 20mg/100ml, 40mg/100ml*	**Acute AP** →50, **heart failure** →56: 5-40µg/min IV; **hypertensive emergency** →48: ini 10-20µg/min IV, incr to max 100µg/min

Nitroglycerin Spray	EHL 2-33min, PRC C, Lact ?
Nitrolingual *Aerosol SL 0.4mg/Spray* **Nitrolingual Pumpspray** *Spray metered SL 0.4mg/Spray*	**Acute AP** →50: 0.4-0.8mq SL, rep prn, max 1.2mg in 15min
Nitroglycerin Sublingual	EHL 2-33min, PRC C, Lact ?
Nitrostat *Tab (SL) 0.3mg, 0.4mg, 0.6mg*	**Acute AP** →50: 0.3-0.6mg SL or in the buccal pouch, rep prn q5min up to 3 doses in 15min; **angina PRO**: 0.3-0.6mg 5-10min before activities which might precipitate an acute attack; DARF: not req
Nitroglycerin Extended Release	EHL 2-33min, PRC C, Lact ?
Nitroglyn *Cap ext.rel 2.5mg, 6.5mg, 9mg, 13mg*	**AP PRO** →50: ini 2.5mg PO bid-tid, incr prn; mind a daily dose-free interval of 10-14h to avoid nitrate tolerance; DARF: not req
Nitroglycerin Transdermal	EHL 2-33min, PRC C, Lact ?
Minitran *Film (ext.rel, TD) 0.1, 0.2, 0.4, 0.6mg/h* **Nitro-Dur** *Film (ext.rel, TD) 0.1, 0.2, 0.3, 0.4, 0.6mg/h* **Transderm-Nitro** *Film (ext.rel, TD) 0.1, 0.2, 0.4, 0.8, 0.8mg/h* **Generics** *Film (ext.rel, TD) 0.2, 0.4, 0.6, 0.8mg/h*	**AP PRO** →50: 0.2-0.4mg/h; patch should remain for 12-14h and then be removed

2 A.13 Antiarrhythmics

Class IA antiarrhythmics (quinidine, disopyramide, procainamide)
MA/EF: inflow of Na^+ blocked ⇒ delayed depolarization, conduction velocity ↓ (neg. dromotropic), threshold potential of the AV node ↑ (excitability ↓), neg. inotropic, K^+-outflow blocked ⇒ action potential length ↑, refractory time ↑
AE: GI impairment, dizziness, confusion, dysopias, BP ↓, AV block, tachycardia
AE (disopyramide): urinary retention, constipation, accommodation impaired, dry mouth
CI: bradycardia, disturbance in conduction, digitalis overdose

Class IB antiarrhythmics (lidocaine, mexiletine, tocainide)
MA: Na^+ inflow ↓, K^+ outflow ↑, slowed phase 4 depolarization
EF: excitability ↓, especially in the ventricles, action potential duration and refractory time in Purkinje fibers ↓, in atria and ventricles ↑; high-frequency excitations are filtered out (premature contractions), possible AV conduction time ↑, negative inotropic effect smaller than class Ia, in high concentrations neg. dromotropic, neg. inotropic
AE (lidocaine hydrochloride): bradycardia, hypotension, dizziness, nausea
AE (mexiletine): dizziness, heartburn, lightheadedness, N/V, nervousness, tremors
AE (tocainide): appetite loss, dizziness, lightheadedness, N/V
CI (lidocaine hydrochloride): AV block II°-III°, asystolia

Class IC antiarrhythmics (flecainide, moricizine, propafenone)
MA: conduction and refractory time ↑ (AV node and ventricle), no vagolysis
AE: hypotension, AV block, nausea, pro-arrhythmias, cholestatic hepatitis
CI: cardiac insufficiency, sick sinus, serious asthma

Class II antiarrhythmics see Beta Blockers →23

Class III antiarrhythmics (amiodarone, bretylium, ibutilide, dofetilide, sotalol)
MA/EF: blockage of K^+ channels $\Rightarrow$ action potential length $\uparrow$
AE (amiodarone): cornea depositions, pulmonary fibrosis, hepatic damage, photosensitivity, dysopias, erythema nodosum, hypo- and hyperthyroidism
AE (sotalol): see Beta Blockers $\rightarrow$23
CI (amiodarone): AV block II° -III°, bradycardia, thyroid diseases, iodine allergy
CI (sotalol): see Beta Blockers $\rightarrow$23

Class IV antiarrhythmics (verapamil) see Calcium Channel Blockers - Non-Dihydropyridines $\rightarrow$29

Other Antiarrhythmics (adenosine, atropine, digoxin $\rightarrow$40, epinephrine $\rightarrow$22)
MA/EF (adenosine): brief blockage of the AV node $\Rightarrow$ termination of re-entry tachycardias, neg. chronotropic at the sinus node
MA/EF (atropine): compet. antagonism at muscarinic rec. $\Rightarrow$ tachycardia, antispasmodic, tear production $\downarrow$; sputum, sweat and bronchial secretion $\downarrow$, mydriasis, blurred vision
AE (adenosine): flush, dyspnea, bronchospasm, nausea; **AE** (atropine): decrease of sweat production, urinary retention, restlessness, hallucinations, oral dryness, acute glaucoma
CI (adenosine): AV block II°-III°, sick-sinus, atrial fibrillation, asthma, QT interval $\uparrow$
CI (atropine): glaucoma, micturition disturbances, tachyarrhythmias

Adenosine	Class IA, EHL < 10s, PRC C, Lact:?
Adenocard *Inj 3mg/ml* **Adenoscan** *Inj 3mg/ml*	**SVT** $\rightarrow$61: 6mg IV as rapid bolus; if tachycardia persists after 1–2min then 12mg IV; **CH SV arrhythmias conversion**: ini 0.05mg/kg IV as rapid bolus, then 0.05-0.1mg/kg IV, max 12mg/dose; DARF: not req
Amiodarone	Class III, EHL 28-107 days, PRC D, Lact -
Cordarone *Tab 200mg, Inj 50mg/ml* **Pacerone** *Tab 200mg* **Generics** *Tab 200, 400mg*	**Ventricular arrhythmias** $\rightarrow$62: ini 150mg IV over 10min, then 360mg over 6h (1mg/min), then 540mg IV over 18h (0.5mg/min); or 800-1600mg PO qd for 1-3 wk, then 600-800mg qd for 1 mo, then maint 200-400mg qd; DARF: not req
Atropine	EHL 4h, PRC C, Lact ?
Atropen *Inj 2mg sulfate/0.7ml*	**Bradycardia, bradyarrhythmia** $\rightarrow$63: 0.5-1.0mg IV, max 2mg IV; **CH** 0.02mg/kg IV, minimum 0.1mg, max 0.5mg IV
Bretylium	Class III, EHL 6-13.5h, PRC C, Lact ?
Generics *Inj 50mg/ml, 100mg/100ml, 200mg/100ml, 400mg/100ml*	**VF** $\rightarrow$62: ini 5mg/kg IV, then 10mg/kg if arrhythmia persists, max 30mg/kg IV; continuous suppression: 1-2mg/min IV
Digoxin	EHL 1.3-2.2 days, PRC C, Lact +
Digoxin pediatric *Inj 0.1mg/ml* **LanoxiCap** *Cap 0.05mg, 0.1mg, 0.2mg* **Lanoxin** *Tab 0.125, 0.25mg, Inj 0.25mg/ml* **Lanoxin pediatric** *Inj 0.1mg/ml* **Generics** *Tab 0.125, 0.25mg, Inj 0.25mg/ml*	**AF** $\rightarrow$60, **heart failure** $\rightarrow$56: ini 0.5mg IV, then 0.25mg q6h for 2 doses; maint 0.125–0.375mg PO/IV qd; **CH** 5-10 y: ini 20-35µg/kg PO div q6-8h, maint 25-35% of loading dose; DARF: see Prod Info

Disopyramide | Class IA, EHL 4-10h, PRC C, Lact +

Norpace *Cap 100mg, 150mg*
Norpace CR *Cap 100, 150mg, Cap ext.rel 100mg, 150mg*
Generics *Cap ext.rel 100mg, 150mg*

Ventricular arrhythmias →62: 150mg PO qid; ext.rel: 300mg PO bid; DARF: GFR (ml/min) >40: 100mg qid or 200mg bid; 30-40: 100mg tid; 15-30: 100mg bid; <15: 100mg qd

Dofetilide | Class III, EHL 7.5-10h, PRC C, Lact -

Tikosyn *Cap 0.125mg, 0.25mg, 0.5mg*

AF →60: 0.5mg PO bid; DARF: GFR (ml/min) >60: 100%, 40-60: 0.25mg bid, 20-40: 0.125 mg bid, <20: contraind.

Epinephrine | EHL no data, PRC C, Lact ?

Epi E Zpen Jr *Inj (IM) 0.15mg/delivery*
Epipen *Inj (IM) 0.3mg/delivery*
Epipen E Z Pen *Inj (IM) 0.3mg/delivery*
Epipen Jr. *Inj (IM) 0.15mg/delivery*
Sus-phrine Sulfite-free *Inj 1.5mg/amp, 5mg/ml*

Cardiac arrest →20: 0.5-1mg IV/ET, rep.ed prn q3-5min; anaphylaxis: 0.3-0.5 mg SC/IM, rep.ed prn q10-15min; **CH cardiac arrest**: 0.01mg/kg IV; 0.1mg/kg ET rep.ed prn with 0.1mg/kg IV/ET q3-5min; **anaphylaxis** →21: 0.01mg/kg SC/IM; 0.1mg/kg IV if response is inadequate; IV: use 1:10.000 Sol; SC/IM: use 1: 1000 sol

Flecainide | Class IC, EHL 14h, PRC C, Lact +

Tambocor *Tab 100mg, 150mg, 50mg*

SV + O1/ventricular arrhythmias →62: 200-400mg/d PO div bid; **CH** >6 mo: 100-200mg/m²/d PO; DARF: GFR (ml/min) <35: 50mg PO bid

Ibutilide | Class III, EHL 2-12h, PRC C, Lact ?

Corvert *Inj 0.1mg/ml*

Conversion of AF →61: >60kg: 1mg IV over 10min; <60kg: 0.01mg/kg; rep equal dose if no response after 10min; DARF: not req

Isoproterenol | Group II, EHL 3-7h, PRC C, Lact ?

Isuprel *Inj 0.2mg/ml*
Generics *Aerosol 0.12mg/Inh, Inj 0.2mg/ml; 0.02mg/ml*

Third degree AV block: ini 0.02-0.06mg IV, then 2-10 µg/min; **CH third degree AV block**: 0.1-1µg/kg/min IV ; →62

Lidocaine →285 | Class IB, EHL 1.5-2h, PRC B, Lact +

Generics *Inj 0.5%, 1%, 1.5%, 2%, 4%, 10%, 20%, Inj 200mg/100ml, 400mg/100ml, 800mg/100ml*

Ventricular arrhythmia →62: ini 50-100mg IV, then 1-4mg/min continuous inf; **CH ventricular arrhythmia**: ini 1mg/kg IV, then 20-50µg/kg/min as continuous inf; **anesthesia**

Mexiletine | Class IB, EHL 6-17h, PRC C, Lact +

Mexitil *Cap 150mg, 200mg, 250mg*
Generics *Cap 150mg, 200mg, 250mg*

Ventricular arrhythmia →62: ini 400mg PO, maint 200mg PO q8h

Moricizine | Class IC, EHL 6.4-13.1 h

Ethmozine *Tab 200mg, 250mg, 300mg*

Ventricular arrhythmias →62: 600-900mg/d PO div q8h

Procainamide	Class IA, EHL 2.5-8h, PRC C, Lact ?
Procanbid *Tab ext.rel 500mg, 1g* **Pronestyl** *Tab 250mg, 375mg, 500mg, Cap 250mg, 375mg, 500mg, Inj 100mg/ml, 500mg/ml* **Pronestyl–SR** *Tab ext.rel 500mg* **Generics** *Tab ext.rel 250mg, 500mg, 750mg, 1g, Cap 250mg, 375mg, 500mg, Inj 100mg/ml, 500mg/ml*	**Ventricular arrhythmias** →62: ini 100mg slow IV q5min, max 1g or until arrhythmia is supressed, then 2-6mg/min as continuous inf; 50mg/kg/d PO div q3h (immediate-release products), q6h (sustained release products), q12h (Procanbid)
Propafenone	Class IC, EHL 5-8h, PRC C, Lact ?
Rythmol *Tab 150mg, 225mg, 300mg* **Generics** *Tab 150mg, 225mg*	**Paroxysmal SVT, paroxysmal AF** →60, **ventricular arrhythmias** →62: ini 150mg PO q8h, incr q3-4d to 225mg q8h, max 900mg/d; DARF: not req
Quinidine Gluconate	Class IA, EHL no data, PRC C, Lact ?
Quinaglute *Tab ext.rel 324mg*	**Maintenance after conversion of AF**: 324-648 mg PO q8-12h; DARF: not req
Quinidine Sulfate	Class IA, EHL no data, PRC C, Lact ?
Quinidex *Tab ext.rel 300mg* **Generics** *Tab 100mg, 200mg, 300mg, Tab ext.rel 300mg*	**Maintenance after conversion of AF**: 200-400mg PO q4-6h; 300-600mg PO q8-12h (ext.rel); **CH** 6mg/kg PO q4-6h; DARF: not req
Sotalol	Class III, EHL 7-18h, PRC B, Lact ?
Betapace *Tab 80mg, 120mg, 160mg, 240mg* **Betapace AF** *Tab 80mg, 120mg, 160mg* **Generics** *Tab 80mg, 120mg, 160mg, 240mg*	**AF** →60, **ventricular arrhythmia** →62: ini 80mg PO bid, maint 160-320mg/d div bid; DARF: see Prod Info
Tocainide	Class IB, EHL 11-22.8h, PRC C, Lact ?
Tonocard *Tab 400mg, 600mg*	**Ventricular arrhythmias** →62: 400-600mg PO q8h; DARF: max 1200mg/d

2 A.14 Cardiac Glycosides

MA: inhibition of active Na^+-K^+-transport into heart muscle cells $\Rightarrow$ intracellular Na^+ ↑ $\Rightarrow$ Na^+-Ca^{2+} exchange $\Rightarrow$ intracellular Ca^{2+} ↑, vagal nerve activity ↑, sympathetic activity ↓
EF: pos. inotropic, stroke volume ↑, higher efficiency of the insufficient heart, tissue perfusion ↑, coronary perfusion ↑, neg. chronotropic and dromotropic, refractory time at S-A node ↑, at the myocardial ↓, $\Rightarrow$ activation of ectopic pacemakers, pos. bathmotropic
AE: AV block, arrhythmias, extrasystoles, N/V, diarrhea, color dysopias, confusion
CI: AV block II°-III°, WPW-syndrome, VT, carotid sinus syndrome, hypertrophic obstructive cardiomyopathy, hypercalcemia, hypokalemia, thoracic aortic aneurysm

Digitoxin	EHL 4-9d, PRC C, Lact +
Crystodigin *Inj 0.2mg/vial, Tab 0.05mg, 0.1mg, 0.15mg, 0.2mg* **Digitaline Nativelle** *Tab 0.1mg, 0.2mg* **Generics** *Tab 0.1mg, 0.2mg*	**AF** →60, **heart failure** →56: ini 0.6-1.2mg PO tid, maint 0.05-0.3mg PO qd; IV doses 75%-100% of PO dose; **CH** 1-2y: load 0.04 mg/kg PO/IV/IM tid; >2y: load 0.03 mg/kg PO/IV/IM tid; DARF req

Digoxin	EHL 1.3-2.2d, PRC C, Lact +
Digoxin pediatric *Inj 0.1mg/ml* **LanoxiCap** *Cap 0.05mg, 0.1mg, 0.2mg* **Lanoxin** *Tab 0.125mg, 0.25mg,* *Inj 0.25mg/ml* **Lanoxin pediatric** *Inj 0.1mg/ml* **Generics** *Tab 0.125, 0.25mg, Inj 0.25mg/ml*	**AF** →60, **heart failure** →56: ini 0.5mg IV, then 0.25mg q6h for 2 doses; maint 0.125-0.375mg PO/IV qd; **CH** 5-10 y: ini 20-35µg/kg PO div q6-8h, maint 25-35% of loading dose; DARF: see Prod Info
Digoxin-Immune Fab	EHL 15-20h, PRC C, Lact +
Digibind *Inj 38mg/vial*	**Digoxin/digitoxin-intoxication** →477: average-dose: 400mg IV; 40mg will bind 0.5-0.6mg digoxin or digitoxin

2 A.15 Phosphodiesterase Inhibitors

MA: inhibition of phosphodiesterase $\Rightarrow$ intracellular accumulation of cAMP $\Rightarrow$ intracellular Ca^{++} ↑ $\Rightarrow$ myocardial contractility ↑, **EF:** pos. inotropic effect (stroke volume, cardiac output ↑), pos. chronotropic effect, vasodilation (preload ↓, afterload ↓), bronchodilation
AE: cholestasis, nausea, hypotension, tachyarrhythmias, thrombocytopenia, splenomegaly, vasculitis, myositis, lung infiltration
CI: severe hypovolemia, continuous arrhythmia, thrombocytopenia, renal insufficiency

Inamrinone (Amrinone)	EHL 4.8-8.3h, PRC C, Lact ?
Amrinone *Inj 5mg/ml* **Inocor** *Inj 5mg/ml*	**Heart failure** →56: ini 0.75mg/kg IV over 2-3min, maint 5-10mg/kg/min; after 30min additional 0.75mg/kg IV prn
Milrinone	EHL 1-3h, PRC C, Lact ?
Primacor *Inj 1mg/ml, 20mg/100ml*	**Heart failure** →56: ini 50µg/kg IV over 10min, maint 0.375-0.75µg/kg/min; DARF: GFR (ml/min). 41-50: 0.43*, 31-40: 0.38, 21-30: 0.33*, 11-20: 0.28*, 6-10: 0.23*, <5: 0.2* (* = µg/kg/min); →54

2 A.16 Antilipidemics
2 A.16.1 Bile Acid Sequestrants

MA/EF: intestinal binding of bile acids $\Rightarrow$ interruption of the biliary cycle $\Rightarrow$ bile acid production from cholesterol ↑ $\Rightarrow$ serum cholesterol ↓; LDL-receptor activity ↑ $\Rightarrow$ LDL-resorption of the liver ↑ $\Rightarrow$ serum cholesterol ↓
AE: constipation, abdominal discomfort/pain, nausea, diarrhea, resorption failure of drugs and fat-soluble vitamins; **AE (colesevelam)**: dyspepsia, constipation; **AE (colestipol)**: constipation, fat soluble vitamin deficiency, N/V, flatulence, abdominal distention; **AE (cholestyramine)**: constipation, abdominal discomfort/pain, flatulence, N/V, bleeding tendencies due to hypoprothrombinemia
CI: bile duct obstruction; **CI (colesevelam)**: bowel obstruction, hypersensitivity to colesevelam; **CI (colestipol)**: hypersensitivity to colestipol products; **CI (cholestyramine)**: complete biliary obstruction, hyperlipidemia types III, IV, or V, hypersensitivity to bile-sequestering resins

Colesevelam	EHL no data, PRC B, Lact ?
Welchol *Tab 625mg*	**Hypercholesterolemia** →169: 3 Tab PO bid or 6 Tab qd

Colestipol	EHL no data, PRC , Lact +
Colestid *Tab 1g, Gran (oral) 5g/pkt, 5g/scoopful* **Flavored Colestid** *Gran (oral) 5g/pkt, 5g/scoopful*	**Hypercholesterolemia** →169: Tab: ini 2g PO qd/bid, max 16g/d; Gran: ini 5g PO qd/bid, incr by 5g increments at 1-2 mo intervals, max 30g/d; DARF: not req

Cholestyramine	EHL no data, PRC C, Lact ?
Locholest *Powder (oral) 4g/9g* **Locholest Light** *Powder (oral) 4g/5g* **Prevalite** *Powder (oral) 4g/5g* **Questran** *Powder (oral) 4g/9g* **Questran Light** *Powder (oral) 4g/5g* **Generics** *Powder (oral) 4g/5g, 4g/9g*	**Hypercholesterolemia** →169: ini 4g PO qd/bid, maint 8-16g/d div bid/qid, max 24g/d; DARF: not req

2 A.16.2 Cholesterol Absorption Inhibitors

MA/EF (ezetimib): inhibition of the intestinal absorption of cholesterol ad related phytosterols
AE (ezetimib): fatigue, pharyngitis, sinusitis, abd. pain, diarrhea, back pain, arthralgia, cough, viral infection; **CI** (ezetimib): hypersensitivity to e., hepatic dysfunction

Ezetimib	EHL 22h, PRC C, Lact -
Zetia *Tab 10mg*	**Primary hypercholesterolemia** →169, **homozyg. fam. hyperchol., homozyg. sitosterolemia**: 10mg PO qd, may be administered with an HMG-CoA reducatse inhibitor; DARF: not req

2 A.16.3 HMG–CoA Reductase Inhibitors ("Statins")

MA/EF: competitive inhibition of HMG CoA reductase ⇒ intracellular cholesterol synthesis↓, LDL↓, HDL↑;
AE: skin reactions, myopathy, vasculitis, headache, abdominal pain, transaminases↑, dyssomnia;
AE (atorvastatin): headache, liver enzymes↑, abdominal pain; **AE** (fluvastatin): dyspepsia, diarrhea, abdominal pain, nausea, headache; **AE** (lovastatin): headache, rhabdomyolysis, diarrhea, hepatotoxicity;
AE (pravastatin): GI disturbances, liver enzymes↑, headache, weakness, flu-like symptoms;
AE (simvastatin): headache, GI upset, rhabdomyolysis, transient hypotension, liver dysfunction
CI: hepatic diseases, cholestasis, myopathy, hypersensitivity to product ingredients

Atorvastatin	EHL 14h, PRC X, Lact -
Lipitor *Tab 10mg, 20mg, 40mg, 80mg*	**Hypercholesterolemia, mixed dyslipidemia** →169: ini 10mg PO qd, maint 10-80mg PO qd, DARF: not req

Fluvastatin	EHL < 3 h, PRC X, Lact -
Lescol *Cap 20mg, 40mg*	**Hypercholesterolemia** →169: ini 20-40mg PO qd, max 80mg/d, give 80mg in div doses bid

Lovastatin	EHL no data, PRC X, Lact -
Altocor *Tab ext. rel. 10, 20, 60mg* **Mevacor** *Tab 10mg, 20mg, 40mg*	**Hypercholesterolemia** →169: ini 20mg PO qd, maint 10-80mg/d PO

Lovastatin + Niacin	EHL no data, PRC X, Lact -
Advicor *Tab ext.rel 20 + 500mg, 20 + 750mg, 20 + 1000mg*	**Hypercholesterolemia** →169: ini 20 + 500mg PO qd, maint 20-40 + 500-2000mg/d PO

Pravastatin	EHL 2.6-3.2 h, PRC X, Lact -
Pravachol *Tab 10mg, 20mg, 40mg*	**Hypercholesterolemia** →169: ini 10-20mg PO qd, maint 10-40mg/d; DARF: ini 10mg PO qd
Simvastatin	EHL no data, PRC X, Lact -
Zocor *Tab 5mg, 10mg, 20mg, 40mg, 80mg*	**Hypercholesterolemia** →169: ini 20-40mg PO qd, maint 5-80mg/d; DARF: ini 5mg PO qd

2 A.16.4 Fibric Acids

MA/EF: lipoprotein lipase activity↑ ⇒ triglycerides↓, LDL↓, HDL↑
AE: myalgia, rhabdomyolysis, N/V, transaminases↑, cholelithiasis, ventricular dysrhythmia, blood count changes; **AE** (clofibrate): diarrhea, flatulence, headache;
AE (fenofibrate): rash, LFT↑;
AE (gemfibrozil): epigastric pain, xerostomia, diarrhea, myopathy, hepatotoxicity
CI: primary biliary cirrhosis, great caution in children; **CI** (clofibrate): renal/liver disease, hypersensitivity to clofibrate; **CI** (fenofibrate): severe hepatic or renal disease, gallbladder disease, hypersensitivity to fenofibrate; **CI** (gemfibrozil): hypersensitivity to gemfibrozil, gallbladder disease/biliary cirrhosis, severe liver/kidney disease

Clofibrate	EHL 14-35h, PRC C, Lact -
Atromid-S *Cap 500mg* **Generics** *Cap 500mg*	**Hyperlipidemia** →169: ini and maint doses of 2g daily in div doses; some patients may respond to a lower dose; DARF: contraind. in clinically significant RF; see Prod Info
Fenofibrate	EHL 20-22h, PRC C, Lact -
Tricor *Cap 67mg, 134mg, 200mg; Tab 54mg, 160mg*	**Hypertriglyceridemia** →170: ini 54-67mg PO qd, maint 134-200mg PO qd
Gemfibrozil	EHL 1.5 h, PRC C, Lact -
Lopid *Tab 600mg* **Generics** *Tab 600mg*	**Hypertriglyceridemia** →170: 600mg PO bid

2 A.16.5 Nicotinic Acid

MA/EF: blockage of the triacylglycerol lipase ⇒ lipoprotein lipase activity↑ ⇒ triglycerides↓, cholesterol↓
AE: flush, a sensation of warmth in face, neck, and ears, GI disturbances, glucose tolerance↓, fasting blood sugar↑, pruritus, hepatotoxicity, feeling of restlessness, headache, hypotension, rash, tingling, itching, and dry skin
CI: acute CVS failure, hypersensitivity to niacin, active liver/peptic ulcer disease

Niacin	EHL 10h, PRC C, Lact ?
Niacor *Tab 500mg* **Niaspan** *Tab ext.rel. 375mg, 500mg, 750mg* **Nicolar** *Tab 500mg* **Generics** *Tab 500mg*	**Hyperlipoproteinemia/hyperlipidemia** →169: ini 100mg PO tid incr slowly to 3g/d, max 6g/d; ext.rel.: 375mg PO qd for 1wk, then 500mg PO qd for 1wk, then 750mg PO qd for 1wk, then 1000mg PO qd; max 2g/d

2 B. Cardiovascular – Therapies

Debabrata Mukherjee, MD
Assistant Professor, UMHS Cardiovascular Center
University of Michigan, Ann Arbor, MI

2 B.1   Hypertension
2 B.1.1   JNC VII Hypertension Guideline

Classification and management of blood pressure for adults*

BP Classification	SBP* (mmHg)	DBP* (mmHg)	Lifestyle Modification	Initial Drug Therapy	
				Without Compelling Indications	With Compelling Indications (see Table 5)
Normal	< 120	and < 80	Encourage	No antihypertensive drug indicated.	Drug(s) for compelling indications***
Prehypertension	120 – 139	or 80 – 89	Yes		
Stage 1 Hypertension	140 – 159	or 90 – 99	Yes	Thiazide-type diuretics for most. May consider ACEI, ARB, BB, CCB, or combination	Drug(s) for the compelling indications. Other antihypertensive drugs (diuretics, ACEI, ARB, BB, CCB) as needed.
Stage 2 Hypertension	≥ 160	or ≥ 100	Yes	Two-drug combination for most** (usually thiazide-type diuretic and ACEI or ARB or BB or CCB).	

DBP: diastolic blood pressure; SBP: systolic blood pressure; ACEI: angiotensin converting enzyme inhibitor; ARB: angiotensin receptor blocker; BB: beta-blocker; CCB: calcium channel blocker.

*   Treatment determined by highest BP category.
**   Initial combined therapy should be used cautiously in those at risk for orthostatic hypotension.
*** Treat patients with chronic kidney disease or diabetes to BP goal of < 130/80 mmHg.

Identifiable causes of hypertension

- Sleep apnea
- Drug-induced or related causes
- Chronic kidney disease
- Primary aldosteronism
- Renovascular disease
- Chronic steroid therapy and Cushing's syndrome
- Pheochromocytoma
- Coarctation of the aorta
- Thyroid or parathyroid disease

Cardiovasular risk factors

Major Risk Factors	Target Organ Damage

• Hypertension*
 • Cigarette smoking
 • Obesity* (body mass index $\geq$ 30 kg/m^2)
 • Physical inactivity
 • Dyslipidemia*
 • Diabetes mellitus*
 • Microalbuminuria GFR < 60 mL/min
 • Age (> 55 years for men, > 65 years for woman)
 • Family history of premature cardiovascular disease (men < 55 years or woman < 65 years)
	• Heart
	   - Left ventricular hypertrophy
	   - Angina or prior myocardial infarction
	   - Prior coronary revasularization
	   - Heart failure
	 • Brain
	   - Stroke or transient ischemic attack
	 • Chronic kidney disease
	 • Peripheral arterial disease
	 • Retinopathy

GFR: glomerular filtration rate., * components of the metabolic syndrome.

Lifestyle modifications to manage hypertension

Modification	Recommendation*, **	Approximate SBP Reduction (Range)
Weight reduction	Maintain normal body weight (body mass index 18.5 - 24.9 kg/m^2)	5 - 20 mmHg/ 10 kg weight loss
Adopt DASH eating plan	Consume a diet rich in fruits, vegetables, and lowfat dairy products with a reduced content of saturated and total fat	8 - 14 mmHg
Dietary sodium reduction	Reduce dietary sodium intake to no more than 100 mmol per day (2.4 g sodium or 6 g sodium chloride)	2 - 8 mmHg
Physical activity	Engage in regular aerobic physical activity such as brisk walking (at least 30 min per day, most days of the week)	4 - 9 mmHg
Moderation of alcohol consumption	Limit consumption to no more than 2 drinks (1 oz or 30 mL ethanol; e.g., 24 oz beer, 10 oz wine, or 3 oz 8o-proof whiskey) per day in most men and to no more than 1 drink per day in woman and lighter weight persons	2 - 4 mmHg

DASH: Dietary Approaches to Stop Hypertension
* For overall cardiovascular risk reduction, stop smoking.
** The effects of implementing these modifications are dose and time dependent, and could be greater for some individuals.

Clinical trial and guideline basis for compelling indications for individual drug classes

Compelling Indication*	Recommended Drugs**						Clinical Trial Basis***
	Diuretic	BB	ACEI	ARB	CCB	Aldo ANT	
Heart failure	x	x	x	x		x	ACC/AHA Heart Failure Guideline, MERIT HF, COPERNICUS, CIBIS, SOLVD, AIRE, TRACE, ValHEFT, RALES
Postmyocardial infarction		x	x			x	ACC/AHA Post-MI Guideline, BHAT, SAVE, Capricorn, EPHESUS

High coronary disease risk	x	x	x		x		ALLHAT, HOPE, ANBP$_2$, LIFE, CONVINCE
Diabetes	x	x	x	x	x		NKF-ADA Guideline, UKPDS, ALLHAT
Chronic kidney disease			x	x			NKF Guideline, Captopril Trial, RENAAL, IDNT, REIN, AASK
Recurrent stroke prevention	x		x				PROGRESS

* Compelling indications for antihypertensive drugs are based on benefits from outcome studies or existing clinical guidelines; the compelling indication is managed in parallel with the BP.

** Drug abbreviations: ACEI, angiotensin converting enzyme inhibitor; ARB, angiotensin receptor blocker; Aldo ANT, aldosterone antagonist; BB, beta-blocker; CCB, calcium channel blocker.

*** Conditions for which clinical trials demonstrate benefit of specific classes of antihypertensive drugs.

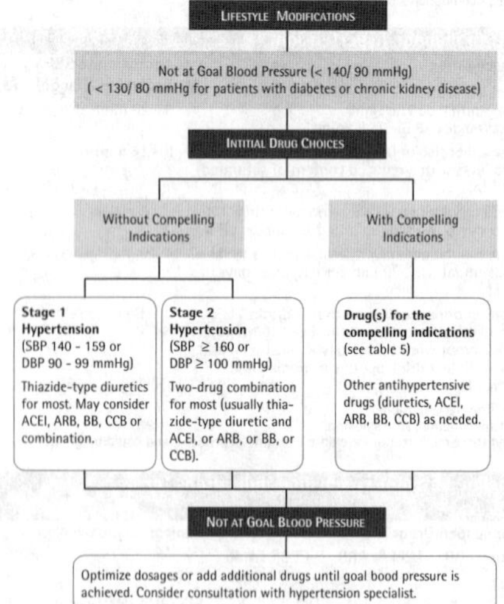

DBP, diastolic blood pressure; SBP, systolic blood pressure.
Drug abbreviations: ACEI, angiotensin converting enzyme inhibitor; ARB, angiotensin receptor; BB, beta-blocker; CCB, calcium channel blocker

JNC VII, Joint National Committee on High BLood Pressure, May 2003

2 B.1.2   Monotherapy

Diuretic

	Thiazide diuretic →33 (renal H_2O/Na^+Cl^- loss, endog. vasoconstrictive stimuli ↓)	**Hydrochlorothiazide** (Esidrix, Hydrodiuril, Microside, Oretic, Gens)	*12.5-50mg PO qd*
poss	**Potassium-sparing diuretic** →34 (renal H_2O/Na^+Cl^- loss, K^+ secretion ↓)	**Triamterene** (Dyrenium)	*50mg PO bid (1-1-0)*
		Amiloride (Midamor, Gens)	*5mg PO qd*
		Spironolactone (Aldactone, Gens)	*25–100mg PO qd*

Renal Na^+Cl^- mobilization, Caution: only effective if creatinine < 2mg/dl

Beta blocker

	Beta-1-selective blocker →23 (CO ↓, neg. chronotropic, neg. inotropic, renin secretion ↓, central sympathetic activity ↓)	**Metoprolol** (Lopressor, Toprol-xl, Gens)	*50-100mg PO qd-bid*
		Atenolol (Tenormin, Gens)	*25–100mg PO qd*
		Bisoprolol (Zebeta, Gen.)	*2.5–10mg PO qd*

Caution: Uncontrolled heart failure, high grade AV-block, bronchial asthma

Calcium channel blocker (CCB)

	CCB - non-dihydropyridine →29 (chrono-, dromo-, inotropic ↓, afterload ↓)	**Diltiazem** (Cardizem, Cartia XT, Tiamate, Tiazac, Gens)	*60-90mg PO tid, 90-180mg SR PO bid, 240mg SR PO qd*
or		**Verapamil** (Calan, Covera-HS, Isoptin, Verelan, Gens)	*80-120mg PO tid, 120-240mg SR PO bid*
or	**CCB - dihydropyridine** →28 (chrono-, dromo-, inotropic ↓, afterload ↓)	**Nifedipine** (Adalat, Adalat cc, Procardia, Procardia XL, Gens)	*20mg SR PO bid, 10mg PO tid*
or		**Amlodipine** (Norvasc)	*5-10mg PO qd*

ACE inhibitor

	ACE inhibitor →25 (vasodilation ↑, renal perfus. ↑, aldosterone ↓, catecholamine ↓)	**Captopril** (Capoten, Gens)	*Incr slowly to 12.5-50mg PO bid-tid*
or		**Enalapril** (Lexxel, Vaseretic, Vasotec, Gens)	*Incr slowly to 5-20mg PO qd*
or		**Lisinopril** (Prinivil, Zestril)	*Incr slowly to 2.5–40mg PO qd*
or		**Ramipril** (Altace)	*Incr slowly to 2.5–10mg PO qd bid*

Angiotensin receptor blocker

	ARB →27 (specific blockade of angiotensin-II type 1 receptor ⇒ angiotensin effects ↓)	**Losartan** (Cozaar)	*50mg PO qd, max 100mg/d*
or		**Candesartan** (Atacand)	*8–32mg PO qd*
or		**Valsartan** (Diovan)	*80-320mg PO qd*
or		**Irbesartan** (Avapro)	*150-300mg PO qd*

Alpha–1 blocker

Alpha–1–Blocker →30 (vasodilation ↑, afterload ↓, preload ↓)	**Prazosin** (Minipress, Minipress XL, Gens)	*1–5mg PO bid-tid, 4–6mg SR PO qd*
or	**Doxazosin** (Cardura, Gens)	*2–8mg PO qd, max 16mg PO qd*

2 B.1.3   Double Therapy (Two Drug Combination)

Diuretic	**CCB**	**ACE-inhibitor**
+ **Beta blocker or** + CCB or + ACE inhibitor or + ARB	+ Beta blocker or + ACE inhibitor	+ ARB

2 B.1.4   Triple Therapy (Three Drug Combination)

Diuretic	**Diuretic**	**Diuretic**
+ Beta blocker + Vasodilator	+ ACE inhibitor + CCB	+ Antisympathotonic + Vasodilator

Vasodilator: CCB, ACE inhibitor, alpha-1 blocker, hydralazine

2 B.2   Hypertensive Emergency
2 B.2.1   In General

First measures

Nitrate →36 (pre-/afterload ↓, venous pooling)	**Nitroglycerin** (Nitrolingual, Nitrostat)	*0.4mg SL, rep prn q5min up to 3 doses in 15min*

If persistent

	Central alpha 2- Agonist →30 (norepinephrine release ↓, periph. sympathetic tone ↓, renin ↓)	**Clonidine** (Catapres, Catapres-TTS, Gens)	*Ini 0.1–0.2mg PO, then 0.05–0.2mg qh until total dose of 0.5–0.7mg*
or	**ACE inhibitor** →25 (vasodilation ↑, renal perfus. ↑, aldosterone ↓, catecholamine ↓) →25	**Captopril** (Capoten, Gens)	*12.5–25mg PO*
or	**Beta blocker** →23 (neg. ino-, chronotropic ⇒ cardiac output ↓)	**Labetalol** (Normodyne, Trandate, Gens)	*0.5–2mg/min slowly IV up to total of 50–200mg*
		Esmolol (Brevibloc)	*Loading dose 250–500µg/kg IV over 1min, then 50–100µg/kg/min for 4min, sos rep prn*
or	**Direct vasodilator** →31 (peripheral resistance ↓, afterload ↓)	**Hydralazine** (Apresoline, Gens)	*5–10mg IV (range: 5–20mg) q20–30min prn*

In pulmonary edema additionally

	Loop diuretic →33 (excretion of H_2O, Na^+, Cl^-, K^+, Ca^+, Mg^+↑)	**Furosemide** (Lasix, Gens)	*20-40mg IV, poss rep after 30min*
plus	**Opioid** →282 (analgesic, sedative)	**Morphine sulfate** (Astramorph, Avinza, Duramorph, Infumorph, Kadian, Numorphan, Roxanol, Gens)	*5-10mg IV (diluted 1:10)*
plus	**Gas** (blood oxygenation)	**Oxygen**	*2-4l/min nasal cannula*

If therapy fails

poss	**Direct vasodilator** →31 (peripheral resistance↓, afterload↓)	**Diazoxide** (Hyperstat, Proglycem)	*50-150mg IV, rep q5-15min, or 15-30mg/min IV Inf to max 600mg*
poss	**Direct vasodilator** →31 (pre-/afterload↓)	**Nitroprusside sodium** (Nipride, Nitropress)	*0.25-10mg/kg/min IV*

2 B.2.2   In Pheochromocytoma

	Alpha blocker →30 (vasodilation↑, afterload↓, preload↓)	**Phentolamine** (Regitine, Rogitine, Gens)	*5-10mg IV, then 0.25-1mg/min Inf*
or		**Phenoxybenzamine** (Dibenzyline)	*1mg/kg over 2-4h in 200ml NS*
poss plus	**Beta blocker** →23: use only after primary treatment with alpha blocker. **Caution: serious blood pressure elevation without concomitant alpha-blockade!**		
	(CO↓, neg. chronotropic, neg. inotropic, renin secretion↓, central sympathetic activity↓)	**Propranolol** (Inderide LA, Gens)	*1mg slowly IV, rep prn, 40-80mg PO bid-tid*
		Metoprolol (Lopressor, Toprol, Gens)	*5mg IV, rep prn, 50-200mg XL PO qd*

2 B.3   Hypotension and Syncope

In neurally mediated syncope

poss	**Methylxanthine** →97 (Phosphodiesterase inhibition ⇒ cAMP↑ ⇒ central stimulation of respiration, positive inotropic/chronotropic, vasodilation)	**Theophylline** (Aerolate, Elixophyllin, Slo-bid, Slo-Phyllin, Theo-24, Theo-DurUni-Dur, Uniphyl, Gens)	*6-12mg/kg/d*
poss	**Beta-1-selective blocker** →23 (CO↓, neg. chronotropic, neg. inotropic, renin secretion↓, central sympathetic activity↓)	**Metoprolol** (Lopressor, Toprol)	*50-200mg PO qd*
		Atenolol (Tenormin, Gens)	*25-200mg PO qd*

In decreased sympathetic tone

	Alpha-beta-adrenergic agonist →22	**Pseudoephedrine** (Sudafed, Afrin)	*60mg q4-6h*
poss	(vasoconstriction, CO↑ ⇒ BP↑)	**Ephedrine** (Gens)	*25mg PO qd-qid*

Consider atrioventricular pacing in refractory cases

In hypocortisolism, diabetic autonomic neuropathy

Drug therapy should be used only after nondrug therapies e.g., support hose, increased sodium intake, lifestyle modifications and fluid expansion have failed.

poss	**Mineralocorticoid** →148 (H_2O and Na^+ resorption $\Rightarrow$ circulating volume ↑)	**Fludrocortisone** (Florinef)	*0.1–1.0mg PO qd*
poss	**Vasopressor** →22 (alpha-adrenergic agonist $\Rightarrow$ vasoconstriction)	**Midodrine** (ProAmatine)	*2.5mg PO bid-tid*

2 B.4 Coronary Artery Disease
2 B.4.1 Acute Angina Pectoris

	Nitrate →36 (pre-/afterload ↓, venous pooling)	**Nitroglycerin** (Nitrolingual, Nitrostat)	*0.4mg SL, rep prn q5min up to 3 doses in 15min*
plus	**Gas** (blood oxygenation)	**Oxygen**	*2-4l/min nasal cannula*
plus	**Antiplatelet drug** →74 (phosphodiesterase/platelet aggregation-adhesion inhibition)	**Aspirin – ASA** (Ascriptin, Aspergum, Asprimox, Bayer Aspirin, Bufferin, Easprin, Ecotrin, Empirin, Genprin, Halfprin, St. Joseph Pain Reliever, Zorprin, Gens)	*325mg PO chewed*
plus	**Opioid** →282 (analgesic, sedative)	**Morphine sulfate** (Astramorph, Avinza, Duramorph, Infumorph, Kadian, Numorphan, Roxanol, Gens)	*5-10mg IV (diluted 1:10)*
plus	**Beta-1-selective blocker** →23 (CO ↓, neg. chronotropic, neg. inotropic, O_2 consumption ↓, central sympathetic activity ↓)	**Metoprolol** (Lopressor, Toprol-xl, Gens)	*5-10mg slowly IV, titrate to HR and BP*
		Atenolol (Tenormin, Gens)	*5mg IV, rep prn*
		Bisoprolol (Ziac, Gens)	*2.5-10mg PO qd*

Under relative contraindication: calcium channel blockers, digitalis glycosides

2 B.4.2 Chronic Stable Angina Pectoris

In general

	Antiplatelet drug →74 (phosphodiesterase/platelet aggregation-adhesion inhibition)	**Aspirin – ASA** (Ascriptin, Asprimox, Bayer Aspirin, Bufferin, Easprin, Ecotrin, Empirin, Genprin, Halfprin, St. Joseph Pain Reliever, Zorprin, Gens)	*81–325mg PO qd*
or	**Antiplatelet drug** →74 (blockage of platelet ADP-receptors)	**Clopidogrel** (Plavix)	*75mg PO qd*

plus	**Nitrate** →36 (pre-/afterload ↓, venous pooling, coronary spasmolysis, O_2-consumption ↓)	**Isosorbide mononitrate** (Imdur, ISMO, Monoket, Gens)	*20-40mg PO bid (1-1-0), 40-100mg SR PO qd*
or / poss plus	**Beta-1-selective blocker** →23 (CO↓, neg. chronotropic, neg. inotropic, O_2 consumption ↓, central sympathetic activity ↓)	**Metoprolol** (Lopressor, Toprol-xl, Gens)	*50-100mg PO qd-bid*
		Atenolol (Tenormin, Gens)	*25-100mg PO qd*
		Bisoprolol (Ziac, Gens)	*1 x 2.5-10mg PO*

Prinzmetal's angina

	Nitrate →36 (pre-/afterload ↓, venous pooling, coronary spasmolysis, O_2-consumption ↓)	**Isosorbide mononitrate** (Imdur, ISMO, Monoket, Gens)	*20-40mg PO bid (1-1-0), 40-100mg SR PO qd*
plus	**CCB** →28, →29 (chrono-, dromo-, inotropic ↓, afterload ↓, O_2-consumption ↓)	**Diltiazem** (Cardizem, Cartia XT, Tiamate, Tiazac, Gens)	*60-90mg PO tid, 90-180mg SR PO bid, 240mg SR PO qd*
		Amlodipine (Norvasc)	*5-10mg PO qd*
poss	**Beta-1-selective blocker** →23 (CO↓, neg. chronotropic, neg. inotropic, O_2 consumption ↓, central sympathetic activity ↓)	**Metoprolol** (Lopressor, Toprol-xl, Gens)	*50-100mg PO qd-bid*
		Atenolol (Tenormin, Gens)	*25-100mg PO qd*

Poss antihypertensive therapy in CAD

	Beta-1-selective blocker →23 (CO ↓, neg. chronotropic, neg. inotropic, O_2-consumption ↓)	**Metoprolol** (Lopressor, Toprol-xl, Gens)	*50-100mg PO qd-bid*
		Atenolol (Tenormin, Gens)	*25-100mg PO qd*
or	**ACE inhibitor** →25 (vasodilation ↑, renal perfusion ↑, aldosterone release ↓, catecholamine release ↓)	**Captopril** (Capoten, Gens)	*Incr slowly to 12.5-25mg PO bid*
		Enalapril (Lexxel, Vaseretic, Vasotec, Gens)	*2.5-20mg PO qd, max 40mg qd; IV ini 1.25mg, then 1.25-2.5mg IV qid*
		Lisinopril (Prinivil, Zestril)	*2.5-40mg PO qd*
		Ramipril (Altace)	*1.25-5mg PO qd-bid max 20mg qd*
or	**CCB** →28 (O_2-consumption ↓, inotropic ↓, afterload ↓)	**Amlodipine** (Norvasc)	*5-10mg PO qd*

Acute coronary syndrome without ST-elevation

	Heparin, unfractionated →70 (coagulation factor inhibition ↑, embolism prophylaxis)	**Heparin** (Gens)	*5000 U IV bolus, then 1000 U/h; aim for aPTT ratio of 1.5-2.5*
or	**Heparin-low-molecular weight** →71 (LMWH)	**Enoxaparin** (Lovenox)	*30mg IV bolus, then 1mg/kg SC bid*

plus	**Antiplatelet drug** →74 (phosphodiesterase/platelet aggregation–adhesion inhibition)	**Aspirin – ASA** (Ascriptin, Asprimox, Bayer Aspirin, Bufferin, Easprin, Ecotrin, Empirin, Genprin, Halfprin, St. Joseph Pain Reliever, Zorprin, Gens)	*325mg PO chewed*
plus	**Antiplatelet drug** →74 (blockage of platelet ADP-receptors)	**Clopidogrel** (Plavix)	*300mg loading dose then 75mg PO qd*
plus	**Nitrate** →36 (pre-/afterload ↓, venous pooling, scientifically disputed)	**Nitroglycerin** (Nitrolingual, Nitrostat)	*0.4mg SL, rep prn q5min up to 3 doses in 15min*
plus	**Opioid** →282 (analgesic, sedative)	**Morphine sulfate** (Astramorph, Avinza, Duramorph, Infumorph, Kadian, Numorphan, Roxanol, Gens)	*5-10mg IV (diluted 1:10)*
plus	**Beta–1–selective blocker** →23 (CO↓, neg. chronotropic, neg. inotropic, O_2 consumption↓, central sympathetic activity↓)	**Metoprolol** (Lopressor, Toprol-xl, Gens)	*5mg IV x 3; Caution: BP↓, HR↓*
		Atenolol (Tenormin, Gens)	*5mg IV, rep prn*
plus	**HMG–CoA–reductase inhibitor** →42 (intracell. cholesterol synthesis ↓, LDL ↓, HDL ↑)	**Atorvastatin** (Lipitor)	*10-20mg PO qd*
		Pravastatin (Pravachol)	*10-20 mg PO qd*

2 B.5   Myocardial Infarction
2 B.5.1   First Measures

	Antiplatelet drug →74 (phosphodiesterase/platelet aggregation–adhesion inhibition)	**Aspirin – ASA** (Ascriptin, Asprimox, Bayer Aspirin, Bufferin, Easprin, Ecotrin, Empirin, Genprin, Halfprin, St. Joseph Pain Reliever, Zorprin, Gens)	*325mg PO chewed*
plus	**Nitrate** →36 (pre-/afterload ↓, venous pooling, scientifically disputed)	**Nitroglycerin** (Nitrolingual, Nitrostat)	*0.4mg SL, rep prn q5min up to 3 doses in 15min*
poss	**Opioid** →282 (analgesic, sedative)	**Morphine sulfate** (Astramorph, Avinza, Duramorph, Infumorph, Kadian, Numorphan, Roxanol, Gens)	*5-10mg IV (diluted 1:10)*
plus	**Heparin, unfractionated** →70 (coagulation factor inhibition ↑, embolism prophylaxis)	**Heparin** (Gens)	*5000-10000 U IV*
plus	**Gas** (blood oxygenation)	**Oxygen**	*2-6l/min nasal cannula*

poss	**Benzodiazepine** →330 (sedative, anxiolytic, muscle relaxing)	**Diazepam** (Diazepam Intensol, Valium, Gens)	*5-10mg IV sos*
poss	**ACE inhibitor** →25 (vasodilation ↑, renal perfus. ↑, aldosterone ↓, catecholamine ↓)	**Captopril** (Capoten)	*6.25–25mg PO tid*
		Enalapril (Vasotec)	*2.5–20mg PO qd*
		Lisinopril (Zestril)	*2.5–10mg PO qd*
		Ramipril (Altace)	*2.5–5mg PO bid*
poss only if CV-stable	**Beta–1–selective blocker** →23 (CO ↓, neg. chronotropic, neg. inotropic, O_2 consumption ↓, central sympathetic activity ↓)	**Metoprolol** (Lopressor, Toprol-xl, Gens)	*5mg IV; Caution: BP↓, HR↓*
		Atenolol (Tenormin, Gens)	*5mg IV, rep prn*

2 B.5.2 Revascularization Therapy

Primary percutaneous transluminal coronary angioplasty (PTCA)

	Thrombolytic →73 (plasminogen activation ⇒ fibrin proteolysis, recanalization, limitation of myocard necrosis, mortality ↓)	**Streptokinase** (Streptase)	*1.5 M IU over 1h IV*
or		**rt-PA** (Alteplase)	*15mg IV as bolus, then 0.75mg/kg (max 50mg) over 30min, then 0.5mg/kg (max 35mg) over 1h*
or		**Reteplase** (Retevase)	*10 U as bolus IV, rep after 30min*
or		**Tenecteplase** (TNKasc)	*30–50mg IV over 5sec, dose based on body weight*
plus	**Heparin, unfractionated** →70 (coagulation factor inhibition ↑, embolism prophylaxis)	**Heparin** (Gens)	*Concomitant heparin: 5000 U IV bolus, then 1000 U/h (no heparin with streptokinase)*

If possible: primary angioplasty, ICU admission. IV Heparin not necessary with Streptokinase. SC heparin may be used in these patients for thromboprophylaxis.
CI of thrombolytics: severe HTN, aortic aneurysm, endocarditis, GI ulcers, pancreatitis, advanced malignant tumors, pathologic hemostasis, head trauma, internal bleeding, operation or puncture < 10d, IM injection < 7d, esophageal varices; CI of anistreplase/streptokinase: hypersensitivity to these products.

2 B.5.3 Therapy of Complication

Ventricular tachyarrhythmias

poss	**Antiarrhythmic, class Ib** →37	**Lidocaine** (Xylocaine)	*Ini 50-100mg IV, then Inf at 2-4mg/min*
	Antiarrhythmic, class Ia →37	**Procainamide** (Pronestyl)	*17mg/kg bolus, then Inf at 1-4mg/min*
or poss	**Antiarrhythmic, class III** →37 (blockage of K^+ channels ⇒ action potential length ↑, refractory time ↑)	**Amiodarone** (Cordarone, Pacerone, Gens)	*IV 150mg over 30min, then 1mg/min for 6h Inf, then 0.5mg/min for 18h, or d1-10: 1000mg PO div in 5 doses, then 200mg/d*

Atrial fibrillation

	Beta-1-select. blocker →23 ($CO\downarrow$, neg. chronotropic, neg. inotropic, renin secretion $\downarrow$, central sympathetic activity $\downarrow$)	**Metoprolol** (Lopressor, Toprol-xl, Gens)	*50-100mg PO qd-bid*
		Atenolol (Tenormin, Gens)	*25–100mg PO qd*
plus	**Antiarrhythmic, class III** →37 (blockage of K^+ channels $\Rightarrow$ action potential length $\uparrow$, refractory time $\uparrow$)	**Amiodarone** (Cordarone, Pacerone, Gens)	*d1-10: 1000mg PO div in 5 doses, then 200mg qd*

Sos cardioversion!

or	**CCB – non-dihydropyridine** →29 (chrono-, dromo-, inotropic $\downarrow$, afterload $\downarrow$, O_2-consumption $\downarrow$)	**Diltiazem** (Cardizem, Cartia XT, Tiamate, Tiazac, Gens)	*15–25mg IV bolus, then 10mg/h Inf*
		Verapamil (Calan, Covera-HS, Isoptin, Verelan, Gens)	*5mg slowly IV, then 5-10mg/h, max 100mg/d*

Bradycardia

	Antiarrhythmic →37 (parasympatholytic, chronotropic $\uparrow$)	**Atropine** (Atropen)	*0.5-1mg IV*

Sos pacemaker!

Heart Failure

poss	**Loop diuretic** →33 (excretion of H_2O, Na^+, Cl^-, K^+, Ca^+, $Mg^+\uparrow$)	**Furosemide** (Lasix, Gens)	*20-40mg IV*
plus	**Nitrate** →36 (pre-/afterload $\downarrow$, venous pooling)	**Nitroglycerin** (Nitro-Bid, Nitrolingual, Nitrostat, Tridil, Gens)	*0.4mg SL, rep prn q5min up to 3 doses in 15min; IV Inf 5-200µg/min*
plus	**Gas** (blood oxygenation)	**Oxygen**	*2-4l/min nasal cannula*
plus	**ACE inhibitor** →25 (vasodilation $\uparrow$, renal perfus. $\uparrow$, aldosterone $\downarrow$, catecholamine $\downarrow$)	**Captopril** (Capoten)	*Incr slowly to 12.5–25mg PO bid*
		Enalapril (Vasotec)	*2.5–20mg PO qd*
		Lisinopril (Zestril)	*2.5–40mg PO qd*

Cardiogenic shock

Primary therapy goal: placement of intra-aortic balloon pump, revascularization with angioplasty or surgery.

	Gas (blood oxygenation)	**Oxygen**	*2-4l/min nasal cannula*
plus	**Loop diuretic** →33 (excretion of H_2O, Na^+, Cl^-, K^+, Ca^+, $Mg^+\uparrow$)	**Furosemide** (Lasix, Gens)	*20–80mg IV qd*

poss	**Vasopressor** →22 (dose-dependent dopamine-, beta-alpha-adrenergic agonism ⇒ inotropia↑, CO↓, renal vasodilation, vasoconstriction)	**Dopamine** (Intropin, Gens)	*Ini 2-5µg/kg/min, incr by 1-4µg/kg/min q10-30min, max 50µg/kg/min; renal dose. 0.5-5µg/kg/min, beta-stimulation at 5-10µg/kg/min, alpha stim. at 10-20µg/kg/min*
poss	**Phosphodiesterase inhibitor** →41 (intracell. cAMP↑ ⇒ Ca^{++}↑ ⇒ chrono-/ inotropia↑, CO↑, vasodilation)	**Milrinone** (Primacor)	*50µg/kg IV over 10 min, maint 0.5µg/kg/min Inf*
poss	**Vasopressor** →22 (primarily beta-adrenergic agonist, inotropia↑, no vasoconstriction)	**Dobutamine** (Dobutrex, Gens)	*Ini 0.5-1µg/kg/min IV, incr to 2.5-20µg/kg/min*

2 B.5.4   Secondary Prophylaxis after Infarction

	Antiplatelet drug →74 (phosphodiesterase/platelet aggregation-adhesion inhibition)	**Aspirin – ASA** (Ascriptin, Asprimox, Bayer Aspirin, Bufferin, Easprin, Ecotrin, Empirin, Genprin, Halfprin, St. Joseph Pain Reliever, Zorprin, Gens)	*81-325mg PO qd*
or	**Antiplatelet drug** →74 (blockage of platelet ADP-receptors)	**Clopidogrel** (Plavix)	*75mg PO qd*
plus	**Beta-1-selective blocker** →23 (CO↓, neg. chronotropic, neg. inotropic, renin secretion↓, central sympathetic activity↓)	**Metoprolol** (Lopressor, Toprol-xl, Gens)	*50-100mg PO qd-bid*
		Atenolol (Tenormin, Gens)	*25-100mg PO qd*
		Bisoprolol (Ziac, Gens)	*2.5-10mg PO qd*
plus	**ACE inhibitor** →25 (vasodilation↑, renal perfusion↑, aldosterone↓, catecholamine↓)	**Captopril** (Capoten, Gens)	*Incr slowly to 12.5-25mg PO bid*
		Lisinopril (Zestril)	*2.5-40mg PO qd*
		Enalapril (Lexxel, Vaseretic, Vasotec, Gens)	*2.5-20mg PO qd, max 40mg qd; IV ini 1.25mg, then 1.25-2.5mg IV qid*
		Ramipril (Altace)	*1.25-5mg PO qd max 10mg qd*
plus	**HMG-CoA-reductase inhibitor** →42 (intracell. cholesterol synthesis↓, LDL↓, HDL↑)	**Atorvastatin** (Lipitor)	*10-20mg PO qd*
		Pravastatin (Pravachol)	*10-20 mg PO qd*

2 B.6   Heart Failure

Determine Heart Failure Stage

ACC/AHA Stage	A	B	C	D
Definition	At high risk for heart failure but without structural heart disease or symptoms of HF	Structural heart disease but without symptoms of HF	Structural heart disease with prior or current symptoms of HF	Refractory HF requiring specialized interventions
e.g. Patients with	- Hypertension - CAD - Diabetes mell. - FHx CM or Patients using cardiotoxins	- Previous MI - LV systolic dysfunction - Asymptomatic valvular disease	- Known struct. heart disease - Shortness of breath, fatigue, reduces exercise tolerance	- Marked symptoms at rest despite maximal medical Tx; frequently hospitalized **(1)**

Stage	NYHA I	NYHA II	NYHA III	NYHA IV
Symptoms	no symptoms	during ordinary physical strain	during slight physical strain	symptoms during rest
CO	normal	normal	during physical strain ↓	at rest ↓
LVEDP	during physical strain ↑	at rest ↑	at rest ↑	at rest ↑

Classification after NYHA (= New York Heart Association)
CO = Cardiac output, LVEDP = Left ventricular end-diastolic pressure

Evaluation of Heart Failure + Concomitant Disorders

Concomitant DOs	Evaluation

Cardiovascular
  Hypertension
  Hyperlipidemia
  Diabetes mellitus
  CAD
  Supraventr. arrhythmias
  Ventr. arrhythmias
  Prevention of sudden death
  Prevention of thrombotic events
	Thorough **H+P** (identify cardiac and noncardiac DO)

	Assess patient's ability to perform routine and desired **activities of daily living** (initial, ongoing)
	Volume status (initial, ongoing)
	Initial labor atory : CBC, UA, serum electrolytes (incl. Ca^{++}, Mg^{+}), BUN, serum cr eatinine, blood glucose, LFT s, TSH (initial)
	Serial labor atory: serum electrolytes, renal function

Noncardiovascular
  Renal insufficiency
  Pulmonary disease
  Cancer
  Thyroid disease   **(1)**
	Initial 12-lead **ECG** and chest **X–ray**

	Initial 2-dimensional **echocardiography** with **Doppler** *or* **radionuclide ventriculography** (assess left ventr. syst. function)
	Cardiac catheterization with **coronary arteriography** in patients with angina who are candidates for revascularization. **(1)**

Start Therapy

Therapy	A	B	C	D
General Measures + Pharmacologic Treatment of Heart Failure + Treatment of Concomitant Disorders	- Encourage smoking cessation and regular exercise - Discourage alcohol intake, illicit drug use - Treat **hypertension** - Treat **lipid** DO - ACE inhibitors in appropriate patients[a] - Control HR in supraventricular tachyarrhythmias - Treat **thyroid** DO - Evaluate periodically for heart failure	**All measures under stage A +** - ACE inhibitors in appropriate patients[b] - Beta-blockers in appropriate patients[c] - Valve replacement or repair for patients with significant valvular stenosis or regurgitation - Evaluate regularly for heart failure	**All measures under stage A +** - Dietary salt restriction - Diuretics in patients with fluid retention - ACE inhibitors in all patients unless CI - Beta-blockers in all stable patients unless CI - Digitalis for Tx of symptoms of HF unless CI - Withdrawal of drugs known to adversely affect HF (e.g. CCBs)	**All measures under stages A, B and C +** - Control of fluid retention - Mechanical assist devices - Referral for cardiac transplantation in eligible patients - Continuous IV inotropic infusion for palliation - Hospice care

a) with a Hx of atherosclerotic vascular disease, diabetes mellitus, or hypertension and associated cardiovascular risk factors
b) with a recent or remote history of myocardial infarction regardless of ejection fraction OR in patients with a reduced ejection fraction, whether or not they have experienced a myocardial infarction.
c) with a recent myocardial infarction regardless of ejection fraction. OR in patients with a reduced ejetion fraction, whether or not they have experienced a myocardial infarction. **(1)**

Therapy Goals

Decrease mortality
Stop progression

Improve symptoms (quality of life)
Decrease hospitalization rate

Drug Class	Decrease in Mortality	Inhibition of Progression	Symptom. Improvem.	Decrease in Hospitaliz. Rate	Improved Hemodyn. Parameters
ACE Inhib.	A	A	A	A	A
Beta Blocker	A	A	A	A	A
Diuretic Loop	C	C	B	B	B
Aldost.antag.	B	B	B	B	B
Glycoside	C	C	B	B	B
ARB	B	B	A	A	B

A: Several randomized controlled clinical studies; **B:** one randomized controlled clinical study or good evidence through clinical experience; **C:** no sure study results that prove beneficial or damaging effects;
D: negative results based on one or more clinical studies **(1)**

Pharmacologic Treatment of Heart Failure

Drug Class	Drug	Initial Dose	Max. Dose
ACE Inhib.	Captopril	6.25–12.5 mg tid	450 mg/d
		Monitor blood pressure. Increase gradually depending on patient's response	
	Enalapril	2.5 mg qd	20 mg bid
		Monitor blood pressure, renal function. Uptitrate as tolerated over a few days or weeks.	
	Lisinopril	5 mg qd	40 mg qd
		Monitor blood pressure. Increase by no greater than 10 mg, at intervals of at least 2 weeks to the highest tolerated dose up to max. 40 mg/d.	
	Quinapril	5 mg bid	20 mg bid
		If well tolerated titrate at weekly intervals until effective dose is reached.	
Beta Blocker	Carvedilol	3.125 mg bid	25 mg bid; >85 kg: 50 mg bid
		Individualize dosage and monitor closely during up-titration! If well tolerated increase to 6.25, 12.5, and 25 mg over successive intervals of at least two weeks to the highest tolerated dose. *Carvedilol has demonstrated improved survival compared to metoprolol in one randomized trial* [COMET].	
	Metoprolol succinate	12.5–25 mg qd	200 mg qd
		Monitor closely during up-titration. Double dose very 2 weeks to the highest dosage level tolerated by the patient or up to max. 200 mg/d.	
Diuretic (loop)	Bumetanide	0.5–2 mg qd	10 mg qd
		Uptitrate by giving 2nd or 3rd dose at 4–5h intervals up to max. 10 mg/d.	
	Ethacrynic acid	50 mg qd	100–200 mg bid
		After diuresis has been achieved give minimally effective dose.	
	Furosemide	20–80 mg as single dose	600 mg qd
		If needed repeat same dose after 6–8h or increase. Raise by increments of 20–40 mg and administer not sooner than 6–8h after previous dose. Give individually determined single dose qd or bid. Titrate up to max. 600 mg/d.	
	Torsemide	10–20 mg qd	200 mg qd
		Uptitrate by approx. doubling until desired diuretic response is obtained.	
Diuretic (thiazide)	Hydrochloro-thiazide	25 mg qd	25–100 mg qd
		Many patients respond to intermittent therapy e.g. on alternate days.	
	Metolazone	5 mg qd	20 mg qd
		Titrate to gain an initial therapeutic response and to determine the minimal dose possible to maintain the desired therapeutic response.	
Diuretic (aldost.antag.)	Spironolactone	25 mg qd (100 mg qd)	200 mg qd
		If an adequate diuretic effect has not occurred after five days, add second diuretic that acts more proximally in the renal tubule.	
	Eplerenone	25 mg qd	50 mg qd
		Monitor serum K^+! Titrate to target dose of 50 mg/d within 4 wks as tolerated.	
Glycoside	Digoxin	Digitalization, e.g.: **ini 0.4–0.6 mg IV**, then 0.1–0.3 mg q6–8h until adequate effect; **maint 0.125 (0.0625)–0.5 mg qd**	
		Titrate according to the patient's age, lean body weight, and renal function.	
ARB (angiotensin rec. blocker)	Valsartan	40 mg bid	160 mg bid
		Uptitrate to the highest dose (to 80 mg bid and 160 mg bid), as tolerated by the patient.	

(1) Hunt SA, Baker DW, Chin MH, Cinquegrani MP, Feldman AM, Francis GS, Ganiats TG, Goldstein S, Gregoratos G, Jessup ML, Noble RJ, Packer M, Silver MA, Stevenson LW. ACC/AHA guidelines for the evaluation and management of chronic heart failure in the adult. 2001. American College of Cardiology

	Drug class	Drug	Dosing
	ACE inhibitor →25 (vasodilation↑, renal perfus.↑, aldosterone ↓, catecholamines↓)	**Captopril** (Capoten, Gens)	*Incr slowly to 12.5-25mg PO bid*
		Lisinopril (Zestril)	*2.5–40mg PO qd*
		Enalapril (Lexxel, Vaseretic, Vasotec, Gens)	*2.5-20mg PO qd, max 40mg qd; IV ini 1.25mg, then 1.25-2.5mg IV qid*
		Ramipril (Altace)	*1.25-10mg PO qd-bid, max 20mg qd*
	Beta-1-selective blocker →23 (CO↓, neg. chronotropic, neg. inotropic, renin secretion↓, central sympathetic activity↓)	**Metoprolol** (Lopressor, Toprol-xl, Gens)	*50-100mg PO qd-bid, ini with very small doses, then slowly incr*
		Atenolol (Tenormin, Gens)	*25–100mg PO qd*
		Bisoprolol (Ziac, Gens)	*2.5-10mg PO qd*
	Thiazide diuretic →33 (renal H_2O/Na^+Cl^- loss, endog. vasoconstrictive stimuli ↓)	**Hydrochlorothiazide** (Esidrix, Hydrodiuril, Microside, Oretic, Gens)	*12.5-50mg PO qd (caution: only effective if creatinine < 2mg/dl, then furosemide)*
	Loop diuretic →33 (excretion of H_2O, Na^+, Cl^-, K^+, Ca^+, Mg^+↑)	**Furosemide** (Lasix)	*20–80mg IV qd*
		Torasemide (Demadex)	*2.5-10mg PO qd-bid, 10-20mg IV qd-tid, max 200mg PO/IV qd*
or	**Aldosterone antagonist** →34 (renal H_2O/Na^+Cl^- loss, K^+ secretion↓)	**Spironolactone** (Aldactone, Gens)	*d1-5: 50-100mg bid-qid, then 50-100mg PO qd-bid*
	Cardiac glycoside →40 (chrono-, dromo-↓, inotropic↑, AV node refract. time↑, economy of coronary work↑)	**Digoxin** (Digoxin pediatric, Lanoxi Cap, Lanoxin, Lanoxin pediatric, Gens)	*Ini 0.5mg IV, then 0.25mg q6h for 2 doses, (total 1mg), then 0.25mg PO qd*
	Nitrate →36 (pre-/afterload↓, venous pooling, coronary spasmolysis, O_2-consumption↓)	**Isosorbide mononitrate** (Imdur, ISMO, Monoket, Gens)	*20-40mg PO bid (1-1-0), 30-120mg SR PO qd*

2 B.7   Arrhythmias

2 B.7.1   Sinus Tachycardia

Find cause i.e hypovolemia, anxiety

Drug class	Drug	Dosing
Beta-1-selective blocker →23 (CO↓, neg. chronotropic, neg. inotropic, renin secretion↓, central sympathetic activity↓)	**Metoprolol** (Lopressor, Toprol-xl, Gens)	*50-100mg PO qd-bid*
	Atenolol (Tenormin, Gens)	*25–100mg PO qd*

2 B.7.2   Atrial Flutter

Heart rate control

poss	**Cardiac glycoside** →40 (chrono-, dromo-↓, inotropic↑, AV node refract. time↑, economy of coronary work↑)	**Digoxin** (Digoxin pediatric, LanoxiCap, Lanoxin, Lanoxin pediatric, Gens)	*Ini 0.5mg IV, then 0.25mg q6h for 2 doses, (total 1mg), then 0.25mg PO qd*
plus	**Beta–1–selective blocker** →23 (CO↓, neg. chronotropic, neg. inotropic, renin secretion↓, central sympathetic activity↓)	**Metoprolol** (Lopressor, Toprol-xl, Gens)	*50-100mg PO qd-bid*
		Atenolol (Tenormin, Gens)	*25-100mg PO qd*
or	**CCB – non–dihydropyridine** →29 (chrono-, dromo-, inotropic↓, afterload↓, O_2-consumption↓)	**Verapamil** (Calan, Covera-HS, Isoptin, Verelan, Gens)	*5mg slowly IV, then 5-10mg/h, max 100mg/d*
		Diltiazem (Cardizem, Cartia XT, Tiamate, Tiazac, Gens)	*IV 15–25mg bolus, then 10mg/h Inf; 60-90mg PO tid, 90-180mg SR PO bid, 240mg SR PO qd*

Catheter ablation

2 B.7.3   Atrial Fibrillation

Embolism prophylaxis

poss	**Heparin, unfractionated** →70 (coagulation factor inhibition↑, embolism prophylaxis)	**Heparin** (Gens)	*5000 U IV bolus, then 1000 U/h; aim for a PTT ratio of 1.5–2.5*
plus	**Antiplatelet drug** →74 (phosphodiesterase/platelet aggregation-adhesion inhibition)	**Aspirin – ASA** (Ascriptin, Asprimox, Bayer Aspirin,Bufferin Easprin, Ecotrin, Empirin, Genprin, Halfprin, St. Joseph Pain Reliever, Zorprin, Gens)	*325mg PO qd*
or	**Oral anticoagulant** →72 (vit. K antagonism ⇒ clotting factors II, VII, IX, X↓ ⇒ longterm anticoag.)	**Warfarin** (Coumadin, Gens)	*2-10mg PO qd to keep INR 2-2.5 times normal*

Heart rate control

poss	**Cardiac glycoside** →40 (chrono-, dromo-↓, inotropic↑, AV node refract. time↑, economy of coronary work↑)	**Digoxin** (Digoxin pediatric, LanoxiCap, Lanoxin, Lanoxin pediatric, Gens)	*Ini 0.5mg IV, then 0.25mg q6h for 2 doses, (total 1mg), then 0.25mg PO qd*
plus	**Beta–1–selective blocker** →23 (CO↓, neg. chronotropic, neg. inotropic, renin secretion↓, central sympathetic activity↓)	**Metoprolol** (Lopressor, Toprol-xl, Gens)	*50-100mg PO qd-bid*
		Atenolol (Tenormin, Gens)	*25-100mg PO qd*

or	CCB – non–dihydropyridine →29 (chrono-, dromo-, inotropic ↓, afterload ↓, O_2-consumption ↓)	Verapamil (Calan, Covera-HS, Isoptin, Verelan, Gens)	*5mg slowly IV, then 5-10mg/h, max 100mg/d; 80-120mg PO tid-qid*
		Diltiazem (Cardizem, Cartia XT, Tiamate, Tiazac, Gens)	*IV 15–25mg bolus, then 10mg/h Inf; 60-90mg PO tid, 90-180mg SR PO bid, 240mg SR PO qd*

Restoration of sinus rhythm

Primary method: DC cardioversion

poss	Antiarrhythmic, class III →37 (blockage of K^+ channels ⇒ action potential length ↑, refractory time ↑)	Amiodarone (Cordarone, Pacerone, Gens)	*150mg IV over 30min, then 1mg/min Inf for 6h, then 0.5mg/min for 18h*
		Ibutilide (Corvert)	*1mg IV, rep once prn*
or	Antiarrhythmic, class III →37 (blockage of K^+ channels + beta-receptor blocker ⇒ refractory time ↑)	Sotalol (Betapace, Betapace AF, Gens)	*80-160mg PO bid; Caution: contraindicated in CAD*

Urgent restoration of normal sinus rhythm only indicated in patients with hypotension, shock, heart failure

2 B.7.4   Relapse Prophylaxis

poss	Antiarrhythmic, class III →37 (blockage of K^+ channels ⇒ action potential length ↑, refractory time ↑)	Amiodarone (Cordarone, Pacerone, Gens)	*d1-10: 1000mg PO div in 5 doses, then 200mg qd*
or	Antiarrhythmic, class III →37 (blockage of K^+ channels + beta-receptor blockage ⇒ refractory time ↑)	Sotalol (Betapace, Betapace AF, Gens)	*80-160mg PO qd-bid; Caution: proarrhythmic*
or	Antiarrhythmic, class IC →37 (Na^+ influx block ⇒ conduction ↑, refractory time ↑)	Propafenone (Rythmol, Gens)	*150mg tid or 300mg bid PO; Caution: proarrhythmic*

Ablation is possible in selected cases

2 B.7.5   Supraventricular Tachycardia in WPW Syndrome, AV Node Tachycardia

Attack

If appl. radiofrequeny ablation (frequently first choice)

poss	Antiarrhythmic →37 (short-term blockade of AV node)	Adenosine (Adenocard)	*6mg IV bolus, then 12-18mg IV prn*
poss	CCB – non–dihydropyridine →29 (chrono-, dromo-, inotropic ↓, afterload ↓, O_2-consumption ↓)	Diltiazem (Cardizem, Cartia XT, Tiamate, Tiazac, Gens)	*15–25mg IV bolus, then 10mg/h Inf; Not in atrial fibrillation!*
		Verapamil (Calan, Covera-HS, Isoptin, Verelan, Gens)	*5mg slowly IV, then 5-10mg/h, max 100mg/d; Not in atrial fibrillation!*

Prophylaxis

poss	**Antiarrhythmic, class III** →37 (blockage of K^+ channels + beta-receptor blocker ⇒ refractory time ↑)	**Sotalol** (Betapace, Betapace AF, Gens	*80-160mg PO bid-tid; Caution: proarrhythmic*
or	**Antiarrhythmic, class Ic** →37 (Na^+ influx block ⇒ conduction ↑, refractory time ↑)	**Flecainide** (Tambocor)	*100-200mg PO bid Caution: proarrhythmic*
or	**Antiarrhythmic, class III** →37 (blockage of K^+ channels ⇒ action potential length ↑, refractory time ↑)	**Amiodarone** (Cordarone, Pacerone, Gens)	*d1-10: 1000mg PO div in 5 doses, then 200mg qd; Caution: proarrhythmic*

Radiofrequency ablation is curative!

2 B.7.6   Ventricular Tachycardia

Attack

	Antiarrhythmic, class Ib →37 (conduction, refr. time ↑)	**Lidocaine** (Gens)	*Ini 50-100mg IV, then 2-4mg/min Inf*
or poss	**Antiarrhythmic, class III** →37 (blockage of K^+ channels ⇒ action potential length ↑, refractory time ↑)	**Amiodarone** (Cordarone, Pacerone, Gens)	*150mg IV over 30min, then 1mg/min for 6h Inf, then 0.5mg/min for 18h, or d1-10: 1000mg PO div in 5 doses, then 200mg/d*

DC cardioversion if evidence of hemodynamic compromise.

Prophylaxis

	Antiarrhythmic, class III →37 (blockage of K^+ channels ⇒ action potential length ↑, refractory time ↑)	**Amiodarone** (Cordarone, Pacerone, Gens)	*d1-10: 1000mg PO div in 5 doses, then 200mg qd*
or	**Antiarrhythmic, class III** →37 (blockage of K^+ channels + beta-receptor blocker ⇒ refractory time ↑)	**Sotalol** (Betapace, Betapace AF, Gens	*80-160mg PO qd-bid*
poss plus	**Beta-1-selective blocker** →23 (CO↓, neg. chronotropic, neg. inotropic, renin secretion↓, central sympathetic activity↓)	**Metoprolol** (Lopressor, Toprol-xl, Gens)	*25-200mg PO qd-bid; Caution: not with Sotalol*
		Atenolol (Tenormin, Gens)	*25-100mg PO qd; Caution: not with Sotalol*

Sos consider implantable defibrillator, especially if LVEF < 35%

2 B.7.7   Torsades De Pointes

Usually **sign of proarrhythmic effects** of other antiarrhythmics - discontinue.
Consider pacemaker to increase heart rate and decrease QTc.

Attack

	Magnesium →140 (antiarrhytmic)	**Magnesium Sulfate** (Gens)	*1-6g IV over several min, then 3-20mg/min IV for 5-48h*

poss plus	**Beta–adrenergic agonist** →39 (chronotropic↑, inotropic↑, HR↑, CO↑, peripheral vasodilatation)	**Isoproterenol** (Isuprel, Gens) — *Ini 0.02–0.06mg IV bolus, then Inf at 2–10µg/min*

Prophylaxis

1. Choice: discontinue antiarrhythmics
2. Sos stimulation
3. Poss pacemaker

2 B.7.8   Extrasystoles

Supraventricular Extrasystoles

Beta–1–selective blocker →23 (CO↓, neg. chronotropic, neg. inotropic, O_2 consumption↓, central sympathetic activity↓)	**Metoprolol** (Lopressor, Toprol-xl, Gens)	*5–10mg slowly IV, max 20mg IV; 25–100mg PO qd-bid, 100–200mg SR PO qd*
	Atenolol (Tenormin, Gens)	*25–100mg PO qd*

Mg^{2+}, K^+ replacement, treat cause, e.g. hyperthyroidism

Ventricular Extrasystoles

Beta–1–selective blocker →23 (CO↓, neg. chronotropic, neg. inotropic, O_2 consumption↓, central sympathetic activity↓)	**Metoprolol** (Lopressor, Toprol-xl, Gens)	*25–100mg PO qd-bid, 100–200mg SR PO qd, 5–10mg slowly IV, max 20mg IV*
	Atenolol (Tenormin, Gens)	*25–100mg PO qd*
Electrolytes →140 (symptomatic)	**Mg^+-K^+ supplement** (Mag-ox, Gens)	*400mg PO bid-tid*

Mg^{2+}, K^+ replacement, treat cause. Antiarrhythmics NOT indicated!

2 B.7.9   Bradycard Arrhythmias

poss	**Parasympatholytic** →37 (chronotropic↑)	**Atropine** (Atropine sulfate) — *0.5–1mg IV*

Usually pacemaker

2 B.8   Infective Endocarditis
2 B.8.1   Rheumatic Fever

Acute Rheumatic Fever

	Penicillin →187 (antibiotic)	**Benzathine Penicillin** (Bicillin L-A, Permapen) — *1.2 M U IM as single dose*
or		**Penicillin V** (Betapen-VK, Ledercillin-VK, Pen-vee K, Uticillin VK, V-cillin VK, Gens) — *250–500mg PO tid for 10d*
plus	**NSAID – salicylate** →264 (antiinflammatory, antipyretic)	**Aspirin – ASA** (Ascriptin, Asprimox, Bayer Aspirin, Bufferin, Easprin, Fortrin, Empirin, Genprin, Halfprin, St. Joseph Pain Reliever, Zorprin, Gens) — *2–3g qd PO (until infection signs ↓)*

plus	**Glucocorticoid** →148 (anti-inflammatory, immunosuppressive)	**Prednisone** (Deltasone, Meticorten, Prednisone Intensol, Gens)	*1-2mg/kg PO qd slowly decreasing (until infection signs↓)*
Relapse prophylaxis			
	Penicillin →187 (antibiotic)	**Benzathine Penicillin** (Bicillin L-A, Permapen)	*1.2 M U IM q3wk (until 25years of age)*
or	In penicillin allergic patients:		
	Macrolide →199	**Erythromycin** (e-Base, E-mycin, Eryc, Ery-tab, Ilosone, Ilotycin, PCE, Gens)	*250mg PO bid (until 25years of age)*

2 B.8.2   Bacterial Endocarditis

Streptococci			
	Benzylpenicillin →187 (antibiotic)	**Penicillin G** (Penicillin, Penicillin G Potassium, Pfizerpen, Gens)	*12–18 M U IV per 24h*
or	In penicillin allergic patients:		
	Glycopeptide →198 (antibiotic)	**Vancomycin** (Vancocin HCT, Vancoled, Gens)	*30mg/kg IV q24h, div in 2 doses*
plus	**Aminoglycoside** →200 (antibiotic)	**Gentamicin** (Garamycin, U-gencin, Gens)	*1mg/kg IV tid or 3mg/kg qd for 2wk*
Staphylococci			
	Isoxazylpenicillin →188 (antibiotic)	**Oxacillin** (Bactocill)	*2g q4h for 6wk*
or	**Glycopeptide** →198 (antibiotic)	**Vancomycin** (Vancocin HCT, Vancoled, Gens)	*30mg/kg IV q24h div in 2 doses*
plus	**Aminoglycoside** →200 (antibiotic)	**Gentamicin** (Garamycin, U-gencin, Gens)	*1mg/kg tid or 3mg/kg qd for 6wk*
Enterococci			
	Aminopenicillin →189 (antibiotic)	**Ampicillin** (Omnipen, Omnipen-N, Principen, Totacillin, Totacillin-N, Gens)	*12g cont IV over 24h or in six divided doses for 4-6wk*
or	**Glycopeptide** →198 (antibiotic)	**Vancomycin** (Vancocin HCT, Vancoled, Gens)	*30mg/kg IV q24h in two divided doses for 4-6wk*
plus	**Aminoglycoside** →200 (antibiotic)	**Gentamicin** (Garamycin, U-gencin, Gens)	*1mg/kg IV tid or 3mg/kg IV qd for 4-6wk*
Pneumococci			
	Benzylpenicillin →187 (antibiotic)	**Penicillin G** (Penicillin, Penicillin G Potassium, Pfizerpen, Gens)	*12-18 M U/24h cont IV or div in 6 doses*

2 B.9 Endocarditis Prophylaxis

2 B.9.1 No Penicillin Allergy – Normal risk (e.g. rheumatic valve defect, HOCM)

Oropharynx, GI, Urogenital

Aminopenicillin →189 (antibiotic)	**Amoxicillin** (Amoxil, Larotid, Trimox, Wymox, Gens)	*2g PO 1h before procedure*

2 B.9.2 No Penicillin Allergy – Higher risk (e.g. artificial heart valve, after bacterial endocarditis)

Oropharynx, GI, Urogenital

	Aminopenicillin →189 (antibiotic)	**Amoxicillin** (Amoxil, Larotid, Trimox, Wymox, Gens)	*2g PO (or 2g IV) 1h before, and 1g PO each 8 + 16h after procedure*
plus	Aminoglycoside →200 (antibiotic)	**Gentamicin** (Garamycin, U-gencin, Gens)	*1.5mg/kg IV 1h before, and 1mg/kg IV each 8 + 16h after procedure*

Skin

Isoxazylpenicillin →188 (antibiotic)	**Cloxacillin** (Cloxacillin sodium)	*2g PO 1h before, and 500mg PO each 8 + 16h after procedure*
	Cefazolin (Ancef)	*1g IV before, and 1g IV each 8 and 16 h after procedure*

2 B.9.3 In Penicillin Allergy – Normal Risk (e.g. rheumatic. valve defect, HOCM)

Oropharynx, Skin

Lincosamide →201 (antibiotic)	**Clindamycin** (Cleocin, Gens)	*600mg PO 1h before procedure*

GI, Urogenital

Glycopeptide →198 (antibiotic)	**Vancomycin** (Vancocin HCT, Vancoled, Gens)	*1g IV 1h before procedure*

2 B.9.4 In Penicillin Allergy – Higher Risk (e.g. artificial heart valve, after bacterial endocarditis)

Oropharynx

Lincosamide →201 (antibiotic)	**Clindamycin** (Cleocin, Gens)	*600mg PO 1h before, and 300mg PO each 8 + 16h after procedure*

GI, Urogenital, Skin

Glycopeptide →198 (antibiotic)	**Vancomycin** (Vancocin HCT, Vancoled, Gens)	*1g IV 1h before, and 1g IV each 8 + 16h after procedure*

2 B.10 Pericarditis
2 B.10.1 Bacterial

Antibiotics only after testing, think of tuberculosis!

2 B.10.2 Dressler's Syndrome (after myocardial infarctions, cardiac operations)

poss	**NSAID acid derivative** →265, →266 (anti-inflammatory, analgesic)	**Diclofenac** (Voltaren, Voltaren-XR, Gens)	*50mg PO qd-tid, 100mg SR PO qd, 75mg IM qd*
		Ibuprofen (Advil, Ibu, Motrin, Gens)	*600–800mg PO tid*
poss	**Glucocorticoid** →148 (antiinflammatory antiallergic, immunosuppressive)	**Prednisone** (Deltasone, Meticorten, Prednisone Intensol, Gens)	*Depending on clinical signs 5–20mg PO qd*

2 B.11 Intermittent Claudication
2 B.11.1 Stage II: Walking Regimen

More important is prevention of cardiovascular morbidity and mortality with appropriate use of statins, antiplatelet drugs and beta blockers

	Antiplatelet drug →74 (phosphodiesterase/platelet aggregation-adhesion inhibition)	**Aspirin – ASA** (Ascriptin, Asprimox, Bayer Aspirin, Bufferin, Easprin, Ecotrin, Empirin, Genprin, Halfprin, St. Joseph Pain Reliever, Zorprin, Gens)	*81–325mg PO qd*
poss plus	**Antiplatelet drug** →74 (blockage of platelet ADP-receptors)	**Clopidogrel** (Plavix)	*75mg PO qd*
or / poss plus	**Hemorheologic** →77 (erythrocyte flexibility↑, rheology↑)	**Pentoxifylline** (Pentoxil, Trental, Gens)	*400mg PO tid*
		Cilostazol (Pletal)	*100mg PO bid*

2 B.11.2 Stage III/IV in Inoperability, Buerger's Disease

	Angiogenic growth factors (experimental protocols)	**Vascular endothelial growth factor** (VEGF$_{165}$)	*Gene therapy*

2 B.12 Superficial Vein Thrombosis
2 B.12.1 In General

poss	**Salicylate – antiplatelet drug** →74 (phosphodiesterase/platelet aggregation-adhesion inhibition, anti-inflammatory)	**Aspirin – ASA** (Ascriptin, Asprimox, Bayer Aspirin, Bufferin, Easprin, Ecotrin, Empirin, Genprin, Halfprin, St. Joseph Pain Reliever, Zorprin, Gens)	*325-1950mg PO bid-tid*

2 B.12.2 In Great Saphenous Vein Thrombosis

poss	**Heparin-low-molecular-weight** →71 (LMWH, coagulation factor inhibition ↑)	**Dalteparin** (Fragmin)	*2850 U SC qd*
		Enoxaparin (Lovenox)	*30mg SC bid*

2 B.13 Deep Vein Thrombosis
2 B.13.1 In Popliteal Vein Thrombosis

	Heparin, unfractionated →70 (coagulation factor inhibition ↑, embolism prophylaxis)	**Heparin** (Gens)	*5000 U IV bolus, then 1000 U/h; aim for a PTT ratio of 1.5–2.5*
then	**Oral anticoagulant** →72 (vit. K antagonism ⇒ clotting factors II, VII, IX, X↓ ⇒ longterm anticoag.)	**Warfarin** (Coumadin, Gens)	*2–10mg PO qd to achieve INR of 2–2.5*

2 B.13.2 In Extensive Cases

	Thrombolytic →73 (plasminogen activation → fibrin proteolysis)	**Streptokinase** (Streptase, Kabikinase)	*250,000 U over 30min, then 100,000 U/h x 24h*
or		**Urokinase** (Abbokinase)	*4400 U/kg IV over 10min, then 4400 U/kg/h IV for 12h*
or		**rt-PA** (Alteplase)	*100mg IV Inf over 2h*
then	**Oral anticoagulant** →72 (vit. K antagonism ⇒ clotting factors II, VII, IX, X↓ ⇒ longterm anticoag.)	**Warfarin** (Coumadin, Gens)	*2–10mg PO qd to achieve INR of 2–2.5 for 6mo*

2 B.14 Thrombosis Prophylaxis
2 B.14.1 Thrombosis Risk Factor Assessment

Each Risk Factor Represents 1 Point

- Age 41 to 60 years
- Minor surgery planned
- History of prior major surgery (<1mo)
- Varicose veins
- Inflammatory Bowel Disease
- Swollen legs (current)
- Obesity (BMI > 25)

Each Risk Factor Represents 2 Points

- Age 60-74 years
- Malignancy (present or previous)
- Major surgery (>45 min)
- Laparoscopic surgery (>45 min)
- Patient confined to bed (>72h)
- Immobilizing plaster cast (<1mo)
- Central venous access

Each Risk Factor Represents 3 Points

- Age over 75 years
- History of DVT/PE
- Family history of thrombosis
- Major surgery with additional risk factors such as myocardial infarction, congestive heart failure, sepsis, serious lung disease, or abnormal pulmonary function, such as COPD
- Medical patient with additional risk factors, such as stroke, myocardial infarction, etc.
- Factor V Leiden
- Prothrombin 20210A
- Serum homocysteine
- Lupus anticoagulant
- Anticardiolipin antibodies
- Other congenital or acquired thrombophilia; If yes: Type: ....
- Other risk factors ....

Each Risk Factor Represents 5 Points

- Elective major lower extremity arthroplasty
- Hip, pelvis or leg fracture (<1mo)
- Stroke (<1mo)
- Multiple trauma (<1mo)
- Acute spinal cord injury (paralysis, <1mo)

For Women Only (Each Represents 1 Point)

- Oral contraceptives or hormone replacement therapy
- Pregnancy or postpartum (<1mo)
- History of stillborn infant, spontaneous abortion, premature birth with toxemia or placental insufficiency

Total Risk Factor Score

2 B.14.2 Prophylaxis Regimen

Total Risk Factor Score	Incidence of DVT	Risk Level	Prophylaxis Regimen
0-1	<10%	Low Risk	No specific measures, early ambulation
2	10-20%	Moderate Risk	**ES** or **IPC** or **LDUH** or **LMWH**
3-4	20-40%	High Risk	**IPC** or **LDUH** or **LMWH**
5 or more	40-80%	Highest Risk	Pharmacological: **LDUH, LMWH, Warfarin,** or **Fac X*** alone or in combination with **ES** or **IPC**

ES - Elastic Stockings; **IPC** - Intermittent Pneumatic Compression; **LDUH** - Low Dose Unfractionated Heparin; **LMWH** - Low Molecular Weigth Heparin; **Fac X** - Factor X Inhibitor
*For use with total hip replacement, total knee replacement and hip fracture

© Evanston Northwestern Healthcare, JA Caprini, www.venousdisease.com;
Based on:
1. Geerts WH et al: Prevention of Venous Thromboembolism. Chest 2001; 119:132S-175S;
2. Nicolaides AN et al: 2001 International Consensus Statement: Prevention of Venous Thromboembolism, Guidelines According to Scientific Evidence;
3. Caprini JA, Arcelus JI et al: State-of-the-Art Venous Thromboembolism Prophylaxis. Scope 2001; 8: 228-240;
4. Oger E: Incidence of Venous Thrombembolism: A Community-based Study in Western France. Thromb Haemost 2000; 657-660; and
5. Turpie AG, Bauer KA, Ericsson BI, et al. Fondaparinux vs. Enoxaparin for the Prevention of Venous Thromboembolism in Major Orthopedic Surgery: a Meta-analysis of 4 Randomized Double-blind Studies. Arch Intern Med 2002; 162(16):1833-40.

2 B.15 Acute Aortic Dissection

Beta blocker →23 (to reduce sheer stress, negative inotrope, negative chronotrope)	**Labetalol** (Normodyne, Trandate, Gens)	*0.5-2mg/min IV Inf, total dose 50-200mg*
	Esmolol (Brevibloc)	*Ini IV loading dose 250-500µg/kg over 1min, then 50-100µg/kg/min for 4min, sos rep prn*

If beta blockers are contraindicated, consider negative chronotrope CCBs

CCB – non–dihydropyridine →29 (chrono-, dromo-, inotropic↓, afterload↓)	**Diltiazem** (Cardizem, Cartia XT, Tiamate, Tiazac, Gens)	*15–25mg IV bolus, then 10mg/h Inf*
	Verapamil (Calan, Covera-HS, Isoptin, Verelan, Gens)	*5mg slowly IV, then 5-10mg/h, max 100mg/d*
then **Direct vasodilator** →31 (pre-/afterload↓)	**Nitroprusside sodium** (Nipride, Nitropress)	*0.25-10mg/kg/min; Caution: use after beta blocker admin*

Emergent surgical repair is indicated for Type A dissection

3 A. Hematology – Drugs

3 A.1 Plasma Expanders

MA/EF (dextran): high molecular weight polysaccharides with water-binding capability and intravascular retention ⇒ plasma volume ↑
MA/EF (hetastarch): oncotic ⇒ retaining fluid in intravascular space ⇒ plasma volume ↑
AE (albumin): hypersensitivity (shaking, chills, urticaria);
AE (dextran): allergic to anaphylactic reactions, great amounts of low-molecular-weight dextran can be nephrotoxic;
AE (hetastarch): coagulopathy
CI (blood plasma substitutes): states of hyperhydration, hypervolemia, serious cardiac insufficiency, pulmonary edema, known allergy to active ingredients;
CI (dextran): hypersensitivity to dextran or corn products, hemostatic defects, cardiac decompensation
CI (albumin): hypersensitivity to albumin, severe anemia, heart failure
CI (hetastarch): hypersensitivity to hetastarch, severe RF, CHF, bleeding DO

Albumin	EHL 15-20d, PRC C
Albuminar *Inj 5%, 25%* **Plasbumin** *Inj 5%, 25%*	**Shock** →161: 500ml of 5% Sol IV infused as rapidly as tolerated, rep prn in 30min; **hypoproteinemia**: 200–300ml of 25% Sol IV

Dextran	EHL 41min, PRC C, Lact ?
Rheomacrodex *Inj 10%, 32%*	**Shock, hypovolemia** →161: Dextran 40, 10% Sol: ini 10ml/kg IV as rapid inf, max 20ml/kg on the 1st d, thereafter 10ml/kg/d for max 4d

Hetastarch (Hydroxyethyl starch = HES)	EHL 1.4h, PRC C, Lact ?
Hespan *Inj 6%*	**Shock, hypovolemia** →161: 500-1000ml IV, max 20ml/kg/d; **DARF GFR (ml/min) <10**: usual ini dose, then 20-50%

3 A.2 Anticoagulants
3 A.2.1 Unfractionated Heparin

MA/EF: forming complexes with antithrombin-III ⇒ inhibiting effect of antithrombin-III ↑ (by a factor of 1000) ⇒ inhibition of thrombin, factors Xa, XIa, XIIa, and callicrein ⇒ thrombin activated conversion of fibrinogen to fibrin ↓; activation of the lipoprotein lipase
AE: hemorrhage complications, allergic reactions, anaphylaxis, osteoporosis, cutaneous necrosis, hair loss, thrombocytopenia
CI: heparin allergy, heparin induced thrombocytopenia (type II), blood dyscrasias, active bleeding, imminent abortion, lumbar puncture, epidural anesthesia

Heparin	EHL 2.13h, PRC C, Lact +
Generics *Inj 10U/ml, 100 U/ml, 1000 U/ml, 2500 U/ml, 5000 U/ml, 10000 U/ml, 20000 U/ml*	**DVT** →67, **pulmonary embolism Tx** →112: ini 80 U/kg IV, maint 18 U/kg/h IV, adjust dose based on PTT; **DVT PRO**: 5000 U SC q8-12h; **CH** ini 50 U/kg IV, maint 10-25 U/kg/h IV, adjust dose based on PTT

3 A.2.2 Low-Molecular-Weight Heparins, Heparinoids

MA/EF (low-molecular-weight heparins): molecular weight↓ ⇒ thrombin inhibition↓, factor Xa inhibition↑; effect on blood platelet function↓, antithrombotic effect↑, danger of hemorrhage↓; neutralization↓ through platelet factor 4; when used subcutaneously bioavailability↑, half-life↑;
MA/EF: (argatroban, bivalirudin): specific and reversible direct thrombin inhibitor;
MA/EF: (danaparoid):
= heparinoid, factor Xa inhibition;
MA/EF: (fondaparinux): selectivly binding to antithrombin III ⇒ activation of the innate neutralization of factor Xa; **MA/EF:** (lepirudin): = recombined hirudin, direct inhibition of thrombin, prevention of thromboembolic diseases
AE/CI (low-molecular-weight heparins): see heparin →70
AE (argatroban): bleeding, hypotension, fever, cardiac arrest, ventricular tachycardia, diarrhea, nausea, allergic reactions; **AE** (bivalirudin): bleeding, backpain, headache, nausea, hypotension; **AE** (danaparoid): bleeding, tachycardia, chest pain, hyperkalemia, inj site hematoma; **AE** (fondaparinux): bleeding, anemia, fever, edema, local irritation;
AE (lepirudin): bleeding, anemia, abnormal LFT, allergic reactions
CI (argatroban): active major bleeding, hypersensitivity to argatroban
CI (bivalirudin): active major bleeding, hypersensitivity to bivalirudin
CI (danaparoid): hypersensitivity to danaparoid, severe hemorrhagic diathesis/states
CI (fondaparinux): severe renal impairment, endocarditis, weight <50kg, thrombocytopenia
CI (lepirudin): hypersensitivity to hirudin products

Ardeparin	EHL 1.2-3.3h, PRC C, Lact ?
Normiflo *Inj 5000 U/0.5ml, 10000 U/0.5ml*	**DVT PRO** →68, **knee replacement:** 50 U/kg SC q12h up to 14d; DARF caution in severe RF
Argatroban	EHL 39-51min, PRC B, Lact ?
Argatroban *Inj 100mg/ml*	**DVT PRO** →68 **and Tx in heparin–associated thrombocytopenia:** 2µg/kg/min, adjust dose based on aPTT, max 10µg/kg/min; DARF not req
Bivalirudin	EHL 25min, PRC B , Lact ?
Angiomax *Inj 250mg/vial*	**Anticoagulation with PTCA** →53: ini 1mg/kg IV, then 2.5mg/kg/h for 4h, may be continued prn at 0.2mg/kg/h upto 20h; DARF: GFR (ml/min) 30-59: 80%; 10-29: 40%; Dialysis: 10%
Dalteparin	EHL 2-5h, PRC B, Lact ?
Fragmin *Inj 2500 U/0.2ml, 5000 U/0.2ml, 10000 U/ml*	**DVT PRO** →68, **hip replacement:** ini 2500 U SC 2h preop, then 2500 U 6h after first dose, then 5000 U SC qd for 14d; **DVT PRO, abdominal surgery:** ini 2500 U SC 1-2h preop, then 2500 U qd postop for 5-10d; **unstable angina or NQWMI** →51: 120 U/kg max 10000 U SC q12h for 5-8d; **anticoagulation, dialysis:** 5000 U into the arterial line
Danaparoid	EHL 1h, PRC B, Lact ?
Orgaran *Inj 750U/0.6ml*	**DVT PRO** →68, **hip replacement:** ini 750 U SC 1-4h preop, then 750 U SC q12h for 7-10d; **anticoagulation, dialysis:** 34 U/kg into the arterial line; DARF req

Enoxaparin — EHL 4.5h (range 3-6h), PRC B, Lact ?

Lovenox *Inj 30mg/0.3ml, 40mg/0.4ml, 60mg/0.6ml, 80mg/0.8ml, 100mg/ml*

DVT PRO →68, **hip/knee replacement**: 30mg SC q12h ini 12-24h postop for 14d; **DVT PRO, abdominal surgery**: ini 40mg SC 2h preop, then 40mg SC qd for 12d; **Tx of DVT without pulmonary embolism, outpatient**: 1mg/kg SC q12h; **Tx of DVT with or without pulmonary embolism, inpatient**: 1mg/kg SC q12h or 1.5mg/kg SC q24h; **unstable angina or NQWMI** →51: 1mg/kg SC q12h for 2-8d; DARF req

Fondaparinux — EHL 17-21h, PRC B, Lact ?

Arixtra *Inj 2.5mg/0.5ml*

DVT PRO →68, **hip/knee replacement**: ini 2.5mg SC6-8h postop, then 2.5mg qd; DARF: GFR (ml/min) <30: contraind.

Lepirudin — EHL 1.3h, PRC B, Lact ?

Refludan *Inj 50mg/vial*

Heparin-associated thrombocytopenia: ini 0.4mg/kg bolus IV, max 44mg, maint 0.15mg/kg/h IV, max 16.5mg/h; DARF ini 0.2mg/kg bolus IV, then GFR (ml/min): 45-60: 0.075mg/kg/h; 30-44: 0.045mg/kg/h; 15-29: 0.0225mg/kg/h; <15, dialysis: 0.1mg/kg IV qod

Tinzaparin — EHL 3-4h, PRC B, Lact ?

Innohep *Inj 20000 U/ml*

DVT Tx with or without pulmonary embolism →67: 175U/kg SC qd; DARF req caution

3 A.2.3   Heparin Antidote

MA/EF: forming of a salt-like bond with heparin ⇒ inactivation of heparin
AE: hypotension, bradycardia, hypersensitivity reactions; **CI**: hypersensitivity to protamine products;
Note: severe hypotension/anaphylactoid reaction with too rapid administration; allergic reactions in fish allergy, previous exposure to protamine (including insulin); risk of allergy unclear in infertile/vasectomized men with anti-protamine antibodies

Protamine — EHL no data, PRC C, Lact ?

Generics *Inj 10mg/ml*

Heparin overdose (usual rule) →480: 1mg antagonizes approx. 100 U of heparin, give at a rate < 50mg/10min; max 1x dose 50mg

3 A.2.4   Oral Anticoagulants

MA/EF: inhibition of the vitamin K negotiated carboxylation of Ca^{2+} dependant blood clotting factors (II, VII, IX, X) in the liver
AE: hemorrhage complications, skin necrosis, urticaria
CI: serious thrombocytopenia, GI ulcers, retinopathy, arterial brain aneurysms, severe HTN

Dicumarol — EHL 1-4 d, PRC D, Lact +

Generics *Tab 25mg*

Anticoagulation: 25-200mg PO qd, adjust dose to PT (1.2-1.5 times control)

Warfarin	EHL 20-60h, PRC X, Lact +
Coumadin *Tub 1mg, 2mg, 2.5mg, 3mg, 4mg, 5mg, 6mg, 7.5mg, 10mg,* **Generics** *Tab 1mg, 2mg, 2.5mg, 3mg, 4mg, 5mg, 6mg, 7.5mg, 10mg*	**Anticoagulation**: ini 2-5mg PO qd for 2-4d, maint 2-10mg/d PO, adjust dose to PT/INR (PT: 1.2-2 times control); →60, →67, →112

3 A.3   Thrombolytics

MA/EF: activation of plasminogen ⇒ formation of plasmin ⇒ Plasmin proteolyses fibrin ⇒ dissolution of not yet fully organized blood clots (Streptokinase forms a streptokinase-plasminogen-complex ⇒ free plasminogen ⇒ plasmin)
AE: hemorrhage, allergic reactions, head-/backache, arrhythmias, hypotension, bleeding
CI: severe HTN, aortic aneurysm, endocarditis, GI ulcers, pancreatitis, advanced malignant tumors, pathologic hemostasis, head trauma, internal bleeding, operation or puncture < 10d, intramuscular injection < 7d, esophageal varices
CI (anistreplase, streptokinase): hypersensitivity to anistreplase products/streptokinase

Alteplase	EHL 26.5-46min, PRC C, Lact ?
Activase I.V. *Inj 50mg/vial, 100mg/vial*	**Acute MI** →53: >67kg: 15mg IV bolus, then 50mg over 30min, then 35mg over 1h; <67kg: 15mg IV bolus, then 0.75mg/kg over 30min, then 0.5mg/kg over 1h; **acute ischemic stroke** →308: 0.9mg/kg, max 90mg, over 60min IV, with 10% of total dose administered as IV bolus over 1min; **pulmonary embolism** →112: 100mg IV over 2h

Anistreplase	EHL 70-120min, PRC C, Lact ?
Eminase *Inj 30 U/vial*	**Acute MI** →53. 30 U IV over 2-5min

Reteplase	EHL 13-16min, PRC C, Lact ?
Retavase *Inj 10.4 U/vial*	**Acute MI** →53: 10 U IV over 2min, rep dose in 30min

Streptokinase	EHL 18-83min, PRC C, Lact ?
Streptase *250,000 U/vial, 750,00 U/vial, 1,500,000 U/vial*	**Acute MI** →53: 1.5 million U IV over 1h; intracoronary: 20,000 U bolus, then 2000 U/min for 1h; **pulmonary embolism** →112: 250,000 U IV over 30min, then 100,000 U/h IV for 24h; **deep vein thrombosis** →67: 250,000 U IV over 30min, then 100,000 U/h IV for 72h; DARF not req

Tenecteplase	EHL 17-20min, PRC C, Lact ?
TNKase *Inj 50mg vial*	**Acute MI** →53: single bolus IV: < 60kg: 30mg; 60-69kg: 35mg; 70-79kg: 40mg; 80-89 kg: 45mg; > 90kg: 50mg

Urokinase	EHL < 20min, PRC B, Lact ?
Abbokinase *Inj 250,00 U/vial*	**Pulmonary embolism** →112: 4400 U/kg IV over 10min, then 4400 U/kg/h for 12h; occluded IV catheter: 5000 U instilled into catheter, remove after 5min

3 A.4 Antiplatelets
3 A.4.1 Glycoprotein IIb-IIIa Inhibitors

MA/EF: antagonist of the glycoprotein IIb-IIIa-receptor on blood platelets ⇒ inhibition of platelet aggregation
AE (abciximab, tirofiban): hemorrhage complications, thrombocytopenia, nausea, fever, headaches;
AE (eptifibatide): bleeding
CI (abciximab, tirofiban): cerebrovascular complications during the last 2 years, operations and traumas during the last 2mo, thrombocytopenia, vasculitis, aneurysm, AV anomalies, retinopathy of hypertensive or diabetic origin
CI (eptifibatide): bleeding DO/surgery/CVA, hypersensitivity to eptifibatide products, severe renal dysfunction, platelet count < 100,000/mm(3)

Abciximab	EHL < 10min, PRC C, Lact ?
ReoPro *Inj 2mg/ml*	**Percutaneous coronary intervention** →53: 0.25mg/kg IV over 1min 10-60min before procedure, then 0.125µg/kg/min, max 10µg/min for 12h; **unstable angina not responding to conventional Tx**: 0.25mg/kg IV over 1min, then 10µg/min for 18-24h concluding 1h after PTCA

Eptifibatide	EHL 1.13-2.5h, PRC B, Lact ?
Integrilin *Inj 0.75mg/ml, 2mg/ml*	**Acute coronary syndrome** →50: ini 180µg/kg IV, then 2µg/kg/min up to max 72h; **percutaneous coronary intervention** →53: ini 135µg/kg IV before procedure, then 0.5µg/kg/min IV for 20-24h after the procedure; DARF serum-creatinine (mg/ml) <2: 100%; 2-4: ini max 135µg/kg IV, then 0.5µg/kg/min

Tirofiban	EHL 90-180min, PRC B, Lact ?
Aggrastat *Inj 0.05mg/ml, 0.25mg/ml*	**Acute coronary syndrome** →50: ini 0.4µg/kg/min IV for 30min, then 0.1µg/kg/min for 48-108h or until 12-24h after coronary intervention; DARF GFR (ml/min) <30: 50%

3 A.4.2 Phosphodiesterase/Platelet Aggregation-Adhesion Inhibitors

MA (aspirin): inhibition of cyclooxygenase ⇒ synthesis of thromboxane A2 ↓ (aggregation activator for blood platelets), synthesis of prostacyclin ↓ (aggregation inhibitor in endothelium); **MA** (clopidogrel, ticlopidine): blockage of the ADP-receptor of blood platelets; **MA** (anagrelide, cilostazol, dipyridamole): inhibition of cAMP phosphodiesterase ⇒ cAMP in platelets ↑ ⇒ inhibition of platelet aggregation
EF: inhibition of platelet aggregation
AE (anagrelide): headache, thrombocytopenia, orthostatic hypotension
AE (aspirin): allergic reactions, gastric ulcers, skin reactions, dizziness, tinnitus, dysopias, nausea, bronchospasm, alkalosis, acidosis; **AE** (cilostazol): palpitations/tachycardia, edema, dizziness, diarrhea, headache; **AE** (clopidogrel): dyspepsia, abdominal pain, constipation, bleeding
AE (dipyridamole): dizziness, headache, rash, abdominal distress, exacerbation of angina pectoris;
AE (ticlopidine): agranulocytosis, pancytopenia, allergic skin reactions
CI: hypersensitivity to the drug; **CI** (clopidogrel) active bleeding, **CI** (cilostazol) CHF
CI (aspirin): GI ulcers, hemorrhagic diathesis, great caution with children
CI (ticlopidine): complete blood count changes

Anagrelide	EHL 76h, PRC C, Lact ?
Agrylin *Cap 0.5mg, 1mg*	**Essential thrombocythemia** →83: ini 0.5mg PO qid or 1mg PO bid, after 7d incr dose prn, not > 0.5mg/d in any 1wk, max 10mg/d or 2.5mg as single dose
Aspirin	EHL 4.7-9h, PRC D, Lact ?
Aspergum *Chewing Gum 227mg* **Bayer Aspirin** *Tab 81mg, 163mg, 325mg, 500mg, 650mg, 975mg, Tab (chew) 81mg* **Easprin** *Tab 975mg* **Ecotrin** *Tab 81mg, 325mg, 500mg* **Genacote** *Tab 325mg, 500mg* **Halfprin** *Tab 81mg, 162mg* **Sureprin** *Tab 81mg, 162mg* **Zorprin** *Tab (ext.rel.) 800mg* **Generics** *Tab 81,325, 500, 650, 975, Tab (chew) 81mg, Supp 60, 120, 200, 300, 325, 600, 650mg*	**Ischemic stroke, TIA** →308: 50-325mg PO qd; **PRO of recurrent MI** →55, **unstable angina pectoris** →50: 75-325mg PO qd
Aspirin + Dipyridamole	
Aggrenox *Cap ext.rel 25mg + 200mg*	**Prevention of stroke/TIA** →309: 1 Cap PO bid
Cilostazol	EHL 11-13h, PRC C, Lact ?
Pletal *Tab 50mg, 100mg*	**Intermittent claudication** →66: 100mg PO bid, 30min ac or 2h pc
Clopidogrel	EHL 7-8h, PRC B, Lact ?
Plavix *Tab 75mg*	**Recent stroke** →308, **recent MI** →55; **peripheral arterial disease** →66: 75mg PO qd; **acute coronary syndrome** →50: 1st d 300mg PO, then 75mg PO qd; DARF not req
Dipyridamole	EHL alpha: 40min, beta: 10h, PRC C, Lact ?
Persantine *Tab 25mg, 50mg, 75mg* **Generics** *Tab 25mg, 50mg, 75mg*	**Prevention of thromboembolism after cardiac valve replacement** →309: 75-100mg PO qid in combination with warfarin
Ticlopidine	EHL 12.6h, PRC B, Lact ?
Ticlid *Tab 250mg* **Generics** *Tab 250mg*	**Prevention of stroke** →309: 250mg PO bid

3 A.5 Antifibrinolytics

MA/EF (aminocaproic acid, tranexamic acid): inhibition of plasminogen activation
AE (aminocaproic acid): hypotension, rash, weakness, myopathy, N/V
AE (tranexamic acid): thromboembolic events, N/V, diarrhea, giddiness, hypotension
CI (aminocaproic acid): disseminated intravascular coagulation, thrombosis prone
CI (tranexamic acid): acquired defective color vision, subarachnoid hemorrhage, active intravascular clotting

Aminocaproic Acid	EHL 1–5h, PRC C, Lact ?
Amicar *Syr 1.25g/5ml, Inj 250mg/ml* **Generics** *Tab 500mg, Syr 1.25g/5ml, Inj 250mg/ml*	**To improve hemostasis when fibrinolysis contributes to bleeding:** 4–5g IV/PO over 1h, then 1g/h for 8h or prn; DARF suggested; →79
Tranexamic Acid	EHL 2h, PRC B, Lact ?
Cyklokapron *Inj 100mg/ml*	**Prevention of hemorrhage in hemophilia during tooth extraktion** →79: 10mg/kg IV; DARF Creatinine (µmol/l) 120–250: 10mg/kg bid; 250–500: 10mg/kg qd; >500: 5mg/kg qd;

3 A.6 Hematopoietic Drugs

MA/EF: darbepoetin, erythropoietin ⇒ production of red cells in bone marrow ↑
MA/EF: filgrastim is a granulocyte colony-stimulating factor (G-CSF) ⇒ activation of hematopoietic elements; **MA/EF:** oprelvekin (human interleukin-11) is a thrombopoietic growth factor ⇒ hematopoietic stem cells ↑, megakaryocyte maturation ↑ ⇒ platelet production ↑; **MA/EF:** sargramostim is a granulocyte macrophage colony-stimulating factor (GM-CSF) ⇒ activation of hematopoietic elements
AE (erythrop.): HTN, headache, arthralgias; **AE** (filgrastim) bone pain, flu-like symptoms;
AE (oprelvekin) edema, tachycardia, dyspnea; **AE** (sargramostim) arthralgia, chills, rash
CI: hypersensitivity to the drug; **CI** (erythropoietin): uncontrolled HTN, children < 2;
CI (sargramostim): excess leukemic myeloid blasts, concomitant chemo/radiotherapy
Note: not for immediate correction of anemia; Monitor, control BP in chronic RF, monitor hematocrit twice weekly in chronic RF, once weekly in HIV-infected and CA patients until stable. Consider iron deficiency if no response

Darbepoetin alfa	EHL IV: 21h; SC: 49h, PRC C, Lact ?
Aranesp *Inj 25µg/ml, 40µg/ml, 60µg/ml, 100µg/ml, 200µg/ml*	**Anemia (chronic RF)** →82: ini 0.45µg/kg SC/IV qwk, incr dose 25% if hemoglobin response <1g/dl over 4wk; decr. dose 25% if hemoglobin response >1g/dl over 2wk; max target hemoglobin 12g/dl
Erythropoietin	EHL IV: 4–13h in CRF; SC: 27h, PRC C, Lact ?
Epogen *Inj 2000 U/ml, 3000 U/ml, 4000 U/ml, 10000 U/ml, 20000 U/ml, 40000 U/ml* **Procrit** *Inj 2000 U/ml, 3000 U/ml, 4000 U/ml, 10000 U/ml*	**Anemia (chronic RF)** →82: ini 50–100 U/kg IV/SC tiw, adjust dose to maintain target hematocrit (doses range 12.5–525U/kg tiw); **anemia of zidovudine Tx:** 100 U/kg IV/SC tiw x 8wk.; may be incr thereafter prn by 50–100 U/kg tiw up to 300 U/kg tiw; adjust dose based on AZT + hematocrit; **anemia in chemotherapy patients** →82: ini 150U/kg SC tiw x 8wk, incr thereafter prn up to 300 U/kg tiw; DARF: see Prod Info; →85

Filgrastim	EHL 2-7h, PRC C, Lact ?
Neupogen *Inj 300µg/ml*	**Neutropenia - chemotherapy induced:** 5µg/kg/d SC, incr prn in increments of 5µg/kg/d for each cycle according to the duration and severity of the absolute neutrophil count (ANC) nadir; **CH** see Prod Info; →82, →85, →85, →92
Oprelvekin	EHL 2h (1x IV inf), 7h (1x SC inf), PRC C, Lact ?
Neumega *Inj 5mg/vial*	**Prevention of severe thrombocytopenia in high-risk patients after chemo for nonmyeloid malignancies:** 50µg/kg SC qd, starting 6-24h after completion of chemotherapy, continued for 14-21d or until post-nadir platelet count is ≥ 50,000 cells/mcl; not rec beyond 21d per Tx cycle; DARF: see Prod Info
Pegfilgrastim	EHL 15-80h, PRC C, Lact ?
Neulasta *Inj 6mg/syringe*	**Neutropenia - chemotherapy induced:** 6mg SC as single dose once per chemo-Tx cycle; never give in period between 14d before and 24h after administr. of chemo-Tx: →82, →85, →86, →92
Sargramostim	EHL 1.5-2.7h, PRC C, Lact ?
Leukine *Inj 250µg/vial, 500µg/vial*	Special dosage in leukemia, bone marrow transplantation; →82, →85, →85, →92

3 A.7 Hemorheologics

MA/EF: blood viscosity↓, erythrocyte flexibility↑, microcirculatory flow↑, tissue O_2 concentrations↑
AE: GI disturbances, CNS depression, headaches; **CI:** hypersensitivity to pentoxifylline, recent surgery/cerebral/retinal bleeding, coagulation defects, bleeding diathesis

| **Pentoxifylline** | EHL 0.4-1h, PRC C, Lact ? |
| **Pentoxil** *Tab ext.rel 400mg* **Trental** *Tab ext.rel 400mg* **Generics** *Tab ext.rel 400mg* | **Intermittent claudication** →66: 400mg PO bid-tid with meals; beneficial effects may occur within 2-4wk (continue Tx for at least 8wk to determine efficacy) |

3 A.8   Other Hematologics

MA/EF, AE, CI (desmopressin): →159
MA/EF (drotrecogin alfa): recombinant activated protein C; inhibiting factors Va + VIIIa ⇒ antithrombotic effect; TNF-production ↓, leukocyte adhesion to selectins ↓, thrombin-induced inflammatory responses ↓ ⇒ antiinflammatory effect
AE (drotrecogin alfa): bleeding
CI (drotrecogin alfa): active internal bleeding, hemorrhagic stroke within the last 3mo, intracranial or intraspinal surgery or severe head trauma within the last 2mo, trauma with an increased risk of life-threatening bleeding, presence of an epidural catheter, intracranial neoplasm or mass lesion, or evidence of cerebral herniation, known hypersensitivity
Note (factor VIII, IX): risk of HIV/hepatitis transmission varies by product; factor VIII: reduced response with development of factor VIII inhibitors, hemolysis with
large/rep.ed doses in A, B, AB blood type; factor IX: products that contain factors II, VII, and X may cause thrombosis in at-risk patients, stop infusion if signs of DIC

Desmopressin	EHL IV 75.5min, PRC B, Lact ?
Concentraid *Sol (nasal) 0.01%* **DDAVP** *Tab 0.1, 0.2mg, Sol (nasal) 0.01%, Spray (nasal) 0.01mg/Spray,* *Inj 0.004mg/ml, 0.015mg/ml* **Stimate** *Spray (nasal) 0.15mg/Spray* **Generics** *Spray (nasal) 0.01mg/Spray,* *Inj. 0.004mg/ml*	**Hemophilia A** →79, **von Willebrand's disease** →80: 300µg intranasally for patients ≧ 50 kg (<50kg: 150µg); 0.3µg/kg IV over 15-30min; **CH** 0.3µg/kg IV over 15-30min; **diabetes insipidus** →159; **enuresis:** →427
Drotrecogin alfa	EHL no data, PRC C, Lact. ?
Xigris *Inj 5mg/vial, 20mg/vial*	**Severe sepsis:** 24µg/kg/h IV for 96h; DARF: not req
Factor VIII, Factor IX	EHL 12-17h, PRC B, Lact. ?
Generics	**Hemophilia A** →79: individualize factor VIII dose, **CH** individualize factor VIII dose; **hemophilia B** →79: individualize factor IX dose, **CH** individualize factor IX dose

3 B. Hematology – Therapies

Tracey Walsh, Pharm.D., BCOP
Cesar O. Freytes, MD, FACP
Adult Bone Marrow Transplant Program,
University of Texas Health Science Center at San Antonio &
South Texas Veterans Health Care System, TX

3 B.1   Hemophilia

3 B.1.1   Hemophilia A

Mild to moderate form

	Vasopressin analogue →78 (release of factor VIII from endothelial cells ⇒ factor VIII ↑ 2-4 fold)	**Desmopressin** (Concentraid, DDAVP, Stimate, Gens)	*0.3µg/kg IV/SC or nasal spray 150 µg (<50kg), 300µg (>50 kg) q12-24h; no more therapeutic response after 3-5 doses*
or	**Antifibrinolytic** →76 (inhibits systemic and local fibrinolysis at sites of vascular injuries)	**E-aminocaproic acid** (Amicar, Gens)	*h1 5g IV/PO, then 1.0-1.25q/h IV for 8h or until bleeding stops; max 30g/d; DARF: red by 15-25%*
		Tranexamic acid (Cyklokapron)	*10mg/kg IV prior surgery, then 25 mg/kg tid-qid for 2-8d; DARF: adj dose*

Severe form

	Coagulation factor →78 (substitution)	**Recombinant Factor VIII** (Helixate FS, Kogenate FS, Recombinate, ReFacto, Bioclate, Kogenate)	*Factor VIII dose: (target Factor VIII — baseline Factor VIII) x weight in kg/2 IV; target factor level in hemarthrosis 40%, in tooth extraction 60-80%, in minor surgery 60-80%, in major surgery 100%; rep dose q12h*
or	**Coagulation factor** →78 (substitution)	**Plasma-derived concentrates** (Alphanate, Hemofil M, Koate-DVI, Monoclate P)	

3 B.1.2   Hemophilia B

	Coagulation factor →78 (substitution)	**Recombinant Factor IX** (BeneFix)	*Factor IX dose: (target factor IX — baseline Factor IX) x weight in kg IV; target Factor IX level similar to Hemophilia A; rep dose q24h*
or	**Coagulation factor** →78 (substitution)	**Plasma-derived concentrates** (Mononine, AlphaNine SD, Profilnine DS, Bebulin VH)	

3 B.1.3   Hemophilia with Inhibitors

	Coagulation factor →78 (substitution)	**Porcine factor VIII** (Hyate C)	*For Factor VIII inhibitor only: 100-160 U/kg IV if antibody level < 50 Bethesda U; rep q6-8h*

or	**Coagulation factor** →78 (substitution)	**Recombinant Factor VIIa** (NovoSeven)	*For Factor VIII or IX inhibitor 90µg/kg IV q2h until hemostasis*
or	**Coagulation factor** →78 (substitution)	**Anti-inhibitor coagulant complex** (Autoplex T, Feiba VH Immuno)	*25-100 U/kg IV prn, rep in 12h sos*

Immune tolerance induction should be considered in severe cases.

6.   Kroll MH. Hemophilia and other coagulation disorders in: Manual of Coagulation Disorders, Blackwell Science, Williston, 2001, 196-209.
7.   Shapiro AD. Coagulation factor concentrates in:Goodnight SH and Hathaway WE, Disorders of Hemostasis and thrombosis, McGraw-Hill, New York, 2001, 505-16.

3 B.2   Von Willebrand's Disease

Non–transfusional Tx in mild cases and before minor surgery

	Vasopressin analogue →78 (release of factor VIII from endothelial cells ⇒ factor VIII ↑ 2-4 fold)	**Desmopressin** (Concentraid, DDAVP, Stimate, Gens)	*0.3µg/kg IV/SC or nasal spray 150 µg (<50kg), 300µg (>50 kg) q12-24h; no more therapeutic response after 3-5 doses.*
	Note: desmopressin effective in type 1, contraindicated in type 2B		
or	**Antifibrinolytic** →76 (inhibits systemic and local fibrinolysis at sites of vascular injuries)	**E-aminocaproic acid** (Amicar, Gens)	*h1 5g IV/PO, then 1.0-1.25g/h IV for 8h or until bleeding stops; max 30g/d; DARF: red by 15-25%*
		Tranexamic acid (Cyklokapron)	*10mg/kg IV prior surgery, then 25 mg/kg tid-qid for 2-8d; DARF: adj dose*
or	**vWF-enriched preparations** (substitution)	**vWF** (Humate-P)	*25-100 U/kg IV prn, rep in 12h sos*

8.   Kroll MH. Hemophilia and other coagulation disorders in: Manual of Coagulation Disorders, Blackwell Science, Williston, 2001, 196-209.
9.   Shapiro AD. Coagulation factor concentrates in: Goodnight SH and Hathaway WE, Disorders of Hemostasis and thrombosis, McGraw-Hill, New York, 2001, 505-16.
10.   Mannucci PM. How I treat patients with von Willebrand disease. Blood 2001;97: 1915-9.

3 B.3   Anemias
3 B.3.1   Iron Deficiency

	Iron preparation →141 (substitution)	**Ferrous Sulfate** (Feosol, Feratab, Fer-In-Sol, Fer-Iron, Slow FE, ED-IN-SOL, Fe^{50}, Fergensol, Gens)	*300mg PO tid, preferably on an empty stomach for 3–6mo*

11.   Brittenham GM. Disorders of iron metabolism in: Hematology Basic Principles and Practice, 3rd ed., Churchill Livingstone, New York, 2000, 397-427.

3 B.3.2 Megaloblastic Anemia

Vitamin B12 deficiency (pernicious anemia)

	Vitamin B12 →145 (substitution)	**Hydroxocobalamin** (Hydro Cobex, Hydro –Crysti-12, LA-12, Gens)	*wk1: 1000µg IM qd, wk2: 1000µg IM tiw wk3-6: 1000µg IM qwk, then 1000µg qmo for life*
or		**Cyanocobalamin** (Crystamine, Cristi 1000, Cyanoject, Cyomin, Rubesol-1000, Gens)	*wk1: 1000µg IM qd, wk2: 1000µg IM biw wk3-6: 1000µg IM qwk, then 1000µg qmo for life*

12.   Antony AC. Megaloblastic anemias in: Hematology Basic Principles and Practice, 3rd ed., Churchill Livingstone, New York, 2000, 397-427.

Folic acid deficiency

	Folic acid →147 (substitution)	**Folic acid** (Folvite, Gens)	*1–5mg PO qd*

Therapeutic doses of folate will partly correct the abnormalities of B12 deficiency, but neurologic manifestations will progress. It is essential to also evaluate patients for B12 deficiency.

13.   Antony AC. Megaloblastic anemias in: Hematology Basic Principles and Practice, 3rd ed., Churchill Livingstone, New York, 2000, 397-427.

3 B.3.3 Hemolytic Anemias

Beta-Thalassemia major

	Antidote →470 (complexes with ferric ions ⇒ renal elimination)	**Deferoxamine** (Desferal)	*1–2g IV or SC qd over 8 12h (long-term Tx)*

14   Brittenham GM. Disorders of iron metabolism in: Hematology Basic Principles and Practice, 3rd ed., Churchill Livingstone, New York, 2000, 397-427.

3 B.3.4 Autoimmune Hemolytic Anemia

IgG warm autoantibodies

	Glucocorticoid →148 (anti-inflammatory, immunosuppressive)	**Prednisone** (Deltasone, Orasone, Liquid Pred, Sterapred DS, Panasol-S, Meticorten, Prednicen-M, Gens)	*1–2mg/kg PO qd, red slowly when adequate Hb level achieved*
poss.	**Alkylating agent** (immunosuppressive)	**Cyclophosphamide** (Cytoxan, Neosar, Gens)	*2 mg/kg/d PO (for patients unresponsive to prednisone)*
or	**Purine antagonist** →260 (immunosuppressive)	**Azathioprine** (Imuran, Gens)	*1.5mg/kg/d PO*

IgM cold autoantibodies (cold agglutinins)

	Alkylating agent (immunosuppressive)	**Cyclophosphamide** (Cytoxan, Neosar, Gens)	*2mg/kg/d PO*
or		**Chlorambucil** (Leukeran)	*0.1mg/kg/d PO*

15.   Schwartz RS et al. Autoimmune hemolytic anemias in: Hematology Basic Principles and Practice, 3rd ed., Churchill Livingstone, New York, 2000, 611-30.

3 B.3.5 Anemia of Chronic Renal Failure

	Erythrocyte colony stimulating factor →76 (RBC production↑, maturation, activation↑)	Erythropoietin (Epogen, Procrit)	*50-100 U/kg SC or IV tiw*
or		Darbepoetin alfa (Aranesp)	*0.45µg/kg/wk SC, target dose to maint Hb at 12g/dl*

16. Dainiak N. Hematologic complications of renal disease in: Hematology Basic Principles and Practice, 3rd ed., Churchill Livingstone, New York, 2000, 2357-73.

3 B.3.6 Anemia in Non-myeloid Cancer Patients on Chemotherapy

	Erythrocyte colony stimulating factor →76 (RBC production↑, maturation, activation)	Erythropoietin (Epogen, Procrit)	*40,000-60,000 U SC qwk*

17. Gabrilove JL, et al. Clinical evaluation of once-weekly dosing of epoetin alfa in chemotherapy patients: improvements in hemoglobin and quality of life are similar to three-times-weekly dosing. J Clin Oncol 2001;19(11):2875-82.

3 B.3.7 Aplastic Anemia

	Anti-lymphocyte antibodies (immunosuppressive)	Lymphocyte immune globulin (ATGAM)	*40mg/kg/d IV for 4d*
plus	Glucocorticoid →148 (anti-inflammatory, immunosuppressive)	Prednisone (Deltasone, Orasone, Liquid Pred, Sterapred DS, Panasol-S, Meticorten, Prednicen-M, Gens))	*60–100mg/d PO for 2wk, taper dose to discontinue on d30*
plus	Inhibition of interleukin-2 activation of T-lymphocytes →260 (immunosuppressive)	Cyclosporine (Gengraf, Neoral, Sandimmune, SangCya, Gens)	*10-12mg/kg/d PO for 6mo to maintain serum levels of 200-400ng/ml*

18. Rosenfeld SJ et al. Intensive immunosuppression with antithymocyte globulin and cyclosporine as treatment of severe acquired aplastic anemia. Blood 1995;85:3058-65.

3 B.4 Agranulocytosis

	Granulocyte colony stimulating factor →76 (neutrophil production↑, maturation, activation↑)	Filgrastim (Neupogen)	*5.75-11.5µg/kg/d SC until ANC ≥ 1500/mm³ (then maint Tx)*
poss.			

19. Dale DC, et al. A randomized controlled phase III trial of recombinant human granulocyte colony-stimulating factor (filgrastim) for treatment of severe chronic neutropenia. Blood 1993:81(10):2496-2502.
20. Welte K, Boxer LA. Severe chronic neutropenia: pathophysiology and therapy. Seminars in Hematology 1997:34(4):267-78.

3 B.5 Idiopathic Thrombocytopenic Purpura
3 B.5.1 In General

	Glucocorticoid →148 (anti-inflammatory, immunosuppressive)	Prednisone (Deltasone, Orasone, Liquid Pred, Sterapred DS, Panasol-S, Meticorten, Prednicen-M, Gens	*1-1.5mg/kg/d PO qd for 3wk then taper slowly*

or	**Anti–D immune globulin** (saturate spleen capacity to clear antibody coated platelets)	**Anti–D immune globulin** (WinRho SDF)	*Ini 50µg/kg IV, then 40-60µg/ kg; only in non-splenectomized, Rh (D) positive patients*
or	**Immune globulin** →258 (Fc receptor saturation of reticuloendothelial system)	**Immune globulin** (Gamimune N, Gammagard S/D, Gammar- P IV, Iveegam, Panglobulin, Polygam S/D, Venoglobulin-S, Sandoglobulin)	*1g/kg IV qd for 2-3d*

3 B.5.2 For Patients Resistant to Prednisone Administration after Splenectomy

	Androgen →452 (platelet clearance↓)	**Danazol** (Danocrine, Gens)	*10-15mg/kg/d PO; maint dose as low as 50mg/d*
or	**Decreases platelet clearance** →209	**Dapsone** (Gens)	*75mg/d PO*
or	**Anti–CD20 monoclonal antibody** (immunomodulation)	**Rituximab** (Rituxan)	*375mg/m² IV qwk for 2-4wk*
or	**Purine antagonist** →260 (immunosuppression)	**Azathioprine** (Imuran, Gens)	*1-4mg/kg PO qd*
or	**Alkylating agent** (immunosuppression)	**Cyclophosphamide** (Cytoxan, Neosar, Gens)	*1-2mg/kg/d PO*

21. Cines DB et al. Immune thrombocytopenic purpura. N Engl J Med 2002;346:995-1008.

3 B.6   Polycythemia Vera

poss	**Antiplatelet drug** →74 (phosphodiesterase/platelet aggregation-adhesion inhibition)	**Aspirin – ASA** (Ascriptin, Asprimox, Bayer Aspirin, Bufferin, Easprin, Ecotrin, Empirin, Genprin, Halfprin, St. Joseph Pain Reliever, Zorprin, Gens)	*81-325mg PO qd; only for Tx of erythromealgia*
poss	**Interferon** →212 (immune modulation)	**INF-alpha-2a/b** (Roferon A, Intron A)	*2-5 M U SC tiw; only to control intractable pruritus, thrombocytosis and extramedullary hematopoiesis*
poss	**Cytostatic** →74 (phospholipase A2 inhibition)	**Anagrelide** (Agrylin)	*0.5mg PO qid; incr dose by 0.5mg/d qwk prn; usual dose 2-2.5mg/d; only in patients with erythromelalgia*

22. Spivak JL. The optimal management of polycythaemia vera, Br J Hematol 2002;116:243-54.

3 B.7   Essential Thrombocytosis

poss.	**Cytostatic** →74 (phospholipase A2 inhibition)	**Anagrelide** (Agrylin)	*In younger patients: 0.5mg PO qid; incr dose by 0.5mg/d qwk prn; usual dose 2-2.5mg/d*
poss.	**Interferon** →212 (immunomodulation)	**INF-alpha-2a/b** (Roferon A, Intron A)	*In younger patients: 2-5 M U SC tiw*

poss.	**Cytostatic** (ribonucleotide diphosphate reductase inhibition)	**Hydroxyurea** (Hydrea, Droxia, Mylocel)	*1 g PO qd; adj according to platelet count*

23. Hoffman R, Primary Thrombocythemia in: Hematology Basic Principles and Practice, 3rd ed., Churchill Livingstone, New York, 2000, 1188-1204.

3 B.8   Chronic Myeloid Leukemia
3 B.8.1   Chronic Phase

	Tyrosine kinase inhibitor (white blood cells ↓)	**Imatinib mesylate** (Gleevec)	*400mg PO qd*
or	**Interferon** →212 (immunostimulation, modulation)	**IFN–alpha–2a/b** (Roferon A, Intron A)	*5 x 10^6 U/m^2 SC qd (long-term Tx)*
+/-	**Cytostatic** (purine antagonist)	**Cytarabine** (Cytosar-U, Cytosine Arabinoside, Ara-C)	*20mg/m^2 IV qd for 10d (q4wk)*
or	**Cytostatic** (ribonucleotide diphosphate reductase inhibition)	**Hydroxyurea** (Hydrea, Droxia, Mylocel)	*40-50 mg/kg PO qd*
poss.	**Xanthine oxidase inhibitor** →138 (uric acid production ↓)	**Allopurinol** (Aloprim, Zyloprim, Gens)	*300-600mg PO/IV qd*
poss.	**Urine hydration + alkalinization** →18 (solubility of uric acid ↑)	**Hydration +/– Sodium bicarbonate**	*150-200ml/h; start 24-48h prior to chemo-Tx*

3 B.8.2   Accelerated/Blast Phase

	Tyrosine kinase inhibitor	**Imatinib mesylate** (Gleevec)	*600mg PO qd*
or	**Interferon** →212 (immunostimulation, modulation)	**IFN–alpha–2a/b** (Roferon A, Intron A)	*5 x 10^6 U/m^2 SC qd (long-term Tx)*
+/-	**Cytostatic** (ribonucleotide diphosphate reductase inhibition)	**Hydroxyurea** (Hydrea, Droxia, Mylocel)	*40-50mg/kg PO qd*
poss.	**Xanthine oxidase inhibitor** →138 (uric acid production ↓)	**Allopurinol** (Aloprim, Zyloprim, Gens)	*300-600mg PO/IV qd*
poss.	**Urine hydration + alkalinization** →18 (solubility of uric acid ↑)	**Hydration +/– Sodium bicarbonate**	*150-200ml/h; start 24-48h prior to chemo-Tx*

24. Guilhot F, et al. Interferon alfa-2b combined with cytarabine versus interferon alone in chronic myelogenous leukemia. N Engl J Med 1997;337:223-9.
25. Silver RT, et al. An evidence-based analysis of the effect of busulfan, hydroxyurea, interferon, and allogeneic bone marrow transplantation in treating the chronic phase of chronic myeloid leukemia: developed for the American Society of Hematology. Blood 1999;94(5):1517-36.
26. Kantarjian HM, et al. Imatinib mesylate (STI571) therapy of Philadelphia chromosome-positive chronic myeloid leukemia in early chronic phase (Ph+ CML Early CP). Blood 2001;98(11):137a (abstract #577).
27. Talpaz M, et al. Imatinib induces durable hematologic and cytogenetic responses in patients with accelerated phase chronic myeloid leukemia: results of a phase 2 study. Blood 2002;99(6):1928-37.

3 B.9 Myelofibrosis with Myeloid Metaplasia

poss.	**Interferon** →212 (immunomodulation)	**INF–alpha–2a/b** (Roferon A, Intron A)	*2-5 M U SC tiw*
poss.	**Cytostatic** (ribonucleotide diphosphate reductase inhibition)	**Hydroxyurea** (Hydrea, Droxia, Mylocel)	*20-30mg/kg PO biw or tiw*
poss.	**Androgen** →452 (erythropoiesis↑)	**Danazol** (Danocrine, Gens)	*200mg PO bid or tid*
poss.	**Anabolic steroid** (erythropoiesis↑)	**Oxymetholone** (Anadrol-50)	*50mg PO tid*

28. Tefferi A et al. Myelofibrosis with myeloid metaplasia. N Engl J Med 2000;342: 1255-65.

3 B.10 Myelodysplastic Syndromes

poss.	**Antidote** →470 (complexes with ferric ions and eliminated through kidneys)	**Deferoxamine** (Desferal)	*2g IV after each unit of blood + 1-2g SC over 8-24h qd or 1g SC bid*
poss.	**Erythrocyte colony stimulating factor** →76 (RBC production↑, maturation, activation)	**Erythropoietin** (Epogen, Procrit)	*150-300 U/kg SC tiw or 40,000-60,000 U SC qwk*
poss.	**Granulocyte colony stimulating factor** →76 (neutrophil production↑, maturation, activation↑)	**Filgrastim** (Neupogen)	*0.3-5µg/kg/d SC*

29. Franchini M, Gandini G, de Gironcoli M, et al. Safety and efficacy of subcutaneous bolus injection of deferoxamine in adult patients with iron overload. Blood 2000;95(9):2776-9.
30. Hellstrom-Lindberg E. Efficacy of erythropoietin in the myelodysplastic syndromes: meta-analysis of 205 patients from 17 studies. Br J Haematol 1995;89:67-71.
31. Negrin RS, Haeuber DH, Nagler A, et al. Maintenance treatment of patients with myelodysplastic syndromes using recombinant human granulocytic colony-stimulating factor. Blood 1990;76(1):36-43.
32. Ozer H, Armitage J, Bennett C, et al. 2000 Update of recommendations for the use of hematopoietic colony-stimulating factors: evidence-based, clinical practice guidelines. J Clin Oncol 2000;18(20):3558-85.

3 B.11 Acute Leukemia
3 B.11.1 Acute Myelogenous Leukemia (AML)

Induction (7+3)

	Antimetabolite (purine antagonist)	**Cytarabine** (Cytosar-U, Tarabine PFS)	*100mg/m²/d continuous IV Inf d1-7*
plus	**Anthracycline** (DNA intercalation, topoisomerase II inhibition)	**Daunorubicin** (Cerubidine)	*45-60mg/m²/d IV d1-3 (may consider other anthracyclines)*
poss.	**Granulocyte colony stimulating factor** →76 (neutrophil production↑, maturation, activation↑)	**Filgrastim** (Neupogen)	*5µg/kg SC qd beginning 24h after chemo-Tx through neutrophil recovery*

or	**Granulocyte and macrophage colony stimulating factor** →76 (neutrophil/macrophage production↑, maturation, activation)	**Sargramostim** (Leukine)	*250μ/m^2 SC qd beginning 24h after chemo-Tx through neutrophil recovery*
poss.	**Xanthine oxidase inhibitor** →138 (uric acid production↓)	**Allopurinol** (Aloprim, Zyloprim, Gens)	*300-600mg PO/IV qd*
poss.	**Urine hydration + alkalinization** →18 (solubility of uric acid↑)	**Hydration +/– Sodium bicarbonate**	*150-200ml/h; start 24-48h prior to chemo-Tx*

Consolidation (histone deacetylase, HDAC)

	Antimetabolite (purine antagonist)	**Cytarabine** (Cytosar-U, Tarabine PFS)	*1-3g/m^2 IV q12h on d1, d3, and d5; rep q28d*

33. Arlin Z, Case D, Moore J, et al. Randomized multicenter trial of cytosine arabinoside with mitoxantrone or daunorubicin in previously untreated adult patients with acute nonlymphocytic leukemia (ANLL). Leukemia 1990;4(3):177-183.
34. Mayer RJ, Davis RB, Schiffer CA, et al. Intensive post-remission chemotherapy in adults with acute myeloid leukemia. N Engl J Med 1994;331:896-903.

3 B.11.2 Acute Lymphocytic Leukemia (except B–ALL)

Induction (Linker)

	Anthracycline (DNA intercalation, topoisomerase II inhibition)	**Daunorubicin** (Cerubidine)	*50mg/m^2/d IV d1-3*
plus	**Antimitotic** (Mitotic spindle poison)	**Vincristine** (Oncovin, Vincasar PFS, Gens)	*2mg IV d1, d8, d15, and d22*
plus	**Glucocorticoid** →148 (anti-inflammatory, immunosuppressive, lympholytic)	**Prednisone** (Deltasone, Orasone, Liquid Pred, Sterapred DS, Panasol-S, Meticorten, Prednicen-M, Gens)	*60 mg/m^2 PO d1-28*
plus	**Enzyme** (asparagine deamination, ⇒ protein synthesis↓)	**L-asparaginase** (Elspar)	*6000 U/m^2 IM d17-28 (test dose prior to 1st dose)*
poss.	**Granulocyte colony stimulating factor** →76 (neutrophil production↑, maturation, activation↑)	**Filgrastim** (Neupogen)	*5μg/kg SC qd beginning 24h after chemo-Tx through neutrophil recovery*
or		**Sargramostim** (Leukine)	*250μg/m^2 SC qd; start 24h after chemo-Tx through neutrophil recovery*
poss.	**Xanthine oxidase inhibitor** →138 (uric acid production↓)	**Allopurinol** (Aloprim, Zyloprim, Gens)	*300-600mg PO/IV qd*
poss.	**Urine hydration + alkalinization** →18 (solubility of uric acid↑)	**Hydration +/– Sodium bicarbonate**	*150-200ml/h; start 24-48h prior to chemo-Tx*

Consolidation (Linker – cycle 1,3,5,7)

	Anthracycline (DNA intercalation, topoisomerase II inhibition)	**Daunorubicin** (Cerubidine)	*50mg/m^2/d IV d1-2*
plus	**Antimitotic** (Mitotic spindle poison)	**Vincristine** (Oncovin, Vincasar PFS, Gens)	*2mg IV d1, d8*
plus	**Glucocorticoid** →148 (anti-inflammatory, immunosuppressive, lympholytic)	**Prednisone** (Deltasone, Orasone, Liquid Pred, Sterapred DS, Panasol-S, Meticorten, Prednicen-M, Gens)	*60mg/m^2 PO d1-14*
plus	**Enzyme** (asparagine deamination, resulting in decreased protein synthesis)	**L-asparaginase** (Elspar)	*12000U/m^2 IM d2,4,7,9,11,14*

Consolidation (Linker – cycle 2,4,6,8)

	Topoisomerase II inhibition	**Etoposide** (VePesid, Etopophos, Toposar) – takes place of teniposide	*100mg/m^2 IV d1,4,8,11*
plus	**Antimetabolite** (purine antagonist)	**Cytarabine** (Cytosar-U, Tarabine PFS)	*300mg/m^2 IV d1,4,8,11*

Consolidation (Linker – cycle 9)

	Antimetabolite →263 (folic acid antagonist)	**Methotrexate** (Gens)	*690mg/m^2 IV over 42h x 1 dose*
plus	**Reduced folate** (normal cell rescue)	**Leucovorin** (Wellcovorin, Follnic acid)	*15mg/m^2 IV q6h x12h beginning h 42 (adj based on MTX levels)*

Maintenance (Linker)

	Antimetabolite →263 (folic acid antagonist)	**Methotrexate** (Rheumatrex, Gens)	*20mg/m^2 PO q wk until 30mo of CR*
plus	**Antimetabolite** (purine antagonist)	**6-Mercaptopurine** (Purinethol)	*75mg/m^2 PO qd until 30mo of CR*

Note: Consolidation treatments given approximately monthly

35.   Linker CA, Levitt LJ, O'Donnell M, et al. Treatment of adult acute lymphoblastic leukemia with intensive cyclical chemotherapy: a follow-up report. Blood 1991;78(11):2814-22.

3 B.11.3 Acute Lymphocytic Leukemia (B-ALL)

Induction/Consolidation (hyperCVAD - cycle 1,3,5,7)

	Alkylating agent (DNA cross-linking)	**Cyclophosphamide** (Cytoxan, Neosar, Gens)	*300mg/m^2 IV q12h x 6 doses, d1-3*
plus	**Antimitotic** (Mitotic spindle poison)	**Vincristine** (Oncovin, Vincasar PFS, Gens)	*2mg IV d4, d11*
plus	**Anthracycline** (DNA intercalation, topoisomerase II inhibition)	**Doxorubicin** (Adriamycin PFS, Adriamycin RDF, Rubex, Gens)	*50mg/m^2 IV d4*

plus	**Glucocorticoid** →148 (anti–inflammatory, immunosuppressive, lympholytic)	**Dexamethasone** (Decadron, Dexameth, Dexone, Hexadrol, Gens)	*40mg/d PO d1-4, d11-14*

Induction/Consolidation (hyperCVAD – cycle 2,4,6,8)

	Antimetabolite →263 (folic acid antagonist)	**Methotrexate** (Gens)	*200mg/m² IV over 2h, then 800mg/m² IV over 22h x1 dose on d1*
plus	**Reduced folate** (normal cell rescue)	**Leucovorin** (Wellcovorin, Folinic acid)	*15 mg IV/PO q6h x 8 doses. Begin 24h after MTX complete (adj based on MTX levels)*
plus	**Antimetabolite** (purine antagonist)	**Cytarabine** (Cytosar-U, Tarabine PFS)	*3g/m² IV q12h x 4 doses on d2-3*
plus	**Glucocorticoid** →148 (anti–inflammatory, immunosuppressive)	**Methylprednisolone** (Solu-Medrol, A-Methapred)	*50mg IV q12h d1-3*
poss.	**Granulocyte colony stimulating factor** →76 (neutrophil production ↑, maturation, activation ↑)	**Filgrastim** (Neupogen)	*5µg/kg SC qd; start 24h after chemo-Tx through neutrophil recovery*
or	**Granulocyte and macrophage colony stimulating factor** →76 (neutrophil/macrophage production ↑, maturation, activation)	**Sargramostim** (Leukine)	*250µ/m² SC qd; start 24h after chemo-Tx through neutrophil recovery*
poss.	**Xanthine oxidase inhibitor** →138 (uric acid production ↓)	**Allopurinol** (Aloprim, Zyloprim, Gens)	*300-600mg PO/IV qd*
poss.	**Urine hydration + alkalinization** →18 (solubility of uric acid ↑)	**Hydration +/- Sodium bicarbonate**	*150-200ml/h; start 24-48h prior to chemo-Tx*

Note: Subsequent treatments given upon WBC and platelet recovery per protocol.

36.   Garcia-Manero G, Kantarjian HM. The Hyper-CVAD regimen in adult acute lymphocytic leukemia. Hematol Oncol Clin North Am 2000;14(4):1381-96.

Central nervous system IT therapy

poss.	**Antimetabolite** (folic acid antagonist)	**Methotrexate** (Methotrexate LPF)	*12-15mg intrathecal (lower doses for age < 3y old)*
poss.	**Antimetabolite** →263 (purine antagonist)	**Cytarabine** (Cytosar-U, Tarabine PFS)	*50-100mg intrathecal (lower doses for age < 3y old)*
poss.	**Glucocorticoid** →148 (anti–inflammatory, immunosuppressive)	**Hydrocortisone acetate** (preservative-free)	*12-35mg intrathecal (lower doses for age < 3y old)*

Note: Frequency of therapy depends on protocol and if patient has active CNS involvement of leukemia.

37.   Hoelzer D. Treatment of acute lymphoblastic leukemia. Semin Hematol 1994;31:1-15.
38.   Steinherz PG. CNS leukemia: problem of diagnosis, treatment, and outcome. J Clin Oncol 1995;13(2):310-13.

3 B.11.4 Acute Promyelocytic Leukemia (APL, M3 AML)

Induction

	Retinoid →348 (APL cell maturation, cytodifferentiation, decreases proliferation)	**Tretinoin** (Vesanoid, ATRA, All-*trans*-retinoic acid)	*45mg/m²/d PO (divided bid)*
plus	**Anthracycline** (DNA intercalation, topoisomerase II inhibition)	**Daunorubicin** (Cerubidine)	*60mg/m²/d IV d1-3 (may consider other anthracyclines)*

Consolidation (cycle 1)

	Retinoid →348 (APL cell maturation, cytodifferentiation, decreases proliferation)	**Tretinoin** (Vesanoid, ATRA, All-*trans*-retinoic acid)	*45mg/m²/d PO (divided BID)*
plus	**Anthracycline** (DNA intercalation, topoisomerase II inhibition)	**Daunorubicin** (Cerubidine)	*60mg/m²/d IV d1-3 (may consider other anthracyclines)*
poss.	**Granulocyte colony stimulating factor** →76 (neutrophil production ↑, maturation, activation ↑)	**Filgrastim** (Neupogen)	*5µg/kg SC qd; start 24h after chemo-Tx through neutrophil recovery*
or	**Granulocyte and macrophage colony stimulating factor** →76 (neutrophil/macrophage production ↑, maturation, activation)	**Sargramostim** (Leukine)	*250µ/m² SC qd; start 24h after chemo-Tx through neutrophil recovery*
poss.	**Xanthine oxidase inhibitor** →138 (uric acid production ↓)	**Allopurinol** (Aloprim, Zyloprim, Gens)	*300-600mg PO/IV qd*
poss.	**Urine hydration + alkalinization** →18 (solubility of uric acid ↑)	**Hydration +/- Sodium bicarbonate**	*150-200ml/h; start 24-48h prior to chemo-Tx*

Consolidation (cycle 2)

	Retinoid →348 (APL cell maturation, cytodifferentiation, decreases proliferation)	**Tretinoin** (Vesanoid, ATRA, All-*trans*-retinoic acid)	*45mg/m²/d PO (divided BID)*
plus	**Anthracycline** (DNA intercalation, topoisomerase II inhibition)	**Daunorubicin** (Cerubidine)	*60mg/m²/d IV d1-3 (may consider other anthracyclines)*
+/-	**Antimetabolite** (purine antagonist)	**Cytarabine** (Cytosar-U, Tarabine PFS)	*1-2g/m² IV q12h d1-4*

Maintenance

	Retinoid →348 (APL cell maturation, cytodifferentiation, decreases proliferation)	**Tretinoin** (Vesanoid, ATRA, All–trans-retinoic acid)	*45mg/m² /d PO for 15d (q3mo x 2y)*
+/–	**Antimetabolite** (purine antagonist)	**6-Mercaptopurine** (Purinethol)	*90mg/m² /d PO (x2y)*
+/–	**Antimetabolite** →263 (folic acid antagonist)	**Methotrexate** (Rheumatrex, Gens)	*15mg/m² /wk PO(x2y)*

39. Fenaux P, Chastang C, Chevret S, et al. A randomized comparison of all transretinoic acid (ATRA) plus chemotherapy and the role of maintenance therapy in newly diagnosed acute promyelocytic leukemia. Blood 1999;94(4):1192-1200.
40. Sanz MA, Martin G, Rayon C, et al. A modified AIDA protocol with anthracycline-based consolidation results in high antileukemia efficacy and reduced toxicity in newly diagnosed PML/RARa-positive acute promyelocytic leukemia. Blood 1999;94(9):3015-21.
41. Tallman MS, Nabhan C, Feusner JH, et al. Acute promyelocytic leukemia: evolving therapeutic strategies. Blood 2002;99(3):759-67.

3 B.12 Non-Hodgkin Lymphoma
3 B.12.1 Low-grade

Single agent

	Alkylating agent (DNA cross-linking)	**Chlorambucil** (Leukeran)	*6-14mg PO qd until symptoms improve, then cont as intermittent Tx: 0.7mg/kg PO over 2-4d; rep q3wk until stabilized*

COP (repeat every 21 days)

	Alkylating agent (DNA cross-linking)	**Cyclophosphamide** (Cytoxan, Neosar, Gens)	*800mg IV on d1*
plus	**Antimitotic** (Mitotic spindle poison)	**Vincristine** (Oncovin, Vincasar PFS, Gens)	*1.4mg/m² IV on d1 (max 2mg)*
plus	**Glucocorticoid** →148 (anti-inflammatory, immunosuppressive, lympholytic)	**Prednisone** (Deltasone, Orasone, Liquid Pred, Sterapred DS, Panasol-S, Meticorten, Prednicen-M, Gens)	*60mg/m² PO, d1-5*

Rituximab

	Anti-CD20 monoclonal antibody (antineoplastic)	**Rituximab** (Rituxan)	*375mg/m² IV qwk x 4 wk*

42. Roeser HP, et al. Advanced non-Hodgkin's lymphomas: response to treatment with combination chemotherapy and factors influencing prognosis. Br J Haematol 1975;30(2):233-47.
43. McLaughlin et al: Rituximab chimeric anti-CD20 monoclonal antibody therapy for relapsed indolent lymphoma: half of patients respond to a four-dose treatment program. J Clin Oncol 1998;16:2825-33.

3 B.12.2 Chronic Lymphocytic Leukemia, Small Lymphocytic Lymphoma

	Alkylating agent (DNA cross-linking)	**Chlorambucil** (Leukeran)	*0.1mg/kg/d PO until counts improve or symptoms subside*
OR	**Alkylating agent** (DNA cross-linking)	**Chlorambucil** (Leukeran)	*0.3mg/kg/d PO qd x 5d; rep q28 d*
plus	**Glucocorticoid** →148 (anti-inflammatory, immunosuppressive, lympholytic)	**Prednisone** (Deltasone, Orasone, Liquid Pred, Sterapred DS, Panasol-S, Meticorten, Prednicen-M, Gens)	*40mg/m^2 PO qd x 5d; rep q28 d*
OR	**Antimetabolite** (purine antagonist)	**Fludarabine** (Fludara)	*25 mg/m^2 IV qd x 5d; rep q28 d*
OR	**Monoclonal antibody** (inhibition of CD52 and subsequent cell lysis)	**Alemtuzumab** (Campath)	*Taper slowly over 3-7d: ini 3mg/d until tolerated, then 10mg/d until tolerated, then 30 mg/d; max single dose 30mg, max cumulative dose 90 mg; maint Tx 30 mg IV tiw on alternate days for up to 12wk*

44. Dighiero G et al: Chlorambucil in indolent chronic lymphocytic leukemia, N Engl J Med 1998; 338:1506-14.
45. Rai KR et al: Fludarabine compared with chlorambucil as primary therapy for chronic lymphocytic leukaemia. N Engl J Med 2000;343:1750-7.
46. Keating MJ et al: Therapeutic role of alemtuzumab (Campath IH) in patients who failed fludarabine: results of a large international study. Blood 2002;99:3554-61.

3 B.12.3 Intermediate-grade Lymphoma

CHOP (repeat every 21 days)

	Alkylating agent (DNA cross-linking)	**Cyclophosphamide** (Cytoxan, Neosar, Gens)	*750mg/m^2 IV on d1*
plus	**Anthracycline** (DNA intercalation, topoisomerase II inhibition)	**Doxorubicin** (Adriamycin PFS, Adriamycin RDF, Rubex, Gens)	*50mg/m^2 IV on d1*
plus	**Antimitotic** (Mitotic spindle poison)	**Vincristine** (Oncovin, Vincasar PFS, Gens)	*1.4mg/m^2 IV (max 2mg) on d1*
plus	**Glucocorticoid** →148 (anti-inflammatory, immunosuppressive, lympholytic)	**Prednisone** (Deltasone, Orasone, Liquid Pred, Sterapred DS, Panasol-S, Meticorten, Prednicen-M, Gens)	*40mg/m^2 qd x 5d*
+/-	**Anti-CD20 monoclonal antibody** (antineoplastic)	**Rituximab** (Rituxan)	*375mg/m^2 IV on d1*

Note: Addition of rituximab recommended for elderly patients.

47. Coiffier B et al: CHOP chemotherapy plus rituximab compared with CHOP alone in elderly patients with diffuse large-B-cell lymphoma, N Engl J Med 2002;346:235-42.

3 B.12.4 High-grade Lymphoma

Induction/Consolidation (hyperCVAD – cycle 1,3,5,7)

	Alkylating agent (DNA cross-linking)	**Cyclophosphamide** (Cytoxan, Neosar, Gens)	*300mg/m² IV q12h x 6 doses, d1-3*
plus	**Antimitotic** (Mitotic spindle poison)	**Vincristine** (Oncovin, Vincasar PFS, Gens)	*2mg IV d4, d11*
plus	**Anthracycline** (DNA intercalation, topoisomerase II inhibition)	**Doxorubicin** (Adriamycin PFS, Adriamycin RDF, Rubex, Gens)	*50mg/m² IV d4*
plus	**Glucocorticoid** →148 (anti-inflammatory, immunosuppressive, lympholytic)	**Dexamethasone** (Decadron, Dexameth, Dexone, Hexadrol, Gens)	*40mg/d PO d1-4, d11-14*

Induction/Consolidation (hyperCVAD – cycle 2,4,6,8)

	Antimetabolite →263 (folic acid antagonist)	**Methotrexate** (Gens)	*200mg/m² IV over 2h, then 800mg/m² IV over 22h x1 dose on d1*
plus	**Reduced folate** (normal cell rescue)	**Leucovorin** (Wellcovorin, Folinic acid)	*15mg IV/PO q6h x 8 doses. Begin 24h after MTX complete (adj based on MTX levels)*
plus	**Antimetabolite** (purine antagonist)	**Cytarabine** (Cytosar-U, Tarabine PFS)	*3g/m² IV q12h x 4 doses on d2-3*
plus	**Glucocorticoid** →148 (anti-inflammatory, immunosuppressive, lympholytic)	**Methylprednisolone** (Solu-Medrol, A-Methapred)	*50mg IV q12h d1-3*
poss.	**Granulocyte colony stimulating factor** →76 (neutrophil production ↑, maturation, activation ↑)	**Filgrastim** (Neupogen)	*5ug/kg SC qd; start 24h after chemo-Tx through neutrophil recovery (dose modification from publication)*
or	**Granulocyte and macrophage colony stimulating factor** →76 (neutrophil/macrophage production ↑, maturation, activation)	**Sargramostim** (Leukine)	*250μ/m² SC qd; start 24h after chemo-Tx through neutrophil recovery*
poss.	**Xanthine oxidase inhibitor** →138 (uric acid production ↓)	**Allopurinol** (Aloprim, Zyloprim, Gens)	*300-600mg PO/IV qd*
poss.	**Urine hydration + alkalinization** →18 (solubility of uric acid ↑)	**Hydration +/– Sodium bicarbonate**	*150-200ml/h; start 24-48h prior to chemo-Tx*

Note: Subsequent treatments given upon WBC and platelet recovery per protocol.

48.   Thomas DA, et al. Hyper-CVAD program in Burkitt's-type adult acute lymphoblastic leukaemia. J Clin Oncol 1999;17(8):2461-70.

3 B.13 Hodgkin Disease
3 B.13.1 ABVD

Repeat cycle every 28 days

	Anthracycline (DNA intercalation, topoisomerase II inhibition)	**Doxorubicin** (Adriamycin PFS, Adriamycin RDF, Rubex, Gens)	*25mg/m² IV d1 and d15*
plus	**Antitumor antibiotic**	**Bleomycin** (Blenoxane)	*10 U/m² IV d1 and d15 (1 U test dose prior to 1ˢᵗ dose)*
plus	**Antimitotic** (mitotic spindle poison)	**Vinblastine** (Velban)	*6mg/m² IV d1 and d15*
plus	**Pseudo–alkylating agent**	**Dacarbazine** (DTIC-Dome)	*375mg/m² IV d1 and d15*

49. Canellos GP, et al. Chemotherapy of advanced Hodgkin's disease with MOPP, ABVD, or MOPP alternating with ABVD. N Engl J Med 1992;327:1478-84.
50. Duggan D, et al. MOPP/ABV versus ABVD for advanced Hodgkin's disease – a preliminary report of CALGB 8952 (with SWOG, ECOG, NCIC). Proc Amer Soc Clin Oncol 1997;16:12a.

3 B.14 Multiple Myeloma
3 B.14.1 General Therapy

Repeat after 14d rest

	Glucocorticoid →148 (anti-inflammatory, immunosuppressive)	**Dexamethasone** (Decadron, Dexameth, Dexone, Hexadrol, Gens)	*20mg/m² PO qd d1-4, 9-12, and 17-20*

Or VAD, repeat cycle every 28 days

	Antimitotic (Mitotic spindle poison)	**Vincristine** (Oncovin, Vincasar PFS, Gens)	*0.4mg/d continuous IV Inf d1-4*
plus	**Anthracycline** (DNA intercalation, topoisomerase II inhibition)	**Doxorubicin** (Adriamycin PFS, Adriamycin RDF, Rubex, Gens)	*9mg/m²/d continuous IV Inf d1-4*
plus	**Glucocorticoid** →148 (anti-inflammatory, immunosuppressive)	**Dexamethasone** (Decadron, Dexameth, Dexone, Hexadrol, Gens)	*40mg PO qd d1-4, 9-12, and 17-20*

Or MP, repeat cycle every 28 days

	Alkylating agent	**Melphalan** (Alkeran)	*8-10mg/m² PO qd d1-4*
plus	**Glucocorticoid** →148 (anti-inflammatory, immunosuppressive)	**Prednisone** (Deltasone, Orasone, Liquid Pred, Sterapred DS, Panasol-S, Meticorten, Prednicen-M, Gens)	*60mg/m² PO qd d1-4*

Or Thalidomide +/- Dexamethasone

	Immunomodulator	**Thalidomide** (Thalomid)	*200-800mg/d PO*
+/-	**Glucocorticoid** →148 (anti-inflammatory, immunosuppressive)	**Dexamethasone** (Decadron, Dexameth, Dexone, Hexadrol, Gens)	*Variable dosing strategies, e.g. 20mg/m² PO qd d1-5, d15-18 (rep qmo)*

poss.	**Bisphosphonate** →143 (osteoclast inhibition)	**Pamidronate** (Aredia)	*90mg IV qmo (long term)*
or poss.	**Biphosphonate** →143 (osteoclast inhibition)	**Zolendronate** (Zometa)	*4mg IV qmo (long term)*
poss.	**Erythrocyte colony stimulating factor** →76 (RBC production↑, maturation, activation)	**Erythropoietin** (Procrit, Epogen)	*150 U/kg SC tiw or 40000 U SC qwk; DARF: lower doses*

51. Alexanian R, Dimopoulos M, Delasalle K, et al. Primary dexamethasone treatment of multiple myeloma. Blood 1992;80(4):887-90.
52. Alexanian R, Barlogie B, Tucker S, et al. VAD-based regimens as primary treatment for multiple myeloma. Am J Hematol 1990;33:86-9.
53. Tricot G, Multiple myeloma and other plasma cell disorders in: Hematology Basic Principles and Practice, 3rd ed., Churchill Livingstone, New York, 2000, 1398-1416.
54. Singhal S, Mehta J, Desikan R, et al. Antitumor activity of thalidomide in refractory multiple myeloma. N Engl J Med 1999;341:1565-71.
55. Weber DM, Rankin K, Gavino M, et al. Thalidomide with dexamethasone for resistant multiple myeloma. Blood 2000;96(11):167a (abstract #719).
56. Berenson JR, Lichtenstein A, Porter L, et al. Efficacy of pamidronate in reducing skeletal events in patients with advanced multiple myeloma. N Engl J Med 1996;334:488-93.

4 A. Respiratory – Drugs

4 A.1 Bronchodilators
4 A.1.1 Systemic Beta Adrenergic Agonists

MA/EF: stimulation of β_2-receptors $\Rightarrow$ bronchial muscles relax, mucociliar clearance ↑
AE: tachyarrhythmias, extrasystoles, angina pectoris, tremors
CI: hyperthyroidism, pheochromocytoma, hypertrophic obstructive cardiomyopathy, glaucoma, severe coronary heart disease, tachycardic arrhythmias

Albuterol (Salbutamol)	EHL 4h, PRC C, Lact ?
Proventil *Tab 2mg, 4mg, Tab ext.rel. 4mg, Syr 2mg/5ml* **Ventolin** *Tab 2mg, 4mg* **Volmax** *Tab ext.rel. 4mg, 8mg* **Generics** *Tab 2mg, 4mg, Syr 2mg/5ml*	**Asthma** →101: 2-4mg PO tid-qid, max 8mg PO qid; ext.rel.: 4-8mg PO q12h, max 32mg/d; **CH asthma** 2-6 y: 0.1-0.2mg/kg PO tid, max 12mg/d; 6-14 y: 2mg PO tid-qid, max 24mg/d

Metaproterenol	EHL no data, PRC C, Lact -
Alupent *Tab 10mg, 20mg, Syr 10mg/5ml* **Generics** *Tab 10mg, 20mg, Syr 10mg/5ml*	**Asthma** →101: 20mg PO tid-qid

Terbutaline	EHL 11-26h, PRC B, Lact +
Brethine *Tab 2.5mg, 5mg, Inj 1mg/ml*	**Asthma** →102: 2.5-5mg PO q6h, max 15mg/d; 0.25mg SC, max 0.5mg/4h, **CH** 12-15 y: 2.5mg PO q6h, max 7.5mg/d

4 A.1.2 Inhaled Beta Adrenergic Agonists

MA/EF: see Systemic Beta Adrenergic Agonists →95; **AE:** nervousness/tremors, tachycardia, coughing, nausea, headache; **CI:** hypersensitivity to the drug. **Note:** formoterol, salmeterol: long-acting β_2-sympathomimetic, not for Tx of acute asthmatic reaction

Albuterol	EHL 4h, PRC C, Lact ?
Proventil-HFA *MDI 0.09mg/puff* **Proventil** *Sol (inhal) 0.083%, 0.5%, MDI 0.09mg/puff* **Ventolin-HFA** *MDI 0.09mg/puff* **Ventolin** *Sol (inhal) 0.083%, 0.5%, MDI 0.09mg/puff* **Ventolin rotacaps** *Cap (inhal) 0.2mg* **Generics** *Sol (inhal) 0.083%, 0.5%, MDI 0.09mg/puff*	**Asthma** →101: MDI: 1-2 puffs q4-6h, max 12 puffs/d; Sol (inhal): 2.5mg diluted in 3ml NS tid-qid; Cap inhal.: 200-400µg q4-6h via Rotahaler; **PRO of exercise-induced asthma** →103: 180µg (2 inhal) by MDI 15min prior to exercise; **CH asthma** MDI >4 y: 1-2 puffs q4-6h; Sol (inhal): 0.1mg/kg diluted in 3ml NS, max 2.5mg tid-qid; Cap inhal.: > 4 y: 200-400µg q4-6h via Rotahaler

Bitolterol	EHL no data, PRC C, Lact ?
Tornalate *Sol (inhal) 0.2%, MDI 0.37mg/puff*	**Bronchospasm:** MDI: 2 puffs at an interval $\geq$ 1-3min, third puff prn; **prevention of bronchospasm:** 2 puffs q8h; Sol (inhal): 0.5-1.5mg tid via intermittent flow, max 8mg/d, 1.5-3.5mg tid via continuous flow, max 14mg/d; **CH** > 12 y: see adults

Formoterol — EHL 10h, PRC C, Lact ?

Foradil *Cap (inhal) 12µg*
Asthma →105, **COPD** →104: 1 inhal (12µg) bid, max 24µg/d; **CH** >5 y: see adults; **PRO of exercise-induced asthma:** 1 inhal (12µg) 15min prior to exercise

Isoetharine — EHL no data, PRC C, Lact ?

Beta-2 *Sol (inhal) 1%*
Generics *Sol (inhal) 0.08%, 0.143%, 0.167%, 0.2%, 1%*
Asthma (Sol for inhal via hand nebulizer) →101: 3-7 inhalations q4h

Levalbuterol — EHL 3.3 h, PRC C, Lact ?

Xopenex *Sol (inhal) 0.021%, 0.042%*
Asthma →103: 0.63-1.25mg nebulized q6-8h; **CH** >12 y: see adults

Metaproterenol — EHL no data, PRC C, Lact -

Alupent *Sol (inhal) 0.4%, 0.6%, 5%, MDI 0.65mg/puff*
Generics *Sol (inhal) 0.4%; 0.6%*
Asthma →101: Sol (inhal) (5%): 0.2-0.3ml diluted in 2.5ml NS, max q4h

Pirbuterol — EHL 2-3h, PRC C, Lact ?

Maxair *MDI 0.2mg/puff*
Asthma →101: 1-2 puffs q4-6h, max 12 puffs/d

Salmeterol — EHL 5.5h, PRC C, Lact ?

Serevent *MDI 0.021mg/puff*
Serevent Diskus *Powder (inhal) 0.046mg/inhal.*
Asthma →101, **COPD** →104: MDI: 2 puffs q12h; **PRO of exercise-induced asthma:** MDI: 2 puffs 30-60min before exercise; **CH** > 4 y: diskus 1 inhal. q12h, > 12 y: MDI: 2 puffs q12h

4 A.1.3   α-β-Adrenergic Agonists

MA/EF (→22): stimulation of alpha- and beta-adrenergic receptors ⇒ bronchodilation; vasoconstriction, cardiac output ↑ ⇒ BP ↑
AE (ephedrine): CNS stimulation, HTN, palpitations, tremor, N/V
AE (epinephrine →22): HTN, N/V, headache, arrhythmias
CI: (ephedrine): hypersensitivity to ephedrine, angle closure glaucoma, anesthesia with cyclopropane or halothane, thyrotoxicosis, DM, HTN (in pregnancy), other CVS DO
CI (epinephrine →22): cardiac dilatation/coronary insufficiency, narrow angle glaucoma, hypersensitivity to epinephrine, shock, intra-arterial injection, labor

Ephedrine — EHL 3-6h, PRC C, Lact ?

Generics *Cap 25mg, Spray 0.25%, Inj 50mg/ml*
Asthma →103: 25-50mg q3-4h or 25-50mg SC or 5-25mg/dose slow IV, max 150mg/d

Epinephrine — PRC C, Lact ?

Epipen Jr. *Inj (IM) 0.15mg/delivery*
Epi E Z Pen Jr. *Inj (IM) 0.15mg/delivery*
Epipen E Z Pen *Inj (IM) 0.3mg/delivery*
Epipen *Inj (IM) 0.3mg/delivery*
Sus-phrine Sulfite-free *Inj 1.5mg/amp, 5mg/ml*
Asthma →103: 0.2-0.5ml of 1:1000 Sol (0.2-0.5mg) SC q2h prn, rep q20min for a max of 3 doses. MDI: inhalation of 0.1% to 1% Sol prn

4 A.1.4   Inhaled Anticholinergics

MA/EF: anticholinergic $\Rightarrow$ bronchodilating
AE: dry mouth, bitter taste, epistaxis, nasal dryness/congestion
CI: hypersensitivity to the drug

Ipratropium	EHL no data, PRC B, Lact ?
Atrovent *MDI 0.018mg/puff, Sol (inhal) 0.02%,* **Generics** *Sol (inhal) 0.02%*	**COPD** →104, **bronchospasms:** MDI: 2 puffs qid, max 12 puffs/d; Sol (inhal): 500µg nebulized qid

4 A.1.5   Xanthines

MA: inhibition of intracellular phosphodiesterase $\Rightarrow$ cAMP ↑
EF: bronchial spasmolysis, central stimulation of respiration, positive inotropic and chronotropic, vasodilation (except for brain vessels), diuresis ↑
AE: N/V, tremors, tachycardia, convulsions
CI: restricted use in acute myocardial infarction, hyperthyroidism, convulsions

Aminophylline	EHL no data, PRC C, Lact ?
Generics *Tab 100mg, 200mg, Sol (oral) 105mg/5ml, Inj 25mg/ml, 100mg/100ml, 200mg/100ml*	**Bronchospasm, asthma** →103: ini 6mg/kg IV, maint 0.5-0.7mg/kg/h IV inf; 16mg/kg/d PO div q6-8h

Theophylline	PRC C, Lact +, serum level: 10-20 µg/ml
Aerolate III, jr, sr *Cap ext.rel. 65mg, 130mg, 260mg* **Elixophyllin** *Elixir 80mg/15ml* **Slo-bid** *Cap ext.rel. 50mg, 75mg, 100mg, 125mg, 200mg, 300mg* **Slo-Phyllin** *Tab 100mg, 200mg, Syr 80mg/15ml* **Theo-24** *Cap ext.rel. 100mg, 200mg, 300mg, 400mg* **Theo-Dur** *Tab ext.rel. 100mg, 200mg, 300mg, 450mg* **Uni-Dur** *Tab ext.rel. 400mg, 600mg* **Uniphyl** *Tab ext.rel. 400mg, 600mg* **Generics** *Cap ext.rel. 100mg, 125mg, 200mg, 300mg, Elixir (oral) 80mg/15ml, Inj 4mg/ml, 40mg/100ml, 80mg/100ml, 160mg/100ml, 200mg/100ml, 320mg/100ml, 400mg/100ml*	**Asthma** →102: 10-16mg/kg/d PO in div doses; adjust dose based on serum level; DARF not req

4 A.2   Inhaled Corticosteroids

EF: suppression of inflammatory reactions $\Rightarrow$ β_2-receptor sensitivity ↓
AE: hoarseness, oral and pharyngeal candidosis
CI: lung tuberculosis, fungal or bacterial respiratory tract infections

Beclomethasone	EHL 3h, PRC C, Lact ?
Beclovent *MDI 0.042mg/puff* **QVar 40, 80** *MDI 0.04mg/puff, 0.08mg/puff* **Vanceril** *MDI 0.042mg/puff* **Vanceril DS** *MDI 0.084mg/puff*	**Asthma** →101: 0.084mg tid-qid or 0.168mg bid; **CH** 6-12 y: 0.042-0.084mg tid-qid, >12 y: see adults

Budesonide	EHL 2-3h, PRC C, Lact ?
Pulmicort Turbuhaler *Powder (inhal) 200µg/inhal*	**Asthma** →101: 1-2 puffs bid, max 4 puffs bid; **CH** >6 y: 1 puff (max 2 puffs) bid
Flunisolide	EHL 1-2h, PRC.: C , Lact ?
AeroBid *MDI 0.25mg/puff*	**Asthma** →101: 2 puffs bid, max 4 puffs bid; **CH** 6-15 y: 2 puffs bid
Fluticasone	EHL 7.8h, PRC C, Lact ?
Flovent *MDI 44, 110, 220µg/puff, Powder (inhal) 50, 100, 250µg/inhal*	**Asthma maint** →101: MDI: 88-220µg bid; Diskus: 100-500µg bid, max 1000µg bid; **CH** 4-11 y: Diskus: 50µg bid, max 100µg bid
Triamcinolone Acetonide	EHL no data, PRC C, Lact ?
Azmacort *MDI 0.1mg/puff*	**Asthma** →101: 2 puffs tid-qid or 4 puffs bid, max 16 puffs/d; **CH** 6-12 y: 1-2 puffs tid-qid or 2-4 puffs bid; max 12 puffs/d

4 A.3   Asthma/COPD Combinations

Fluticasone + Salmeterol	
Advair Diskus *Powder (inhal) 0.1+0.05mg/inhal., 0.25+0.05mg/inhal., 0.5+0.05mg/inhal.*	**Asthma** →101: maint inhalation of 0.1-0.5 + 0.05mg q12h
Ipratropium + Albuterol	EHL no data, PRC C, Lact ?
Combivent *MDI 0.018 + 0.09mg/puff* **Duoneb** *Sol (inhal) 0.017% + 0.083%*	**COPD** →104, **bronchospasms:** MDI: 2 puffs qid, max 12 puffs/d; Sol (inhal): 3ml nebulized qd-tid

4 A.4   Leukotriene Inhibitors

MA: blockage of leukotriene receptors
EF: bronchial dilatation, decrease of bronchial hyperreactivity
AE: headache, fever, diarrhea, nausea, sinusitis

Montelukast	EHL 2.7-5h, PRC B, Lact -
Singulair *Tab 10mg, Tab (chew) 4mg, 5mg*	**Asthma** →101: 10mg PO qd; **CH** 2-5 y: 4mg PO qd; 6-14 y: 5mg PO qd
Zafirlukast	EHL 10h, PRC B, Lact -
Accolate *Tab 10mg, 20mg*	**Asthma** →101: 20mg PO bid (1h ac or 2h pc) **CH** 7-11 y: 10mg PO bid (1h ac or 2h pc), >12 y: see adults
Zileuton	EHL 2-2.5h, PRC C, Lact -
Zyflo *Tab 300mg, 600mg*	**Asthma** →101: maint 600mg PO qid

4 A.5 Mucolytics, Expectorants

MA/EF (acetyl cysteine): splits disulfide bridges in protein part of mucus molecules ⇒ sputum viscosity ↓
AE (acetyl cysteine): allergic skin reactions, nausea, heartburn
AE (guaifenesin): dizziness, headache, N/V, rash, urticaria
CI (acetyl cysteine): restricted use in children < 1
CI (guaifenesin): hypersensitivity to guaifenesin products

Acetylcysteine	EHL 11min-2.27h, PRC B, Lact ?
Mucomyst *Sol (inhal) 10%, 20%* **Mucosil** *Sol (inhal) 10%, 20%* **Generics** *Sol (inhal) 10%, 20%*	**Mucolytic** →114: nebulization of 1-10ml (20%) or 2-20ml (10%) q2-6h prn; intratracheal instillation: 1-2ml ET (10-20%) prn up to qh

Guaifenesin	EHL 1h, PRC C, Lact ?
Humibid *Tab 600mg, Cap 300mg* *Cap ext.rel (pediatric) 300mg* **Robitussin** *Syr 100mg/5ml* **Generics** *Tab 200mg, Tab ext.rel 600mg, 1200mg,* *Sol (oral) 100mg/5ml* *Liquid (oral) 100mg/5ml*	**Expectorant:** 100-400mg PO q4h or 600-1200mg PO q12h (ext.rel), max 2.4g/d; →419 **CH** >12y: adult dose, 6-11y: 100-200mg PO q4h or 600mg PO q12h (ext.rel), max 1.2g/d, 2-5y: 50-100mg PO q4h or 300mg PO q12h (ext.rel), max 600mg/d

4 A.6 Mast Cell Stabilizers

MA/EF: stabilization of mast cell membranes ⇒ mediator release ↓
AE: bad taste, nausea, ocular burning, nasal congestion, cough
CI: hypersensitivity to the drug

Cromolyn Sodium	EHL 80-90min, PRC B, Lact ?
Intal *MDI 0.8mg/puff, Sol (inhal) 10mg/ml* **Generics** *Sol (inhal) 10mg/ml*	**Asthma** →101: MDI. 2-4 puffs qid; Sol (inhal): 20mg nebulized qid

Nedocromil	EHL 1.5-3.3h, PRC B, Lact ?
Tilade *MDI 1.75mg/puff*	**Asthma** →101: 2 puffs qid, reduce dose after improvement; **CH** > 6 y: 2 puffs qid, reduce dose after improvement

4 A.7 Antitussives
4 A.7.1 Antitussives – Single Ingredient Drugs

MA/EF (benzonatate): local anesthetic effect ⇒ blocking cough reflex
MA/EF (dextromethorphan): acts on cough center in medulla oblongata ⇒ threshold for coughing ↑
AE (benzonatate): drowsiness, sedation, dizziness, nausea, headache, numbness of mouth/throat
AE (dextromethorphan): restlessness, hallucination, GI symptoms and skin reactions
CI (benzonatate): hypersensitivity to benzonatate
CI (dextromethorphan): advanced respiratory insufficiency, advanced hepatic disease

Benzonatate	EHL no data, PRC C, Lact ?
Tessalon *Cap 100mg*	**Cough:** 100mg tid, q4h prn, max 600mg/d

Dextromethorphan

EHL 1.5-4h, PRC C, Lact +

Benylin *Sol (oral) 7.5mg/5ml, 15mg/5ml*
Delsym *Susp (ext.rel) 30mg/5ml*
Diabe–Tuss DM *Sol (oral) 15mg/5ml*
Hold *Lozenge 5mg*
Pertussin *Sol (oral) 3.5mg/5ml, 15mg/5ml*
Sucrets *Lozenge 15mg*
Vicks *Sol (oral) 10mg/5ml*

Cough: 10-20mg q4h or 30mg q6-8h, max 120mg/d; →419

4 A.7.2   Antitussives – Combinations

Guaifenesin + Codeine

PRC C, Lact ?

Robitussin AC *Syr 100mg/5ml + 10mg/5ml*

Cough: 10ml PO q4h, max 60ml/d; →419
CH >12y: adult dose, 6-11y: 5ml PO q4h, max 30ml/d

Guaifenesin + Dextromethorphan

PRC C, Lact ?

Benylin *Sol (oral) 100mg/5ml + 15mg/5ml, Liquid (oral) 100mg/5ml + 5mg/5ml*
Humibid DM *Tab 600mg + 30mg, Cap 300mg + 15mg*
Robitussin DM *Sol (oral) 100mg/5ml + 15mg/5ml, Syr 100mg/5ml + 10mg/5ml*

Cough: 10ml PO q4h, max 60ml/d or 1-2 Tab PO q12h, max 4 Tab/d; →419
CH >12y: adult dose, 6-11y: 5ml PO q4h, max 30ml/d or 1 Tab PO q12h, max 2 Tab/d,
2- 5y: 2.5ml PO q4h, max 15ml/d or ½ Tab PO q12h, max 1 Tab/d

Homatropine + Hydrocodone

PRC C, Lact -

Hycodan *Tab 1.5mg + 5mg, Syr 1.5mg/5ml + 5mg/5ml*
Hydrocodone compound *Syr 1.5mg/5ml + 5mg/5ml*
Mycodone *Syr 1.5mg/5ml + 5mg/5ml*
Tussigon *Tab 1.5mg + 5mg*
Generics *Tab 1.5mg + 5mg, Syr 1.5mg/5ml + 5mg/5ml*

Antitussive: 1 Tab or 5ml PO q4-6h, max 6 doses/d;
CH >12y: use adult dose,
6-12y: 2.5mg (based on hydrocodone) PO q4-6h prn, max 15mg/d

4 A.8   Other Respiratory Drugs

MA/EF: cholinergic (parasympathomimetic) analogue of acetylcholine ⇒ stimulation of muscarinic, parasympathetic receptors ⇒ smooth-muscle contraction of airways, tracheobronchial secretions ↑
AE: cough, dyspnea, throat irritation, headache, lightheadedness
CI: hypersensitivity to methacholine, clinically apparent asthma/wheezing

Methacholine

EHL no data, PRC C, Lact -

Provocholine *Sol (inhal) 100mg/vial*

Diagnosis of bronchial airway hyperreactivity: inhalation of incr serial conc (0.025mg/ml-25mg/ml)

4 B. Respiratory – Therapies

Charles L. Daley, MD
Associate Professor of Medicine
Division of Pulmonary and Critical Care Medicine, SF General Hospital
University of California San Francisco, San Francisco, CA

4 B.1   Asthma
4 B.1.1   Long–Term Therapy and Quick Relief Therapy

Step 1 (mild intermittent)

Beta$_2$–agonist, short acting →95 (bronchodilating)	**Albuterol** (Proventil, Proventil HFA, Ventolin, 90µg/puff; Ventolin Rotacaps, 200µg/puff)	*2 puffs tid-qid prn*
or	**Metaproterenol** (Alupent, 650µg/puff)	*2 puffs tid-qid prn*
or	**Pirbuterol** (Maxair, Maxair Autoinhaler, 200µg/puff)	*2 puffs tid-qid prn*

Step 2 (mild persistent) – Step 1 plus:

Corticosteroid, inhaled, low doses →97 (anti-inflammatory)	**Beclomethasone** (Beclovent, Vanceril, 42µg/puff; Vanceril DS, 84µg/puff)	*168-504µg/d: 4-12 puffs qd (42µg/puff) or 2-6 puffs qd (84µg/puff)*
or	**Budesonide** (Pulmicort Turbohaler, 200µg/dose)	*200-400µg/d: 1-2 inhs qd*
or	**Flunisolide** (Aerobid, Aerobid M, 250µg/puff)	*500-1000µg/d: 2-4 puffs qd*
or	**Fluticasone** (Flovent MD, 44, 110, 220µg/puff; Flovent Rotadisk, 50, 100, 250µg/dose)	*88-264µg/d: 2-6 puffs qd (44µg/puff) or 2 puffs qd (110µg/puff) or 2-6 inhs qd (50µg/puff)*
or	**Triamcinolone acetonide** (Azmacort, 100µg/puff)	*400-1000µg/d: 4-10 puffs qd*
OR	Mast cell stabilizer →99 (mediator release ↓)	**Cromolyn sodium** (Intal, 1mg/puff)	*2-4 puffs tid -qid*
or		**Nedocromil** (Tilade, 1.75mg/puff)	*2-4 puffs bid-qid*
OR	Leukotriene modifiers →98 (bronchodilating)	**Zafirlukast** (Accolate, 20mg)	*20mg PO bid*
or		**Zileuton** (Zyflo, 600mg)	*600mg PO qid*

Step 3 (moderate persistent) – Step 1 plus

Either	**Corticosteroid, inhaled, medium dose** →97 (anti-inflammatory)	**Beclomethasone** (Beclovent, Vanceril, 42µg/puff; Vanceril DS, 84µg/puff)	*504-840µg/d: 12-20 puffs qd (42µg/puff) or 6-10 puffs qd (84µg/puff)*
or		**Budesonide** (Pulmicort Turbohaler, 200µg/dose)	*400-600µg/d: 2-3 inhs qd*
or		**Flunisolide** (Aerobid, Aerobid M, 250µg/puff)	*1000-2000µg: 4-8 puffs qd*
or		**Fluticasone** (Flovent MD, 220µg/puff; Flovent Rotadisk, 250µg/dose)	*264-660µg/d: 2-6 puffs qd (110µg(puff) or 3-6 inhs qd (100µg/puff)*
or		**Triamcinolone acetonide** (Azmacort, 100µg/puff)	*1000-2000µg/d: 10-20 puffs qd*
or	**Corticosteroid, inhaled, low–medium dose** →97 (anti-inflammatory)	**See above**, →101	
plus	**Beta$_2$-agonist, long-acting inhaled** →95 (bronchodilating)	**Salmeterol** (Serevent MDI, 21µg/puff; Serevent Diskus, 50µg/blister)	*MDI: 2 puffs q12h; Diskus: 1 inh q12h*
or		**Formoterol** (Foradil Aerolizer, 12µg/Cap)	*1 inh q12h*
poss	**Methylxanthines** →97 (bronchodilating, central respiratory stimulation)	**Theophylline–sustained release** (multiple preparations)	*Ini dose 10mg/kg/d up to 300mg div over 24h: max 800mg/d; adj dose to serum level (5-15µg/ml)*
or	**Beta$_2$-agonist, long-acting tablets** →95	**Albuterol – sustained release** (Volmax)	*4-8mg PO q12h*
or		**Terbutaline** (Brethine, Gens)	*2.5-5.0mg PO tid*

Step 4 (severe persistent)

	Corticosteroid, inhaled, high dose →97 (anti-inflammatory)	**Beclomethasone** (Beclovent, Vanceril, 42µg/puff; Vanceril DS, 84µg/puff)	*>840 µg/d: >20 puffs qd (42µg/puff) or >10 puffs qd (84µg/puff)*
or		**Budesonide** (Pulmicort Turbohaler, 200µg/dose)	*>600µg/d: >3 inh qd*
or		**Flunisolide** (Aerobid, Aerobid M, 250µg/puff)	*>2000µg/d: >8 puffs qd*
or		**Fluticasone** (Flovent MD, 44, 110, 220µg/puff; Flovent Rotadisk, 50, 100, 250µg/dose)	*>660µg/d: >6 puffs qd (110µg/puff) or >3 puffs qd (220µg/puff) or >6 inhs qd (100µg/dose) or >2 inhs qd (250µg/dose)*
or		**Triamcinolone acetonide** (Azmacort, 100µg/puff)	*>2000µg/d: >20 puffs qd*

and	**Beta₂-agonist, long-acting inhaled** →95 (bronchodilating)	**Salmeterol** (Serevent MDI, 21µg/puff; Diskus, 50µg/blister)	*2 puffs q12h* *1 inh q12h*
or		**Formoterol** (Foradil Aerolizer, 12µg/Cap)	*1 inh q12h*
poss	**Methylxanthines** →97 (bronchodilating, central respiratory stimulation)	**Theophylline–sustained release** (multiple preparations)	*Ini dose 10mg/kg/d up to 300mg in div doses over 24h: max dose 800mg/d; adj dose to serum level (5-15µg/ml)*
or	**Beta₂-agonist, long-acting tablets** →95	**Albuterol - sustained release** (Volmax)	*4-8mg PO q12h*
		Terbutaline (Brethine, Gens)	*2.5-5.0mg PO tid*
and	**Corticosteroid, oral** →148 (anti-inflammatory)	**Methylprednisolone** (Gens) **Prednisolone** (Gens) **Prednisone** (Gens)	*7.5-60mg qd or qid prn OR short-course "burst": 40-60mg qd or div bid for 3-10d*

4 B.1.2   Prophylaxis of Exercise or Irritant-Induced Asthma

	Beta₂-agonist, short acting →95 (bronchodilating)	**Albuterol** (Proventil, Proventil HFA, Ventolin, 90µg/puff; Ventolin Rotacaps, 200µg/puff)	*2 puffs prior to exercise or allergen exposure*
or		**Metaproterenol** (Alupent, 650µg/puff)	*2 puffs prior to exercise or allergen exposure*
or		**Pirbuterol** (Maxair, Maxair Autoinhaler, 200µg/puff)	*2 puffs prior to exercise or allergen exposure*
OR	**Long-acting inhaled beta₂-agonist** →95	**Salmeterol** (Serevent MDI, 21µg/puff; Serevent Diskus, 50µg/blister)	*2 puffs or 1 inh at least 30min prior to excercise*
or		**Formoterol** (Foradil Aerolizer, 12µg/Cap)	*1 inh at least 15min prior to excercise*
OR	**Mast cell stabilizer** →99 (mediator liberation inhibition)	**Cromolyn sodium** (Intal, 1mg/puff)	*2 puffs qid or one puff prior to exercise or allergen exposure*

4 B.1.3   Asthma Exacerbations in Emergency Medical Care or Hospital

	Beta₂-agonist, short acting →95 (bronchodilating)	**Albuterol** (Proventil, Ventolin, Gens; Nebulizer Sol - 5mg/ml, MDI = 90µg/puff)	*2.5-5mg q20min x 3, then 2.5-10mg q1-4h prn or 10-15mg/h cont; 4-8 puffs q20min up to 1h, then q1-4h prn (use spacer device)*
or		**Pirbuterol** (Maxair, Maxair Autoinhaler, 200µg/puff)	
or		**Levalbuterol** (Xopenex)	*0.63-1.25mg nebulized q6-8h*
poss	**Methylxanthines** →97 (bronchodilating, central respiratory stimulation)	**Aminophylline** (Gens)	*5mg/kg as short-inf over 30 min, then 1mg/kg/h, after 12h 0.8mg/kg/h (serum level = 5-15)*

and	**Corticosteroid** →148 (anti-inflammatory) betarecept. ↑)	**Prednisone** (Gens) **Methylprednisolone** (Gens) **Prednisolone** (Gens)	*120-180mg/d in 3-4 div doses for 48h, then 60-80mg/d until PEF 70% of predicted/personal best*
poss	**Beta$_2$-agonist, systemic** →95 (bronchodilating)	**Terbutaline** (Brethine, 1mg/ml)	*0.25mg SC q20min for 3 doses*
or	**Alpha-beta-adrenergic agonist** →96 (bronchodilating)	**Epinephrine** (1:1000, 1mg/ml)	*0.3-0.5mg SC q20min for 3 doses*
poss	**Anticholinergic** →97 (bronchodilating)	**Ipratropium bromide** (Atrovent; nebulizer Sol - 0.25mg/ml, MDI - 18µg/puff)	*0.5mg q30min for 3 doses, then q2-4h prn* *4-8 puffs prn*
and	**Gas** (blood oxygenation)	**Oxygen**	*Prn to maintain O$_2$ saturation of ≥ 90%*

57.   National Institutes of Health. National Heart, Lung, and Blood Institute. Guidelines for the Diagnosis and Management of Asthma. 1997:1-86.

4 B.2   Chronic Obstructive Pulmonary Disease (COPD)

4 B.2.1   In General

Smoking cessation is critical!

Gas (blood oxygenation)	**Oxygen**	*If pO$_2$ < 55mmHg at rest or < 60mmHg with exercise, sleep, chronic cor pulmonale or secondary polycythemia; Caution when pCO$_2$↑*

4 B.2.2   Long-Term Therapy

Stage 1 (mild COPD – FEV$_1$ > 80% predicted)

	Beta$_2$-agonist, short acting →95 (bronchodilating)	**Albuterol** (Proventil, Proventil HFA, Ventolin, 90µg/puff; Ventolin Rotacaps, 200µg/puff)	*2 puffs tid-qid prn*
or		**Metaproterenol** (Alupent, 650µg/puff)	*2 puffs tid-qid prn*
or		**Pirbuterol** (Maxair, Maxair Autoinhaler, 200µg/puff)	*2 puffs tid-qid prn*
OR	**Anticholinergic** →97 (bronchodilating)	**Ipratropium bromide** (Atrovent; MDI, 18µg/puff)	*2-4 puffs tid-qid*
OR	**Beta$_2$-agonist + Parasympatholytic** (bronchodilating)	**Albuterol + Ipratropium bromide** (Combivent, 103µg+18µg/puff)	*2 puffs qid*

Stage 2 (moderate COPD – 30% < FEV$_1$ < 80% predicted) – Stage 1 plus

	Beta$_2$-agonist, long-acting inhaled →95 (bronchodilating)	**Salmeterol** (Serevent MDI, 21µg/puff; Serevent Diskus, 50µg/blister)	*2 puffs q12h* *1 inh q12h*
or		**Formoterol** (Foradil Aerolizer, 12µg/Cap)	*1 inh q12h*
or	**Methylxanthines** →97 (bronchodilating, central respiratory stimulation)	**Theophylline-sustained release** (multiple preparations)	*Ini dose 10mg/kg/d up to 300mg, max 800mg/d; adj dose to serum level (5-15µg/ml)*
poss	**Corticosteroid, inhaled** →97	If significant symptoms and spirometric response or if repeated excerbations; low to moderate doses, see Asthma →101	
and	**Rehabilitation**	Refer for pulmonary rehabilitation if available	

Stage 3 (severe COPD – FEV$_1$ < 30% predicted) – Stage 2 plus

	Gas (blood oxygenation)	**Oxygen**	*If pO$_2$ < 55mmHg at rest or < 60mmHg with exercise, sleep, chronic cor pulmonale or secondary polycythemia; Caution when pCO$_2$↑*
and	**Rehabilitation**	Refer for pulmonary rehabilitation if available	
and	**Surgery**	Consider for surgical treatments	

4 B.2.3 Acute Exacerbations of Chronic Bronchitis

Possible organisms: usually Pneumococci, H. influenzae, Moraxella.
Begin narrow spectrum antibiotic unless drug resistance is known or suspected to be present. All durations are 5–10 days unless specified otherwise

	Aminopenicillin →189	**Amoxicillin** (Amoxil, Gens)	*250-500mg PO qid*
or	**Folate antagonist + p-Aminobenzoic acid antagonist (Co-trimoxazole)** →206	**Trimethoprim + Sulfamethoxazole** (Bactrim, Bactrim DS, Septra, Gens)	*160mg+800mg PO bid*
or	**Tetracycline** →198	**Doxycycline** (Vibramycin, Gens)	*d1: 200mg PO, then 100mg PO qd*

If no response to above or underlying drug resistance known or suspected consider switching to antibiotic with broader spectrum

	Macrolide – advanced generation →199	**Azithromycin** (Zithromax)	*d1: 500mg PO, d2-5: 250mg/d*
		Clarithromycin (Biaxin, Biaxin XL)	*250-500mg PO bid*
or	**Fluoroquinolone** →204	**Levofloxacin** (Levaquin)	*500mg PO qd*
		Moxifloxacin (Avelox)	*400mg PO qd*
		Gatifloxacin (Tequin)	*400mg PO qd*
or	**Penicillin + beta-lactamase Inhibitor** →191	**Amoxicillin + Clavulanate** (Augmentin)	*875/125mg PO bid or 500/125mg PO tid*

or	Oral Cephalosporin →194	**Cefuroxime-Axetil** (Ceftin, Veftin)	*250-500mg PO bid*
		Cefpodoxime (Vantin)	*200mg PO q12h*

58. Pauwels RA, Buist AS, Calverley PMA, Jenkins CR, Hurd SS, Gold Scientific Committee. Global strategy for the diagnosis, management, and prevention of chronic obstructive pulmonary disease. NHLBI/WHO global initiative for chronic obstructive lung disease (GOLD) Workshop Summary. Am J Respir Crit Care Med 2001;163: 1256-1276.

4 B.3   Pneumonia
4 B.3.1   General Measures

poss	**Gas** (blood oxygenation)	**Oxygen**	*Prn to maintain O_2 saturation of $\geq 90\%$*
poss	**Aniline derivative** →269 (anlagesic, antipyretic)	**Acetaminophen** (Tylenol, Gens)	*500-1000mg PO/PR q6-8h*

The recommended dosages are meant for adults with normal renal and hepatic function. The duration of therapy is 7-14 days unless specified otherwise.

4 B.3.2   Community-acquired Pneumonia (CAP)

CAP – Group I

Outpatient with no history of cardiopulmonary disease + no modifying factors
Possible organisms: Streptococcus pneumoniae, Mycoplasma pneumoniae, Chlamydia pneumoniae, Haemophilus influenzae, miscellaneous

	Macrolide -advanced generation →199	**Azithromycin** (Zithromax)	*500mg PO X 1 then 250mg/d days 2-5*
or		**Clarithromycin** (Biaxin, Biaxin XL)	*500mg PO bid or 1.0g XL qd*

OR if allergic to or intolerant of macrolide

	Tetracycline →199	**Doxycycline** (Vibramycin, Gens)	*100mg PO bid*

CAP – Group II

Outpatient with cardiopulmonary disease and/or other modifying factors
Possible organisms: Streptococcus pneumoniae (including DRSP), Mycoplasma pneumoniae, Chlamydia pneumoniae, mixed infections, Hemophilus influenzae, enteric Gram-negatives, miscellaneous

	Oral Cephalosporin →194	**Cefuroxime-Axetil** (Ceftin, Veftin)	*250-500mg PO q12h*
		Cefpodoxime (Vantin)	*200mg PO q12h*
or	**Penicillin** →187	**high-dose Amoxicillin** (Amoxil)	*1g PO q8h*
or	**Penicillin + beta-lactamase Inhibitor** →191	**Amoxicillin + Clavulanate** (Augmentin)	*875/125mg PO bid or 500/125mg PO tid*

or	Macrolide – advanced generation →199	Azithromycin (Zithromax)	*500mg PO X 1 then 250mg/d days 2-5*
		Clarithromycin (Biaxin, Biaxin XL)	*500mg PO bid or 1.0g XL PO qd*
or	Tetracycline →198	Doxycycline (Vibramycin, Gens)	*100mg PO bid*
OR	Antipneumococcal fluoroquinolone (used alone) →204	Levofloxacin (Levaquin)	*500mg PO/IV qd*
		Moxifloxacin (Avelox)	*400mg PO/IV qd*
		Gatifloxacin (Tequin)	*400mg PO/IV qd*

CAP – Group IIIa

Inpatients, not in ICU, cardiopulmonary disease and/or modifying factors including being from a nursing home
Possible organisms: Streptococcus pneumoniae, Haemophilus influenzae, Mycoplasma pneumoniae, Chlamydia pneumoniae, mixed infections, enteric Gram-negatives, aspiration, Legionella spp., miscellaneous

	Cephalosporin →195	Cefotaxime (Claforan)	*1-2.0g IV q4-8h*
		Ceftriaxone (Rocephin)	*1-2.0g IV qd*
or	Penicillin + beta-lactamase inhibitor →191	Ampicillin + Sulbactam (Unasyn)	*1+0.5g - 2+1g IV q6h*
or	Penicillin →187	high-dose Ampicillin (Amoxil)	*500mg IV q6h*
Plus	Macrolide →199	Azithromycin (Zithromax)	*500mg PO/IV qd on d1, then 250mg qd on d2-5*
		Clarithromycin (Biaxin, Biaxin XL)	*500mg PO/IV bid or 1.0g XL PO qd*
or	Tetracycline →198	Doxycycline (Vibramycin, Gens)	*100mg PO/IV bid*
OR	Antipneumococcal fluoroquinolone →204 (used alone)	Levofloxacin (Levaquin)	*500mg PO/IV qd*
		Moxifloxacin (Avelox)	*400mg PO/IV qd*
		Gatifloxacin (Tequin)	*400mg PO/IV qd*

CAP – Group IIIb

Inpatients, not in ICU, no cardiopulmonary disease and no modifying factors
Possible organisms: Streptococcus pneumoniae, Haemophilus influenzae, Mycoplasma pneumoniae, mixed infections, Legionella spp., miscellaneous

	Macrolide →199	Azithromycin (Zithromax)	*500mg IV qd*
or if macrolide intolerant or allergic			
	Tetracycline →198	Doxycycline (Vibramycin, Gens)	*100mg PO/IV bid*
Plus	Cephalosporin →195	Cefotaxime (Claforan)	*1-2.0g IV q4-8h*
		Ceftriaxone (Rocephin)	*1-2.0g IV qd*
or	Penicillin + beta-lactamase inhibitor →191	Ampicillin + Sulbactam (Unasyn)	*1+0.5g - 2+1g IV q6h*
or	Penicillin →189	high-dose Ampicillin (Amoxil)	*500mg IV q6h*
OR	Antipneumococcal fluoroquinolone (used alone) →204	Levofloxacin (Levaquin)	*500mg PO/IV qd*
		Moxifloxacin (Avelox)	*400mg PO/IV qd*
		Gatifloxacin (Tequin)	*400mg PO/IV qd*

CAP – Group VIa

Inpatient in ICU, no risk for Pseudomonas aeruginosa
Possible organisms: Streptococcus pneumoniae, Legionella spp., Hemophilus influenzae, enteric gram negatives, Staphylococcus aureus, Mycoplasma pneumoniae, miscellaneous

	Cephalosporin →195	Cefotaxime (Claforan)	1-2.0g IV q4-8h
		Ceftriaxone (Rocephin)	1-2.0g IV qd
Plus either	Macrolide →199	Azithromycin (Zithromax)	500mg IV qd
or	Fluoroquinolone →204	Levofloxacin (Levaquin)	500-750mg IV qd
		Moxifloxacin (Avelox)	400mg IV qd
		Gatifloxacin (Tequin)	400mg IV qd

CAP – Group IVb

Inpatient in ICU, risks for Pseudomonas aeruginosa

	Cephalosporin – antipseudomonal →197	Cefepime (Maxipime)	1-2.0g IV q12h
or	Carbapenem →197	Imipenem (Primaxin)	500mg IV q6h
		Meropenem (Merrem)	500-1000mg IV q8h
or	Penicillin + beta-lactamase inhibitor →191	Piperacillin + Tazobactam (Zosyn)	3 + 0.375g IV q6h
Plus	Quinolone - antispeudomonal →203	Ciprofloxacin (Cipro)	200-400mg IV q12h
OR	Cephalosporin – antipseudomonal →197	Cefepime (Maxipime)	1-2.0g IV q12h
or	Carbapenem →197	Imipenem (Primaxin)	500mg IV q6h
		Meropenem (Merrem)	500-1000mg IV q8h
or	Penicillin + beta-lactamase inhibitor →191	Piperacillin + Tazobactam (Zosyn)	3 + 0.375g IV q6h
Plus	Aminoglycoside →200	Tobramycin (Nebcin, Gens	2mg/kg/d IV load, then 1.7mg/kg q8h; Caution: DARF, also check peak and trough serum levels to adj dosages
		Gentamycin (Garamycin, Gens)	
Plus either	Macrolide →199	Azithromycin (Zithromax)	500mg IV qd
or	Fluoroquinolone →204	Levofloxacin (Levaquin)	500-750mg IV qd
		Moxifloxacin (Avelox)	400mg IV qd
		Gatifloxacin (Tequin)	400mg IV qd

59. American Thoracic Society. Guidelines for the management of adults with community-acquired pneumonia. Diagnosis, assessment of severity, antimicrobial therapy, and prevention. Am J Respir Crit Care Med 2001;163:1730-1754.

4 B.3.3   Hospital-acquired Pneumonia (HAP)

Mild-to-moderate HAP without risk factors, onset any time or patients with severe pneumonia with early onset
Possible organisms: enteric gram-negatives, Enterobacter species, Escherichia coli, Klebsiella pneumoniae, Proteus spp., Serratia marcescens, Haemophilus influenzae, methicillin-sensitive Staphylococcus aureus, Streptococcus pneumoniae

	Cephalosporin – 2nd gen. →193	**Cefamandole** (Mandol)	*1-2g IV q4-6h*
		Cefotetan (Cefotan)	*1-3g IV q12h*
		Cefoxitin (Mefoxin)	*1-2g IV q4-8h*
		Cefuroxime (Kefurox, Zinacef)	*750mg-1000mg IV q8h*
or	**Cephalosporin – nonpseudomonal 3rd gen.** →195	**Cefotaxime** (Claforan)	*1-2g IV q4-8h*
		Ceftriaxone (Rocephin)	*1-2g IV q12h*
		Ceftizoxime (Cefizox)	*1.0g IV q8-12h to 4.0g IV q8h*
or	**Penicillin + beta-lactamase inhibitor** →191	**Piperacillin + Tazobactam** (Zosyn)	*3+0.375g IV q6h*
		Ampicillin + Sulbactam (Unasyn)	*1+0.5g - 2+1g IV q6h*
		Ticarcillin + Clavulanate (Timentin)	*3+0.1g IV q4-6h*

OR if allergic to penicillin

	Nonpseudomonal fluoroquinolone →204	**Levofloxacin** (Levaquin)	*500-750mg IV qd*
		Moxifloxacin (Avelox)	*400mg IV qd*
		Gatifloxacin (Tequin)	*400mg IV qd*
or	**Lincosamide** →201	**Clindamycin** (Cleocin)	*600-900mg IV q8h*
plus	**Monobactam** →197	**Aztreonam** (Azactam)	*1.0g IV q8h to 2.0g IV q6h*

Mild to moderately severe HAP with risk factors, onset any time
Possible organisms: as above plus anaerobes (recent abdominal surgery, witnessed aspiration)

Previous antibiotics plus

	Lincosamide →201	**Clindamycin** (Cleocin)	*600-900mg IV q8h*
or	**Penicillin + beta-lactamase inhibitor** →191	**Piperacillin + Tazobactam** (Zosyn)	*3+0.375g IV q6h*
		Ampicillin + Sulbactam (Unasyn)	*1+0.5g - 2+1g IV q6h*
		Ticarcillin + Clavulanate (Timentin)	*3+0.1g IV q4-6h*

poss Staphylococcus aureus (coma, head trauma, diabetes mellitus, renal failure)

	Glycopeptide →198	**Vancomycin** (Vancocin, Vancoled, Gens)	*15mg/kg IV q12h until methicillin-resist. Staph. aureus is ruled out; Caution: DARF, also check peak and trough serum levels to adj dose*

poss Legionella spp (high-dose steroids)

	Macrolide →199	**Erythromycin** (Ilosone)	*500mg IV q6h*
		Azithromycin (Zithromax)	*500mg IV qd*
poss	**Antibiotic** →208	**Rifampin** (Rifadin, Rimactane)	*600mg PO/IV qd*

poss Pseudomonas aeruginosa (prolonged ICU stay, steroids, antibiotics, structural lung disease). Treat as severe HAP (see below)

Severe HAP with risk factors, early onset or patients with severe HAP, late onset
Possible organisms: as above plus P. aeruginosa, Acinetobacter spp., consider MRSA

	Aminoglycoside →200	**Tobramycin** (Nebcin, Gens)	*2mg/kg/d IV load, then*
		Gentamycin (Garamycin, Gens)	*1.7mg/kg q8h; Caution: DARF, also check peak and trough serum levels to adj dosages*
or	**Quinolone – antispeudomonal** →203	**Ciprofloxacin** (Cipro)	*200-400mg IV q12h*
Plus	**Penicillin – antipseudomonal** →190	**Mezlocillin** (Mezlin)	*3.0g IV q4h*
		Piperacillin (Pipracil)	*3.0-4.0g IV q4-6h*
		Ticarcillin (Ticar)	*3.0g IV q4-6h*
or	**Penicillin + beta-lactamase inhibitor** →191	**Piperacillin + Tazobactam** (Zosyn)	*3+0.375g IV q6h*
		Ticarcillin + Clavulanate (Timentin)	*3+0.1g IV q4-6h*
or	**Cephalosporin – antipseudomonal** →195	**Ceftazidime** (Fortaz)	*1.0-2.0g IV q8-12h*
		Cefoperazone (Cefobid)	*2.0g IV q12h to 4.0g IV q6h*
or	**Carbapenem** →197	**Imipenem** (Primaxin)	*500mg qIV 6h*
		Meropenem (Merrem)	*1000mg IV q8h*
or	**Monobactam** →197	**Aztreonam** (Azactam)	*1.0g IV q8h to 2.0g IV q6h*
poss	**Glycopeptide** →198	**Vancomycin** (Vancocin, Vancoled, Gens)	*15mg/kg q12h; Caution: DARF, also check peak and trough serum levels to adj doses*

60.   American Thoracic Society. Hospital-acquired pneumonia in adults: diagnosis, assessment of severity, initial antimicrobial therapy, and preventive strategies. Am J Respir Crit Care Med 1995:153:1711-1725.

4 B.4   Pleural Disease
4 B.4.1   Pleurisy

	Aniline derivative →269 (analgesic, antipyretic)	**Acetaminophen** (Tylenol, Gens)	*500-1000mg PO/PR qid*
or	**NSAID** →265 (analgesic, antipyretic)	**Ibuprofen** (Advil, Motrin, Gens)	*400-800mg PO tid-qid*
poss	**Opioid** →270 (antitussive, analgesic)	**Codeine** (Gens)	*30-50mg PO bid, max. 150mg/d prn*

4 B.4.2   Pleural Infections

Empiric Treatment: In general, treat as for pneumonia and alter Tx if a specific pathogen is isolated. Include antibiotics with anaerobic coverage in the Tx regimen unless a specific pathogen is identified. Complicated parapneumonic effusions and empyemas require chest tube drainage and prolonged antibioticTx(e.g.,1+ mo).

	Cephalosporin – 3rd gen. →195	Cefotaxime (Claforan)	*1-2g IV q8h*
		Ceftriaxone (Rocephin)	*1-2g IV q4-8h*
and	Lincosamide →201	Clindamycin (Cleocin)	*900mg IV q8h*

4 B.4.3   Specific Pathogens

Streptococcus pneumoniae

| 1st choice | Benzylpenicillin →187 | Penicillin G (Gens) | *1-2 M U IV q4-6h* |

If penicillin allergic

| | Macrolide →199 | Azithromycin (Zithromax) | *500mg IV qd* |
| or | Glycopeptide →198 | Vancomycin (Vancocin, Vancoled, Gens) | *15mg/kg IV q12h* |

If penicillin resistant

	Fluoroquinolone →204	Levofloxacin (Levaquin)	*500-750mg IV qd*
		Moxifloxacin (Avelox)	*400mg IV qd*
		Gatifloxacin (Tequin)	*400mg IV qd*
or	Cephalosporin →196	Ceftriaxone (Rocephin)	*1-2g IV q12h*
or	Glycopeptide →198	Vancomycin (Vancocin, Vancoled, Gens)	*15mg/kg IV q12h*

Streptococcus spp.

| | Benzylpenicillin →187 | Penicillin G (Gens) | *1-2 M U IV q4-6h* |

Staphylococcus aureus

| 1st choice | Penicillin – 2nd gen. →188 | Nafcillin (Nallpen, Unipen, Gens) | *1-2g IV q4-6h* |

If methicillin resistant

| | Glycopeptide →198 | Vancomycin (Vancocin, Vancoled, Gens) | *15mg/kg IV q12h* |

Pseudomonas aeruginosa

	Cephalosporin – 3rd gen. →195	Ceftazidime (Ceptaz, Fortaz, Tazicef, Tazidime, Gens)	*1-2g IV q8-12h*
or	Carbapenem →197	Imipenem (Primaxin)	*500-1000mg IV q6-8h*
		Meropenem (Merrem)	*1g IV q8h*
plus	Aminoglycoside →200	Tobramycin (Nebcin)	*2-3mg/kg IV loading dose, then 1.0-1.7mg/kg IV q8h*
or	Fluoroquinolone →203	Ciprofloxacin (Cipro)	*200-400mg IV bid*

Haemophilus influenzae

	Aminopenicillin (if beta-lactamase negative) →189	**Ampicillin** (Gens)	*250-500mg IV q6h*
or	**Cephalosporin – 3rd gen.** →195	**Cefotaxime** (Claforan)	*1.0-2.0g IV q4-8h*
		Ceftriaxone (Rocephin)	*1.0-2.0g IV qd*
		Ceftizoxime (Cefizox)	*1.0g IV q8-12h to 4.0g IV q8h*

Klebsiella

	Cephalosporin – 3rd gen. →195	**Cefotaxime** (Claforan)	*1.0-2.0g IV q4-8h*
		Ceftriaxone (Rocephin)	*1.0-2.0g IV qd*
		Ceftizoxime (Cefizox)	*1.0g IV q8-12h to 4.0g IV q8h*

4 B.5   Pulmonary Thromboembolism (PE)
4 B.5.1   General measures

	Gas (blood oxygenation)	**Oxygen**	*Prn to maintain O_2 saturation of $\geq 90\%$*

4 B.5.2   Anticoagulation

	Heparin, low–molecular–weight (LMWH) →71	**Enoxaparin** (Lovenox)	*1mg/kg SC q12h or 1.5mg/kg SC qd; single dose max. 180mg*
		Tinzaparin (Innohep)	*175 anti-Xa IU/kg SC qd*
		Dalteparin (Fragmin)	*200 anti-Xa IU/kg SC qd*
or	**Heparin – unfractionated** →70	**Heparin** (Gens)	*5000 U bolus IV, then maint inf 18 U/kg/h IV; rebolus 80 U/kg IV prn; adj dose based on PTT (2-3) or plasma heparin level (0.2-0.4 U/ml)*
and	**Oral anticoagulant** (carboxylation of coagulation factors in liver ↓) →72	**Warfarin** (Coumadin, Gens)	*Ini 5mg PO, adj dose based on INR (2.0); stop LMWH or UFH, when INR in therapeutic range (INR 2) for 4d*

Continue for 3mo with INR 2.5 (2-3) in first PE with reversible risk or time-limited factors; for 6 mo in first PE without risk factors; or 12mon/permanent after recurrence or continuous risk factor

4 B.5.3   Thrombolysis in PE

The use of thrombolytics in treating PE must be individualized. Thrombolysis is generally indicated in hypotension or other signs of systemic hypoperfusion. In right ventricular dysfunction, consider thrombolysis if there are no contraindications.

	Tissue Plasminogen activator (thrombolytic) →73	**rt-PA** (Alteplase)	*100mg continuous IV inf over 2h; then heparin IV to maintain a PTT of 1.5-2.5*
or	**Plasminogen activator** (thrombolytic) →73	**Streptokinase** (Streptase)	*250,000 U loading dose over 30 min, then 100,000 U/h over 24h; then heparin IV to maintain a PTT of 1.5-2.5*

IVC Filter: Consider with: 1) proximal vein thrombosis or PE or with high risk for these conditions, when anticoagulant therapy has failed or is contraindicated or has resulted in a complication; 2) recurrent thromboembolism that occurs despite adequate anticoagulation, with chronic recurrent embolism and pulmonary hypertension, and with concurrent surgical pulmonary embolectomy or pulmonary thromboendarterectomy)

IVC Filter	IVC filter should be placed by experienced practitioner

61. The American College of Chest Physicians. Sixth ACCP consensus conference on antithrombotic therapy. Chest 2001;119;16-20.

4 B.6   Primary Pulmonary Hypertension
4 B.6.1   In General

Gas (blood oxygenation)	Oxygen	*If pO$_2$ < 55mmHg at rest or < 60mmHg with exercise, sleep, chronic cor pulmonale or secondary polycythemia; Caution when pCO$_2$↑*

4 B.6.2   PPH patients with significant pulmonary vasore4activity

Patients with primary pulmonary hypertension should be assessed for evidence of vasoreactivity by undergoing right heart catheterization with acute vasoreactivity testing (inhaled nitrious oxide, epoprostenol, or adenosine). Responders (e.g., = 10% decrease in mean pulmonary arterial pressure (MPAP) with either no change or an increase in cardiac output and/or a decrease in pulmonary vascular resistance (PVR) of approximately 20%) should have a hemodynamically monitored trial of calcium channel blockers.

	Calcium–channel blocker →28 (inotropic ↓, afterload ↓)	Nifedipine (Procardia, Procardia XL, Gens)	*Ini 20mg, incr dose qh up to a 20% decr in MPAP and PVR; then admin 50% of effective dose q6-8h*
or		Diltiazem (Cardizem CD, Cardizem SR, Gens)	*Ini 60mg, incr dose qh up to a 20% decr in MPAP and PVR, then admin 50% of effective dose q6-8h*

4 B.6.3   PPH patients without pulmonary vasoreactivity

For patients who do not respond to acute vasoreactivity testing, consider other vasodilator drugs. The drugs should be titrated to the desired effect.

	Endothelin receptor antagonist →32 (vasodilation)	Bosentan (Tracleer)	*62.5mg bid PO for 4wk, then incr to maint dose 125mg bid; monitor liver function tests, Hb, HLG*
or	Direct vasodilator →31 (peripheral resistance ↓)	Epoprostenol (Flolan)	*Ini 2 ng/kg/min cont IV inf, then titrate in increments of 2 ng/kg/min q15 min*

| Or poss | **Direct vasodilator** →31 (peripheral resistance ↓) | **Treprostinil** (Remodulin) | *Ini 1.25 ng/kg/min via SC inf pump; adj dose to 0.625 ng/kg/min if inability to tolerate ini dose or in mild/moderate hepatic insuff. or renal impairment; incr inf rate in increments of 0.625ng/kg/min qwk* |
| and | **Oral anticoagulant** →72 (carboxylation of coagulation factors ↓) | **Warfarin** (Coumadin, Gens) | *Ini 5mg PO, adj to maintain INR of 2.0* |

62. Pass SE, Dusing ML. Current and Emerging Therapy for Primary Pulmonary Hypertension. Ann Pharmacother 2002; 36:1430–42

4 B.6.4   Right heart failure

	Aldosterone antagonist →28 (renal H_2O and NaCl loss, K^+ secretion ↓)	**Spironolactone** (Aldactone, Gens)	*25-100mg PO qd or bid*
and/or	**Loop diuretic** →33	**Furosemide** (Lasix, Gens)	*10-240mg PO qd-qid*
and/or	**Cardiac glycoside** →40	**Digoxin** (LanoxiCap, Lanoxin, Gens)	*0.125-0.375mg PO qd; monitor levels*

4 B.7   Cystic Fibrosis (CF)
4 B.7.1   In General

The primary goals of Tx are to **treat infections**, decrease the burden of infections, aid in the clearance of secretions, and improve bronchopulmonary hygiene. **Nutrition** is critical for both the pulmonary and nonpulmonary manifestations of CF.

	Gas (blood oxygenation)	**Oxygen**	*If pO_2 < 55mmHg at rest or < 60mmHg with exercise, sleep, chronic cor pulmonale or secondary polycythemia; Caution when pCO_2↑*
	Mucolytic →99 (sputum viscosity ↓)	**Dornase alpha**	*2.5mg q12-24h via nebulizer*
	Beta$_2$-agonist, short acting →95 (bronchodilating)	**Albuterol** (Proventil, Proventil HFA, Ventolin, 90µg/puff; Ventolin Rotacaps, 200µg/puff)	*2 puffs tid-qid prn*
or		**Metaproterenol** (Alupent, 650µg/puff)	*2 puffs tid-qid prn*
or		**Pirbuterol** (Maxair, Maxair Autoinhaler, 200µg/puff)	*2 puffs tid-qid prn*

4 B.7.2   Infections

Suppressive Regimen

	Aminoglycoside →200	**Tobramycin** (Nebcin, Gens)	*300mg bid via nebulizer x 28d*

4 B.7.3   Acute Infection

For acute infections, a prolonged course of oral antibiotics is recommended. If the patient does not respond or has a severe exacerbation, consider IV antibiotics. The antibiotic regimen should cover for Pseudomonas aeruginosa. If a specific pathogen is identified, that pathogen should be treated based on drug-susceptibility results.

Haemophilus influenzae

	Aminopenicillin →189	**Ampicillin** (Gens)	*2-3g IV q4-6h*
or	**Folate antagonist + p–Aminobenzoic acid antagonist (Co–trimoxazole)** →206	**Trimethoprim + Sulfamethoxazole** (Bactrim, Bactrim DS, Septra, Gens)	*160+800mg PO bid or 5mg/kg IV q8h*

Staphylococcus aureus

	Penicillin – 2nd gen. →188	**Nafcillin** (Nallpen, Unipen, Gens)	*2mg IV q4h*
	Cephalosporin – 1st gen. →191	**Cefazolin** (Ancef, Kefzol, Gens)	*1–2g IV q4–6h*
or	**Glycopeptide (if methcillin resistant)** →198	**Vancomycin** (Vancocin, Vancoled, Gens)	*1g q12h*

Pseudomonas aeruginosa

	Cephalosporin – 3rd/4th gen. →195, →197 (antipseudomonal)	**Ceftazidime** (Ceptaz, Fortaz, Tazicef, Tazidime, Gens)	*2g IV q8h*
or		**Cefepime** (Maxipime)	*2g IV q12h*
or	**Penicillin – antipseudomonal** →190	**Piperacillin** (Pipracil)	*100mg/kg IV q6h*
or		**Ticarcillin** (Ticar)	*100mg/kg IV q6h*
Plus	**Quinolone – antispeudomonal** →203	**Ciprofloxacin** (Cipro)	*400mg IV q8-12h*
or	**Aminoglycoside** →200	**Tobramycin** (Nebcin)	*3mg/kg IVq8h*

4 B.8   Sarcoidosis

4 B.8.1   Relief of Musculoskeletal Symptoms

poss	**NSAID – acetic acid derivative** →266 (analgesic, antipyretic)	**Indomethacin** (Indocin, Indocin SR, Indo-lemmon, Indomethagan, Gens)	*25-50mg PO bid-tid*

4 B.8.2   In Symptomatic Systemic Disease

In cardiac, neurologic, progressive pulmonary disease and eye disease not responding to topical therapy, and in hypercalcemia

	Corticosteroid →148 (anti-inflammatory)	**Prednisone** (Deltasone, Meticorten, Prednisone Intensol, Gens)	*Ini 20-40mg PO qod for 1-3mon: red to 5-10mg qod for 12mon, then reassess*
or/plus	**Immunosuppressant** →263 (cytokine synthesis ↓)	**Methotrexate** (Folex, Rheumatrex, Gens)	*10-25mg/wk PO*
or		**Azathioprine** (Imuran, Gens)	*50-200mg PO qd*
or	**Immunosuppressant** (alkylating agent)	**Cyclophosphamide** (Cytoxan, Neosar)	*50-100mg PO qd or 500-2000mg q2wks IV (more toxic than above drugs)*
poss	**Antirheumatic** →262 (stabilization of lysosome membrane)	**Hydroxychloroquine** (Plaquenil, Gens)	*200-400mg PO qd*

63.   American Thoracic Society. Statement on Sarcoidosis. Am J Respir Crit Care 1999;160:736-755.

5 A. Gastroenterology – Drugs

5 A.1   Antiulcer Drugs
5 A.1.1   H₂ Antagonists

MA: competitive antagonism at H_2-receptor on parietal cells
EF: inhibition of basal and histamine-stimulated acid secretion
AE: exanthema, headache, dizziness, confusion, agranulocytosis, gynecomastia, cholestasis, transaminases ↑
CI: children

Cimetidine	EHL 2h, PRC B, Lact +
Tagamet *Tab 200mg, 300mg, 400mg, 800mg, Sol (oral) 300mg/5ml, Inj 300mg/2ml* **Generics** *Tab 200mg, 300mg, 400mg, 800mg, Sol (oral) 300mg/5ml, Inj 6mg/ml, 90mg/100ml, 120mg/100ml, 180mg/100ml, 240mg/100ml, 300mg/2ml, 360mg/ 100ml, 480mg/100ml*	**Active ulcers** →131: 800mg PO qhs, 400mg PO bid or 300mg PO/IV qid x 4-8wk; **ulcer (maint):** 400mg qhs; **GERD** →130: 800mg PO bid or 400mg PO qid x 12wk; **hypersecretory conditions:** 300mg PO/IV qid or 300mg IM q6-8h, max 2400mg/d; DARF: GFR (ml/min) >50: 100%, 10-50: 75%, <10: 50%
Famotidine	EHL 2.59-4h, PRC B, Lact ?
Pepcid *Tab 20mg, 40mg, Susp 40mg/5ml, Inj 0.4mg/ml, 10mg/ml* **Pepcid RPD** *Tab (orally disint) 20mg, 40mg*	**Active ulcers** →131: 20mg bid PO/IV or 40mg PO qhs x 4-8wk; **ulcer (maint):** 20mg PO/IV qhs; **GERD** →130: 20 PO bid; **esophagitis (due to GERD):** 20-40mg PO bid x 12wk; **hypersecretory conditions:** 20mg PO q6h, max 160mg PO q6h; DARF. CrCl (ml/min) >10: 20-40mg PO qd or 20mg IV q12h, <10: 20mg PO qd or 40mg PO qod or 20mg IV q24h
Nizatidine	EHL 1-2.8h, PRC B, Lact -
Axid *Cap 150mg, 300mg*	**Active ulcers** →131: 300mg PO qhs or 150mg PO bid x 8wk; **ulcer (maint):** 150mg PO qhs; **GERD** →130: 150mg PO bid x 12wk; **heartburn PRO:** prn 75mg PO 1h ac, max 150mg/d; DARF: GFR (ml/min), 20-50: 150mg qd, <20: 150mg qod
Ranitidine	EHL 2-2.5h, PRC B, Lact +
Zantac *Tab 150mg, 300mg, Tab (efferv) 150mg, Cap 150mg, 300mg, Gran (efferv) 150mg/packet, Syr 15mg/ml, Inj 1mg/ml, 25mg/ml* **Generics** *Tab 150mg, 300mg, Cap 150mg, 300mg*	**Active ulcers** →131: 150mg PO bid or 300mg qhs or 50mg IV/IM q6-8h or 6.25mg/h as continuous IV inf, max 400mg/d; **ulcer (maint):** 150mg PO qhs; **GERD** →130: 150mg PO bid; **hypersecretory conditions** →130: 150mg PO bid, max 6g/d; **Zollinger-Ellison syndrome** →184: ini 100mg IV (bolus), then ini 0.5mg/kg/h continuous IV inf, prn incr by 0.5 mg/kg/h, max 4mg/kg/h or 9,000mg/24h; **esophagitis (erosive, active)** →130: 150mg PO qid; **esophagitis (erosive, maint)** →130: 150mg PO bid; DARF: GFR (ml/min) <50: 150mg PO qd or 50mg IV q18-24h

5 A.1.2 Proton Pump Inhibitors

MA/EF: blockage of H^+/K^+-ATPase $\Rightarrow$ greatest suppression of acid production
AE: dizziness, headache, diarrhea, constipation, flatulence, exanthema, liver enz. ↑

Esomeprazole	EHL 1.5h, PRC B, Lact ?
Nexium *Cap ext.rel. 20mg, 40mg*	**GERD** →130, **erosive esophagitis (active, maint):** 40mg PO qd
Lansoprazole	EHL 0.9-1.5h, PRC B, Lact ?
PrevAcid *Cap ext.rel. 15mg, 30mg*	**GERD** →130, **duodenal ulcers** →131: 15mg PO ac qam x 4wk; **gastric ulcers, erosive esophagitis (active)** →131: 30mg PO qd x 8-16wk; **erosive esophagitis (maint):** 15mg PO ac qam; **Zollinger-Ellison syndrome** →184: 60mg PO ac qam, >120mg/d div bid, max 90mg ac bid; DARF: not req
Omeprazole	EHL 0.5-1.5h, PRC C, Lact ?
Prilosec *Cap ext.rel. 10mg, 20mg, 40mg* **Generics** *Cap ext.rel. 10mg, 20mg, 40mg*	**GERD** →130: 20mg PO qd x 4-8 (-12)wk; **active duodenal ulcers** →131: 20mg PO qd x 4-8wk; maint 20mg PO qd; **gastric ulcers** →131: 40mg PO ac qam x 4-8wk; **ulcer PRO:** 20mg PO/NG qd; **erosive esophagitis (active, maint):** 20mg PO qd; **hypersecretory conditions, Zollinger-Ellison syndrome** →184: 60mg PO qd, >80mg div prn, max 120mg PO tid; ini prn 60mg IV q8h; DARF: not req
Pantoprazole	EHL 1h, PRC B, Lact ?
Protonix *Tab ext.rel. 40mg, Inj 40mg/vial*	**Duodenal/gastric ulcer** →131: 40mg PO ac qam x 4-8wk, max 80mg/d; **GERD** →130: 40mg PO ac qam x 8-16wk; 40mg IV qd x 7-10d; **hypersecretory conditions, Zollinger-Ellison syndrome** →184: 80mg IV bid; DARF: max 40mg/d
Rabeprazole	EHL 1-2h, PRC B, Lact ?
Aciphex *Tab ext.rel. 20mg*	**GERD (active, maint)** →130: 20mg PO qd; **duodenal ulcers** →131: 20mg PO qd; **hypersecretory conditions, Zollinger-Ellison syndrome** →184: 60mg PO qd, max 100mg PO qd or 60mg PO bid; DARF: not req

5 A.1.3 Helicobacter pylori Treatment

MA/EF (bismuth): antibacterial activity and protective effects on gastric mucosa
AE (bismuth): black coloration of tongue, teeth and feces; neurological and psychic DO
CI (bismuth): renal insufficiency, children <14

Amoxicillin + Clarithromycin + Lansoprazole	PRC C , Lact ?
Prevpac contains: Prevacid, Cap 30mg (lansoprazole), Trimox, Cap 500mg (amoxicillin), Biaxin, Tab 500mg (clarithromycin)	**Duodenal ulcers associated with H.p.** →132: Prevacid 1 Cap, Trimox 2 Cap, Biaxin 1 Tab PO bid x 10-14d

Bismuth Subsalicylate + Metronidazole + Tetracycline	PRC D, Lact -
Helidac *Tab (chew) 262.4mg (bismuth) + Tab 250mg (metronidazole) + Cap 500mg (tetracycline)*	**Duodenal ulcers associated with H.p.** →132: 2 bismuth Tab + 1 metronidazole Tab + 1 tetracycline Cap PO qid, at meals and hs x 2wk with H2 antagonist

Ranitidine + Bismuth + Citrate	EHL 2.8-3.1h (R.), 11-28d (Bis.), PRC C, Lact ?
Tritec *Tab 400mg (162+128+110mg)*	**Duodenal ulcers associated with H.p.** →132: 400mg PO bid x 4wk (ini + clarithromycin 500mg PO tid x 2wk), DARF: GFR (ml/min) <25: not rec

5 A.1.4 Other Antiulcer Drugs

MA/EF (misoprostol): prostaglandin E_1 analog ⇒ prostaglandin-mediated inhibition of acid secretion, activation of bicarbonate and mucus secretion
MA/EF (clinidium): anticholinergic, bladder capacity↑, urinary frequency↓, gastric acid secretion↓, antispasmodic
MA/EF (sucralfate): forming of an adherent, protective protein complex at ulcer site
MA/EF (chlordiazepoxide): see Benzodiazepines →330
AE (misoprostol): diarrhea, dizziness, headache, metrorrhagia; **AE** (clinidium): urinary retention, constipation, blurred vision, dry mouth, tachycardia, dizziness, headache
AE (sucralfate): constipation, raise of aluminum level in renal insufficiency
CI (misoprostol): children, epilepsy, women of childbearing potential have to use adequate contraception, infectious intestinal illnesses; **CI** (clinidium): hypersensitivity to anticholinergic drugs, Myasthenia gravis, narrow-angle glaucoma, obstructive GI disease, paralytic ileus, reflux esophagitis, ulcerative colitis, obstructive uropathy, unstable CVS status in acute hemorrhage; **CI** (sucralfate): hypersensitivity to sucralfate

Clinidium + Chlordiazepoxide	PRC D, Lact -
Librax *Cap 2.5mg+5mg*	**Irritable bowel syndrome:** 1 Cap PO tid-qid, DARF: 50% in severe RF

Misoprostol	EHL rapid, metabol. 20-40min, PRC X, Lact -
Cytotec *Tab 0.1mg, 0.2mg*	**NSAID-ind. gastric ulcers** (PRO), **peptic ulcers** (Tx) →131: 200 µg PO qid; if not tolerated: 100 µg PO qid; DARF: not req

Sucralfate	PRC B, Lact +
Carafate *Tab 1g, Susp 1g/10ml* **Generics** *Tab 1g*	**Duodenal ulcers** →132: 1g PO qid (1h ac and hs) x 6-8wk; **ulcer (maint):** 1g PO bid; DARF: risk of aluminium accumulation in chronic RF

see Propantheline →127

5 A.2   Antacids

MA/EF: neutralization of stomach acid
AE (aluminium): constipation, ileus, phosphate deficiency; **AE** (magnesium): diarrhea
AE (calcium): kidney stones, hypercalcemia, constipation
CI: hypersensitivity to antacids

Aluminium Hydroxide	PRC B, Lact ?
Alternagel *Liquid (oral) 600mg/5ml* **Alu-tab** *Tab 500mg* **Amphojel** *Tab 300mg, 600mg, Sol (oral) 320mg/5ml*	**GERD** →130, **mild heartburn:** 500-1800mg PO tid-6 times/d between meals and hs; DARF: req in severe RF

Aluminium + Magnesium Hydroxide	PRC B, Lact ?
Maalox *Tab (chew) 200mg+200mg, Susp 225mg/5ml+200mg/5ml*	10-20ml or 1-4 Tab PO qid; DARF: req in severe RF

Calcium Carbonate	PRC B, Lact ?
Mylanta *Tab (chew) 400mg, 750mg, 1g* **Titralac** *Tab 750mg, Tab (chew) 420mg* **Tums** *Tab (chew) 500mg, 750mg, 1g*	0.5-1.5g PO prn, max 8g/d

Magaldrate	PRC B, Lact ?
Riopan *Tab 480mg, Tab (chew) 480mg, Liquid (oral) 1080mg, Susp 540mg/5ml*	400-1080mg qd between meals

5 A.3   Laxatives

MA/EF (bisacodyl, sodium sulfate): resorption and metabolism in liver → biliary excretion, effective in intestine as free diphenyl ⇒ antiresorptive, water binding
MA/EF (lactulose): osmotic effect, fermented to acids through bacteria ⇒ peristaltic ↑
MA/EF (polycarbophil): swelling effect
MA/EF (senna): splitting of contained anthraglycosides through coli bacteria to anthrones/ anthranols ⇒ antiresorptive and water binding effects
AE (laxatives): electrolyte loss (especially K⁺), melanosis coli, albuminuria, hematuria
AE (polycarbophil): abdominal fullness, flatulence
CI (laxatives): ileus, gastroenteritis, acute surgical abdomen, appendicitis, rectal bleeding

Bisacodyl	PRC B, Lact ?
Correctol *Tab 5mg* **Dulcolax** *Tab 5mg, Supp 10mg* **Generics** *Tab 5mg, Supp 5mg, 10mg, Enema 10mg/5ml, 10mg/10ml, 10mg/30ml*	**Constipation, colonic evacuation:** 10-15mg PO hs prn, 10mg PR prn, max 30mg/d; **CH** <2 y: 5mg PR prn, max 5mg/d, **CH** 2-12 y: 5-10mg PR prn, max 10mg/d

Cascara	PRC C, Lact -
Generics *Tab 325mg, Cap 450mg, Sol (oral, aromatic fluid extract), Liquid (oral, aromatic)*	**Constipation:** 325 mg PO hs prn, max 1,000mg/d or 5ml/d aromatic fluid extract PO hs prn, max 6ml/d; **CH** >2 y: 1-3ml/d aromatic fluid extract PO or 150-150mg PO

Castor Oil
PRC N, Lact ?

Purge *Liquid (oral) 95%*
Generics *Liquid (oral) 60%, 100%*

Constipation: 15ml PO prn on empty stomach; **colonic evacuation**: 15-30ml PO prn on empty stomach; **CH** < 2 y: 1-2ml, max 5ml PO, **CH** 2-11 y: 5-15ml PO

Docusate Calcium
PRC C, Lact ?

Surfak *Cap 240mg*
Generics *Cap 240mg, Gel 240mg*

Constipation: 240mg PO prn

Docusate + Casanthranol
PRC C, Lact ?

Peri-Colace *Gel 100mg + 30mg, Syr 20mg/5ml + 10mg/5ml*

Constipation: 1-2 Cap or 15-30ml PO hs prn; **CH** 1-3 tsp PO hs prn

Docusate Sodium
PRC C, Lact ?

Colace *Liquid (oral) 10mg/ml, Gel 50mg, 100mg, Syr 20mg/5ml, Enema 200mg/5ml*
Generics *Tab 100mg, Cap 50mg, 100mg, 250mg, Sol (oral) 20mg/5ml, 100mg/10ml, Liquid (oral)10mg/ml, Gel 100mg, 250mg, Syr 20mg/5ml, 50mg/15ml, 60mg/15ml*

Constipation: 50-400mg/d PO qd-qid; **CH** <3 y: 10-40mg/d PO prn, 3-6 y: 20-60mg/d PO prn, 6-12 y: 40-150mg/d PO prn, >12 y: 50-200mg/d PO prn

Lactulose
PRC B, Lact ?

Cephulac *Sol (oral, rectal) 10g/15ml*
Cholac *Sol (oral, rectal) 10g/15ml*
Chronulac *Sol (oral) 10g/15ml*
Constilac *Sol (oral) 10g/15ml*
Constulose *Sol (oral) 10g/15ml*
Enulose *Sol (oral, rectal) 10g/15ml*
Evalose *Sol (oral) 10g/15ml*
Heptalac *Sol (oral, rectal) 10g/15ml*
Laxilose *Sol (oral) 10g/15ml*

Constipation: 30-45ml PO qd-qid prn; infants: 2.5-10ml/d PO div tid-qid, **CH** adolescents: 40-90ml/d PO div tid-qid; **hepatic encephalopathy** (PRO/Tx) →136: 30-45ml/dose PO q1h until effect, then 30-45ml PO tid-qid or 300ml PR with 700ml water, rep q4-6h prn

Magnesium Citrate
PRC B, Lact +

Generics *Cap 140mg, Sol (oral) 59mg/ml*

Bowel evacuation: 150-300ml PO qd; **CH** 6-12y: 0.5ml/kg PO q4-6h

Magnesium Hydroxide
PRC N, Lact +

Philipps' Milk of Magnesia *Tab (chew) 311mg, Liquid (oral) 400mg/5ml, 800mg/5ml*
Generics *Tab (chew) 311mg, Liquid 375mg/5ml, 400mg/5ml, 800mg/5ml, 2400mg/10ml*

Laxative: 15-40ml PO qd or 6-8 Tab PO/d prn; **CH** <2 y: 0.5ml/kg PO qd, 2-5 y: 5-15ml/d PO qd or 1-2 Tab PO/d prn, 6-11 y: 15-30ml PO qd, 3-4 Tab PO/d prn; DARF: req in severe RF

Methylcellulose
PRC N, Lact ?

Citrucel *Powder (oral) 2g/10.2g, 2g/19g*

Laxative: 1 tablespoon in 8 oz cold water PO qd-tid; **CH** 6-12 y: 50% of adult dose

Mineral Oil
PRC C, Lact ?

Agoral *Emulsion 4.2g/15ml*
Fleet Enema Mineral Oil *Sol (rectal) 130ml/dose*
Kondremul *Liquid (oral) 55% mineral oil*

Laxative: 15-45ml PO or 120ml PR; **CH** 5-11 y: 5-15ml PO, 2-11 y: 30-60ml PR

Polycarbophil — PRC N, Lact ?

Equalactin *Tab (chew) 500mg*
FiberCon *Tab 500mg*
Generics *Tab 625mg, Tab (chew) 500mg, Cap 625mg*

Laxative: 1g PO qd-qid prn; **CH** 3-5 y: 500mg PO qd-bid prn, >6 y: 500mg PO qd-tid prn

---

Polyethylene Glycol — PRC C, Lact ?

Miralax *Powder for Sol (oral) 17g/tablespoon*

Constipation: 1 heaping tsp in 8 oz water PO qd

Polyethylene Glycol with Electrolytes — PRC C, Lact ?

Colyte *Powder for Sol (oral) polyethylene glycol 240g/4L*
Golytely *Powder for Sol (oral) polyethylene glycol 236g/4L*

Bowel preparation: 1.5 l/h PO

Senna — EHL 4.0-12.1h, PRC C, Lact +

Senokot *Tab 8.5mg, 375mg, Sol (oral) 218mg/5ml, Gran 326mg/5ml, Supp 30mg*
Generics *Tab 5.6mg, 8mg, 217mg, Liquid (oral) 33.3mg/ml, Syr 8.8mg/5ml*

Laxative or bowel preparation: 1 tsp gran (15mg) in water or 10-15ml or 2 Tab (8.5mg) PO or 1 supp PR hs; max 4 tsp of gran or 30ml syrup or 8 Tab (34-50mg PO bid) or 2 supp/d; **CH** 6-12 y: 1 Tab or 1/2 tsp PO bid, 2-6 y: 1/2 Tab or 1/4 tsp PO qd

---

Sodium Phosphate — EHL 20h, PRC N, Lact ?

Fleet Enema *Enema 118ml, 59ml*
Fleet Phospho-Soda *Sol (oral) sodium phosphate monohydrate 2.4 g/5ml + sodium phosphate heptahydrate/5ml 0.9 g*

Laxative: 1 adult enema (118ml) PR prn or 20-45ml oral sol PO prn; **CH** 2-11 y: 1 pediatric enema (59ml) PR prn or 5-9 y: 5-10ml oral sol PO prn, 10-11 y: 10-20ml oral sol PO prn; DARF: contraind.

5 A.4   Antidiarrheals

MA/EF (attapulgite): swelling agent ⇒ inhibition of peristalsis
MA/EF (bismuth subsalicylate): direct binding of bacteria toxines ⇒ antimicrobial, antisecretory
MA/EF (loperamide, diphenoxylate): stimulation of peripheral opium rec. ⇒ peristalsis↓
AE (loperamide): headache, tiredness, dizziness, dry mouth, nausea
CI (bismuth): hypersensitivity to salicylates, varicella/influenza infection in children
CI (loperamide): ileus, children <2 y

Atropine + Diphenoxylate — EHL 2.5h (D.), 4h (A.), PRC C, Lact ?

Lomotil *Tab 0.025mg + 2.5mg, Sol (oral) 0.025mg/5ml + 2.5mg/5ml*
Lonox *Tab 0.025mg + 2.5mg*
Generics *Tab 0.025mg + 2.5mg, Cap 0.025mg + 2.5mg, Sol (oral) 0.025/5ml + 2.5mg/5ml*

Diarrhea: 15-20mg PO div tid-qid; **CH** >2 y: 0.3-0.4mg/kg/d div bid-qid

---

Attapulgite — PRC N, Lact ?

Kaopectate *Tab 2mg, 750mg, Liquid (oral) 750mg, 750mg/tablespoon*
Diasorb *Tab 750mg, Liquid (oral) 750mg/5ml, Susp 750mg/15ml*
Donnagel *Tab (chew) 600mg, Susp 600mg/15ml*

Diarrhea: 1,200-1,300mg PO; max 9,000mg/d; **CH** 3-6 y: 300mg/dose PO, max 2,250mg/d, 6-12 y: 600-750mg/dose PO; max 4,500mg/d

Bismuth Subsalicylate	EHL 21-72d, PRC D, Lact -
Pepto–Bismol *Tab (chew) 262mg, Liquid (oral) 262mg/15ml, 525mg/15ml, 525mg/oz, 1050mg/oz* **Generics** *Tab 262mg, Tab (chew) 262mg, Liquid (oral) 262mg/15ml, 130mg/15ml*	**Diarrhea**: 2 Tab or 30ml PO q30-60min max 8 doses/d;**CH** 3-6 y: 1/3 Tab or 5ml q30-60min prn, 6-9 y: 2/3 Tab or 10ml q30-60min prn, 9-12 y: 1 Tab or 15ml q30-60min prn
Loperamide	EHL 7-15h, PRC B, Lact +
Imodium *Tab 2mg, Tab (chew) 2mg Cap 2mg, Sol (oral) 1mg/5ml* **Generics** *Tab 2mg, Cap 2mg, Sol (oral) 1mg/5ml*	**Diarrhea**: 4mg PO ini, then 2mg after each loose stool, max 16mg/d; →185 **CH** 2-5 y: 1mg tid, 6-8 y: 2mg bid, 8-12 y: 2mg tid

5 A.5   Antiemetics
5 A.5.1   Antiemetics – 5-HT3 Receptor Antagonists

MA/EF: selective blockage of central 5-HT$_3$-receptors ⇒ antiemetic
AE: headache, constipation, tiredness; **CI:** children

Dolasetron	EHL <10min, PRC B, Lact ?
Anzemet *Tab 50mg, 100mg, Inj 20mg/ml*	**N/V with chemo** →453: 1.8mg/kg or 100mg IV 30min before chemo or 100mg PO 60min before chemo; **CH** 2-16 y: 1.8mg/kg, max 100mg IV/PO; **postoperative N/V**: 12.5mg IV, 100mg PO 2h prior to surgery; **CH** 2-16 y: 0.35mg/kg IV, max 12.5mg or 1.2mg/kg PO, max 100mg 2h before surgery; DARF not req
Granisetron	EHL 10-11h, PRC B, Lact ?
Kytril *Tab 1mg, Inj 1mg/ml*	**N/V with chemo** →453: 10µg/kg IV 30min before chemo or 1mg PO 1h before and 12h after chemo; **CH** 2-16y: 10µg/kg IV 30min before chemo; **postop N/V**: 1-3mg IV; DARF: not req
Ondansetron	EHL 3h, PRC B, Lact ?
Zofran *Tab 4mg, 8mg, 24mg, Tab (orally disint) 4mg, 8mg, Sol (oral) 4mg/5ml, Inj 2mg/ml*	**N/V with chemo** →453: 8mg IV, rep in 8h or 8mg PO 30min before chemo, rep in 8h; **CH** >4 y: 0.15mg/kg IV, rep in 4h and 8h after first dose, 4-11 y: 4mg PO, rep in 4h and 8h after first dose; **N/V with radiation**: 8mg PO tid; **postop N/V**: 4mg IV

5 A.5.2 Antiemetics – Antihistamines

MA/EF: inhibition of histamine receptors ⇒ antiemetic (see antihistamines →331, →408, →409)
AE (dimenhydrinate): sedation, glaucoma, urination difficulties
AE (promethazine): drowsiness, xerostomia, dizziness
CI (dimenhydrinate): eclampsia, epilepsy, prostate adenoma, glaucoma, alcohol abuse, cerebrovascular insuff.

Dimenhydrinate	PRC B, Lact +
Dramamine *Tab 50mg, Tab (chew) 50mg, Liquid (oral) 12.5mg/4ml* **Marmine** *Tab 50mg, Inj 50mg/ml* **Generics** *Tab 25mg, 50mg, Cap 25mg, 50mg, Inj 50mg/ml*	**PRO of motion sickness**: 50-100mg PO 30min prior to travel, q4-6h; **nausea**: 50-100mg/dose PO/IM/IV q4-6h; DARF: not req; →422
Meclizine	EHL 6h, PRC B, Lact ?
Antivert *Tab 12.5mg, 25mg, 50mg, Tab (chew) 25mg* **Bonine** *Tab (chew) 25mg* **Dizmiss** *Tab (chew) 25mg* **Dramamine II** *Tab (chew) 25mg* **D-Vert** *Tab 15mg, 30mg* **Generics** *Tab 12.5mg, 25mg, 50mg, Tab (chew) 25mg*	**Motion sickness**: 25-50mg PO 1h prior to travel, rep q24h prn; **vertigo**: 25-100mg PO qd-qid; **pregnancy-induced vomiting**: 25-50mg/d; **radiation sickness**: 25-100mg/d div qd-qid; →422
Promethazine	EHL 7-15h, PRC C, Lact ?
Phenergan *Tab 12.5mg, 25mg, 50mg, Supp 12.5mg, 25mg, 50mg, Inj 25mg/ml, 50mg/ml*	**Nausea** →453, **motion sickness**: 12.5-25mg PO/IM/PR q4-6h prn; DARF: not req
Trimethobenzamide	PRC C, Lact ?
Tigan *Cap 100mg, 250mg, Supp 200mg, Inj 100mg/ml*	**Nausea** →453: 250mg PO tid-qid or 200mg PR/IM tid-qid; **CH** <13.6kg (except neonates): 100mg PR tid-qid, 13.6-40.9kg: 100-200mg PO/PR tid-qid

5 A.5.3 Antiemetics – Anticholinergics

MA/EF: antimuscarinic ⇒ antiemetic
AE: tachycardia, dizziness, hallucinations, dry mouth, constipation, blurred vision
CI: primary glaucoma, hypersensitivity to scopolamine products

Scopolamine	PRC C, Lact +
Hypodermic *Tab 0.4mg, Tab 0.6mg* **Transderm Scop** *Film (ext.rel, TD) 1mg/72h* **Transderm-V** *Film (ext.rel, TD) 1mg/72h* **Generics** *Inj 0.3mg/ml, 0.33mg/ml, 0.43mg/ml, 0.65mg/ml, 1mg/ml*	**Motion sickness, postop vomiting** →453: 0.6-1mg PO/SC, 1 patch behind ear q3d; **pre-med**: 1mg IM/IV/SC 1-4h prior to anesthesia or 0.4-0.6mg IM/IV/SC 45-60min prior to anesthesia

5 A.5.4   Other Antiemetics

MA/EF (aprepitant): selective antagonism of substance P/neurokinin receptors ⇒ antiemetic
MA/EF (metoclopramide, prochlorperazine): inhibition of dopamine receptors ⇒ antiemetic
AE (aprepitant): asthenia, fatigue, anorexia, diarrhea, constipation, hiccups
AE (metoclopramide): tiredness, headache, dizziness, dyskinesias (children), parkinsonism, diarrhea, prolactin ↑; **AE** (prochlorperazine): EPS, drowsiness, postural hypotension
CI (aprepitant): combination with pimozide, terfenadine, astemizole, cisapride
CI (metoclopramide): pheochromocytoma, mechanic ileus, epilepsy, extra pyramidal motor impairment, combination with MAO inhibitors, caution with children <14, and RF

Aprepitant	EHL 9-13h, PRC B, Lact ?
Emend *Cap 80mg, 125mg*	**Acute and delayed N/V with chemo** →453: 125mg PO 1h prior to chemo, then 80mg qd on days 2 and 3; give with corticosteroid and $5HT_3$-antagonist; DARF: not req
Dronabinol	EHL 19-36h, PRC C, Lact ?
Marinol *Cap 2.5mg, 5mg, 10mg*	**Postop nausea**: 5-15mg/m2 PO q3-6h; **chemo-induced nausea** →453: 5mg/m2 PO 1-3 h prior to chemo, then 5mg/m2/dose q2-4h after chemo for 4-6 doses/d; DARF: not req
Metoclopramide	EHL 2.5-5h, PRC B, Lact ?
Metoclopramide Intensol *Conc (oral) 10mg/ml* **Reglan** *Tab 5mg, 10mg, Sol (oral) 5mg/5ml, Inj 5mg/ml* **Generics** *Tab 5mg, 10mg, Sol (oral) 5mg/5ml, Inj 5mg/ml*	**GERD** →130: 10-15mg PO qid; **postop nausea**: 10mg IV/PO; **chemo-induced nausea** →453: 1-2mg/kg/dose IV q2-4h; DARF: GFR (ml/min) >50: 100%, 10-50: 75%, <10: 50%
Prochlorperazine	EHL 6.8-9h, PRC C, Lact -
Compazine *Supp 2.5mg, 5mg, 25mg, Inj 5mg/ml* **Compro** *Supp 25mg* **Generics** *Supp 25mg*	**Nausea** →453: 5-10mg PO/IM tid/qid, max 40mg/d or 25mg PR bid or 5-10mg IM q3-4h prn

5 A.6   Anti-Inflammatory Drugs, Bowel

MA: influence on prostaglandin biosynthesis, inhibition of leukotriene synthesis
EF: locally anti-inflammatory
AE: headache, dizziness, nausea, agranulocytosis, pancytopenia, allergic reactions, renal function impairment; **CI:** severe hepatic and renal impairment

Balsalazide	EHL 1h, PRC B, Lact ?
Colazal *Cap 750mg*	**Ulcerative colitis** →133: 2,250mg PO tid x 8wk, maint 3-4g/d div bid
Mesalamine	EHL 0.6-1.4h, PRC B, Lact ?
Asacol *Tab ext.rel. 400mg* **Canasa** *Supp 500mg* **Pentasa** *Cap ext.rel. 250mg* **Rowasa** *Enema 4g/60ml*	**Ulcerative colitis** →133: 800mg Tab PO tid or 1g Cap PO qid or 500mg Supp PR bid or 4g (60ml) Susp PR qhs, maint 1,600mg/d PO in div doses; →132

Olsalazine	EHL 0.9h, PRC C , Lact ?
Dipentum *Cap 250mg*	**Ulcerative colitis** →133: 500mg PO bid
Sulfasalazine	EHL 7.6h , PRC B , Lact ?
Azulfidine *Tab 500mg,* *Susp 250mg/5ml* **Azulfidine EN–tabs** *Tab ext.rel. 500mg* **Generics** *Tab 500mg*	**Ulcerative colitis** →133: ini 500-1000mg PO qid, maint 500mg PO qid, max 6g/d; →276, →278, →279 **CH** >2 y: 40-60mg/kg/d PO div tid-6 times/d, maint 30mg/kg/d PO div qid, max 2g/d; DARF: use with caution in RF

5 A.7   GI Enzymes

MA/EF (pancreatin, pancrelipase): mixture of amylase, trypsin, and lipase
AE (pancreatin, pancrelipase): skin rash, hypersensitivity, nausea/diarrhea with large doses, hyperuricemia, hyperuricosuria
CI (pancreatin, pancrelipase): hypersensitivity to pork protein

Lactase Enzyme	PRC N, Lact ?
Lactaid *Cap (original strength) 3,000 FCC U of enzyme, Cap (extra strength) 4,500 FCC U of enzyme, Cap (ultra) 9,000 FCC U of enzyme, Cap (ultra, chew) 9,000 FCC U of enzyme, Gtt*	**Lactose intolerance**: 3 Cap PO (original strength), 2 Cap PO (extra strength), 1 Cap PO (ultra), swallow Cap with first bite of dairy foods or 5-7 Gtt, max 15gtt PO/quart of milk
Pancreatin	PRC C, Lact ?
Creon 5, Creon 10, Creon 20 *Cap (Lipase + Protease + Amylase)* **Donnazyme** *Tab (Lipase + Protease + Amylase) 500mg* **Ultrase** *Cap (Lipase + Protease + Amylase)* **Ultrase MT12, MT18, MT20** *Cap (Lipase + Protease + Amylase)*	**Pancreatic enzyme deficiency** →134: 1-2 Tab/Cap PO with each meal
Pancrelipase	PRC C, Lact ?
Cotazym *Cap 30000 U, 8000 U, 30000 U*	**Pancreatic enzyme deficiency** →134: 1-3 Cap PO; **CH** 6-12mo 2000 U lipase, 1-6y: 4000-8000 U lipase, 7-12y: 4000-12000 U lipase (always with meals, feedings)

5 A.8   Antiflatulents

MA/EF: altering surface tension of gas bubbles, antifoaming; **AE**: mild diarrhea, regurgitation ;
CI: known or suspected GI obstruction/perforation

Simethicone	PRC B, Lact ?
Gas–X *Tab (chew) 80mg, 125mg, Cap 125mg, Liquid (oral) 50mg/5ml* **Mylicon** *Tab 40mg, Tab (chew) 80mg, 125mg, Gtt 20mg/0.3ml* **Generics** *Tab ext.rel 60mg, 95mg, Tab (chew) 125mg, 166mg, Cap 125mg, 166mg, Gtt 40mg/0.6ml, Liquid (oral) 62.5mg/5ml*	**Gastric bloating**: 40-125mg PO qid prn, max 480mg/d; **CH** <2 y: 20mg PO qid, 2-12 y: 40mg PO qid

5 A.9   Gallstone Dissolving Drugs

MA/EF: Inhibition of biliary cholesterol secretion and intestinal cholesterol resorption; inhibition of HMG-CoA-reductase $\Rightarrow$ cholesterol synthesis $\downarrow \Rightarrow$ dissolving of cholesterol stones; **AE:** diarrhea, transaminases↑
CI: infx of the gall bladder and ducts, common bile duct or cystic duct occlusion, disturbed contractility of the gall bladder, calcified gall stones

Ursodiol (Ursodeoxycholic acid)	PRC B, Lact ?
Actigall *Cap 300mg* **Urso** *Tab 250mg*	**Gallstone dissolution**: 8-10mg/kg/d PO div bid-tid, maint 250mg qhs x 0.5-1y

5 A.10   Antispasmodics (Parasympatholytics)

MA/EF (dicyclomine): antimuscarinic $\Rightarrow$ antispasmodic, smooth muscle relaxation
MA/EF (hyoscyamine): competitive inhibition of muscarinic acetylcholine receptors $\Rightarrow$ antisecretory (exocrine glands, intestinal mucosa), smooth muscle relax, vagolytic effects
MA/EF (propantheline): anticholinergic, antispasmodic, bladder capacity↑, urinary frequency↓, gastric acid secretion↓
AE (dicyclomine, hyoscyamine): urinary retention, constipation, blurred vision, dry mouth, tachycardia, dizziness, headache, nausea
AE (propantheline). urinary retention, constipation, blurred vision, dry mouth, tachycardia, dizziness, headache, sexual dysfunction
CI (dicyclomine, hyoscyamine): obstructive uropathy, GI obstruction, ulcerative colitis, glaucoma, children (<6 mo dicyclomine, <2 y hyoscyamine)
CI (hyoscyamine): hepatic, renal, or pulmonary insufficiency, intestinal atony in elderly or debilitated patients, myasthenia gravis, cardiospasm, unstable CVS status
CI (propantheline): hypersensitivity to anticholinergic drugs, myasthenia gravis, narrow-angle glaucoma, obstructive GI disease, paralytic ileus, reflux esophagitis, ulcerative colitis, obstructive uropathy, unstable CVS status in acute hemorrhage

Dicyclomine	EHL 1.8h, PRC B, Lact ?
Bentyl *Tab 20mg, Cap 10mg, Syr 10mg/5ml, Inj 10mg/ml* **Generics** *Tab 20mg, Cap 10mg*	**Functional bowel syndrome**: 20mg PO 15min ac qid, max 40mg PO qid, 20mg IM qid (max 2d); **CH** 6 mo-2 y: 5-10mg PO 15min ac tid-qid, max 40mg/d, 2-12 y: 10mg/d PO tid

Hyoscyamine	EHL 3.5h, PRC C, Lact -
Cystospaz *Tab 0.15mg,* *Cap ext.rel. 0.375mg* **Levbid** *Tab ext.rel. 0.375mg* **Levsin** *Tab 0.125mg, Tab ext.rel. 0.125mg, Gtt 0.125mg/ml, Inj 0.5mg/ml* **Levsinex** *Cap ext.rel. 0.375mg*	**GI hypermotility, functional bowel syndr.**: 0.125-0.25mg PO/SL q4h or prn, max 1.5mg/d or 0.375-0.75mg PO q12h, max 1.5mg/d (ext. rel); **CH** 2-12 y: 0.0625-0.125mg q4h prn or 0.375mg (ext. rel) PO q12h, max 0.75mg/24h, >12 y: adult dose; **UT** →423

Propantheline	EHL (biphasic) 57.9min, 2.93h, PRC C, Lact ?
Pro-Banthine *Tab 7.5mg, 15mg* **Generics** *Tab 7.5mg, 15mg*	**GI antispasmodic, peptic ulcer** →131: 15mg tid 30min ac, 30mg qhs; **UT** →423

5 A.11 Other GI Drugs

MA (alosetron): selective antagonism of serotonin 5-HT3 receptor ⇒ modulation of the enteric nervous system; **MA** (budesonide): high topical glucocorticosteroid activity, 80-90% first past metabolism; **MA** (infliximab): monoclonal antibody specifically binding to TNF; **MA/EF** (octreotide): similar to somatostatin ⇒ secretory inhibition of some anterior pituitary hormones (growth hormone), suppression of pancreatic endocrine and exocrine function, inhibition of gastric acid and GI hormone secretion, suppression of serotonin secretion, inhibition of GI motility and splanchnic blood flow; **MA** (tegaserod): agonist at neuronal 5HT-4 receptors ⇒ stimulation of peristaltic reflex and intestinal secretion, inhibition of visceral sensitivity; **MA** (vasopressin): stimulation of smooth muscle receptors ⇒ vasoconstriction
AE (alosetron): headache, constipation, ileus, perforation, ischemic colitis
AE (budesonide): headache, dizziness, dyspepsia, abdominal pain, resp. tract infection
AE (infliximab): dyspnea, urticaria, flushing, headache, infections, recurrent malignancies
AE (octreotide): N/V, diarrhea, stomachache, hepatitis
AE (tegaserod): abdom. pain, diarrhea, nausea, flatulence, headache, dizziness, back pain
AE (vasopressin): tremor, sweating, vertigo, N/V, metabolic acidosis, cardiac arrhythmias
CI (alosetron): history of constipation, intest. obstruction, ischemic colitis, Crohn's disease, ulcerative colitis, diverticulitis; **CI** (budesonide): known hypersensitivity to budesonid; **CI** (infliximab): heart failure NYHA III-IV, hypersensitivity to murine proteins; **CI** (tegaserod): history of bowel obstruction, symptom. gallbladder disease, sphincter of Oddi dysfunction, abdom. adhesions, moderate or severe hepatic impairment, severe renal impairment; **CI** (vasopressin): chronic nephritis with nitrogen retention, use with caution in epilepsy, migraine, asthma, heart failure, vascular diseases

Alosetron	EHL 1.5h, PRC B, Lact ?
Lotronex *Tab 1mg*	**Severe diarrhea-predominant irritable bowel syndrome:** 1mg PO qd, may incr. to 1mg bid after 4wk;
Budesonide	EHL 2-3.6h , PRC C, Lact -
Entocort EC *Cap 3mg*	**Crohn's disease involving ileum or ascending colon** →132: 9mg PO qd for up to 8wk; DARF: not req
Infliximab	EHL 8-9.5d, PRC B, Lact ?
Remicade *Inj 100mg/20ml vial*	**Crohn's disease** →132: 5mg/kg IV; **fistulizing Crohn's disease**: 5mg/kg IV at 0, 2, and 6wk
Neomycin	EHL 3h, PRC C, Lact ?
Mycifradin *Sol (oral) 87.5mg/5ml* **Neo-rx** *Powder, for rx compounding 100%* **Generics** *Tab 350mg*	**Bowel-preparation**: 1g PO 19, 18 and 9h prior to surgery; **CH** 90mg/kg/d div q4h **hepatic coma** →136: 4-12g/d PO div q6h; **CH** 2.5-7g/m2/d x 5-6d div q4-6h, max 12g/d; DARF: GFR (ml/min): > 50: q6, 10-50: q12-18h, <10: q18-24h

Octreotide	EHL 1.5h, PRC B, Lact ?
Sandostatin *Inj 0.05mg/ml, 0.1mg/ml, 0.2mg/ml, 0.5mg/ml, 1mg/ml* **Sandostatin Lar Depot** *Inj 10mg, 20mg, 30mg/vial*	**Acromegaly** ›183: 50 100µg SC tid, depot 20mg IM q4wk x 3mo, then q4wk according to GH level; **carcinoid tumors** →185: 100-600µg/d SC bid-qid or depot 20mg IM q4wk x 2 mo, then q4wk prn; **vipomas** →184: 200-300µg/d SC bid-qid or depot 20mg IM q4wk x 2 mo, then q4wk prn; also in **esophageal varices, bleeding**; DARF: req in severe RF
Secretin	EHL no data, PRC C
SecreFlo *Inj. 16µg/vial*	**Diagnosis of pancreatic exocrine dysfunction:** 0.2µg/kg over 1 min IV; **diagnosis of gastrinoma:** 0.4µg/kg over 1 min IV
Tegaserod	EHL 11h, PRC B, Lact ?
Zelnorm *Tab 2mg, 6mg*	**Irritable bowel syndrome, women**: 6mg PO bid for 4-6wk; DARF: contraind. in severe RF
Vasopressin	EHL 10-20min, PRC C, Lact ?
Pitressin *Inj 20 U/ml*	**GI hemorrhage/esophageal varices**: ini 0.2-0.4 U/min IV, incr by 0.2 U/min q1h, max 0.9 U/min; **diabetes insipidus** →183: 5-10U SC/IM bid-tid prn →159

Drug pocket 2005 for PDA (460 kb, US $ 16.95)
Drug Therapy pocket for PDA (840 kb, US $ 16.95)
Homeopathy pocket for PDA (2040 kb, US $ 16.95)
ICD-9-CM 2004 pocket for PDA
(5323 kb, US $ 24.95)
Medical Abbreviations pocket for PDA
(1279 kb, US $ 16.95)
Medical Spanish pocket for PDA
(670 kb, US $ 16.95)
Medical Spanish Dictionary pocket for PDA
(2343 kb, US $ 16.95)
Medical Spanish pocket plus
(2487 kb, US $ 24.95)
Differential Diagnosis pocket
(867 kb, US $ 24.95)
ECG pocket (670 kb, US $ 24.95)
coming soon: Normal Values pocket
(5323 kb, US $ 16.95)

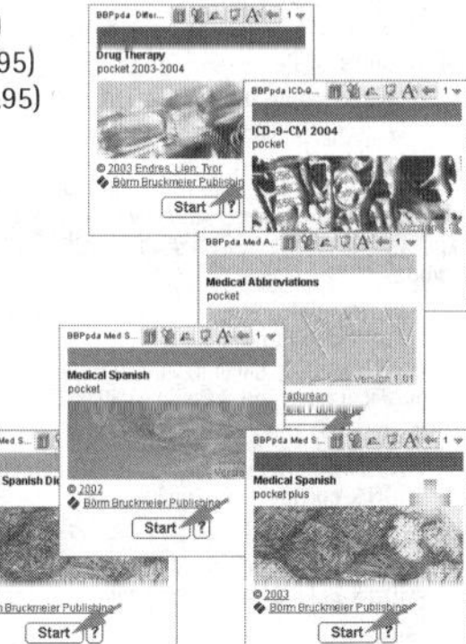

 Online-Shop, PDA demo files, FAQs...

http://pda. **media4u** .com

5 B.   Gastroenterology – Therapies

Stefan Endres, MD
Chief, Division of Clinical Pharmacology
University of Munich, Munich, Germany

5 B.1   Esophagitis

5 B.1.1   Gastroesophageal Reflux Disease (GERD)

Grade I/II (endoscopy: erythema–non-confluent erosions)

	Antacid →120 (acid binding)	**Al Hydroxide + Mg Hydroxide** (Maalox)	*10ml PO qid-6x/d prn*
or	**Proton pump inhibitor** →118 (acid secretion ↓)	**Omeprazole** (Prilosec, Gens)	*20mg PO qd for 4wk, if ineffective for another 4wk; in relapse 40mg qd*
		Lansoprazole (PrevAcid)	*30mg PO qd for 4-8wk*

Grade III/IV (endoscopy: confluent erosions – ulcer, stricture)

	Proton pump inhibitor →118 (acid secretion ↓)	**Omeprazole** (Prilosec, Gens)	*20-40mg PO qd for 8-12wk*

64.   DeVault KR, Castell DO. Updated guidelines for the diagnosis and treatment of gastroesophageal reflux disease. Am J Gastroenterol 1999;94:1434-42
65.   Galmiche JP, Letessier E, Scarpignato C. Treatment of gastro-oesophageal reflux disease in adults. BMJ 1998; 316: 1720-1723
66.   Moss SF, J Clin Gastroenterol 1998, 27, 6-12

Maintenance of Remission

	Proton pump inhibitor →118 (acid secretion ↓)	**Omeprazole** (Prilosec, Gens)	*20mg PO qd, max 40mg qd; try to red after 6mo, sometimes life-long Tx*

67.   Venables TL, Scand J Gastroenterol, 1997, 32(7), 627-32

5 B.1.2   Infectious Esophagitis

Candida

	Antifungal →217 (azole derivative)	**Fluconazole** (Diflucan)	*d1: 200mg PO qd, then: 100mg PO qd for 14d*

68.   Rex JH, Walsh TJ, Sobel JD, et al. Practice guidelines for the treatment of candidiasis. Infectious Diseases Society of America. Clin Infect Dis. 2000;30:662-678

Herpes simplex

	Antiviral →209 (DNA-polymerase inhib.)	**Famciclovir** (Famvir)	*250mg PO tid for 14d*

Cytomegaly virus

	Antiviral →209 (DNA-polymerase inhib.)	**Ganciclovir** (Cytovene)	*5mg/kg IV bid for 14d*

5 B.2   Achalasia (Dysphagia)

poss	Ca^{++} channel blocker →28 (muscle relaxation)	Nifedipine (Adalat, Procardia, Gens)	*20mg SL ac prn*
poss	Nitrate →36 (muscle relaxation)	Isosorbide dinitrate (Isordil, Sorbitrate, Gens)	*10mg SL ac prn*
poss	Muscle relaxant (acetylcholine release ↓)	Botulinum toxin (Botox)	*Endoscopic Inj of the LES prn, see Prod Info*
poss	**Surgical intervention**: Graded pneumatic dilation or Surgical myotomy		

69.   Vaezi MF, Richter JE. Diagnosis and Management of Achalasia. Am J Gastroenterol 1999;94:3406-3412

5 B.3   Gastritis
5 B.3.1   Acute Erosive Gastritis

	Antacid →120 (acid binding)	Al Hydroxide + Mg Hydroxide (Maalox)	*10ml PO qid-6x/d for a few days*
poss	H$_2$ Antagonist →117 (acid secretion ↓)	Ranitidine (Zantac, Gens)	*300mg PO qpm for a few days*

5 B.3.2   Stress Lesion Prophylaxis

	Antiulcer drug →117 (formation of a film ⇒ mucosa protection)	Sucralfate (Carafate, Gens)	*1g PO qid*

5 B.3.3   Type A in Pernicious Anemia

poss	Vitamin B12 →145 (substitution)	Cyanocobalamin (Rubramin PC, Vibisone, Gens)	*1000µg/wk IM for 1-3wk, then 1000µg/mo IM (lifelong)*

5 B.4   Peptic Ulcer Disease (PUD)
5 B.4.1   PUD without Proof of Helicobacter

Uncomplicated

	H$_2$ Antagonist →117 (acid secretion ↓)	Ranitidine (Zantac)	*300mg PO qpm for 3-6wk*

Complicated (hemorrhage, obstruction, perforation)

	Proton pump inhibitor →118 (acid secretion ↓)	Omeprazole (Prilosec, Gens)	*80mg as short IV inf over 30min, then 200mg IV qd for 3d, then 20mg PO qd for 3wk*
or		Lansoprazole (PrevAcid)	*30mg PO qd*

Maintenance of Remission

	H$_2$ Antagonist →118 (acid secretion ↓)	Ranitidine (Zantac)	*150mg PO qpm*

70.   Schattalitzky de Muckadell OB, Scand J Gastroenterol, 1997, 32(4), 320-7

5 B.4.2   PUD with Proof of Helicobacter

„Italian" triple therapy

	Proton pump inhibitor →118 (acid secretion ↓)	**Omeprazole** (Prilosec, Gens)	*20mg PO bid (1h ac) for 14d*
or		**Lansoprazole (PrevAcid)**	*30mg PO bid (1h ac) for 14d*
plus	**Macrolide** →199 (HP eradication)	**Clarithromycin** (Biaxin)	*500mg PO bid for 14d*
plus	**Nitroimidazole** →118 (HP eradication)	**Metronidazole** (Protostat, Gens)	*500mg PO bid for 14d*

„French" triple therapy as second therapy in failure

	Proton pump inhibitor →118 (acid secretion ↓)	**Omeprazole** (Prilosec, Gens)	*20mg PO bid (1h ac) for 10-14d*
or		**Lansoprazole (PrevAcid)**	*30mg PO bid (1h ac) for 10-14d*
plus	**Macrolide** →118 (HP eradication)	**Clarithromycin** (Biaxin)	*500mg PO bid for 10-14d*
plus	**Aminopenicillin** →118 (HP eradication)	**Amoxicillin** (Amoxil, Larotid, Trimox, Wymox, Gens)	*1g PO bid for 10-14d*

Eradication therapy in patients that cannot be treated orally

	Proton pump inhibitor →118 (acid secretion ↓)	**Omeprazole** (Prilosec)	*200mg IV cont inf qd (switch to PO Tx asap)*
plus	**Nitroimidazole** →118 (HP eradication)	**Metronidazole** (Flagyl, Metro, Gens)	*500mg IV tid (switch to PO Tx asap)*
plus	**Aminopenicillin** →118 (HP eradication)	**Amoxicillin** (Amoxil, Larotid, Trimox, Wymox, Gens)	*1g IV tid (switch to PO Tx asap)*

71.   Salcedo JA, Al-Kawas F: Treatment of Helicobacter pylori infection. Arch Intern Med 1998 Apr 27; 158(8): 842-51
72.   Soll AH: Consensus conference. Medical treatment of peptic ulcer disease. Practice guidelines. Practice Parameters Committee of the American College of Gastroenterology. JAMA 1996 Feb 28; 275(8): 622-9

5 B.5   Diverticular Disease

	Fluoroquinolone →203	**Ciprofloxacin** (Cipro)	*500mg PO bid for 7-10d*
plus	**Nitroimidazole** →206	**Metronidazole** (Flagyl, Gens)	*500mg PO tid for 7-10d*

73.   Sanford, Guide to Antimicrobial Therapy, 30th edition, 2000, page 14

5 B.6   Crohn's Disease
5 B.6.1   Acute Exacerbation

	Glucocorticoid →148 (anti-inflammatory, immunosuppressive)	**Prednisolone** (Onapred, Pediapred, Prelone, Gens)	*60mg PO qd over 6wk, red to 10mg PO qd (wk to mo)*
or	**Cyclooxygenase inhibitor** →125 (anti-inflammatory)	**Mesalamine** (Asacol/Tab, Pentasa/Cap)	*800mg Tab PO tid (Asacol) or 1g Cap PO tid (Pentasa)*

5 B.6.2   Acute Exacerbation with Fistulas

plus	**Nitroimidazole** →206 (antibiotic)	**Metronidazole** (Flagyl, Metromidol, Gens)	*500mg PO tid for <10d*

5 B.6.3   Maintenance of Remission

Cyclooxigenase inhibitor →125 (anti-inflammatory)	**Mesalamine** (Asacol/Tab, Pentasa/Cap)	*800mg Tab PO tid (Asacol) or 1g Cap PO tid (Pentasa) for 1yr*

5 B.6.4   Chronic Active Disease, Refractory Disease

Purine antagonist →260 (immunosuppressive)	**Azathioprine** (Imuran, Gens)	*2mg/kg PO qd (effect after 2-4wk)*

5 B.6.5   Refractory Disease with Fistulas

Immunomodulator →128 (anti-TNFα antibodies)	**Infliximab** (Remicade)	*5mg/kg IV inf over 2h, rep at 2wk and 6wk prn*

74. Hanauer SB and Sandborn W. Management of Crohn's Disease in Adults. Am J Gastroenterol March 2001;96:635-643
75. Schreiber S, et al. Use of anti-tumour necrosis factor agents in inflammatory bowel disease. European guidelines for 2001-2003. Int J Colorectal Dis, 200116:1-11

5 B.7   Ulcerative Colitis
5 B.7.1   Acute Exacerbation

	Cyclooxigenase inhibitor →125 (anti-inflammatory)	**Mesalamine** (Asacol/Tab, Canasa/PR, Pentasa/Cap, Rowasa/PR)	*Pancolitis: 000mg Tab PO tid or 1g Cap (4 x 250mg) PO tid; in distal involvement: 1g PR qd*
In Tx failure plus	**Glucocorticoid** →148 (anti-inflammatory, immunosuppressive)	**Prednisolone** (Onapred, Pediapred, Prelone, Gens)	*40mg PO qd over 6wk, red to 10mg PO qd (red further over wk to mo)*

5 B.7.2   Maintenance of Remission

Cyclooxigenase inhibitor →125	**Mesalamine** (Pentasa/Cap)	*500mg Cap PO tid for 2yr*

5 B.7.3   Refractory Disease

Purine antagonist →260 (immunosuppressive)	**Azathioprine** (Imuran, Gens)	*2.5mg/kg PO qd (effect after 2-4wk)*

76. Kornbluth A, Sachar DB: Ulcerative colitis practice guidelines in adults. American College of Gastroenterology, Practice Parameters Committee. Am J Gastroenterol 1997 Feb;92(2):204-11
77. Sands BE: Therapy of inflammatory bowel disease. Gastroenterology 2000 Feb; 118(2 Suppl 1): S68-82

5 B.8 Pancreatitis
5 B.8.1 Acute Pancreatitis

Basic therapy

	Glucose electrolyte solution (volume substitution)	**Glucose 5% + Ringer's solution (1:1)**	*> 3l/d, according to CVP*
	Opioid →271 (analgesia without spasmogenic effects on Oddi's sphincter)	**Buprenorphine** (Buprenex, Gens)	*0.15mg IV q6h prn*
or		**Meperidine** (Demerol, Gens)	*15-35mg/h IV; 50-150mg IM q3-4h*
poss	**Calcium preparation** →139 (replacement)	**Calcium gluconate 10%** (4.5meq/ml)	*10-20ml slowy IV prn*
poss	**H₂ Antagonist** →117 (stomach acid secretion ↓ ⇒ pancreas secretion ↓)	**Ranitidine** (Zantac, Gens)	*50mg IV tid*

In biliary/necrotizing pancreatitis

	Cephalosporin →195	**Ceftriaxone** (Rocephin)	*1-2g IM/IV qd (or div bid)*
or	**Acylaminopenicillin** →189	**Ampicillin** (Omnipen, Principen, Totacillin, Gens)	*500-1000mg IV q6h*
or	**Acylaminopenicillin + lactamase inhibitor** →191	**Ampicillin + Sulbactam** (Unasyn)	*2+1g IV q6h*

Banks P. Practice guidelines in acute pancreatitis. Am J Gastroenterology. 92(3):377-386, 1997

5 B.8.2 Chronic Pancreatitis

	Exocr. pancreas enzymes →126 (enzyme substitution)	**Pancreatin** (Creon, Donnazyme, Ultrase)	*1-2 Tab/Cap PO with each meal (100.000 IU/d), poss life-long*
poss	**Fat soluble vitamins** →145 (substitution)	**Vitamins A, D, E, K**	*1ml q2wk IM prn*
poss	**Analgesic (aniline)** →269 (inhibits cyclooxygenase)	**Acetaminophen** (Tylenol, Gens)	*1000mg PO qid*
poss	**Opioid (analgesic)** →274	**Tramadol** (Ultram)	*50-100mg PO qid*

78.   Sanford, Guide to Antimicrobial Therapy, 30th edition, 2000

5 B.9 Hepatitis
5 B.9.1 Acute Viral Hepatitis A

poss	**Bile acid sequestrant** →41 (binding of bile acid ⇒ inhibition of pruritus)	**Cholestyramine** (Locholest, Prevalite, Questran, Gens)	*4-16g PO qd prn*
poss	**H₁-Antihistamine** →409 (inhibition of pruritus)	**Loratadine** (Claritin)	*10mg PO qd prn*

5 B.9.2   Chronic Viral Hepatitis B

or	**Alpha-Interferon** →212 (immunostimulating and directly antiviral)	**INF Alpha-2A** (Roferon A) **INF Alpha-2B** (Intron A)	*6 M IU tiw SC for 6mo* *5 M IU tiw SC for 6mo*
or	**Antiviral** →209 (nucleoside analogue)	**Lamivudine** (Epivir-HBV)	*100mg PO qd for 4yr or up to 6mo after anti-HBe seroconversion*

5 B.9.3   Chronic Viral Hepatitis C

	Peginterferon →212 (immunostimulating, antiviral; complexed to increase half-life)	**PEG-IFN Alpha-2A** (Pegasys) **PEG-IFN Alpha-2B** (Peg-Intron)	*180µg SC qwk* *1.5µg/kg SC qwk*
	Admin for 6mo; admin for 12mo, if genotype 1 or >2 risk factors (male, >40yr, signs of liver reorganisation, >3.5 M copies/ml)		
plus	**Antiviral** →209 (nucleoside analogue, immunostimulating and directly antiviral)	**Ribavirin** (Rebetol)	*1000mg PO qd (1200mg in BW >75kg; 800mg in BW <60kg); Dur of Tx see Interferon*

5 B.9.4   Autoimmune Hepatitis

	Glucocorticoid →148 (anti-inflammatory, immunosuppressive)	**Prednisolone** (Onapred, Pediapred, Prelone, Gens)	*40-60mg PO qd over 6wk, red to 10mg PO qd, maint Tx for up to 2yr*
poss	**Immunosuppressant** →260 (purine antagonist)	**Azathioprine** (Imuran, Gens)	*2mg/kg PO qd (effects after 2-4mo)*

79.   Manns MP, McHutchison JG, Gordon SC, et al. Peginterferon alfa-2b plus ribavirin compared with interferon alfa-2b plus ribavirin for initial treatment of chronic hepatitis C: a randomised trial. Lancet 2001 Sep 22;358(9286):958-965

5 B.10   Cirrhosis
5 B.10.1   General Measures

Ascites therapy

	Aldosterone antagonist →28 (volume relief)	**Spironolactone** (Aldactone, Gens)	*d1-5: 50-100mg PO bid-qid, then: 50-100mg qd-bid (max BW ↓ 500g/d)*
poss	**Loop diuretic** →33 (volume relief)	**Furosemide** (Lasix, Gens)	*20-40mg PO qd-bid (max BW ↓ 500g/d)*

Vitamin substitution

poss	**Fat soluble Vitamins** →145 (substitution)	**Vitamins A, D, E, K**	*1ml IM q2wk (in proven deficiency)*
poss	**B-Vitamins** →145 (substitution)	**Vitamins B1 + B6 + B12 + Folic acid** (Gens)	*See Prod Info (in proven deficiency)*

Alcoholism, see Psychiatry →339, →341

5 B.10.2 Primary Biliary Cirrhosis

	Cholic acid derivative →127 (cholesterol secretion ↓, cholesterol resorption ↓)	**Ursodiol (Ursodeoxycholic acid)** (Actigall, Urso)	*15mg/kg PO qd (life-long)*
poss	**Bile acid sequestrant** →41 (binding of bile acid ⇒ inhibition of pruritus)	**Cholestyramine** (Locholest, Prevalite, Questran, Gens)	*4g PO qd-bid prn, alternating with ursodiol and fat soluble vit.)*
or poss	**H₁-Antihistamine** →409 (inhibition of pruritus)	**Loratadine** (Claritin)	*10mg PO qd prn*

Beers MH, Berkow R: Primary Biliary Cirrhosis. The Merck Manual of Diagnosis and Therapy. 1999

5 B.10.3 Primary Sclerosing Cholangitis

	Cholic acid derivative →127 (cholesterol secretion ↓, cholesterol resorption ↓)	**Ursodiol (Ursodeoxycholic acid)** (Actigall, Urso)	*15mg/kg PO qd (life-long)*

5 B.10.4 Portal Hypertension

Primary prophylaxis of bleeding from esophageal varices

poss	**Betablocker** →23 (CO ↓, portal vein pressure ↓)	**Propranolol** (Inderal, Gens)	*Ini 20mg PO tid (goal: HR decrease of 25%)*

Bleeding from esophageal varices

poss	**Somatostatin analogue** →128 (splanchnic vasoconstriction ⇒ portal vein pressure ↓)	**Octreotide** (Sandostatin)	*25µg/h IV*
poss	**Fluoroquinolone** →203 (antibiotic)	**Ciprofloxacin** (Cipro)	*Prophylactic: 500mg PO bid for 7d*

Medical Care
- Initial resuscitation with replacement of blood volume loss
- Endoscopic injection sclerotherapy, balloon-tube tamponade
- Surgical intervention: portal systemic shunts, selective shunts, splenectomy, liver transplantation

80.   Garcia-Tsao G: Current management of the complications of cirrhosis and portal hypertension: variceal hemorrhage, ascites, and spontaneous bacterial peritonitis. Gastroenterology 2001 Feb; 120(3): 726-48

5 B.10.5 Hepatic Encephalopathy, Hepatic Coma

poss	**Osmotic Laxative** →120 (laxative, NH₃ elimination)	**Lactulose** (Cephulac, Cholac, Chronulac, Constilac, Constulose, Enulose, Evalose, Heptalac, Laxilose)	*20-30ml PO tid*
or poss	**Aminoglycoside** →200 (intestinal sterilization)	**Neomycin** (Mycifradin, Neo-rx, Gens)	*2g PO qd-bid*

81.   Blei AT and Córdoba J. Hepatic Encephalopathy. Am J Gastroenterol, 2001;96:1968-1976.

5 B.11   Cholelithiasis
5 B.11.1 Oral Bile Acid Dissolution Therapy

Stone: < 10mm, **not** calcareous, **not** > 2 concrements, contractible gall bladder

Cholic acid derivative →127 (cholesterol secretion↓, cholesterol resorption↓)	**Ursodiol (Ursodeoxycholic acid)** (Actigall, Urso)	*10mg/kg PO qd with food (div qid) for up to 3mo after litholysis*

5 B.11.2 Maintenance of Remission

Cholic acid derivative →127 (cholesterol secretion↓, cholesterol resorption↓)	**Ursodiol (Ursodeoxycholic acid)** (Actigall, Urso)	*300mg PO qd (long-term Tx)*

5 B.12 Biliary Colic

	Analgesic, NSAID →265 (activity of cyclooxygenase↓)	**Ketorolac** (Acular PF, Toradol, Gens)	*Ini 30-60mg IM, then 15-30mg IM q6h; or 15-30mg IV prn; not to exceed 120mg/d*
plus/or	**Analgesic, opioid** →270 (analgesia without spasmogenic effects on Oddi's sphincter)	**Meperidine** (Demerol, Gens)	*50-150mg PO/IV/IM/SC q3-4h prn*
Plus	**Antiemetic** →125 (dopamine rec. antag.)	**Metoclopramide** (Reglan, Gens)	*10mg IV q6h prn*
or	**Antiemetic** →125 (inhibits dopamine receptors)	**Prochlorperazine** (Compazine, Compro, Gens)	*5-10mg IM/PO q6h prn; not to exceed 40mg/d*

5 B.13 Cholecystitis, Cholangitis

Acylaminopenicillin + lactamase inhibitor →191	**Piperacillin + Tazobactam** (Zosyn)	*3 + 0.375g IV tid*
Antiemetic, antidopaminergic →124 (stimuli to brainstem reticular system↓)	**Promethazine** (Phenergan, Gens)	*12.5-25mg PO/IV/IM/PR q4-6h prn*

6 A. Metabolic, Endocrine – Drugs

6 A.1 Antigout Drugs
6 A.1.1 Uricosurics

MA/EF: inhibition of tubular uric acid reabsorption ⇒ uricosuric agent
AE: initial gout attack, N/V, headache, urate calculus, GI distress, rash, blood dyscrasias, nephrotic syndrome
CI: kidney stones, renal insufficiency, hypersensitivity to bromide + probenecid, < 2y, salicylate use, initiation-gouty attack, blood dyscrasias

Probenecid	EHL 3-17h, PRC B, Lact ?
Probalan *Tab 500mg* **Probampacin** *Susp 3.5g/bot, 1g/bot* **Generics** *Tab 500mg*	**Gout** →171: 250mg PO bid for 7d, then 500mg PO bid; penicillin-therapy: 2g/d PO in div doses; **CH** 2-14 y: ini 25mg/kg PO, then 40mg/kg div qid; DARF: GFR (ml/min) >50: 100%, <50: not rec

6 A.1.2 Xanthine Oxidase Inhibitors

MA/EF: inhibition of xanthine oxidase ⇒ uric acid formation ↓ (uricostatic agent)
AE: N/V, allergic reactions, leukopenia, xanthic calculus, pruritus, rash, myelosuppression, hepatotoxicity

Allopurinol	EHL 1-2h, PRC C, Lact ?
Alloprin *Inj 500mg/vial* **Lopurin** *Tab 100mg, 300mg* **Zyloprim** *Tab 100mg, 300mg* **Generics** *Tab 100mg, 300mg*	**Mild gout** →171: 200-300mg PO qd; **moderate – severe gout**: 400-600mg PO qd; **secondary hyperuricemia**: 100-200mg qd, max 800mg/d; **calcium oxalate stones** →433: 200-300mg PO qd; **chemotherapy with expected cell lysis**: ini 200-400mg/square meter IV qd or div bid or qid; **CH hyperuricemia**: 10mg/kg/d PO div tid; **secondary hyperuricemia**: <6y: 150mg PO qd; 6-10y: 300mg PO qd; DARF: GFR (ml/min): 10-20: 200mg/d, <10: 100mg/d

6 A.1.3 Other Antigout Drugs

MA/EF (colchicine): prevention of phagocytosis of deposited urate crystals by leukocytes which release of inflammatory agents ⇒ antimitotic agent
AE (colchicine): diarrhea, N/V, epigastric pain, leukopenia, myelosuppression, myoneuropathy, alopecia
CI (colchicine): hypersensitivity to colchicine, blood dyscrasias, children < 2y

Colchicine	EHL 4.4h, PRC D, Lact +
Generics *Tab 0.5mg, 0.6mg, Inj 0.5mg/ml*	**Acute gout** →171: ini 1-1.2mg PO, then 0.5- 1.2mg PO q1-2h until symptoms abate or AE occur, max 8mg/d PO; 2mg IV, then 0.5mg IV q6h, max 4mg/d IV

Colchicine + Probenecid	PRC D, Lact +
Colbenemid *Tab 0.5mg + 500mg* **Col-Probenecid** *Tab 0.5mg + 500mg*	**Gout** →171: ini 0.5mg + 500mg PO qd for 7d, then 0.5mg + 500mg bid; DARF: GFR (ml/min) <30: not rec

6 A.2 Ions, Minerals
6 A.2.1 Potassium

AE: N/V, belching, heartburn, flatulence, abdominal pain, diarrhea, mucosal ulcers, GI hemorrhage, ECG changes
CI: hyperkalemia, hyperchloremia, renal insufficiency, Addison's disease, acute dehydration, heat cramps

Potassium Chloride	PRC C, Lact ?
Cena-k, Kaochlor, Kaon Cl, Kay Ciel, **K⁺ Care, K-Dur, K-Lor, Klor-Con, Klotrix, K-lyte,** **Micro-K, Rum-K, Slow-K** *Tab (ext.rel) 6.7mEq, 8mEq, 10mEq, 20mEq, 750mg,* *1500mg,* *Tab (efferv) 20mEq, 25mEq, 50mEq,* *Cap (ext.rel) 600mg, 750mg,* *Powder 15mEq/pkt, 20mEq/pkt, 25mEq/pkt, Liquid* *20mEq/15ml, 30mEq/15ml, 40mEq/15ml,* *45mEq/15ml*	**Hypokalemia Tx** →163: 40-100mEq/d PO; 40-300mEq/d IV, max 40mEq/liter, max 15mEq/h; **hypokalemia PRO:** 20-40mEq/d PO qd-bid

6 A.2.2 Calcium

AE (calcium IV): sensation of heat, fits of perspiration, BP o, N/V, arrhythmias
CI (calcium IV): hypercalcemia, nephrocalcinosis, digitalis intoxication, severe renal insuff.

Calcium Acetate	PRC C, Lact ?
PhosLo *Tab 667mg, Cap 667mg (169mg Ca)* **Generics** *Inj 0.5mEq/ml*	**Hyperphosphatemia in end-stage RF** →432: ini 2 Tab PO tid with each meal, adjust dose based on serum phosphate; most patients require 3-4 Tab with each meal

Calcium Carbonate	PRC C, Lact +
Alka-Mints *Tab (chew) 340mg* **Calci-Chew** *Tab (chew) 500mg* **Calci-Mix** *Cap 500mg* **Caltrate** *Tab 600mg* **Chooz** *Tab (chew) 200mg* **Liqui-Cal** *Cap 240mg* **Mallamint** *Tab (chew) 168mg* **Nephro-Calci** *Tab 600mg* **Os-Cal** *Tab 500mg, Tab (chew) 500mg* **Titralac** *Tab (chew) 168mg, 300mg* **Tums** *Tab (chew) 200, 300, 400, 500mg* **Generics** *Susp 500mg/5ml, Tab 260mg, 500mg,* *Tab (chew) 500mg*	**Hypocalcemia** →164: 1-2g PO qd; **osteoporosis PRO** →172: 1-1.5g PO qd; **RDA:** 1200mg PO qd
Calcium Chloride	PRC C, Lact ?
Generics *Inj 10% (1.36 mEq/ml)*	**Hypocalcemia** →164: 500-1000mg IV q1-3d; **magnesium intoxication** →165: 500mg IV; **hyperkalemia** →163: dose must be titrated by ECG-changes
Calcium Citrate	PRC C, Lact ?
Citracal *Tab 200mg, Tab (efferv) 500mg*	→164
Calcium Gluceptate	PRC C, Lact ?
Generics *Inj 22% (0.9mEq/ml)*	→164
Calcium Gluconate	PRC C, Lact ?
Generics *Tab 45mg, 58.5mg, 90mg;* *Inj 10% Sol (0.46mEq/ml)*	**Hypocalcemia** →164: 0.5-2g slowly IV; 500-1000mg PO bid-qid

6 A.2.3 Magnesium

AE: sleepiness, diarrhea, CNS disturbances, arrhythmias, muscle weakness, respiratory depression, flushing, hypotension
CI: restricted use in case of depressed renal function, 2 hrs preceding delivery, heart block; IV: AV block, myasthenia gravis

Magnesium Gluconate	PRC A, Lact +
Magonate *Tab 500mg (27mg Mg), Liquid 54mg* *Mg/5ml*	**Hypomagnesemia** →165: 100-600mg/d elemental magnesium PO div tid
Magnesium Oxide	PRC B, Lact ?
Mag-Ox *Tab 400mg [241.3mg Mg (19.86mEq)]* **Uro-Mag** *Cap 140mg, [84.5mg Mg (6.93 mEq)]* **Generics** *Cap 400mg [84.5mg Mg (6.93 mEq)],* *420mg*	**Hypomagnesemia** →165: 100-600mg/d elemental magnesium PO div tid

Magnesium Sulfate | PRC A, Lact +

Generics *Inj 80mg/ml, 500mg/ml, Inj 1g/100ml, 2g/100ml , 4g/100ml*

Ventricular arrhythmias →62: 1–6g IV over several min, then 3–20mg/min IV for 5–48h; **preeclampsia, eclampsia**: 4g IV, simultaneously 4–5g IM each buttock; preterm labor: 4–6g IV over 20min, then 1–3g/h IV

6 A.2.4   Fluoride

AE: N/V, diarrhea
CI: areas where water fluoride content is greater than 0.7ppm

Fluoride | PRC no data currently available , Lact ?

Flura–Drops *Sol 5mg/ml*
Flura–Tab *Tab 1mg*
Flura–Loz *Tab (chew) 0.25mg*
Fluoritab *Sol 5mg/ml,*
Tab (chew) 25mg, 0.5mg, 1mg
Luride *Sol 0.5mg/ml,*
Tab (chew) 0.25mg, 0.5mg, 1mg
Pediaflor *Sol 0.5mg/ml*

Osteoporosis →172: 25mg PO bid (in combination with calcium citrate 400mg bid)

6 A.2.5   Phosphorous

Phosphorous | PRC no data, Lact no data

K–Phos *Tab phosphorus/sodium/potassium 250mg/298mg/45mg, Tab 500mg (phosphorus/ potassium 114mg/144mg)*

Severe hypophosphatemia (< 1mg/dl): 1–3g PO/PR; **CH** 2–4mmol/kg/d PO

6 A.2.6   Iron

AE: N/V, diarrhea, constipation, dark-colored stools, when used intravenously: headaches, thrombophlebitis, allergic reactions, collapse
CI: hemochromatosis, chronic hemolysis, iron utilization impairment, peptic ulcers, ulcerative colitis

Ferrous Fumarate | PRC C, Lact +

Feostat *Susp 45mg(15mg iron)/0.6ml, 100mg (33mg iron)/5ml, Tab (chew) 100mg (33mg iron)*
Ircon *Tab 200mg (66mg iron)*
Hemocyte *324mg (106mg iron)*
Nephro–Fer *Tab 350mg (115mg iron)*
Generics *Tab 325mg (107mg iron)*

Iron deficiency →80: 2–3mg/kg/d elemental iron PO div bid–tid

Ferrous Gluconate | PRC C, Lact +

Fergon *Tab 240mg (27mg iron), 320mg (37mg iron)*
Generics *Tab 300mg (35mg iron), 325mg (38mg iron)*

Iron deficiency →80: 2–3mg/kg/d elemental iron PO div bid–tid

Ferrous Polysaccharide	PRC C, Lact +
Ferrex *Cap 150mg* **Fe-Tinic** *Cap 150mg* **Hytinic** *Cap 150mg* **Niferex** *Tab 50mg, Cap 150mg, Sol 100mg/5ml* **Nu-Iron** *Cap 150mg, Sol 100mg/5ml*	**Iron deficiency** →80: 2-3mg/kg/d elemental iron PO div bid-tid
Ferrous Sulfate	PRC C, Lact +
Feosol *Sol 220mg(44mg iron)/5ml,* *Tab 325mg (65mg iron), 200mg (65mg iron),* *Caplet 45mg iron/caplet* **Fer-Gen-Sol** *Sol 125mg(25mg iron)/ml,* **Fer-In-Sol** *Sol 90mg(18mg iron)/5ml, 125mg* *(25mg iron)/ml, Tab 325mg (65mg iron), Cap 190mg* *(60mg iron)* **Fero-Gradumet** *Tab 525mg (105mg iron)* **Mol-Iron** *Tab 195mg (39ng iron)* **Generics** *Sol 300mg(60mg iron)/5ml,* *Cap (ext.rel) 150mg (30mg iron), 250mg* *(50mg iron), Tab 300mg (60mg iron), 325mg* *(65mg iron)*	**Iron deficiency** →80: 2-3mg/kg/d elemental iron PO div bid-tid
Iron Dextran	PRC C, Lact +
DexFerrum *Inj 50mg/ml* **InFed** *Inj 50mg/ml* **Generics** *Inj 50mg/ml*	**Iron deficiency anemia** →80: total dose (ml) = 0.0442 x (desired Hb – observed Hb) x kg + [0.26 x kg] IV
Iron Sucrose	PRC C, Lact +
Venofer *Inj 100mg (iron)/5ml*	**Iron deficiency anemia in chronic hemodialysis** →80: 100mg IV 1-3x/wk up to a total of 1g, rep prn
Sodium Ferric Gluconate	PRC C, Lact +
Ferrlecit *Inj 62.5mg (iron)/5ml*	**Iron deficiency anemia in chronic hemodialysis** →80: 10ml (125mg iron) diluted in 100ml 0.9% NaCl IV over 1h; rep. for a total of 8 dialysis sessions (1g of iron)

6 A.3   Drugs Affecting Electrolyte Imbalances
6 A.3.1   Biphosphonates

MA/EГ: osteoclastic activity ↓ ⇒ osteal release of calcium ↓, bone degradation ↓
AE: allergic skin reactions, hypocalcemia, GI DO; **AE** (alendronate): abdominal pain, musculoskeletal pain, headache, diarrhea, constipation; **AE** (etidronate): loss of taste, osteomalacia, GI complaints, bone pain; **AE** (pamidronate): myelosuppression, HTN, thrombophlebitis, malaise, N/V; **AE** (risedronate): flu like syndrome, diarrhea, arthralgia, headache, abdominal pain, rash; **AE** (tiludronate): N/V/diarrhea, skin reactions, edema, chest pain; **CI:** renal insuff., acute GI inflamm., CH; **CI** (alendronate): hypersensitivity to alendronate products, hypocalcemia, esophageal DO, inability to stand or sit upright for 30min; **CI** (etidronate): hypersensitivity to etidronate products, osteomalacia; **CI** (pamidronate): hypersensitivity to biphosphonates; **CI** (risedronate): hypocalcemia, hypersensitivity to risedronate products ; **CI** (tiludronate): hypersensitivity to tiludronate products

Alendronate	EHL up to 10y, PRC C, Lact ?
Fosamax *Tab 5mg, 10mg, 35mg, 40mg, 70mg*	**Postmenopausal osteoporosis PRO** →172: 5mg PO qd or 35mg qwk; **postmenopausal osteoporosis Tx**: 10mg PO qd or 70mg qwk; **steroid-induced osteoporosis Tx**: 5mg PO qd (men and pre-menopausal women) or 10mg PO qd (postmenopausal women not taking estrogen); **Paget's disease** →174: 40mg PO qd for 6mo; DARF: GFR (ml/min) 35-60: 100%, <35: not rec
Etidronate	EHL 1-6h (nr); 6.3 G.7h (IV), PRC C, Lact -
Didronel *Tab 200mg, 400mg, Inj 50mg/ml*	**Paget's disease** →174: 5-10mg/kg/d PO for 6mo or 11-20mg/kg/d PO for 3mo; **heterotopic ossification with hip replacement**: 20mg/kg/d PO 1mo before and 3mo after surgery; **heterotopic ossification with spinal cord injury**: 20mg/kg/d PO for 2wk, then 10mg/kg/d PO for 10wk; **hypercalcemia** →164: 7.5mg/kg IV for 3d, then 20mg/kg/d for 30d; DARF: creatinine >5mg/dl: not rec
Ibandronate	EHL no data
Boniva *Tab 2.5mg*	**Postmenopausal osteoporosis**: →172 2.5mg PO qd
Pamidronate	EHL no data, PRC C, Lact ?
Aredia *Inj 30mg/vial, 60mg/vial, 90mg/vial*	**Moderate hypercalcemia** (Ca = 12-13.5mg/dl) →164: 60-90mg IV over 24h as single dose; **severe hypercalcemia** (Ca >13.5mg/dl): 90mg IV single dose over 24h, rep. prn after at least 7d; **Paget's disease** →174: 30mg IV over 4h qd for 3d; **osteolytic bone lesions**: 90mg IV over 4h q4wk; DARF: not req in patients who receive 90mg monthly; →93, →164

Risedronate	EHL 1.5h, PRC C, Lact ?
Actonel *Tab 5mg, 30mg*	**Paget's disease** →174: 30mg PO qd for 2 mo; **postmenopausal and steroid-induced osteoporosis** →172: 5mg PO qd; DARF: GFR (ml/min): >30: 100%, <30: not rec
Tiludronate	EHL 43-150h, PRC C, Lact ?
Skelid *Tab 200mg*	**Paget's disease** →174: 400mg PO qd for 3 mo; DARF: GFR (ml/min): >30: 100%, <30: not rec
Zoledronate	EHL 1.5h, PRC D, Lact -
Zometa *Inj 4mg/vial*	**Hypercalcemia of malignancy, multiple myeloma, osteolytic bone lesions** →93, →164: 4mg IV over 15min, rep. q3-4wk

6 A.3.2   Calcitonin

MA/EF: calcium and phosphate uptake in bone ↑, renal calcium and phosphate excretion ↑
AE: sensation of heat, flush, N/V, diarrhea, rash, depression, flu-like symptoms
CI: hypocalcemia, hypersensitivity to salmon calcitonin products

| **Calcitonin-Salmon** | EHL 1h, PRC C, Lact ? |
| **Calcimar** *Inj 200 U/ml*
 Miacalcin *Spray (nasal) 200 U/ml, Inj 200 U/ml* | **Postmenopausal osteoporosis** →172: 100 U SC/IM qd or qod; 200 U intranasal qd; **Paget's disease** →174: 50-100 U SC/IM qd or qod; **hypercalcemia** →164: 4 U/kg SC/IM q12h, incr prn to max 8 U/kg q6-12h |

6 A.3.3   Phosphate Binding Substances

MA: sevelamer is a polymer, free of calcium and aluminum
EF: inhibition of enteral phosphate resorption
AE: pain, N/V, diarrhea, constipation, flatulence, dyspepsia, dyspnea
CI: hypophosphatemia, ileus, bowel obstruction, hypersensitivity to sevelamer products

| **Sevelamer** | PRC C, Lact ? |
| **Renagel** *Cap 403mg* | **Hyperphosphatemia:** 2-4 Cap tid with meals, adjust dose based on serum phosphorus concentration |

6 A.3.4   Potassium Binding Resins

MA: enteral application of an insoluble synthetic material with sulphonic acid as basic structure; exchange of cations for neutralization of acid according to the cation concentrations in the intestinal lumen ⇒ binding and removal of potassium
AE: colonic necrosis, electrolyte abnormalities, constipation, hypocalcemia, N/V
CI: hypersensitivity to sodium polystyrene sulphonate, hypokalemia

Polystyrene Sulfonate	PRC C, Lact +
Kayexalate *Powder (oral, rect) 453.6g/bot* **Kionex** *Powder (oral, rect) 454g/bot* **SPS** *Susp (oral, rect) 15g/60ml* **Generics** *Susp (oral, rect) 15g/60ml, Powder (oral, rect) 454g/bot*	**Hyperkalemia** →163: 15g PO qd-qid; 30-50g retention enema q6h, retain for at least 30-60min

6 A.4   Vitamins
6 A.4.1   Vitamin B Group

AE (thiamine/vitamin B1): IV injection site reaction
AE (riboflavin/vitamin B2): urine discoloration
AE (pyridoxine/vitamin B6): neuropathy, N/V
CI: hypersensitivity product ingredients
CI (cyanocobalamin/vitamin B12): diarrhea, urticaria, pruritus, rash

Vitamin B1 (Thiamine)	EHL , PRC A, Lact +
Generics *Tab 25mg, 50mg, 100mg, 500mg, Inj 100mg/ml*	**RDA:** 1-1.6mg PO qd; **Wernicke's encephalopathy:** ini 100mg IV, then 50-100mg IV/IM qd; **beriberi:** 10-20mg IM tid for 2wk, then 5-30mg PO qd; **wet beriberi with heart failure:** 10-30mg IV tid
Vitamin B2 (Riboflavin)	EHL 1.4h, PRC A, Lact +
Generics *Tab 10mg*	**RDA:** 1.2-1.8mg PO qd; **riboflavin deficiency:** 5-25mg/d PO qd
Vitamin B6 (Pyridoxine)	EHL 15-20d, PRC A, Lact +
Generics *Tab 10mg, 25mg, 50mg, 100mg, 250mg*	**RDA:** 1.6-2.5mg PO qd; **pyridoxine deficiency:** 10-20mg PO qd for 3wk, then 2-5mg PO qd; **PRO of isoniazid neuropathy** →235: 25-50mg PO qd; **Tx of isoniazid neuropathies** →235: 50-200mg PO qd
Vitamin B12 (Cyanocobalamin)	PRC A, Lact +
Rubramin PC *Inj 1mg/ml* **Vibisone** *Inj 1mg/ml* **Generics** *Tab 1mg, Inj 0.1mg/ml, 1mg/ml*	**RDA:** 2µg PO qd; **vitamin B12 deficiency** →81: 25-250µg qd PO/intranasal; **pernicious anemia** →81: 100µg/d IM/SC for 6-7d, then 100µg/d IM/SC qod for 7d, then 100µg/d IM/SC q3-4d for 2-3wk, then 100µg qmo IM/SC

6 A.4.2   Vitamin C

AE: occasional osmotic diarrhea, kidney stones, renal insufficiency
CI: restricted use in oxaluric urolithiasis, thalassemia and hemochromatosis, hypersensitivity to vitamin C products

Ascorbic Acid (Vitamin C)	EHL , PRC C, Lact ?
Tab 100mg, 250mg, 500mg, Inj 500mg/ml	**RDA:** 60-95mg/d PO; **scurvy:** 300mg/d IV/PO for 7d, then 100mg PO qd

6 A.4.3 Vitamin D

AE (calcitriol): hypercalcemia, N/V, polydipsia, polyuria
AE (dihydrotachysterol): hypercalcemia, renal impairment, N/V
AE (doxercalciferol): headache/malaise, edema, dyspnea, hypercalcemia
CI (calcitriol): hypercalcemia, vitamin D toxicity, hypersensitivity to calcitriol products
CI (dihydrotachysterol): hypercalcemia, hypersensitivity to dihydrotachysterol products
CI (doxercalciferol): hypercalcemia or vitamin D toxicity

Calcitriol	EHL 5-8h, PRC C, Lact ?
Calcijex *Inj 1µg/ml, Inj 2µg/ml* **Rocaltrol** *Cap 0.25µg, Cap 0.5µg,* *Sol (oral) 1µg/ml*	**Hypocalcemia in dialysis patients** →432: ini 0.25µg PO qd, incr by 0.25µg q4–8 wk until normocalcemic, most dialysis patients respond to 0.5–1µg/d PO or 1–2µg IV tiw; **hypoparathyroidism** →181: 0.25µg PO qd; incr prn q2–4wk up to 2µg/d
Dihydrotachysterol (Vitamin D)	EHL no data, PRC C, Lact ?
DHT *Tab 0.125mg, 0.2mg, 0.4mg* *Sol (oral) 0.2mg/5ml*	**Hypoparathyroidism** →181: ini 0.8–2.4mg PO qd for several d, maint 0.2–1mg PO qd
Doxercalciferol	EHL alpha,25-(OH)2D2 32–37h, PRC B, Lact ?
Hectorol *Cap 2.5µg, Inj 2µg/ml*	**Secondary hyperparathyroidism** →181: 10µg PO tiw

6 A.4.4 Vitamin D Analogs

AE: N/V
CI: hypersensitivity to vitamin D analogs, hypercalcemia, vitamin D toxicity

Paricalcitol	EHL 5-7h, PRC C, Lact ?
Zemplar *Inj. 5µg/ml*	**Secondary hyperparathyroidism** →181: 0.04–0.1µg/kg IV tiw

6 A.4.5 Vitamin E

AE: bleeding DO
CI: hypersensitivity to vitamin E products, IV use in low birth-weight infants, caution in coagulation DO or anticoagulant Tx, topical use in recent chemical peel or dermabrasion

Tocopherol (Vitamin E)	EHL , PRC A, Lact +
Generics *Tab, Cap, Susp, Oint*	**RDA:** 8–10mg PO qd; **vitamin E deficiency**: 4–5 times the RDA

6 A.4.6 Vitamin K

AE: when given intravenously anaphylactic reactions with apnea, dermatitis at injection site, hemolytic anemia with excessive doses
CI: hypersensitivity to Vitamin K, menadione (K3) administration in individuals with glucose-6-phosphate dehydrogenase deficiency

Phytonadione (Vitamin K)	EHL 26-193h, PRC C, Lact +
Aquamephyton *Inj 1mg/0.5ml, 10mg/ml* **Mephyton** *Tab 5mg* **Vitamin K1** *Inj 1mg/0.5ml, 10mg/ml* **Generics** *Inj 1mg/0.5ml*	**Hypoprothrombinemia**: 2.5-25mg PO/IM/SC; **anticoagulant-induced hypoprothrombinemia**: 2.5-10mg PO/SC/IM; **haemorrhagic disease of the newborn**: PRO: 0.5-1mg IM 1h after birth; Tx: 1mg SC/IM

6 A.4.7 Folic Acid

MA: required for nucleoprotein synthesis
AE: occasional CNS impairment, GI impairment, irritability, urticaria, pruritus
CI: megaloblastic anemia due to vit. B_{12} deficiency, hypersensitivity to folic acid products

Folic Acid	EHL , PRC A, Lact +
Folicet *Tab 1mg* **Folvite** *Inj 5mg/ml* **Generics** *Tab 1mg, Inj 5mg/ml*	**RDA:** 0.18-0.4mg PO qd; **megaloblastic anemia** →81: 1mg PO/IM/SC/IV qd;

6 A.5 Sex hormones

6 A.5.1 Androgens, Anabolic Steroids

MA/EF: development and upkeep of secondary male sexual characteristics, regulation of spermatozoon production, libido, potentia coeundi, protein anabolism, sebum production
AE (androgens): cholestasis, inhibited spermatogenesis, accelerated bone maturation, virilization in women
AE (fluoxymesterone): irregular menses, hirsutism, LFT ↑
AE (methyltestosterone): liver dysfunction, HTN, CNS effects, gynecomastia, anaphylaxis
AE (nandrolone decanoate): edema, HTN, virilization, hypoglycemia, lipid abnormalities
AE (testosterone): scrotal itching (Testoderm), clotting factor suppression, cholestatic jaundice
CI (androgens): prostate CA
CI (fluoxymesterone, methyltestosterone): hypersensitivity to product ingredients, male breast CA, known/suspected prostate CA, severe cardiac, hepatic, or renal disease
CI (nandrolone decanoate): hypersensitivity to nandrolone products, male breast/prostate CA, metastatic female breast CA with hypercalcemia, nephrosis/nephrotic phase of nephritis, severe liver disease
CI (testosterone): prostate/breast CA, hypersensitivity to testosterone products, women of child-bearing potential

Fluoxymesterone	EHL 9.2h, PRC X, Lact ?
Halotestin *Tab 2mg, 5mg, 10mg* **Generics** *Tab 10mg*	**Male hypogonadism**: 5-20mg PO qd or div tid-qid; **palliative Tx in advanced breast CA** →455: 10-40mg/d PO; **delayed puberty in males**: 2.5-10mg PO qd for 4-6mo

Methyltestosterone	EHL 10-100min, PRC X, Lact ?
Android *Tab 10mg, Tab 25mg* **Oreton** *Tab (buccal) 10mg* **Testred** *Cap 10mg* **Virilon** *Cap 10mg* **Generics** *Tab 10mg, 25mg, Tab (buccal/SL) 10mg*	**Male hypogonadism, postpuberal cryptorchidism**: 10-50mg PO qd; **palliative Tx in advanced breast CA** →455: 50-500mg/d PO
Nandrolone Decanoate	EHL 6-8d, PRC X, Lact ?
Deca-Durabolin *Inj 50mg/ml, 100mg/ml,* *200mg/ml*	**Anemia due to chronic RF** →82: women: 100-200mg IM qwk
Testosterone	EHL 10-100min (IM: approx. 8d), PRC X, Lact ?
Androderm *Film (ext.rel, TD) 2.5mg/24h, 5mg/24h* **Androgel** *Gel 1%* **Delatestryl** *Inj 200mg/ml* **Depo-Testosterone** *Inj 100mg/ml, 200mg/ml* **Testoderm** *Film (ext.rel, TD) 4mg/24h, 5mg/24h,* *6mg/24h* **Testim** *Gel 1%*	**Hypogonadism**: 50-400mg IM q2-4wk; 5mg patch qd ; **androgen replacement Tx** →182: 6mg patch qd; 5-7.5g Gel qd

6 A.5.2   Female Sex Hormones

see **Gynecology, Obstetrics** →437

6 A.6   Systemic Corticosteroids

EF: activation of gluconeogenesis, protein catabolism and lipolysis, inhibition of mesenchymal reactions (inflammation, exudation, proliferation), immunosuppression and anti-allergic effects (lymphopenia, eosinopenia, atrophy of lymphoid tissue, suppression of B and T cell activity); see also side effects
AE (corticosteroids): Diabetogenic EF: hyperglycemia, glucosuria, steroid diabetes; **Catabolic EF:** negative nitrogen balance, growth inhibition, osteoporosis; **DO in fat metabolism:** truncal obesity, moon face, serum fatty acids ↑; **Complete blood count:** thrombocytes↑, erythrocytes↑, neutrophils↑, eosinophils↓, basophils↓, lymphocytes↓; **Ulcerative EF:** gastric acid ↑, gastric mucus protection ↓; **Eyes:** corneal ulcer, glaucoma, cataract; **Skin:** atrophy, striae rubrae, acne; **Capillary fragility**↑: petechiae, ecchymosis, purpura; **Mineralocorticoid EF:** H_2O + Na^+ retention, hypokalemia, BP ↑, alkalosis; **Immunodeficiency:** susceptibility to infections ↑, reactivation of tuberculosis; **Endocrine neuropsychologic DO:** euphoria, depression, confusion, hallucinations; **Muscles:** weakness, atrophy; **Suprarenal gland atrophy**: withdrawal syndrome (weakness, dizziness, shock);**AE (fludrocortisone):** HTN, CHF, edema, hypokalemia; **CI** (corticosteroids, when used for longer periods): GI ulcerations, severe osteoporosis, acute viral and bacterial infx, systemic mycosis, glaucoma, history of psychiatric diseases
CI (fludrocortisone): hypersensitivity to fludrocortisone, systemic fungal infections

Betamethasone	EHL 5.6h, PRC C, Lact -	**Glu**	**Min**
Celestone Soluspan *Inj 3mg/ml* **Generics** *Inj 3mg /ml*	**Inflamm. disease**: 0.5-9mg qd IV/IM, intraarticular or into soft tissue; **fetal lung** **maturation, maternal antepartum**: 12mg IM q24h x 2 doses	25	0

		Glu	Min
Cortisone	EHL 30min, PRC C, Lact ?		
Cortone *Tab 25mg, Inj 25mg/ml, 50mg/ml* **Generics** *Tab 5mg, 10mg, 25mg*	**Adrenal insufficiency** →179, **inflamm. disease:** 25-300mg PO qd or 25-150mg IM q12-24h; **CH adrenal insufficiency:** 0.5-0.75mg/kg/d PO; **CH inflamm. disease:** 2.5-10mg/kg/d PO; DARF not req	0.8	0.8
Dexamethasone	EHL 200min, PRC C, Lact -	30	0
Dexamethasone Intensol *Conc (oral)1mg/ml* **Decadron** *Tab 0.25mg, 0.5mg, 0.75mg, 1.5mg, 4mg, 6mg, Elixir 0.5mg/5ml, Inj 4mg/ml, 8mg/ml, 10mg/ml, 24mg/ml* **Hexadrol** *Tab 4mg, Elixir·0.5mg/5ml, Inj 4mg/ml, 10mg/ml* **Mymethasone** *Elixir 0.5mg/5ml* **Generics** *Tab 0.25mg, 0.5mg, 0.75mg, 1mg 1.5mg, 2mg, 4mg, 6mg, Sol (oral) 0.5mg/5ml, Elixir 0.5mg/5ml, Inj 4mg/ml, 8mg/ml, 10mg/ml, 16mg/ml*	**Inflamm. disease:** 0.75-9mg/d PO/IM/IV div bid-qid; **cerebral edema:** ini 10mg IV, then 4mg IM q6h or 2mg PO bid-tid; **CH inflamm. disease:** 0.08-0.3mg/kg/d PO/IM/ IV div bid-qid; **CH cerebral edema:** ini 1.5mg/kg IV, then 1.5mg/kg/d IV div q4-6h; **fetal lung maturation, maternal antepartum:** 6mg IM q12h x 4 doses; DARF: not req		
Fludrocortisone	EHL 3.5h, PRC C, Lact ?	10	125
Florinef *Tab 0.1mg*	**Adrenal insufficiency** →179: 0.1-0.2mg PO qd **salt-losing adrenogenital syndrome:** 0.1- 0.2mg PO qd		
Hydrocortisone	EHL 1-2h, PRC C, Lact -	1	2
A-Hydrocort *Inj 100mg/vial, 250mg/vial, 500mg/vial, 1g/vial* **Cortef** *Tab 5mg, 10mg, 20mg, Susp 10mg/5ml* **Solu-Cortef** *Inj 100mg/vial, 250mg/vial, 500mg/vial, 1g/vial* **Generics** *Tab 20mg, Inj 100mg/vial*	**Adrenal insufficiency** →179: 5-30mg PO bid-qid; **inflamm. disease:** 10-320mg/d PO div tid-qid or 100-500mg IV/IM q12h; **CH adrenal insufficiency:** 0.5-0.75mg/kg/d PO div tid; **CH inflamm. disease:** 2.5-10mg/ kg/d PO div tid-qid; DARF: not req		
Methylprednisolone	EHL 2-3h, PRC C, Lact ?	5	0
Medrol *Tab 2mg, 4mg, 8mg, 16mg, 24mg, 32mg* **Depo-Medrol** *Inj (M.-acetate) 20mg/ml, 40mg/ml, 80mg/ml* **Solu-Medrol** *Inj (M.-succinate) 40mg/vial, 125mg/vial, 500mg/vial, 1g/vial* **Generics** *Tab 4mg, 8mg, 16mg, 24mg, 32mg*	**Inflamm. disease:** 10-250mg IV/IM q4h; 4-48mg PO qd; 4-80mg intraarticular (methylprednisolone acetate), may be repeated after 1-5wk; **spinal cord injury:** ini 30mg/kg IV over 15min, then 5.4mg/kg/h IV for 23h; **lupus nephritis** →431: 1g IV qd for 3d; **CH inflamm. disease:** 0.5-1.7mg/kg/d PO/IV/IM div q6-12h, **CH spinal cord injury:** see adults; DARF: not req		

Prednisolone	EHL 2.6-3h, PRC C, Lact ?	**Glu**	**Min**
Orapred *Sol (oral) 15mg/5ml* **Pediapred** *Sol (oral) 5mg/5ml* **Prelone** *Syr 5mg/ml, 15mg/ml* **Generics** *Tab 1mg, 2.5mg, 5mg, Syr 15mg/ml,* *Inj (P. acetate) 25mg/ml, 50mg/ml*	**Inflamm. disease**: 5-60mg PO/IV/IM qd; **CH** 0.1-2mg/kg/d PO/IV div qd-qid; DARF: not req	4	1
Prednisone	EHL 2.6-3h, PRC C, Lact +	3.5	1
Deltasone *Tab 2.5mg, 5mg, 10mg, 20mg,* *50mg,* **Meticorten** *Tab 1mg* **Prednisone Intensol** *Sol (oral) 5mg/ml* **Generics** *Tab 1mg, 2.5mg, 5mg, 10mg, 20mg,* *50mg, Sol (oral) 5mg/5ml*	**Inflamm. disease**: 5-60mg/d PO qd or div bid-qid; **CH** 0.05-2mg/kg/d div qd-qid; DARF: not req		
Triamcinolone	EHL no data, PRC C, Lact +	5	0
Aristocort *Tab 1mg, 2mg, 4mg, 8mg* **Kenacort** *Tab 4mg, 8mg* **Kenalog** *Inj (T.acetonide) 10mg/ml, 40mg/ml* **Generics** *Tab 4mg, Inj (T. acetonide) 3mg/ml,* *40mg/ml*	**Inflamm. disease**: 4-48mg/d PO div qd-qid; 2.5-15mg, max 40mg intraarticular (triamcinolone acetonide); DARF: not req		

Glu: relative glucocorticoid potency, **Min**: relative mineralocorticoid potency

6 A.7   Oral Antidiabetics
6 A.7.1   Sulfonylureas – 1st Generation

MA/EF: blockage of ATP-dependent K^+ channels $\Rightarrow$ release of insulin from pancreatic β-cells ↑, sensitivity of peripheral tissues to insulin ↑
AE (sulfonylureas): N/V, hypoglycemia, cholestatic jaundice, pancytopenia
AE (chlorpropamide): hypoglycemia, N, allergic skin reactions
AE (tolazamide, tolbutamide): hypoglycemia, N, heartburn, allergic skin reactions
CI (sulfonylureas): type 1 DM, ketosis, renal insufficiency; **CI** (chlorpropamide, tolazamide, tolbutamide): hypersensitivity to product ingredients, DKA or IDDM as sole therapy

Chlorpropamide	EHL 25-48h, PRC C, Lact -
Diabinese *Tab 100mg, 250mg* **Generics** *Tab 100mg, 250mg*	**DM** →168: ini 100-250mg PO qd, maint 100-500mg, max 750mg PO qd; DARF: GFR (ml/min) >50: 50%, <50: not rec
Tolazamide	EHL 7h, PRC C, Lact ?
Tolinase *Tab 100mg, 250mg, 500mg* **Generics** *Tab 100mg, 250mg, 500mg*	**DM** →168: ini 100-250mg PO, maint 250-500mg PO qd, max 1g/d; doses >500mg/d: div bid
Tolbutamide	EHL 4.5-6.5h, PRC C, Lact ?
Orinase *Tab 500mg* **Generics** *Tab 500mg*	**DM** →168: ini 1g PO qd, maint 250mg-2g PO qd, max 3g/d

6 A.7.2   Sulfonylureas - 2nd Generation

MA/EF: see Sulfonylureas - 1st Generation →150
AE (glimepiride): hypoglycemia, N; **AE** (glipizide): hypoglycemia, GI distress, allergic skin reactions,
dizziness; **AE** (glyburide): hypoglycemia, N, heartburn, allergic skin reactions
CI (glimepiride): hypersensitivity to glimepiride products, DKA or IDDM as sole therapy complicated by DM;
CI (glipizide, glyburide): hypersensitivity to product ingredients, DKA

Glimepiride	EHL 5-9h, PRC C, Lact -
Amaryl *Tab 1mg, 2mg, 4mg*	**DM** →168: ini 1-2mg PO qd, maint 1-4mg PO qd, max 8mg/d
Glipizide	EHL 2-5h, PRC C, Lact ?
Glucotrol *Tab 5mg, 10mg* **Glucotrol XL** *Tab ext.rel. 2.5mg, 5mg, 10mg* **Generics** *Tab 5mg, 10mg*	**DM** →168: ini 5mg PO qd, maint 10-15mg/d, max 40mg/d; if >15mg div bid; ext.rel.: ini 5mg PO qd, maint 5-10mg PO qd, max 20mg/d
Glyburide	EHL 5-10h, PRC C, Lact ?
DiaBeta *Tab 1.25mg, 2.5mg, 5mg* **Glynase** *Tab 1.5mg, 3mg, 6mg* **Micronase** *Tab 1.25mg, 2.5mg, 5mq* **Generics** *Tab 1.25mg, 2.5mg, 5mg* **Generics (micronized)** *Tab 1.5mg, 3mg, 4.5mg, 6mg*	**DM** →168: ini 2.5-5mg PO qd, maint 1.25-20mg PO qd or div bid; micronized Tab (Glynase, Micronase): ini 1.5-3mg PO qd, maint 0.75-12mg PO qd, max 12mg/d

6 A.7.3   Oral Antidiabetics - α-Glucosidase Inhibitors

MA (acarbose, miglitol): Inhibition of glucosidase ⇒ intestinal glucose resorption ↓
AE (acarbose, miglitol): diarrhea, abdominal pain, flatulence
CI (acarbose): hypersensitivity to acarbose, DKA, cirrhosis or severe bowel disease, inflammatory intestinal
diseases
CI (miglitol): DKA, chronic intestinal diseases characterized by marked digestive or absorptive DO,
hypersensitivity to miglitol, inflammatory bowel disease or other conditions which may deteriorate with
gas formation ↑, intestinal obstruction

Acarbose	EHL 2h, PRC B, Lact ?
Precose *Tab 25mg, 50mg, 100mg*	**DM** →168: ini 25mg PO tid, incr to 50mg PO tid, max 300mg/d
Miglitol	EHL 2h, PRC B, Lact -
Glyset *Tab 25mg, 50mg, 100mg*	**DM** →168: ini 25mg PO tid, incr to 50mg PO tid after 4-8wk, max 300mg/d

6 A.7.4   Oral Antidiabetics – Meglitinides

MA/EF: stimulates insulin secretion via inhibition (closing) of ATP-sensitive potassium channels in beta cells (⇒ increases in beta-cell calcium influx)
AE: hypoglycemia
CI: diabetic ketoacidosis, type 1 DM, hypersensitivity to repaglinide products

Repaglinide	EHL < 1h, PRC C, Lact ?
Prandin *Tab 0.5mg, 1mg, 2mg*	**DM** →168: 0.5–4mg PO tid within 30min before a meal; max 16mg/d

6 A.7.5   Oral Antidiabetics – Biguanides

MA: cellular glucose uptake ↑, non-oxidative glucose metabolism ↑
AE: lactic acidosis, N/V/D, flatulence, anorexia, complete blood count changes
CI: type 1 DM, renal/hepatic/respiratory/cardiac insufficiency, CHF, febrile diseases, hypersensitivity to metformin, metabolic acidosis, concomitant use of iodinated contrast media

Metformin	EHL 1.5–6.2h, PRC B, Lact ?
Glucophage *Tab 500mg, 850mg, 1g* **Glucophage XR** *Tab ext.rel. 500mg*	**DM** →168: ini 500mg PO qd-bid or 850mg PO qd, incr by 500mg qwk or 850mg q2wk, max 2550mg/d; ext.rel.: ini 500mg PO qd, incr by 500mg/d qwk, max 2000mg/d; DARF: contraind. in RF

6 A.7.6   Oral Antidiabetics – Thiazolidinediones

MA/EF: binding to peroxisome proliferator activated (PPA)-receptor in insulin target tissue ⇒ insulin effectiveness ↑ ⇒ cellular glucose uptake ↑, hepatic gluconeogenesis ↓
AE: edema, weight gain, anemia. Combination with metformin: anemia, hypo- and hyperglycemia, headache, diarrhea, stomachache, N, tiredness, edema. Combination with sulfonylureas: anemia, thrombopenia, hypo- and hyperglycemia, weight gain, edema
CI: heart failure, hepatic function DO, combination with insulin, hypersensitivity to product ingredients

Pioglitazone	EHL 3–7h, PRC C, Lact ?
Actos *Tab 15mg, 30mg, 45mg*	**DM** →168: monotherapy or in combination with sulfonylureas, metformin, or insulin: ini 15–30mg PO qd, max 45mg/d; DARF: not req

Rosiglitazone	EHL 3–4h, PRC C, Lact –
Avandia *Tab 2mg, 4mg, 8mg*	**DM** →168: monotherapy or in combination with metformin or sulfonylureas: ini 4mg PO qd or 2mg bid, incr after 8–12wk to max 8mg/d; DARF: not req

6 A.7.7   Oral Antidiabetics – Combinations

AE (Glucovance): hypoglycemia, lactic acidosis (rare), GI adverse events; **AE** (Avandamet): diarrhea, anemia, upper resp. tract infx, headache, fatigue; **CI** (Glucovance): renal disease, congestive heart failure, hypersensitivity to metformin or glyburide, acute or chronic metabolic acidosis, DKA; **CI** (Avandamet): renal disease, congestive heart failure, acute or chronic metabolic acidosis

Metformin + Glyburide	PRC B, Lact ?
Glucovance *Tab 250mg + 1.25mg, 500mg + 2.5mg, 500mg + 5mg*	**DM** →168: ini 250+1.25mg PO qd or bid, incr prn by 250+1.25mg to max 2000+20mg; DARF: contraind. in RF
Metformin + Rosiglitazone	PRC C, Lact -
Avandamet *Tab 500mg + 1mg, 500mg + 2mg, 500mg + 4mg*	**DM** →168: ini 500+1-2mg PO bid, max 2000+ 8mg/d; DARF: contraind. in RF
Metformin + Glipizide	PRC C, Lact -
Metaglip *Tab 250mg + 2.5mg, 500mg + 2.5mg, 500mg + 5mg*	**DM** →168: ini 250+2.5mg PO qd-bid, incr prn to max 2000+10mg; DARF: contraind. in RF

6 A.8   Insulins
6 A.8.1   Short-Acting Insulins

MA/EF: glucose resorption in muscle and fat cells↑ ⇒ anabolic metabolism↑ (glycogen-, lipid- and protein synthesis), catabolic metabolism↓ (glycogenolysis, lipolysis, proteolysis)
MA/EF: faster resorption because of amino acid changes ⇒ shorter inject eat-interval
AE: hypoglycemia, transient injection site reaction, pain at inj site, lipodystrophy, allergic reactions
CI: current hypoglycemic episode, systemic allergic reaction to insulin (desensitize)

Insulin Aspart	EHL 81min, PRC no data, Lact ?
Novolog *Inj 100 U/ml*	**DM** →166: individualized dosage SC 5-10min ac
Insulin Lispro	EHL 26-52min, PRC B, Lact ?
Humalog *Inj 100 U/ml* **Humalog pen** *Inj 100 U/ml*	**DM** →166: individualized dosage SC within 15min ac
Insulin Regular	EHL 5-15min (IV), PRC B, Lact +
Humulin R *Inj 100 U/ml* **Novolin** *Inj 100 U/ml* **Regular Iletin II** *Inj 100 U/ml*	**DM** →166: individualized dosage SC 30min ac; **diabetic ketoacidosis** →107: ini 0.1 U/kg IV bolus, then 0.1 U/kg/h, decrease when blood glucose falls to < 250mg/dl

6 A.8.2   Intermediate- and Long-Acting Insulins

MA, EF, AE, CI see short-acting insulins →153

Insulin NPH	PRC B, Lact ?
Humulin N *Inj 100 U/ml* **Novolin N** *Inj 100 U/ml* **NPH Iletin I** *Inj 100 U/ml* **NPH Iletin II** *Inj 100 U/ml*	**DM** →166: individualized dosage

Insulin Lente	PRC B, Lact ?
Iletin lente *Inj 100 U/ml* **Novolin L** *Inj 100 U/ml*	**DM** →166: individualized dosage

6 A.8.3   Insulin Glargine

MA/EF (insulin glargine): genetically changed insulin molecule, badly soluble in physiological pH-span ⇒ slow resorption ⇒ longer action
AE: hypoglycemia, injection site pain, lipodystrophy, pruritus, rash, allergic reactions, hypersensitivity
CI: hypoglycemia, prior hypersensitivity to any component of insulin glargine formulation

Insulin Glargine	PRC C, Lact ?
Lantus *Inj 100 U/ml*	**DM** →166: individualized dosage SC qd hs

6 A.8.4   Biphasic Insulins

Insulin Aspart-protamine + Insulin Aspart	
Novolog mix 70/30 *Inj 70 + 30 U/ml*	**DM** →169: individualized dosage

Insulin Lispro-protamine + Insulin Lispro	
Humalog mix 50/50 *Inj 50 + 50 U/ml* **Humalog mix 75/25** *Inj 75 + 25 U/ml*	**DM** →169: individualized dosage SC within 15min ac

Insulin NPH + Insulin Regular	
Humulin 70/30 *Inj 70 + 30 U/ml* **Novolin 70/30** *Inj 70 + 30 U/ml*	**DM** →169: individualized dosage

6 A.9   Antihypoglycemic Drugs

MA/EF (glucagon): cAMP mediated glycogenolysis in the liver ⇒ gluconeogenesis ↑ ⇒ blood glucose ↑
AE (dextrose): thrombophlebitis, rebound hypoglycemia, hypokalemia
AE (diazoxide): hypotension, tachycardia, aggravation of angina, N/V, hyperglycemia
AE (glucagon): N/V
CI (dextrose): anuria, diabetic coma + hyperglycemia, intracranial/intraspinal hemorrhage, delirium tremens in dehydrated patients, glucose-galactose malabsorption syndrome
CI (diazoxide): hypersensitivity to diazoxide products, functional hypoglycemia, pheochromocytoma, CAD
CI (glucagon): pheochromocytoma, glucagonoma, insulinoma, hypersensitivity to glucagon

Dextrose	
B-D Glucose *Tab (chew) 5g* **Insta-Glucose** *liquid (oral) 40%* **Generics** *Inj 50mg/ml, 250mg/ml* *2.5g/100ml, 5g/100ml, 10g/100ml,* *20g/100ml, 30g/100ml, 40g/100ml, 50g/100ml,* *60g/100ml, 70g/100ml*	**Hypoglycemia** →167: 10-25g IV; **hypoglycemia in conscious diabetics:** 10-20g of dextrose PO prn, may repeat prn q10-20min
Diazoxide	EHL 20-36h, PRC C, Lact ?
Proglycem *Cap 50mg,* *Susp 50mg/ml*	**Hypoglycemia** →167: ini 3mg/kg/d PO div tid, maint 3-8mg/kg/d div bid-tid
Glucagon	EHL 8-18min, PRC B, Lact ?
Glucagen *Inj 1mg/vial* **Generics** *Inj 1mg/vial*	**Hypoglycemia** →167: 0.5-1mg IV/SC/IM, may rep. in 5-20min

6 A.10 Obesity Drugs

MA/EF (orlistat): inhibition of gastric and pancreatic lipase ⇒ hydrolysis of triglycerides into free fatty acids and monoglycerides ↓ ⇒ absorption ↓

MA/EF (phentermine): anorexigenic effect ⇒ loss of weight

MA/EF (sibutramine): central inhibition of neuronal reuptake of serotonin (and noradrenaline) ⇒ repletion ↑, body temperature ↑

AE (orlistat): stomachache, fatty stool, flatulence with stool excretion, tenesmus, headache, tiredness, resorption of fat soluble vitamins ↓

AE (phentermine): HTN, tachycardia, psychosis, nervousness, insomnia, dizziness

AE (sibutramine): appetite loss, constipation, dry mouth, sleeplessness, tachycardia, HTN, nausea, dizziness, headache, paresthesia, anxiety, vasodilation

CI (orlistat): chronic malabsorption syndrome, cholestasis

CI (phentermine): hypersensitivity to phentermine, hyperthyroidism, glaucoma, during or within 14 days of MAO inhibitors, CVS disease, advanced arteriosclerosis, HTN, pulmonary hypertension, history of drug abuse, alcoholism, agitated states

CI (sibutramine): anorexia, bulimia, psychiatric diseases, Gilles de la Tourette's syndrome, combined treatment with CNS-effective drugs, coronary heart disease, decompensated heart insufficiency, arrhythmia, arterial occlusive disease, hyperthyroidism

Orlistat	EHL 1-2h, PRC B , Lact ?
Xenical *Cap 120mg*	**Obesity:** 120mg PO tid with meals; DARF: not req
Phentermine	EHL 20h, PRC C, Lact ?
Adipex-P *Tab 37.5mg, Cap 37.5mg* **Fastin** *Cap 30mg* **Ionamin** *Cap ext.rel.15mg, 30mg* **Generics** *Tab 8mg, 30mg, 37.5mg* *Cap 15mg, 18.75mg, 30mg, 37.5mg*	**Obesity:** 8mg PO tid (30min ac) or 15-37.5mg PO qd; DARF: see Prod Info

Sibutramine

EHL 1.1h, PRC C , Lact ?

 Meridia *Cap 5mg, 10mg, 15mg*

Obesity: 10mg PO qd, max15mg/d;
DARF: containdicated in severe RF

6 A.11 Thyroid Drugs
6 A.11.1 Iodine

AE: skin/mucous membrane irritation, headache, weakness, erythema
CI: hypersensitivity to iodine

Iodine

EHL no data, PRC D, Lact ?

 Pima *Sol 325mg/5ml (potassium iodide)*
 Thyro–Block *Tab 130mg (potassium iodide)*
 Generics *Sol 50mg/ml, 100mg/ml, 1g/ml*

Preparation of thyroidectomy →175: 50-250mg PO
10-14d before surgery; **thyroid blocking in
radiation exposure** →176: 130mg PO qd x 3-7d or
as directed by state health officials

6 A.11.2 Thyroid Hormones

MA/EF: growth, physical + mental development ↑, protein synthesis ↑, oxidative breakdown of fats and
carbohydrates ↑ (basal metabolism ↑)
AE: tachycardia, extrasystoles, angina pectoris, weight loss, hyperthermia, diarrhea, nervousness,
sleeplessness, tremors, muscle weakness; **CI:** hyperthyroidism

Levothyroxine (T_4)

EHL 5.3-9.5d, PRC A, Lact ?

 Levo–T *Tab 0.025mg, 0.05mg, 0.075mg, 0.088mg,
0.112mg, 0.125mg, 0.15mg, 0.175mg, 0.1mg, 0.2mg,
0.3mg*
 Levoxyl *Tab 0.025mg, 0.05mg, 0.075mg, 0.088mg,
0.112mg, 0.125mg, 0.137mg, 0.15mg, 0.175mg,
0.1mg, 0.2mg, 0.3mg*
 Synthroid *Tab 0.025mg, 0.05mg, 0.075mg,
0.088mg, 0.112mg, 0.125mg, 0.137mg, 0.15mg,
0.175mg, 0.1mg, 0.2mg, 0.3mg*
 Unithroid *Tab 0.025mg, 0.05mg, 0.075mg,
0.088mg, 0.112mg, 0.125mg, 0.15mg, 0.175mg,
0.1mg, 0.2mg, 0.3mg*

Hypothyroidism →177: ini 50µg PO qd, incr by 25µg
q2-3wk, maint 100-200µg PO qd; **CH** 0-3mo:
10-13µg/kg/d PO, 3-6mo: 8-10µg/kg/d PO, 6-12mo:
6-8µg/kg/d PO, 1-5y: 5-6µg/kg/d PO, 6-12y:
4-5µg/kg/d PO, >12y: 2-3µg/kg/d PO, post-puberty:
1.6µg/kg/d PO

Liothyronine (T_3)

EHL 25h, PRC A, Lact ?

 Cytomel *Tab 0.005mg, 0.025mg, 0.05mg*

Hypothyroidism →177: ini 25µg PO qd, incr by 12.5-
25µg q1-2wk, maint 25-75µg PO qd; **goiter** →175:
ini 5µg PO qd, incr by 5-10µg q1-2wk, maint 75µg
PO qd; **myxedema**: →177 5µg PO qd, incr by 5- 10µg
q1-2wk, maint 50-100µg/d PO; **congenital
hypothyroidism**: ini 5µg PO qd, incrby 5 µg q3-4d
prn

Liotrix (Levothyroxine + Liothyronine)	PRC A, Lact ?
Thyrolar *Tab 0.0125 + 0.0031mg, 0.025 + 0.00625mg, 0.05 + 0.0125mg, 0.1 + 0.025mg, 0.15 + 0.0375mg*	**Hypothyroidism** →177: 0.0125-0.15 + 0.0031-0.0375mg PO qd
Thyroid - dessicated	EHL 2-7d, PRC A, Lact ?
Armour Thyroid *Tab 15mg, 30mg, 60mg, 90mg, 120mg, 180mg, 240mg, 300mg*	**Hypothyroidism** →177: ini 30mg PO qd, incr by 15mg q2-3wk to max180mg/d; **CH** 0-6mo: 4.8-6mg/kg/d PO, 6-12mo: 3.6-4.8mg/kg/d PO, 1-5y: 3.0-3.6mg/kg/d PO, 6-12y: 2.4-3.0mg/kg/d PO, >12y: 1.2-1.8mg/kg/d PO

6 A.11.3 Antithyroid Drugs (Thioamides)

MA/EF: inhibition of thyroid hormone synthesis through inhibition of thyroidal peroxidase ($J^- \rightarrow J$). The incretion of already synthesized hormones is not inhibited. Propylthiouracil: in addition partial inhibition of the conversion of T4 to T3.

AE: agranulocytosis, leukopenia, allergic skin reactions, development of goiter, GI DO, hepatitis, transient cholestasis

AE (propylthiouracil): myelosuppression, lupus-like syndrome, drug fever, N/V, epigastric distress

AE (methimazole): N/V, rash/urticaria, epigastric distress, arthralgia, paresthesia

CI: previous serious hypersensitivity reactions, severe liver diseases

CI (methimazole): hypersensitivity to methimazole products

CI (propylthiouracil): hypersensitivity to antithyroid drugs

Methimazole	EHL 2-28h, PRC D, Lact ?
Tapazole *Tab 5mg, 10mg* **Generics** *Tab 5mg, 10mg*	**Hyperthyroidism** →175: 5-20mg PO tid; **thyrotoxic crisis** →176: 60-120mg/d PO div tid; **CH hyperthyroidism**: ini 0.4mg/kg/d PO div tid, maint 1/2 of ini dose; DARF: not req
Propylthiouracil	EHL 0.9-4.3h, PRC D, Lact ?
Generics *Tab 50mg*	**Hyperthyroidism** →175: ini 300-400mg/d PO div tid, maint 100-300mg/d; **CH** ini 5-7mg/kg/d PO div tid, maint 1/3-2/3 of ini dose

6 A.11.4 Parathyroid Hormone

MA/EF (teriparatide): recombinant human parathyroid hormone
AE: rhinitis, transient hypercalcemia, pain, asthenia, headache, HTN, angina pectoris, syncope, dizziness, depression, insomnia, vertigo, constipation, neck pain, arthralgia
CI: Paget's disease, radiation therapy, bone metastases or skeletal malignancies, hypercalcemia, metabolic bone disease other than osteoporosis; use cautiously in patients with active or recent urolithiasis, in hypotensive patients and in those taking digoxin.

Teriparatide — EHL no data , PRC C, Lact -

  Forteo *Pen 750µg/3ml* — **Osteoporosis in postmenopausal women, primary or hypogonadal Osteoporosis in men** →172: 20µg SC qd

6 A.12 Prolactin Inhibitors

MA: stimulation of hypophyseal dopamine receptors ⇒ inhibition of prolactin release
AE: N/V, GI disturbances, psychomotor- and extrapyramidal motor system DO, hypotension, bradycardia, peripheral vascular perfusion disturbances
AE (bromocriptine): hypotension, periph. vasoconstriction, dyskinesias, fatigue, N/V
AE (cabergoline): dizziness, headache, weakness, fatigue, orthostatic hypotension
CI: limited use in psychiatric DO, gastroduodenal ulcers, serious CVS diseases
CI (bromocriptine): hypersensitivity to bromocriptine products
CI (cabergoline): hypersensitivity to ergot derivates, uncontrolled HTN

Bromocriptine — EHL 50h, PRC C, Lact -

  Parlodel *Cap 2.5mg, 5mg* — **Hyperprolactinemia** →183: 1.25-2.5mg PO qd, incr by 2.5mg q3-7d, maint 2.5-15mg/d div qd-bid, max 50mg/d; **acromegaly** →183: 1.25-2.5mg PO qd for 3d, incr by 1.25-2.5mg q3-7d to 20-30mg/d, max 100mg/d; **lactation suppression postpartum:** 2.5mg PO bid x 4-14d; **Parkinson's** →316; DARF: not req

Cabergoline — EHL 63-69h, PRC B, Lact ?

  Dostinex *Tab 0.5mg* — **Hyperprolactinemia** →183: ini 0.25mg PO biw, incr by 0.25mg biw at 4wk intervals according to response, max 1mg biw

6 A.13 Growth Hormone Receptor Antagonists

MA (pegvisomant): binds selectively to growth hormone receptors ⇒ inhibition of GH binding ⇒ decrease of IGF-1 and IGF-binding proteins
AE (pegvisomant): infection, pain, backpain, nausea, flu syndrome, peripheral edema, diarrhea
CI (pegvisomant): hypersensitivity to p. or to latex

Pegvisomant	EHL 6d, PRC B, Lact ?
Somavert *Inj 10mg, 15mg, 20mg*	**Acromegaly** →183: ini 40mg SC, then 10mg qd, adjust dose after 4-6 wk in 5mg increments/ decrements based on IGF-1 levels, max 30mg/d

6 A.14 Anterior Pituitary Hormones

AE (somatropin): hyperglycemia, hypothyroidism, BP ↑, N/V, edema, retention of H_2O + Na^+, development of antibodies; **AE** (somatrem): development of antibodies, periph. edema
CI (somatropin, somatrem): active intracranial lesions, active malignancy, acute critical illness (post open heart or abdominal surgery; multiple accidental trauma; acute respiratory failure), closed epiphyses, hypersensitivity to growth hormone or product ingredients

Somatotropin (Growth Hormone)	EHL 18min, PRC C, Lact ?
Genotropin *Inj 0.2, 0.4, 0.6, 0.8, 1, 1.2, 1.4, 1.5, 1.6, 1.8, 2, 5.8, 13.8mg/vial* **Humatrope** *Inj 5, 6, 12, 24mg/vial* **Norditropin** *Inj 5mg/1.5ml, 10mg/1.5ml, 15mg/1.5ml, 4mg/vial, 8mg/vial* **Nutropin** *Inj 5mg/vial, 10mg/vial* **Protropin** *Inj 5mg/vial, 10mg/vial* **Saizen** *Inj 5mg/vial, 6mg/vial*	Dosage varies with product, see Prod Info! **somatotropin deficiency** →182: Genotropin: ini 0.04mg/kg/wk SC div 6-7 times/wk, incr prn q4-8wk to max 0.08mg/kg/wk; **CH** Genotropin: 0.16-0.24mg/kg/wk SC div 6-7 times/wk

Clomiphene →447

Menotropins, FSH/LH, Follitropins, FSH, Chorionic Gonadotropins, hCG →447

Cosyntropin	EHL no data, PRC C, Lact ?
Cortrosyn *Inj 0.25mg/vial*	**Adrenal function screening test**: 0.25mg IM/IV over 2min; **CH** <2y: 0.125mg IM/IV over 2min; >2y: see adults

6 A.15 Posterior Pituitary Hormones

MA (desmopressin): renal H_2O resorption ↑, vasoconstriction
AE (desmopressin): flushing, headache, nausea
CI (desmopressin): hypersensitivity to desmopressin products, children < 3mo, Type IIB von Willebrand's

Desmopressin	EHL IV 75.5min, PRC B, Lact ?
Concentraid *Sol (nasal) 0.01%* **DDAVP** *Tab 0.1, 0.2mg, Sol (nasal) 0.01%, Spray (nasal) 0.01mg/Spray, Inj 0.004mg/ml, 0.015mg/ml* **Stimate** *Spray (nasal) 0.15mg/Spray* **Generics** *Spray (nasal) 0.01mg/Spray, Inj. 0.004mg/ml*	**Central diabetes insipidus** →183: 10-40µg (0.1-0.4ml) intranasally qd or div bid-tid; 0.1-1.2mg/d PO qd or div bid-tid; 2-4µg/d SC/IV div bid; **CH central diabetes insipidus**: 3mo - 12y: 5-30µg (0.05-0.3ml) intranasally qd or div bid; 0.05mg PO bid; **hemophilia A** →79; →78; **enuresis**. →427

6 A.16　Therapeutic Enzymes

MA (agalsidase): recombinant human α-galactosidase A enzyme replacement $\Rightarrow$ prevents glycosphingolipid accumulation
MA (laronidase): recombinant alpha–L–iduronidase enzyme replacement $\Rightarrow$ increases glycosaminglycan catabolism
MA (nitisinone): inhibition of 4–hydroxyphenylpyruvate-dioxygenase $\Rightarrow$ prevents the accumulation of toxic tyrosine metabolites
AE (agalsidase): infusion reactions, stroke, pain, ataxia, cardiac arrhythmia, vertigo
AE (laronidase): infusion reactions, upper resp. tract infx., edema, paraesthesia
AE (nitisinone): seizures, brain tumor, encephalopathy, hepatic neoplasm, liver failure
CI (agalsidase, laronidase, nitisinone): no known CI

Agalsidase beta	EHL 45–102min, PRC B, Lact ?
Fabrazyme *Inj 35mg/7ml*	**Fabry disease:** 1mg/kg IV q2wk
Laronidase	EHL 1.5–3.6h, PRC B, Lact ?
Aldurazyme *Inj 2.9mg/5ml*	**Mucopolysaccharidosis I:** 0.58mg/kg IV qwk
Nitisinone	EHL no data, PRC C
Orfadin *Cap 2mg, 5mg, 10mg*	**Hereditary tyrosinemia type 1: CH** 1mg/kg/d PO div bid

6 B. Metabolic, Endocrine – Therapies

Y. Howard Lien, MD Endocrine
Ehud Ur, MB, FRCP
Professor, Section of Nephrology, College of Medicine,
University of Arizona, Tucson, AZ
Head, Division of Endocrinology & Metabolism
Dalhousie University, Halifax, Nova Scotia, Canada

6 B.1   Volume Depletion
6 B.1.1   Isotonic Volume Depletion

Mild

	Saline solution (volume expansion + electrolyte replacement)	Saline or sugar–electrolyte solutions (sport drinks)	*10g Na⁺Cl⁻ in 2–3l PO Recommendation of WHO for diarrhea:* 3.5g Na⁺Cl⁻ + 2.5g Na⁺H⁺CO₃⁻ + 1.5g K⁺Cl⁻ + 20g glucose in 1000ml water PO

Severe

	Isotonic saline solution (volume expansion + electrolyte replacement)	Normal Saline 0.9% (154meq/l)	*IV according to CVP and urine output*
If low K⁺	**Crystalloid plasma expander** (volume expansion + electrolyte replacement)	**Ringer's solution**	*IV according to CVP and urine output*

In oliguria/anuria or renal failure

	Isotonic saline solution (potassium free volume + electrolyte replacement)	Normal Saline 0.9% (154meq/l)	*IV according to CVP and urine output*

In profound circulatory failure

	Colloid plasma expander →70 (volume expansion)	Albumin 5% (Albuminar, Buminate, Plasbumin)	*250–500ml IV*

Only as acute therapy, later replace with saline or Ringer's solution

6 B.1.2   Hypotonic Volume Depletion

Mild

	Saline solution (volume expansion + electrolyte replacement)	Saline or sugar–electrolyte solutions (sport drinks)	*10g Na⁺Cl⁻ in 2–3l PO Recommendation of WHO for diarrhea:* 3.5g Na⁺Cl⁻ + 2.5g NaHCO₃ + 1.5g K⁺Cl⁻ + 20g glucose in 1000ml water PO

Severe (Na$^+$ < 125mmol/l, starting CNS symptoms)

	Isotonic saline solution (volume expansion + electrolyte replacement)	**Normal Saline 0.9%** (154meq/l)	*IV according to CVP* *Keep Na$^+$ increase <10meq/l/d*
(1:1) plus	**Crystalloid plasma expander** (volume expansion + electrolyte replacement)	**Ringer's solution**	*IV according to CVP* *Keep Na$^+$ increase <10meq/l/d*

Emergency (severe CNS symptoms, i.e. seizure and coma)

	Hypertonic saline solution (volume expansion + electrolyte replacement)	**Saline 3%** (513meq/l)	*Correct Na$^+$ 1.5–2meq/l for 3–4h and keep Na$^+$ increase < 10meq/l/d*

Caution: central pontine myelinolysis if hyponatremia corrected too quickly. Rapid correction can be applied when hyponatremia develops within 24h.
Na$^+$ deficit for initial therapy (meq): 10 x 0.6 x kg (man, for woman use 0.5)

6 B.1.3 Hypertonic Volume Depletion

Mild

	Free water replacement (volume expansion)	**Water, tea**	*2–3l PO*

Severe

first	**Isotonic saline solution** (volume expansion)	**Normal Saline 0.9%** (154meq/l)	*1–2l IV according to CVP*
then	**Hypotonic saline solution** (free water replacement)	**Half Saline 0.45%** (77meq/l)	*Slowly IV. Caution: cerebral edema*
or	**Glucose solution** (free water replacement)	**Glucose 5%** (D5W)	*Slowly IV. Caution: cerebral edema*

Water deficit (l) = [(Na/140)–1] x 0.5 x kg (man, for woman use 0.4)
Correction rate <0.5meq/h
Caution: rapid correction may cause cerebral edema

6 B.2 Volume Overload
6 B.2.1 Isotonic Volume Overload

sos	**Loop diuretic** →33	**Furosemide** (Lasix, Gens)	*20mg IV, sos↑ dose*

Poss. + fluid/Na$^+$ restriction

6 B.2.2 Hypotonic Volume Overload

	Fluid restriction	**Reduce free water**	*<1.5 l/d*
	Loop diuretic →33	**Furosemide** (Lasix, Gens)	*20mg IV, sos↑ dose*

Water excess (l) = (1–Na/140) x 0.6 x kg (man, for woman use 0.5)

6 B.2.3   Hypertonic Volume Overload

Na⁺ restriction	Reduce Na⁺ intake	*Remove iatrogenic causes*
Loop diuretics →33	Furosemide (Lasix, Gens)	*20mg IV with D5W*
Hypernatremia due to primary aldosteronism+˙		
Aldosterone antagonist →28	Spironolactone (Aldactone, Gens)	*25-100mg q 8h*

6 B.3   Generalized Edema

Low-dose heparinization →71 (DVT prophylaxis)	Enoxaparin (Lovenox)	*40mg SC qd*
Loop diuretic →33	Furosemide (Lasix, Gens)	*20-40mg PO or IV*
plus sos Thiazide diuretic →33	Metolazone (Zaroxolyn)	*2.5-5mg PO given same time as PO Lasix or IV 30min earlier than Furosemide. Watch K⁺ deficit*
Cir-rhosis Aldosterone antagonist →28	Spironolactone (Aldactone, Gens)	*25-100mg bid-qid*

6 B.4   Hypokalemia
6 B.4.1   Mild Hypokalemia

sos Potassium replacement →139	K⁺Cl⁻ (K-Dur, K-Lor, Micro-K, Ram-K, Slow-K)	*20-80meq PO qd (40meq ➡ approx. K⁺ 0.3meq/l↑)*

6 B.4.2   Severe Hypokalemia (K⁺ deficit: 200meq, if K⁺<3meq/l, and no intracellular K⁺ shift)

Potassium replacement →139	K⁺Cl⁻ solution	*Peripheral line: 20-40meq in 1 l NS IV over 2-4h. Central line: 10-20meq in 50ml NS IV over 1h. ECG monitor*

6 B.5   Hyperkalemia
6 B.5.1   Mild Hyperkalemia

K⁺ restriction	Low K⁺ diet	*<2g/d*

6 B.5.2   Severe Hyperkalemia (> 6meq/l or ECG changes)

Loop diuretic →33 (K⁺ excretion)	Furosemide (Lasix, Gens)	*40-80mg IV*
sos Cation exchangers →144 (remove K⁺ from GI)	Sodium polystyrene sulfonate (Kayexalate)	*20g in 100ml 20% sorbitol every 4-6h prn*
Redistribution (intracellular shift of K⁺)	Glucose 50% + Regular insulin	*50ml + 10units IV over 20min*

plus sos	**Redistribution** →18 (intracellular shift of K⁺)	**Sodium bicarbonate 8.4%** (1meq/ml)	*50ml IV over 5min*
plus sos	**Membrane antagonism** →139 (inhibition of depolarization)	**Calcium gluconate 10%** (4.5meq/ml, Gens)	*10ml IV over 2-3min Caution: digitalis toxicity*
or	**Redistribution** →95 (intracellular shift of K⁺)	**Albuterol** (Proventil, Ventolin, Gens)	*0.5mg IV slowly in 15min or 10-20mg in 4ml saline nasal inhalation over 10min*
sos	**Hemodialysis** (removal of K⁺)	**Hemodialysis**	*Use 1meq/l K⁺ bath and ECG monitoring*

6 B.6   Hypocalcemia
6 B.6.1   Mild Hypocalcemia

	Calcium preparation →139 (replacement)	**Ca⁺⁺ carbonate** (Mylanta, Titralac, Tums)	*1-2g PO qd*
	Vitamin D →146 (increase Ca⁺ absorption)	**Ergocalciferol** (Drisdol, Gens)	*50,000IU PO qd*
sos	**1,25OH Vitamin D** →146 (increase Ca⁺ absorption)	**Calcitriol** (Rocaltrol)	*0.25µg PO tiw*

6 B.6.2   Acute Hypocalcemic Crisis

	Calcium preparation →139 (replacement)	**Ca⁺⁺ gluconate 10%** (4.5meq/ml)	*Ini: 1g slowly IV, then: 1mg/kg/h in D5W Caution: digitalis toxicity*
If low Mg⁺	**Magnesium preparation** →140 (replacement)	**Mg⁺⁺ sulfate 50%** (4meq/ml)	*2g in 100ml D5W IV over 1h*

6 B.7   Hypercalcemia
6 B.7.1   Mild Hypercalcemia

sos	**Isotonic saline solution** →33 (volume expansion)	**Normal Saline 0.9%** (154meq/l)	*1-2l IV*
sos	**Loop diuretic** →33 (Ca excretion)	**Furosemide** (Lasix, Gens)	*20-40mg IV*

6 B.7.2   Hypercalcemic Crisis

	Isotonic saline solution (volume expansion)	**Normal Saline 0.9%** (154meq/l)	*1-2l IV, max. 10l/24h*
sos	**Loop diuretic** →33 (Ca⁺⁺ excretion)	**Furosemide** (Lasix, Gens)	*Only after volume repletion, 20-40mg IV q 4-6h*
sos	**Bisphosphonate** →143 (osteoclast inhibition)	**Pamidronate** (Aredia)	*60 or 90mg IV over 4 or 24h*
sos	**Calcitonin** →144 (osteoclast inhibition)	**Calcitonin** (Calcimar, Miacalcin)	*4IU/kg SC q 12h (only works for a few d)*

sos malig-nancy	**Cytotoxic** (osteoclast inhibition)	**Mithramycin** (Mithracin)	*25µg/kg over 6h. Caution: bone marrow toxicity*
sos malig-nancy	**Glucocorticoid** →148 (inhibition of Vitamin D synthesis)	**Prednisone** (Deltasone, Meticorten, Prednisone Intensol, Gens)	*0.5-1mg/kg qd*

6 B.8   Hypomagnesemia
6 B.8.1   Chronic Hypomagnesemia

	Magnesium preparation →140 (replacement)	**Mg$^+$Cl$^-$** (Slow Mg) **Mg$^+$ lactate** (Mg-Tab) **Mg$^+$ Oxide** (Mag-OX)	*1-2 PO bid*

6 B.8.2   Acute Symptomatic Hypomagnesemia

	Magnesium preparation →140 (replacement)	**Mg$^+$ sulfate 50%** (4meq/ml)	*2g in 100ml D5W IV over 1h*

6 B.9   Hypermagnesemia

	Loop diuretic →33 (Mg$^+$ excretion)	**Furosemide** (Lasix, Gens)	*20-40mg IV*
sos	**Membrane antagonism** →139 (inhibit depolarization)	**Ca^{++} gluconate 10%** (4.5meq/ml)	*10ml slowly IV*
plus sos	**Isotonic saline solution** (volume expansion)	**Normal Saline 0.9%** (154meq/l)	*IV according to CVP*

Require hemodialysis if renal failure

6 B.10   Metabolic Acidosis
6 B.10.1   Chronic Metabolic Acidosis

	Buffer (pH neutralization)	**Na$^+$ citrate and citric acid** (Shohl's solution)	*15-30ml PO bid*
or	**Buffer** →18 (pH neutralization)	**Sodium bicarbonate**	*30-100meq PO qd*

6 B.10.2 Acute Metabolic Acidosis (pH < 7.2 or HCO$_3$ < 12mmol/l)

	Buffer (pH neutralization)	**Sodium bicarbonate 8.4%** (1meq/ml)	*Inl Tx (meq)= (12-bicarb) x 0.7 x kg IV over 4-8h*

6 B.11 Metabolic Alkalosis
6 B.11.1 In General

	Isotonic saline solution (Cl$^-$ replacement)	**Normal Saline 0.9%** (154meq/l)	*1–2l IV*
If low K$^+$	**Potassium chloride solution** →139 (K$^+$ replacement)	**K$^+$Cl$^-$**	*20-40meq in 1l NS at 10-20meq/h*
sos	**Carbonic anhydrase inhibitor** →35 (inhibition of H$^+$CO$_3^-$ reabsorption)	**Acetazolamide** (Diamox, Gens)	*250mg PO qd or bid*
sos	**Acid** (pH neutralization)	**Hydrochloric acid** (150meq/l)	*H$^+$Cl$^-$ (meq buffers 50% bicarb excess) IV via central line over 8-24h*

Na$^+$Cl$^-$ only effective in chloride sensitive forms, not in mineralocorticoid excess

Bicarb excess (meq)= (bicarb-24) x 0.6 x kg (man, use 0.5 for woman)

6 B.11.2 Metabolic Alkalosis due to Primary Aldosteronism

	Aldosterone antagonist →28 (mineralocorticoid steroid effects ↓)	**Spironolactone** (Aldactone, Gens)	*25-100mg q8h*

6 B.12 Diabetes Mellitus
6 B.12.1 Type 1 (formerly IDDM)

Conventional insulin therapy (strict insulin administrations)

e.g.	**Intermediate-acting insulin or biphasic insulins** →154 (glucose resorption in muscle and fat cells ↑ ⇒ anabolism ↑ (glycogen-, lipid- and protein synthesis), catabolism ↓ (glycogenolysis, lipolysis, proteolysis))	**Insulin NPH** (Humulin N, Novolin N) **Insulin NPH + Insulin Regular** (Humulin 70/30, Novolin 70/30)	*2/3 of needs qam, 1/3 qpm (e.g. comb. 2/3 intermediate + 1/3 regular insulin) (outdated approach!)*

Intensive insulin therapy (basal/bolus concept) (specialist may be required!)

e.g.	**Long-acting insulin + regular insulin** →154 (substitution according to circadian rhythm of insulin needs)	**Insulin lente** (Novolin L) **+ Insulin Regular** (Novolin L)	*R= regular insulin, L= long-acting insulin; R: 50% of daily needs, 10-20% of total daily insulin requirement at each meal; L: 50% of the total dose: of this 50% at night, of the other 50%, 30% am and 70% at noon; am: R>L, noon: R<L, pm R, qhs (10pm) L*

Basal needs managed with long-acting insulin (L), with regular insulin at meals (R) according to circadian rhythm of insulin needs. High insulin requirement am and a little less pm, low insulin around noon and from midnight until 4 am.

	Short-acting insulin analogue →153 (monom. insulin anal.)	**Insulin lispro** (Humalog) **Insulin aspart** (Novolog)	*Effect maximum 1h after inj, inj immediately after eating*
	Long-acting insulin analogue →154 (precipitation of insulin Glargine in neutral pH of SC tissue ⇒ release into circulation ↓)	**Insulin Glargine** (Lantus)	*Inj around 10pm, duration of action about 24h, almost constant absorption rate*

82. Bolli B. How to ameliorate the problem of hypoglycemia in intensive as well as non intensive treatment of type 1 diabetes; Diabetes care, 22 Suppl 2 B43-B52, 1999
83. American Diabetes Association: Clinical practice recommendations. Diabetes Care 1998; 21(Supplement 1): s1-s70

Diabetic Ketoacidosis (ICU, specialist required!)

	Isotonic saline solution (volume + electrolyte substitution)	**Saline 0.9%** (if Na > 150mmol/l ⇒ 0.45%)	*1l in 1h, then 500ml/h over the next 6h, then 250ml/h over 4h*
plus	**Insulin** →153 (substitution)	**InsulinRegular**	*0.1U/kg/h in IV; at BS of 250mg/dl add gluc. 5%*
sos	**K⁺Cl⁻ solution** →139 (substitution)	**K⁺Cl⁻ 7.45%** (1ml = 1mmol)	*K⁺< 3mmol/l: 40mmol/h; K⁺< 4mmol/l: 30mmol/h; K⁺< 5mmol/l: 20mmol/h*
sos	**Buffer** →10 (acidosis therapy, pH neutralisation)	**Sodium bicarbonate 8.4%** (100ml = 100mmol HCO3⁻)	*BE x 0.3 x kg = mmol, only give 1/3 of calculated need (starting at pH < 6.9)*
sos	**Phosphate** (substitution)	**Potassium phosphate**	*2mmol/h in 500ml saline 0.9% over 6h (prn)*
sos	**Low-dose heparin** →71 (low-molecular; thrombosis PRO)	**Dalteparin** (Fragmin)	*2850IU SC qd (prn)*

84. Fleckmann AM, Diabetic ketoacidosis, Endocrin Metab Clin North Am, 1993, 22, 181-207
85. Kitabchi AE, Wall BM: Diabetic ketoacidosis. Med Clin North Am 1995 Jan; 79(1): 9-37

Hypoglycemic coma

	Glucose (substitution)	**Glucose 40%, then Glucose 5%**	*20-50ml 40% IV, then 5% (until BS 200mg/dl)*
sos	**Antihypoglycemic** →154 (hepat. glycogenolysis ↑, gluconeogenesis ↑ ⇒BS ↑)	**Glucagon** (GlucaGen, Gens)	*0.5-1mg SC, IM, IV*

86. Service FJ, Hypoglycemic disorders, N Eng J Med, 1995, 332, 1144-52

6 B.12.2 Type 2 (formerly NIDDM)

1. Biguanide and/or Glucosidase inhibitor (if diet is not sufficient)

1sr choice	**Biguanide** →152 (glucose uptake into cell ↑, gluconeogenesis in liver ↓, glucose transport into muscle/fat tissue ↑)	**Metformin** (Glucophage, Glucophage XR)	*500-1500mg PO qam, max. 2500mg/d (tid); Caution: extensive CI, lactic acidosis, creatinine > 130μmol/l*
or / sos plus	**Glucosidase inhibitor** →151 (intestinal glucose release ↓)	**Acarbose** (Precose)	*50-200mg PO tid, incr slowly; Caution: poor compliance due to AE*

Generally Metformin is first choice over Acarbose especially in obese patients.

2. Other Oral Antidiabetics

	Sulfonylurea →151 (blockade of ATP dependent K$^+$ channels, insulin release from pancreas beta-cells ↑)	**Glyburide** (DiaBeta, Glynase, Micronase, Gens)	*Ini 1.25-10mg PO qam, max. 10mg bid; Caution: not > 65y: severe protracted hypoglycemias; Tx break in unstable AP, before PTCA, very acute MI – temporary insulin Tx)*
or	**Sulfonylurea** →151 (frequency of hypoglycemia ↓)	**Glimepiride** (Amaryl)	*1-4mg qd qam*
or	**Meglitinide** →152 (insulin secretagogue, acts like sulfonylureas, short EHL ⇒ admin ac)	**Repaglinide** (Prandin)	*Up to 8mg PO tid within 30min ac; max 16mg/d*
or	**Thiazolidinedione** →152 ("insulin sensitizer" binds to (PPA)-receptor in insulin target tissue ⇒ insulin effectiveness ↑ ⇒ cellular glucose uptake ↑, hepatic glucose output ↓)	**Rosiglitazone** (Avandia)	*4-8mg PO qd or 2-4mg PO bid*
		Pioglitazone (Actos)	*15-45mg PO qd caution: hepatotoxicity, fluid retention, weight gain (especially when combined with insulin)*

3. Useful: combination of Meglitinide (insulin secretagogue) and Thiazolidinedione (insulin sensitizer)

4. Combination therapy: Insulin + Metformin (biguanide) or sulfonylurea

	Intermediate–acting insulin →154	**Insulin NPH** (Humulin N, Novolin N)	*HPH (basal) insulin qhs, sos 2nd insulin inj qam*

5. Insulin monotherapy (if 28IU in comb. with sulfonylureas is not sufficient)

Biphasic insulins →154 (glucose resorption in muscle and fat cells ↑ ⇒ anabolism ↑ (glycogen-, lipid- and protein synthesis), catabolism ↓ (glycogenolysis, lipolysis, proteolysis))	**Insulin NPH + Insulin Regular** (Humulin 70/30, Novolin 70/30)	*0.14-0.24IU/kg qam, 0.07-0.12IU/kg qpm IU according to BS profile, disadvantage: strict system; Intensified insulin Tx: ac admin of regular insulin. Starting total dose = fasting BS x 0.2, div in 3 regular insulin doses ac in relationship 3:1:2 per BU more IU qam 2IU; In increased fasting BS additional NPH Insulin qpm or metformin admin*

87.   Williams G., Management of non-insulin depent diabetes mellitus, Lancet, 1994, 343, 95-100
88.   UK Prospective Diabetes Study Group, Effect of intensive blood-glucose control with metformin on complications in overweight patients with type 2 diabetes, UKPDS 34, Lancet, 1998, 352, 854-65
89.   UK Prospective Diabetes Study Group, Intensive blood-glucose control with sulphonylureas or insulin compared with conventional treatment and risk of complications in patients with type 2 diabetes, UKPDS 33, Lancet, 1998, 352, 837-53

6 B.13 Hyperlipidemias

6 B.13.1 Hypercholesterolemia (Hereditary/Polygenic)

	HMG-CoA-reductase inhibitor →42 (intracell. cholesterol synthesis ↓, LDL ↓, HDL ↑)	**Lovastatin** (Altocor, Mevacor)	*20-40mg PO qd qpm*
		Atorvastatin (Lipitor)	*10-80mg PO qd*
		Fluvastatin (Lescol)	*20-40mg PO qd*
		Pravastatin (Pravachol)	*10-40 mg PO qd*
		Simvastatin (Zocor)	*20-80mg PO qd*
poss.	**Bile acid sequestrant** →41 (intestinal bile acid binding ↑ ⇒ bile acid production from cholesterol ↑ ⇒ serum cholesterol ↓ ⇒ hepat. LDL uptake ↑)	**Cholestyramine** (Locholest, Locholest Light, Prevalite, Questran, Questran Light, Gens)	*4-16g PO qd, incr slowly; Caution: sufficient distance to ingestion of other drugs (e.g. warfarin, digitalis, thiazides)*
sos	**Fat soluble vitamins** →145 (parenteral substitution)	**Vitamins A, D, E, K**	*1ml/2wk IM (prn)*

90.   Illingworth DR: Management of hypercholesterolemia. Med Clin North Am 2000 Jan; 84(1): 23-42

6 B.13.2 Hereditary Lipoprotein Lipase Deficiency

sos	**Fat soluble vitamins** →145 (parenteral substitution)	**Vitamins A, D, E,K**	*1ml/2wk IM (prn)*

6 B.13.3 Hereditary Dysbetalipoproteinemia

	Fibric acid →43 (lipoprotein lipase activity ↑ ⇒ LDL ↓, HDL ↑, triglycerides ↓)	**Fenofibrate** (Tricor)	*67-200 mg PO qd ac*
		Gemfibrozil (Lopid, Gens)	*300-600mg PO bid*

sos	**Nicotinic acid derivative** →43 (triglyceride lipase activity ↓, lipoprotein lipase activity ↑ ⇒ triglycerides ↓, cholesterol ↓)	**Inositol nicotinate** (Hexopal, No-Flush Niacin)	*600-800mg PO bid-tid*
sos	**HMG–CoA–reductase inhibitor** →42 (intracell. cholesterol synthesis ↓, LDL↓, HDL↑)	**Lovastatin** (Mevacor, Altocor)	*20-40mg PO qd qpm*
		Atorvastatin (Lipitor)	*10-80mg PO qd*
		Fluvastatin (Lescol)	*20-40mg PO qd*
		Pravastatin (Pravachol)	*10-40 mg PO qd*
		Simvastatin (Zocor)	*20-80mg PO qd*

Caution if combining HMG-CoA-reductase inhibitors with fibrates due to increased risk of rhabdomyolysis!

6 B.13.4 Hereditary Hypertriglyceridemia

	Fibric acid →43 (lipoprotein lipase activity ↑ ⇒ LDL ↓, HDL ↑, triglycerides ↓)	**Fenofibrate** (Tricor)	*67-200 mg PO qd ac*
		Gemfibrozil (Lopid, Gens)	*300-600mg PO bid*
possibly in combination with	**Nicotinic acid derivative** →43 (triglyceride lipase activity ↓, lipoprotein lipase activity ↑ ⇒ triglycerides ↓, cholesterol ↓)	**Inositol nicotinate** (Hexopal, No-Flush Niacin)	*600-800mg PO bid-tid*

6 B.13.5 Hereditary Combined Hyperlipidemia

	HMG–CoA–reductase inhibitor →42 (intracelluläre cholesterol synthesis ↓, LDL ↓, HDL ↑)	**Lovastatin** (Mevacor, Altocor)	*20-80mg PO qd qpm*
sos	**Fibric acid** →43 (lipoprotein lipase activity ↑ ⇒ LDL ↓, HDL ↑, triglycerides ↓)	**Fenofibrate** (Tricor)	*67-200 mg PO qd ac*
		Gemfibrozil (Lopid, Gens)	*300-600mg PO bid*
sos	**Nicotinic acid derivative** →43 (triglyceride lipase activity ↓, lipoprotein lipase activity ↑ ⇒ triglycerides ↓, cholesterol ↓)	**Inositol nicotinate** (Hexopal, No-Flush Niacin)	*600-800mg PO bid-tid*

91. Betteridge DJ, Management of hyperlipidaemia: guidelines of the British Hyperlipidaemia Association, Postgrad Med J, 1993, 69, 359-69
92. Oster G, Cholesterol-Reduction Intervention study. A randomized trial to assess effectivness and costs in clinical practice, Arch Intern Med, 1996, 156, 731-9

6 B.14 Gout
6 B.14.1 Long-Term Therapy

	Xanthine oxidase inhibitor →138 (Xanthine oxidase inhibition ⇒ uric acid production ↓)	**Allopurinol** (Alloprin, Lopurin, Zyloprim, Gens)	*100-300mg PO qd (UA in serum < 6.5mg/dl)*
	Uricosuric →138 (tubular uric acid reabsorption ↓)	**Probenecid** (Probalan, Probampacin, Gens)	*50-100mg PO qd*
sos	**Urine alkalinization** (uric acid solubility ↑)	**K⁺Na⁺-hydrogen citrate**	*2.5g PO qid, target urine pH 6.5 - 7.5*

6 B.14.2 Acute Gout Attack

	NSAID - acetic acid derivative →266 (cyclooxygenase inhibitor ⇒ anti-inflammatory, analgesic, antipyretic)	**Indomethacin** (Indocin, Indocin SR, Indo-lemmon, Indomethagan, Gens)	*25-50mg PO bid-tid, 75mg/d (SR) PO qd-bid, 50-100mg/d PR qd-bid*
	Other antigout drug →139 (phagocytosis of urate crystals by leukocytes ↓ ⇒release of inflamm. mediators; antimitotic)	**Colchicine** (Gens)	*1mg PO, max 8mg/d in first 4h, qh 1mg PO, then q2h 0.5 -1mg PO*

93. Emmerson BT, The management of gout, N Eng J Med, 1996, 334, 445-51
94. Pittman JR, Bross MH, Diagnosis and management of gout, Am Fam Physician, 1999 Apr 1;59(7):1799-806
95. Shrestha M, Randomized double blind comparison of the analgesic efficacy of IM ketordac and oral indomethacin in the treatment of acute gouty arthritis, Ann Emerg Med, 1995, 26, 682-86
96. Wallace ST, Cholchicine gem in Arthritis, Rheum, 1974, 3, 369-81

6 B.15 Porphyrias
6 B.15.1 Porphyria Cutanea Tarda (Chronic Hepatic)

	Aminoquinoline derivative →222 (builds chloroquine porphyrin complexes ⇒ renal elimination)	**Chloroquine** (Aralen, Gens)	*2 x 125mg/wk (8-12mo)*

6 B.15.2 Acute Intermittent Porphyria (Acute Hepatic; Specialist Required!)

	Delta aminolevulic acid reactivity ↓ (delta-aminolevulic acid ↓, porphobilinogen ↓)	**Glucose 20%**	*2l/d IV*
plus	**Heme analogue** (heme synthesis ↓)	**Hemin** (Panhematin)	*4mg/kg/d as short inf. over 15min for 4d*
plus	**Loop diuretic** →33 (forced diuresis)	**Furosemide** (Lasix, Gens)	*40-80mg IV qd*

sos	**Neuroleptic** →327 (sedation)	**Chlorpromazine** (Sonazide, Sparine, Thorazine, Gens)	*25-50mg PO tid, 25-50mg IM, IV tid after dilution with saline*
sos	**Betablocker** →23 (cardiac output ↓ (neg. chrono-/ inotropic), central sympathetic activity ↓)	**Propranolol** (Inderal, Inderal LA, Gens)	*40-80mg PO bid-tid, 1mg slowly IV qd, max. 10mg IV (prn)*
sos	**Parasympatholytic** →124 (spasmolysis)	**Scopolamine** (Hypodermic, Transderm Scop, Transderm-V, Gens)	*3-5 x 10-20mg/d PO, up to 5 x 20mg slowly IV (prn)*
sos	**Opioid** →270 (analgesia)	**Meperidine** (Demerol, Gens)	*25-100mg PO, PR up to qid, or 25-100mg slowly IV up to qid, max. 500mg/d (prn)*

97. Elder G, The acute porphyrias, Lancet, 1997, 349, 1613-161
98. Sassa S, Diagnosis and therapy of acute intermittent porphyria, Blood Rev, 1996, 10, 53-8

6 B.16   Osteoporosis
6 B.16.1 In General

	Calcium preparation →139 (substitution)	**Calcium** (Alka-Mints, Calci-Chew, Calci-Mix, Caltrate, Chooz, Liqui-Cal, Nephro-Calci, Os-Cal, Titralac, Tums, Gens)	*500-1000mg PO qd*
sos	**Hormone** →144 (mostly analgesia, osteoclast inhibition)	**Calcitonin** (Calcimar, Miacalcin)	*100IU SC, IM or 200IU intranasal (1-2y)*
sos	**Vitamin D** →146 (calcium resorption ↑)	**Vit D3**	*500-2000IU PO qd*
sos	**Biphosphonate** →143 (osteoclast inhibition)	**Alendronate** (Fosamax)	*10mg PO qd (30min before breakfast; optimal duration not known)*
		Etidronate (Didronel)	*400mg qd over 14d, then 1g calcium qd over 11wk (repeat cycle q3mo)*

6 B.16.2 Postmenopausal Patients

	Estrogen →437 (hormone replacement)	**Estrogen, conjugated** (Premarin)	*0.3-1.25mg*
		Estradiol valerate (Delestrogen, Gens)	*1-2mg*
		Estradiol (Estrace)	*2-4mg*
		Estradiol (Estring -ext.rel, vag)	*1mg*

Estrogens in patients with personal or family history of breast CA.

plus sos	**Progesterone** →440	**Medroxyprogesterone acetate** (Depo-provera, Amen, Provera, Gens)	*5mg d1-d10 of calendar month or 2.5mg continuously*
		Progesterone Prometrium	*200-300mg*
	Addition of Progesterone in patients with intact uterus.		
poss.	**Selective estrogen receptor modulator** →439 (bone density ↑, total + LDL cholesterol ↓)	**Raloxifene** (Evista)	*Osteoporosis PRO/Tx: 60mg PO qd; breast CA PRO: 60-120mg PO qd*
sos	**Fluoride preparation** (osteoblast stimulation)	**Sodium fluoride** (Flura-Drops, Fluorodex, Fluoritab, Flura, Pediaflor, Luride, Luride-Sf)	*75mg qpm (plus qam 1g calcium plus 1000IU Vit D; for 3-4y, yearly x-ray controls)*
sos	**Cyclooxygenase inhibitors** (anti-inflammatory, antipyretic, analgesic)	**Diclofenac** (Voltaren, Voltaren-XR, Gens)	*50mg PO, PR qd-tid, 100mg (SR) PO qd, 75mg IM qd (prn)*
sos	**Opioid** →274 (analgesic, sedating, respiratory depressive, antitussive, constipating)	**Tramadol** (Ultram)	*50-100mg PO, IV, IM, SC, up to qid; 100-200mg SR PO qd-bid (prn)*
sos	**Conjugated estrogen-progestogen combination** →441 (calciumresorption ↑, osteoblast activity ↑)	**Conjugated estrogen + Medroxyprogesterone**	*0.6mg estrogen qd + 2.5mg medroxy-progesterone qd for max. 4y*

99. AAC Clinical Practise Guidelines for the Prevention and Treatment of Postmenopausal Osteoporosis 1996 AACE
100. Avioli L, Salmon Calcitonine Nasal Spray (Review), Endocrine, 1996, 2, 115-127
101. Bamighade T, Tramadol hydrochloride. An overview of current use, Hospital Medicine, 5/98, Vol 59, No 5, 373-76
102. Black BM, Randomised trial of effect of alendronate on risk of fracture in women with exsi sting vertebral fractures, Lancet, 1996, 348, 1535-41
103. Gennari C, Use of calcitonin in treatment of bone pain associated with osteoporosis, Calcif Tis sue Int, 1991, 49, Supp 2, 9-13
104. Hanson T, The effect of fluoride and calcium on spinal bone mineral content. a controlled pro spective study (3 years), Calcif Tissue Int, 1987, 40(6), 315-7
105. Recker RR, Correcting calcium nutritional deficiency prevents spine fractures in elderly women, J Bone Miner res, 1996, 11, 1961-6
106. Sahota O. et al, A comparison of continous Atendronate, cyclical Atendronate and cyclical Eti dronate with calcitriol in the treatment of postmenopausal vertebral osteoporosis: A randomi zed Controlled Trial, Osteoporos Int 2000 11: 959-966
107. The Writing Group for the PEPI trial, Effects of hormone therapy on bone mineral density: results from the Postmenopausal Estrogen/Progestin Interventions Trial (PEPI), JAMA, 1996, 276, 1389-90

6 B.17 Osteomalacia
6 B.17.1 In General

	Calcium preparation →139 (substitution)	**Calcium** (Alka-Mints, Calci-Chew, Calci-Mix, Caltrate, Chooz, Liqui-Cal, Mallamint, Nephro-Calci, Os-Cal, Titralac, Tums,Gens)	*1000-1500mg PO qd*

sos	**Vitamin D** →146 (calcium resorption ↑)	**Cholecalciferol**	*Ini 0.25µg PO qid, then 2-3 x 0.25µg/wk (prn, calcitriol in renal osteomalacia)*

6 B.17.2 Anticonvulsive Drug Induced Rickets

	Vitamin D →146 (calcium resorption ↑)	**Cholecalciferol**	*2000-5000IU qd over 5wk, then 1000IU qd*

6 B.17.3 Malabsorbtion Syndrome

	Fat soluble vitamins →145 (parenteral substitution)	**Vitamins A, D, E, K**	*Once a wk IM*

6 B.17.4 Chronic Renal Failure

	1,2 (OH)$_2$D$_3$ →146 (proph.)	**Calcitriol** (Calcijex, Rocaltrol)	*0.25µg qd*
plus	**Phosphate binder** →139	**Calcium carbonate** (Mylanta, Titralac, Tums)	*1-2g qd*

6 B.17.5 Manifest Osteomalacia

	1,25 (OH)$_2$D$_3$ →146	**Calcitriol** (Calcijex, Rocaltrol)	*0.25-1µg qd*
plus	**Phosphate binder** →139	**Calcium carbonate** (Mylanta, Titralac, Tums)	*1-2g qd*

108.   Hutchison F, Osteomalacia and Rickets, Seminars in Nephrology, 1992, Vol 12 (2), 127-45

6 B.18 Paget's Disease of Bone (Osteitis Deformans)

	NSAID – acetic acid derivative →266 (cyclooxygenase inhibitor ⇒ anti-inflammatory, analgesic, antipyretic)	**Indomethacin** (Indocin, Indocin SR, Indo-lemmon, Indomethagan, Gens)	*25-50mg PO bid-tid, 75mg/d (SR) PO qd-bid, 50-100mg PR qd-tid*
sos	**Hormone** →144 (analgesic, osteoclast inhibition)	**Calcitonin** (Calcimar, Miacalcin)	*100IU SC, IM (6wk)*
sos	**Biphosphonate** →143 (osteoclast inhibition)	**Alendronate** (Fosamax)	*40mg PO qd (3-6mo)*

109.   Meunier PJ, Therapeutic Strategy in Paget's disease of bone, Bone, 1995, 17 (5 Suppl), 489S- 91S
110.   Siris E, Comperative study of alendronate versus etidronate for the treatment of Paget's disease of bone, J Clin Endocrinol Metabol, 1996, 81, 961-7
111.   Tiegs RD: Paget's disease of bone: indications for treatment and goals of therapy. Clin Ther 1997 Nov-Dec; 19(6): 1309-29

6 B.19 Wilson's Disease

	Complex builder →471 (copper elimination ↑)	**Penicillamine** (Cuprimine, Depen)	*1-2wk: 150mg PO qd, incr qwk by 150mg up to 450-900mg PO qd; add pyridoxine supplement 25mg qd*
	Complex builder (intestinal copper resorption ↓)	**Zinc**	*75-300mg qd; not in acute hepatic or neurologic symptoms*

112.   Gitlin N, Wilson's disease: the scourge of copper, J Hepatol, 1998, 28, 734-9

6 B.20 Hemochromatosis

sos	**Complex builder** →470 (iron elimination ↑)	**Deferoxamine** (Desferal)	*25-50mg, 1g/kg as SC inf over 24h; Caution: q(1/2)y eye/ear exams*

113. Kirking MH, Treatment of chronic iron overload, Clin Pharm, 1991, 10, 775-83

6 B.21 Nontoxic Goiter
6 B.21.1 In General

	Potassium iodide →156 (substitution)	**Potassium iodide** (iodine)	*200µg PO qd (at first for 6-12mo)*
or	**Thyroid hormone** →156 (hormone substitution ⇒ TSH↓)	**Levothyroxine** (Levo-T, Levoxyl, Unithroid)	*25-100µg PO qd, incr dose up to 200µg PO sos; adj to low normal range 0.3-0.8 mV/l*

Ind: manifest/subclinical hypothyroidism, patients > 40y, patients with evidence of thyroid antibodies, insufficient effects of iodine Tx after 1y

or	**Potassium iodide + thyroid hormone** (substitution of synthesis component + hormone ⇒ TSH ↓)	**Iodine + Levothyroxine** (100µg I⁻ + 100µg T4)	*Iodine: 100-200µg PO qd (at first for 6-12mo) + Levothyroxine: 50-75µg PO qd*

6 B.21.2 Relapse-/Prophylaxis

	Potassium iodide →156 (substitution of synthesis component)	**Potassium iodide** (iodine)	*100-200µg PO qd*

6 B.21.3 Objectives of Therapy with Iodine

- **Children, teens: complete regression of goiter**
- **Adults < 40y: Volume reduction of 30%, sonographic control after 0.5, 1y**

114. Perrild H, Hansen JM, Hegedus L: Triiodothyronine and thyroxine treatment of diffuse non-toxic goiter evaluated by ultrasonic scanning. Acta Endocrinol (Copenh) 1982 Jul; 100(3): 382-7
115. Ross DS: Thyroid hormone suppressive therapy of sporadic nontoxic goiter. Thyroid 1992 Fall; 2(3): 263-9

6 B.22 Hyperthyroidism
6 B.22.1 Grave's Disease, Thyrostatic

	Antithyroid →157 (peroxidase inhibition ⇒ hormone synthesis ↓)	**Methimazole** (Tapazole, Gens)	*Ini 10-20mg PO qd, maint dose 10mg/d PO qd; euthyroid usually after 2-8wk, try to discontinue after 12-18mo; Caution: check blood count due to AE (agranulocytosis 0.1-1%)*
or sos	**Antithyroid** →157 (conversion T4 → T3↓, peroxidase inhibition ⇒ hormone synthesis ↓)	**Propylthiouracil** (Gens)	*Ini 150-400mg div into blu, maint dose 50-150mg qd*

116. Leech NJ, Controversies in the management of Graves' disease, Clinical Endocrinology, 1998, 49, 273-80
117. Reinwein D, A prospective randomized trial of antithyroid drug dose in Grave´disease therapy, J Clin Endocrinol Metabol, 1993, 76, 1516-21
118. Weetman AP: Graves' disease. N Engl J Med 2000 Oct 26; 343(17): 1236-48

6 B.22.2 Functional Autonomy, Thyrostatic

	Antithyroid →157 (peroxidase inhibition ⇒ hormone synthesis ↓)	**Methimazole** (Tapazole, Gens)	*Ini 20mg PO qd-bid, maint dose 5-20mg PO qd*
or sos	**Radio-iodine** beta (90%)/gamma (10%) emission ⇒ destruction of hormone active cells	**I 131 radio-iodine**	*In isolation according to thyroid volume*

6 B.22.3 Symptomatic (Tachycardia, Hypertension)

	Betablocker →23 (conversion T4 → T3 ↓, cardiac output ↓ (neg. chronotropic, neg. inotropic), central sympathic activity ↓)	**Propranolol** (Inderal, Inderal LA, Gens)	*10-40mg PO bid-tid (prn)*

6 B.22.4 Inoperability/Relapse after Operation

	Radio-iodine beta (90%)/gamma (10%) emission ⇒ destruction of hormone active cells	**I 131 radio-iodine**	*In isolation according to thyroid volume*

6 B.22.5 Thyrotoxicosis (Specialist Required!)

1. Thyrostatic

	Antithyroid →157 (peroxidase inhibition ⇒ hormone synthesis ↓)	**Methimazole** (Tapazole)	*40-80mg slowly IV q6-8h*
or sos	**Antithyroid** →157 (conversion T4 → T3 ↓, peroxidase inhibition ⇒ hormone synthesis ↓)	**Propylthiouracil** (Gens)	*Ini 150-400mg div into bid, maint dose 50-150mg qd*

2. Symptomatic

	Calorie substitution (nutrient substitution)	**Glucose 20-50%**	*Approx. 4000-6000KJ/d (prn)*
	Isotonic saline solution, cristalloid plasma expander (volume + electrolyte substitution)	**Saline 0.9%, Ringer's solution**	*Approx. 4-6l/d IV according to CVP (prn)*
	Betablocker →23 (conversion T4 → T3 ↓, cardiac output ↓ (neg. chronotropic, neg. inotropic, central sympathic activity ↓)	**Propranolol** (Inderal, Inderal LA, Gens)	*40mg IV over 6h (prn)*

Benzodiazepine →330 (sedation)	**Diazepam** (Diastat, Diazepam Intensol, Valium, Gens)	*10mg IV (prn)*
Glucocorticoid →148 (manage associated adrenal cortex failure, conversion T4 → T3 ↓)	**Hydrocortisone** (A-Hydrocort, Cortef, Solu-Cortef, Gens)	*100mg as bolus, then 250mg/ 24h IV; emerg. thyroid resection in hyperdynamic shock with multiorgan failure*

6 B.22.6 Prophylaxis of Iodine Induced Hyperthyroidism in Suppressed Basal TSH

	Antithyroid (peroxidase inhibition ⇒ hormone synthesis ↓)	**Perchlorate** (Irenat)	*500mg (= 25gtt) 2-4h before CM admin and 2-4h after CM admin, then 3 x 300mg (=15gtt) over 7- 14d; begin before CM admin over 7-14d*
plus	**Antithyroid** →157 (peroxidase inhibition ⇒ hormone synthesis ↓)	**Methimazole** (Tapazole)	*20mg over 7-14d, start before CM admin*

119.   Gittoes NJ, Franklyn JA: Hyperthyroidism. Current treatment guidelines. Drugs 1998 Apr; 55(4): 543-53

6 B.23   Hypothyroidism
6 B.23.1 Chronic Hypothyroidism

Thyroid hormone →156 (hormone substitution ⇒ TSH↓)	**Levothyroxine** (Levo-T, Levoxyl, Unithroid)	*Ini 50µg PO qd, incr by 25µg q1-3wk up to maint dose: 100-150µg qd; in older patients with CHD ini 25µg, incr q4wk cautiously by 12.5µg*

6 B.23.2 Myxedema Coma (Specialist Required!)

Glucocorticoid →148 (because of possible adrenal cortex failure)	**Hydrocortisone** (A-Hydrocort, Cortef, Solu-Cortef, Gens)	*100-200mg/24h IV*
Thyroid hormone →157 (hormone substitution ⇒ TSH ↓)	**Levothyroxine** (Levo-T, Levoxyl, Unithroid)	*d1: 500µg IV, d2-7: 100µg IV qd, from d8: 100µg PO qd*
Calorie substitution (symptomatic Tx, ICU)	**Glucose 20–40%**	

Electrolyte balance: fluid restriction due to dilution hyponatremia (depending on CVP)

Circulation support: catecholamine admin. possibly relief of a pericardial effusion, slow warming (1°C/h)

120.   Nicoloff JT, Myxedema coma, Endocrin Metabol Clin North Am, 1993, 2, 279-90

6 B.24 Thyroiditis

6 B.24.1 Hashimoto's Thyroiditis (Chronic Lymphocytic Thyroiditis)

sos	**Thyroid hormone** →156 (hormone substitution ⇒ TSH ↓)	**Levothyroxine** (Levo-T, Levoxyl, Unithroid)	*Ini 50-100µg PO qd, maint dose 1.5-2µg/kg qd; Caution: in older patients with CHD incr dose cautiously*

121. Dayan CM, Daniels GH: Chronic autoimmune thyroiditis. N Engl J Med 1996 Jul 11; 335(2): 99-107

6 B.24.2 Riedel's Thyroiditis (Invasive Fibrous Thyroiditis)

	Glucocorticoid →148 (anti-inflammatory, immunosuppressive)	**Prednisolone** (Econopred, Econopred Plus, Pred Forte, Pred Mild)	*80mg PO qd, red gradually to 5mg qd*

122. Vaidya B, Corticosteroid therapy in Riedel's thyroiditis, Postgrad Med J, 1997, 73, 817-9

6 B.24.3 Subacute Thyroiditis (De Quervain's Thyroiditis)

Mild

	NSAID – acetic acid derivative →266 (cyclooxygenase inhibitor ⇒ anti-inflammatory, analgesic, antipyretic)	**Indomethacin** (Indocin, Indocin SR, Indo-lemmon, Indomethagan, Gens)	*25-50mg PO bid-tid, 75mg (SR) PO qd-bid, 50-100mg PR qd-bid*

Severe

sos	**Glucocorticoid** →148 (anti-inflammatory, immunosuppressive)	**Prednisolone** (Econopred, Econopred Plus, Pred Forte, Pred Mild)	*Ini 40mg PO qd for 4-6 wk, then reduce q3d by 8mg until 16mg/d, then qwk by 4mg; sos pulse Tx 500-1000mg on d3 IV*

123. Hamburger JI: The various presentations of thyroiditis. Diagnostic considerations. Ann Intern Med 1986 Feb; 104(2): 219-24

6 B.25 Cushing Syndrome

6 B.25.1 ACTH-Producing Pituitary Tumor

1st choice	**Transsphenoidal surgery**, if failure, bilateral adrenalectomy – preoperative normalisation of hypercortisolism		
	Inhibition of 11-/ and 18-beta-hydroxylase →217 (blocking of cortisone synthesis)	**Ketoconazole** (Nizoral, Gens)	*200-1200mg qd*

6 B.25.2 Ectopic ACTH Production and ACTH Independent Cushing Syndrome

sos	**Inhibition of 3beta-dehydrogenase** (cytotoxic, cortisol synthesis ↓)	**Mitotane** (Lysodren)	*0.5-4g qd (glucocorticoid substitution sos; in LDL cholesterol ↑, HMG-CoA reductase inhibitor)*
sos	**Inhibition of 11-/ and 18-beta-hydroxylase** →217 (blocking of cortisone synthesis)	**Ketoconazol** (Nizoral, Gens)	*200-1200mg qd*

sos	**Inhibition of 11-/ and 18-beta-hydroxylase** (blocking of cortisone synthesis)	**Metyrapone** (Metopirone)	*1.5g PO qd div tid-qid (AE limit use)*
sos	**Aromatase inhibitor** →439 (cortisol synthesis ↓)	**Aminoglutethimide** (Cytadren)	*Adrenal cortex adenoma: 250mg PO bid-tid, in ect. ACTH prod. qid-7x/d*

124. Trainer PJ, Cushing's syndrome. Therapy directed at the adrenal gland, Endocrin Metab Clin North Am, 1994, 23, 571-84
125. Yanovski JA, Cutler GB Jr: Glucocorticoid action and the clinical features of Cushing's syndrome. Endocrinol Metab Clin North Am 1994; 23(3): 487-509

6 B.26 Aldosteronism

sos	**Thiazide diuretic** →33 (elimination of Na$^+$, Cl$^-$, H$_2$O and K$^+$ ↑)	**Hydrochlorothiazide** (Esidrix, Hydrodiuril, Microside, Oretic, Gens)	*12.5-50mg PO qd*
plus	**Aldosterone antagonist** →28 (mineralocorticoid steroid effects ↓)	**Spironolactone** (Aldactone, Gens)	*D1-5: 50-100mg bid-qid, then 50-100mg PO qd-bid*

6 B.27 Adrenal Insufficiency
6 B.27.1 Long-Term Therapy

Primary (Addison disease)

	Glucocorticoid →148 (substitution)	**Hydrocortisone** (A-Hydrocort, Cortef, Solu-Cortef, Gens)	*10-12mg/m² PO bid-qid, adj replacement dose based on cortisol day curve, e.g. 15-5-5mg, 10-10-5mg or 15-10-0mg*
plus	**Mineralocorticoid** →148 (substitution)	**Fludrocortisone** (Florinef)	*50-200µg qd qam*

6 B.27.2 Addison Crisis (Specialist Required!)

	Glucocorticoid →148 (substitution)	**Hydrocortisone** (A-Hydrocort, Cortef, Solu-Cortef, Gens)	*100mg IV q6h, when stabilized 50mg IV q6h; maint dose from d4/d5*
	Isotonic saline solution + glucose (volume + glucose + electrolyte substitution)	**Saline 0.9% + Glucose 40%**	*Ini 500ml saline 0.9% + 40ml glucose 40%, then glucose 5%*
sos	**Low dose heparin** →71 (low molecular heparin, embolism PRO)	**Dalteparin** (Fragmin)	*2850IU SC qd*

126. Werbel S, Acute adrenal insufficiency, Endocrin Metab Clin North Am, 1993, 22, 303-28

6 B.28 Pheochromocytoma
6 B.28.1 Long-Term Therapy, Preoperative Preparation

	Alphablocker, non competitive →30 (vasodilation ↑, afterload ↓, preload ↓)	**Phenoxybenzamine** (Dibenzyline)	*10mg PO bid, max. 30mg tid (sos until OP; hematocrit ↓, normotension)*
plus	**Betablocker** →23 (cardiac output ↓ (neg. chrono-/inotropic), renin secretion ↓, central sympathetic activity ↓)	**Propranolol** (Inderal, Inderal LA, Gens)	*40-80mg PO bid-tid, 80-320mg (SR) PO qd; tachycardia Tx only after sufficiently long alpha-blockade (otherwise paradox BP ↑)*
or sos	**Alphablocker, reversible** →30 (reversible blockage of alpha1-receptor)	**Prazosin** (Minipress, Minipress XL, Gens)	*1mg tid-qid up to 20mg*

6 B.28.2 Hypertensive Crisis

	Alphablocker, imidazole derivative →30 (vasodilation ↑, afterload ↓, preload ↓)	**Phentolamine** (Regitine, Rogitine, Gens)	*5-10mg IV, then 0.25-1mg/min inf, max. dose 120mg/h; duration of BP↓ 20min*
sos plus	**Betablocker** →23 (cardiac output ↓ (neg. chrono-/inotropic), renin secretion ↓, central sympathetic activity ↓)	**Propranolol** (Inderal, Inderal LA, Gens)	*1 x 1mg slowly IV, repeat sos*

127. Bravo E, Pheochromocytoma, Endocrin Metab Clin North Am, 1993, 22, 329-41

6 B.29 Hyperparathyroidism
6 B.29.1 Primary Hyperparathyroidism (Adenoma, Hypertrophy)

Mild

sos	**Isotonic saline solution** (rehydratation)	**Saline 0.9%**	*D1: 4-6l, then 3-4l/d*
sos	**Loop diuretic** →33 (calcium excretion)	**Furosemide** (Lasix, Gens)	*50-100mg IV*

Hypercalcemic crisis

	Isotonic saline solution (rehydratation)	**Saline 0.9%**	*1-2l IV*
sos	**Loop diuretic** →33 (calcium excretion)	**Furosemide** (Lasix, Gens)	*40-120mg IV*
sos	**Potassium chloride solution** →139 (substitution)	K^+Cl^- 7.45% (1ml = 1mmol)	*20-40ml in 1l istotonic sol in 10-20mmol/h, max. 100-200mmol/d (prn)*

sos	**Biphosphonate** →143 (osteoclast inhibition in tumor hypercalcemia)	**Pamidronate** (Aredia)	*60mg as single dose if Ca < 3.38mmol/l, 90mg if Ca > 3.38mmol/l, inf over 4-24h*
		Ibandronate (experimental)	*1mg/ml, 4mg in 500ml saline 0.9% over 2h*
sos	**Glucocorticoid** →148 (resorption ↓, mobilisation ↓)	**Prednisone** (Deltasone, Meticorten, Prednisone Intensol, Gens)	*100-200mg qd*
sos	**Hormone** →144 (osteoclast inhibition, only slightly effective)	**Calcitonin** (Calcimar, Miacalcin)	*Ini 3-4IU/kg slowly IV, then 4IU/kg SC qd*
sos	**Cytostatic** (osteoclast inhibition)	**Mithramycin** (Mithracin)	*25ng/kg IV, final resort*

128. Bilezikian JP: Clinical review 51: Management of hypercalcemia. J Clin Endocrinol Metab 1993 Dec; 77(6): 1445-9
129. Bushinsky DA, Calcium, Lancet, 1998, 352, 306-11
130. Edelson GW, Kleerekoper M: Hypercalcemic crisis. Med Clin North Am 1995 Jan; 79(1): 79-92

6 B.29.2 Secondary Hyperparathyroidism (Circulating Calcium ↓ ⇒ PTH ↑)

In general

	Calcium preparation →139 (substitution)	**Calcium** (Alka-Mints, Calci-Chew, Calci-Mix, Caltrate, Chooz, Liqui-Cal, Mallamint, Nephro-Calci, Os-Cal, Titralac, Tums,Gens)	*700-2000mg PO qd (prn)*

In malabsorbtion

	Vitamin D$_3$ →146	**Vit D3**	*1000IU qd*

In renal genesis

	Vit. D (1,25/ OH$_2$) D$_3$ →146	**Calcitriol** (Calcijex, Rocaltrol)	*0.25-1µg PO qd*

131. Allerheiligen DA, Schoeber J, Houston RE, et al: Hyperparathyroidism. Am Fam Physician 1998 Apr 15; 57(8): 1795-802, 1807-8

6 B.30 Hypoparathyroidism
6 B.30.1 Long-Term Therapy

	Calcium preparation →139 (substitution)	**Calcium carbonate** (Alka-Mints, Calci-Chew, Calci-Mix, Caltrate, Chooz, Liqui-Cal, Mallamint, Nephro-Calci, Os-Cal, Titralac, Tums, Gens)	*1-2g PO qd (prn)*
plus	**Vitamin D analogue** →146 (metabolism influence)	**Dihydrotachysterol** (DHT)	*0.3-1.0mg PO qd (prn)*
or	**Vitamin D3** →146	**Vit D3**	*500-2500µg qd (depending on Ca level)*

132. Schilling T, Current therapy of hypoparathyroidism, a survey of German endocrinology centers, Exp Clin Endocrinal Diabetes, 1997, 105, 237-41

6 B.30.2 Hypocalcemic Crisis

Calcium preparation →139 (substitution)	**Calcium gluconate 10%** (10ml = 2.3mmol)	*ini 2.3-4.5mmol slowly IV over 5-15min, then in glucose 5% inf (hospital)*

6 B.31　Hypopituitarism
6 B.31.1 Long-Term Therapy (Specialist Required!)

In general

	Glucocorticoid →148 (substitution)	**Hydrocortisone** (A-Hydrocort, Cortef, Solu-Cortef, Gens)	*10-12mg/m² qd, e.g. 10-5-10mg at 7am, 11.30am, 17.30pm (chronic)*
plus	**Thyroid hormone** →156 (substitution)	**Levothyroxine** (Levo-T, Levoxyl, Unithroid)	*Ini 50-100µg PO qd, maint dose: 1.5-2µg/kg qd (after Tx start with steroids)*
plus	**Growth hormone** →159 (substitution)	**Somatotropin** (Genotropin, Humatrope, Norditropin, Nutropin, Protropin, Saizen)	*0.04-0.08mg/kg SC qd, incr slowly (if without benefit discontinue slowly after 6mo)*

In women additionally

plus	**Estrogen + progestogen** →441 (substitution)	**Estradiol + Norethindrone**	

Premenopausal: comb. contraceptive with 20 - 35µg ethinyl-estradiol, **postmenopausal**: estradiol valerate 2mg cyclic or cont. with progestogen preparation; if **restitution of fertility** spec. Tx required: pulsatile GnRH inf SC

In men additionally

plus	**Androgen** →147 (substitution)	**Testosterone depot preparation** (Delatestryl, Depo-Testosterone, Testoderm)	*1 x 250mg IM q2-4wk or 5mg patch qd (if restitution of fertility spec. Tx required: pulsatile GnRH inf SC)*

133.　Lamberts SWJ, Pituitary insufficiency, Lancet, 1998, 352, 127-34

6 B.31.2 Pituitary Coma

Adrenal crisis (Specialist Required!)

	Isotonic saline solution + glucose (volume + glucose + electrolyte substitution)	**Saline 0.9% + Glucose 40%**	*Ini 500ml saline 0.9%+ 40ml glucose 40%, then glucose 5%*
plus	**Glucocorticoid** →148 (substitution)	**Hydrocortisone** (A-Hydrocort, Cortef, Solu-Cortef, Gens)	*Ini 100mg IV, then inf 10mg/h or 100mg IM/IV q6h, then 50mg PO qid, decrease slowly*
sos	**Vasopressor** →22 (dose-depend. dopamine-/ β- and α-agonism ⇒ cardiac output↓, vasoconstriction, renal vasodilation	**Dopamine** (Intropin, Gens)	*Renal dose: 0.5-5µg/kg/min IV, perf. (250mg) = 5mg/ml ⇒ 1-3.5ml/h, BP dose: 6-10µg/kg/min IV, perf. (250mg) ⇒ 4.5-9ml/h, max. 18ml/h*

| sos | **(Beta)sympathomimetic** →22 (inotropic) | **Dobutamine** (Dobutrex, Gens) | *2.5-12µg/kg/min IV* |
| sos | **Low-molecular heparin** →71 (coagulation factor ↓, embolism PRO) | **Dalteparin** (Fraxiparin) **Enoxaparin** (Lovenox) | *2850IU SC qd* |

Myxedema coma (see Hypothyroidism, →177)

6 B.32 Hyperpituitarism, Pituitary Tumors
6 B.32.1 Hyperprolactinemia (Specialist Required!)

| | **Prolactin inhibitor** →158 (pituitary dopamine receptor stimulation ⇒ prolactin ↓) | **Bromocriptine** (Parlodel) | *1.25mg PO qhs (in the middle of bedtime snack), incr slowly sos, max 30mg/d in div doses* |
| | | **Cabergoline** (Dostinex) | *0.25mg PO biw, incr slowly sos, max 1mg biw* |

134. Cunnah D, Management of prolactinomas, Clin Endocrinol, 1991, 34, 231-35
135. Serri O: Progress in the management of hyperprolactinemia. N Engl J Med 1994 Oct 6; 331(14): 942-4

6 B.32.2 Acromegaly (Specialist Required!)

| | **Prolactin inhibitor** →158 (pituitary dopamine receptor stimulation ⇒ prolactin ↓, STH ↓) | **Bromocriptine** (Parlodel) | *1.25mg PO qd, incr slowly sos, max 30mg/d div bid; individual dose!* |
| or | **Somatostatin analogue** →128 (STH ↓) | **Octreotide** (Sandostatin, Sandostatin LAR Depot) | *Ini 0.05mg SC, then up to 0.5mg SC tid (according to GH level), then depot 20-30mg IM q4wk x 3mo, then q4wk according to GH level* |

136. Shimon I, Management of pituitary tumors, Ann Intern Med, 1998, 129, 472-83

6 B.33 Diabetes Insipidus
6 B.33.1 Central Diabetes Insipidus

| | **Hormone** →159 (ADH substitution) | **Desmopressin** (Concentraid, DDAVP, Stimate, Gens) | *0.1-0.4mg intranasal tid, SC (chronic)* |

6 B.33.2 Peripheral Diabetes Insipidus

| | **Thiazide diuretic** →33 (GFR ↓, antidiuretic effect) | **Hydrochlorothiazide** (Esidrix, Hydrodiuril, Microside, Uretic, Gens) | *12.5-50mg PO qd* |

137. Robertson GL, Diabetes insipidus, Endocrin Metab Clin North Am, 1995, 24, 49-71

6 B.34 Insulinoma
6 B.34.1 In General (Specialist Required!)

sos	**Hormone** →154 (antihypoglycemic, gluconeogenesis ↑, glycogenolysis ↑)	**Glucagon** (GlucaGen, Gens)	*According to BS*
sos	**K⁺ channel modulation** →154 (insulin secetion ↓, hepatic glucose output ↑)	**Diazoxide** (Proglycem)	*5mg/kg/d PO in 2-3 single doses*
sos	**Somatostatin analogue** →128 (insulin secretion ↓)	**Octreotide** (Sandostatin, Sandostatin LAR Depot)	*Ini 1-2 x 0.05mg SC, then 0.5mg SC up to tid under close supervision, then depot 20-30mg IM q4wk*

6 B.34.2 Cytostatic

	Cytostatic, pyrimidine antagonist (thymidine nucleotide synthesis ↓)	**5-Fluorouracil** (Adrucil)	*400mg/m² IV on d1-d5 (repeat cycle from d43)*
plus	**Cytostatic, alkylating** (nitrosourea analog, inhibits DNA synthesis)	**Streptozocin** (Zanosar)	*500mg/m² IV on d1-d5 (repeat cycle from d43)*
plus	**Cytostatic antibiotic** (DNA damage)	**Doxorubicin** (Adriamycin)	*50mg/m² IV on d1 + d21 (repeat cycle from d43)*

138.   Perry RR, Diagnosis and management of functioning islet-cell tumors, J Endocrin Metab, 1995, 80, 2273

6 B.35 VIPoma

	Somatostatin analogue →128 (VIP secretion ↓)	**Octreotide** (Sandostatin, Sandostatin LAR Depot)	*Ini 1-2 x 0.05mg SC, then 0.5mg SC up to tid under close supervision, then depot 20-30mg IM q4wk*

139.   Arnold R, Management of gastroenteropathic endocrine tumors: The place of Somatostatin Analogues, Digestion, 1994, Suppl 3, 107-13

6 B.36 Gastrinoma (Zollinger-Ellison Syndrome)

sos	**Proton pump inhibitors** →118 (acid secretion ↓)	**Omeprazole** (Prilosec, Gens)	*20-40mg PO qd, up to max.160mg*
sos	**Somatostatin analogue** →128 (gastrin secretion ↓)	**Octreotide** (Sandostatin, Sandostatin LAR Depot)	*Ini 1-2 x 0.05mg SC, then 0.5mg SC up to tid under close supervision, then depot 20-30mg IM q4wk*

140.   Meko JB, Management of patients with Zollinger Ellison syndrome, Ann Rev Med, 1995, 46, 395

6 B.37 Carcinoid Tumor

	Somatostatin analogue →128 (gastrin sekretion ↓)	Octreotide (Sandostatin, Sandostatin LAR Depot)	Ini 1-2 x 0.05mg SC, then 0.5mg SC up to tid under close supervision, then depot 20-30mg IM q4wk
	Serotonin antagonist (serotonine effects ↓)	Methysergide (Sansert)	4mg (SR) PO bid
sos	Interferon →212 (immune stimulation/ -modulation)	IFN-alpha-2a/b (Intron A, Roferon)	3-5 MIU/wk prn
sos	Antidiarrheal →122 (stimulation of peripheral opiod receptors)	Loperamide (Imodium, Gens)	Ini 4mg PO, after each episode 2mg, max: 12mg/d (prn)

141. Kema IP, Willemse PH, De Vries EG: Carcinoid tumors. N Engl J Med 1999 Aug 5; 341(6): 453-4

6 B.38 Gynecomastia

	Antiestrogen →439 (blockade of peripheral estrogen receptors ⇒ estrogen effects ↓)	Tamoxifen (Nolvadex)	20-40mg PO qd (short-term)
sos			

142. Braunstein GD, Gynecomastia, N Engl J Med, 1993, 328, 490-5

7 A. Infections – Drugs

7 A.1   Organism – Antibiotic

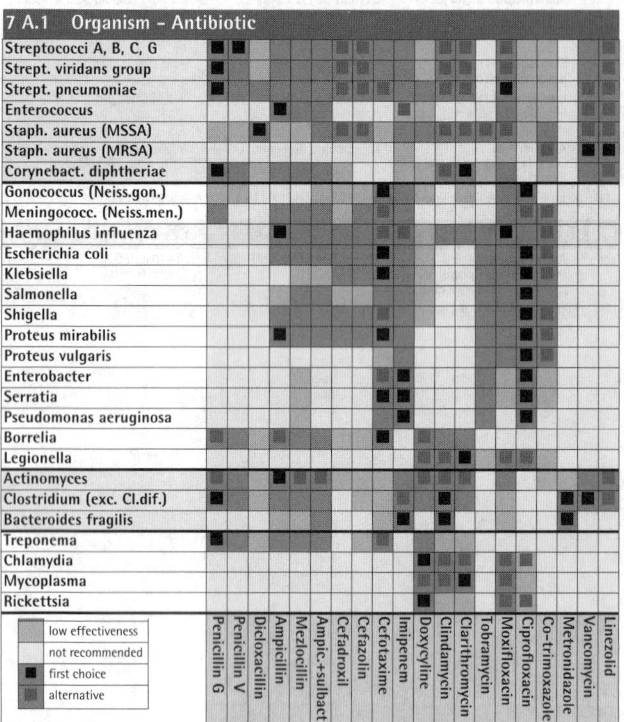

from Antibiotics pocketcard 2004; Hof, Börm Bruckmeier Publishing, ISBN 3-59103-018-8

7 A.2   Penicillins
7 A.2.1   Penicillins – 1st Generation (Benzylpenicillins, Penicillinase-Sensitive)

S: Pneumo-, Strepto-, Meningo-, Staphylococcus, Actinomyces, Leptospira,
C. diphtheria, Treponema, Borrelia, Past. multocida, Fusobacteria, Peptococcus, Clostridia
R: Enteric bacteria, Pseudomonas, B. fragilis, E. faecium, Nocardia, Mycoplasma, Chlamydia, beta-lactamase
producing bacteria, Salmonella, V. cholerae
AE: allergic skin reactions, Lyell-syndrome, anaphylaxis, vasculitis, myoclonia, seizures, oral dryness, N/V,
diarrhea, Herxheimer-reaction, complete blood count changes, hemolytic anemia, interstitial nephritis,
superinfection by multiresistant bacteria or yeasts
CI: hypersensitivity to prod ingredients, penicillins (Pen G procaine: additional sulfites), hx of anaphylaxis,
accelerated or serum sickness reaction to previous penicillin administration

Benzathine Penicillin	EHL 20-50min
Bicillin L-A *Inj 300,000 U/ml, 600,000 U/ml* **Permapen** *Inj 600,000 U/ml*	**Erysipeloid, streptococcal infx**: 1.2 M U IM as single dose; **PRO of rheumatic fever** →64: 1.2 M U IM qmo; **primary, secondary syphilis** →239: 2.4 M U IM as single dose; **late syphilis**: 2.4 M U IM q7d for 3 wk; **CH congenital syphilis**: 50.000 U IM as single dose; **pharyngitis**: <27kg, 300,000-600,000 U IM, > 27kg, 900,000 U IM as single dose

Benzylpenicilloyl polylysine	
Pre-Pen *Inj. 60 umolar*	**Penicillin sensitivity detection**: 0.01-0.03ml intradermally

Penicillin G	EHL 20-50min, PRC B, Lact +
Penicillin *Sol (oral) 200,000 U/5ml, 250,000 U/5ml, 400,000 U/5ml* **Penicillin G Potassium** *Inj 20,000 U/ml, 40,000 U/ml, 60,000 U/ml* **Pfizerpen** *Inj 1,000,000 U/vial, 5,000,000 U/vial, 20,000,000 U/vial* **Generics** *Tab 200,000 U, 250,000 U, 400,000 U, 500,000 U, 800,000 U* *Inj 1,000,000 U/vial, 5,000,000 U/vial, 10,000,000 U/vial, 20,000,000 U/vial*	**Streptococcal, pneumococcal, meningococcal infx**: 1-5 M U/d IV div q4-6h; **streptococcal or staphylococcal endocarditis** →64: 12-18 M U/d IV div q4h; **enterococcal endocarditis** →64: 18-30 M U/d continuous IV inf or div q4h with aminoglycoside; **meningococcal meningitis**: 20-40 M U/d IV div q2-4h; **CH** <12y: 25,000-400,000 U/kg/d IV div q4-6h, neonates: see Prod Info

Penicillin V	EHL 30-40min, PRC B, Lact +
Beepen-VK *Tab 250mg, 500mg,* *Sol (oral) 125mg/5ml, 250mg/5ml* **Betapen-VK** *Tab 250mg, 500mg* **Ledercillin VK** *Tab 250mg, 500mg,* *Sol (oral) 125mg/5ml, 250mg/5ml* **Pen-vee K** *Tab 250mg, 500mg,* *Sol (oral) 125mg/5ml, 250mg/5ml* **Uticillin VK** *Tab 250mg* **V-cillin K** *Tab 125mg, 250mg, 500mg, Sol (oral)* *125mg/5ml, 250mg/5ml* **Veetids** *Tab 250mg, 500mg,* *Sol (oral) 125mg/5ml, 250mg/5ml* **Generics** *Tab 250mg, 500mg,* *Sol (oral) 125mg/5ml, 250mg/5ml,* *Susp 125mg/5ml, 250mg/5ml*	**Streptococcal infx**: 250-500mg PO qid; **secondary PRO of rheumatic fever** →64: 250mg PO bid; **PRO of endocarditis** →65: 2g 1h before procedure, 1g 6h later; **CH** <12y: 25-50mg/kg/d PO div tid or qid, max 3g/d

Procaine Penicillin	EHL 20-30min
Pfizerpen-as *Inj 300,000 U/ml,* *600,000 U/ml* **Wycillin** *Inj 300,000 U/ml, 600,000 U/ml* **Generics** *Inj 300,000 U/vial, 1,500,000 U/vial*	**Streptococcal, staphylococcal infx**: 0.6-1.0 M U IM qd for 7-10d **neurosyphilis** →239: 2.4 M U IM qd + probenecid 500mg PO q6h for 10-14d; **CH** 300.000 U IM qd; **congenital syphilis**: 50.000 U/kg IM qd for 10d; DARF: GFR (ml/min): 10-50: 75%, <10: 20-50%

Procaine + Benzathine Penicillin	
Bicillin C-R *Inj 150,000 U/ml + 150,000 U/ml,* *300,000 U/ml + 300,000 U/ml* **Bicillin C-R 900/300** *Inj 900,000 U/2ml* *+ 300,000 U/2ml*	**Scarlet fever, erysipelas, upper-respiratory, skin and soft-tissue infx due to group A streptococci**: 2.4 M U IM as single dose; **pneumococcal infx except meningitis**: 1.2 M U IM q2-3d until temperature normal for 48h; **CH scarlet fever, erysipelas, upper-respiratory, skin and soft-tissue infx due to group A streptococci**: >27kg: 2.4 M U IM; 13.6-27kg: 900.000-1.2 M U IM; <13kg: 600.000 U IM; **pneumococcal infx except meningitis**: 600.000 U IM q2-3d until temperature normal for 48h

7 A.2.2   Penicillins – 2nd Generation (Penicillinase-Resistant)

S/R: highly effective against beta-lactamase producing S. aureus; otherwise very narrow spectrum + lower activity against all other gram-positive bacteria than penicillin G
AE/CI: see benzylpenicillins →187
AE (cloxacillin): fever, rash, N/V, diarrhea, hepatotoxicity; **AE** (dicloxacillin): diarrhea, N/V; **AE** (nafcillin): neutropenia, interstitial nephritis; **AE** (oxacillin): N/V, diarrhea, rash
CI: hypersensitivity to product ingredients/penicillins

Cloxacillin	EHL 0.5-1h, PRC B, Lact ?
Cloxacillin sodium *Cap 250mg, 500mg,* *Sol (oral) 125mg/5ml*	**Staphylococcal infx**: 250-500mg PO qid; **CH** > 20kg: see adults; <20kg: 50-100mg/kg/d PO div qid; DARF: not req

Dicloxacillin
EHL 0.7h, PRC B, Lact ?

Dycill *Cap 250mg, 500mg*
Pathocil *Cap 250mg, 500mg, Susp 62.5mg/5ml*
Generics *Cap 125mg, 250mg, 500mg,*
Susp 62.5mg/5ml

Upper respiratory, skin and soft-tissue infx:
125mg PO qid; **severe infx:** 250-500mg PO qid;
CH >40kg: see adults, <40kg: 12.5-25mg/kg/d PO
div qid; DARF: not req

Nafcillin
EHL 0.5-1h, PRC B, Lact ?

Nallpen *Inj 20mg/ml, 2g/100ml, 500mg/vial,*
1g/vial, 2g/vial, 10g/vial
Unipen *Inj 500mg/vial, 1g/vial, 2g/vial, 4g/vial,*
10g/vial
Generics *Inj 500mg/vial, 1g/vial, 1.5g/vial, 2g/vial,*
4g/vial, 10g/vial

Staphylococcal infx: 500mg IM q4-6h or 500mg-1g
IV q4h; **severe infx:** 1-2g IV q4h; **CH** 50-100mg/kg/d
IM/IV div qid;
DARF: not req

Oxacillin
EHL 23-45min, PRC B, Lact +

Bactocill *Cap 250mg, 500mg*
Sol (oral) 250mg/5ml

Staphylococcal infx: 500-1000mg PO q4-6h or
250-500mg IM/IV q4-6h; **severe infx:** 1-2g IV
q4-6h; **CH** >40kg: see adults, <40kg: 50-100mg/kg/d
PO div qid; DARF: not req

7 A.2.3 Penicillins - 3rd Generation (Aminopenicillins)

S: compared to penicillin G additional action against Enterococcus, H. influenza,
E. coli, Listeria, P. mirabilis, Salmonella, Shigella
R: B. fragilis, Pseudomonas, E. faecium, Nocardia, Mycoplasma, Chlamydia, beta-lactamase producing
bacteria, Klebsiella, Yersinia
AE/CI: see benzylpenicillins →187
CI: infectious mononucleosis

Amoxicillin
EHL 1-2h, PRC B, Lact +

Amoxil *Tab 500mg, 875mg, Tab (chew) 125mg,*
200mg, 250mg, 400mg, Cap 250mg, 500mg, Susp
50mg/ml, 125mg/5ml, 200mg/5ml, 250mg/5ml,
400mg/5ml
Larotid *Susp 125mg/5ml, 250mg/5ml*
Trimox *Cap 250mg, 500mg, Susp 50mg/ml,*
125mg/5ml, 250mg/5ml
Wymox *Cap 250mg, 500mg, Susp 125mg/5ml,*
250mg/5ml
Generics *Tab 500mg, 875mg, Tab (chew) 125mg,*
200mg, 250mg, 400mg, Cap 250mg, 500mg,
Susp 50mg/ml, 125mg/5ml, 250mg/5ml

Respiratory tract, ENT, genitourinary tract, skin,
infx: 250-500mg PO q8h or 500-875mg PO q12h;
endocarditis PRO →65: 2g PO 1h before the
procedure, **CH** > 3mo: 20-45mg/kg/d PO div bid or
tid; DARF: GFR (ml/min) <10: 250-500mg PO q24h

Ampicillin
EHL 1-1.8 h and 15-20 h, PRC B, Lact +

Omnipen *Susp 100mg/ml, 125mg/5ml, 250mg/5ml*
Omnipen-N *Inj 125mg/vial, 250mg/vial,*
500mg/vial 1g/vial, 2g/vial
Principen *Cap 250mg, 500mg, Susp 100mg/ml,*
125mg/5ml, 250mg/5ml
Totacillin *Cap 250mg, 500mg,*
Susp 125mg/5ml, 250mg/5ml
Totacillin-N *Inj 125mg/vial, 250mg/vial,*
500mg/vial 1g/vial, 2g/vial, 10g/vial
Generics *Cap 250mg, 500mg,*
Susp 125mg/5ml, 250mg/5ml
Inj 125mg/vial, 250mg/vial, 500mg/vial, 1g/vial,
2g/vial, 10g/vial

Respiratory tract, GI infx, UTI: 250-500mg PO/IV/
IM q6h; **meningitis**: 8-14g/d IV div q3-4h;
endocarditis PRO →65: 2g IM/IV 30min. before the
procedure;
endocarditis Tx →63: 3g IV q6h in combination with
an aminoglycoside;
CH >20kg: see adults; <20kg: 50-100mg/kg/d PO div
q6-8h; 50-200mg/kg/d IV div q6h; DARF: GFR
(ml/min) >50: q6h,
10-50: q6-12h, <10: q12-16h

7 A.2.4   Penicillins – 4th Generation (Extended Spectrum, Antipseudomonal)

S/R: similar to aminopenicillins, but highly effective against Ps. aeruginosa
AE/CI: see benzylpenicillins →187
AE (mezlocillin): bleeding time ↑, fever, rash, hypokalemia, thrombophlebitis, interstitial nephritis
AE (piperacillin): fever, headache, rash
AE (ticarcillin): convulsions, nephritis, anemia, thrombophlebitis, rash, anaphylaxis
CI (mezlocillin, piperacillin, ticarcillin): hypersensitivity to product ingred./penicillins

Mezlocillin
EHL 0.7-1.1h, PRC B, Lact ?

Mezlin *Inj 1g/vial, 2g/vial, 3g/vial,*
4g/vial, 20g/vial

**Respiratory tract, urinary tract, intra-abdominal,
skin, gynecologic infx, febrile neutropenia:**
2-4g IV q4-6h, **CH** 1mo-12y: 75mg/kg IV/IM q8-12h;
DARF: GFR (ml/min): 10-30: 3g IV q8h;
<10: 2g IV q8h

Piperacillin
EHL 3.33h, PRC B, Lact +

Pipracil *Inj 2g/vial, 3g/vial, 4g/vial*

Sepsis, nosocomial pneumonia →109, **intra-
abdominal, urinary tract, skin and soft tissue
infx: serious infx:** 12-18g/d IV/IM div q4-6h,
max 24g/d; **uncomplicated UTI:** 6-8g/d IV/IM div
q6-12h; DARF: GFR (ml/min): 20-40: 4g q8h,
<20: 4g q12h

Ticarcillin
EHL 1.2h, PRC B, Lact +

Ticar *Inj 1g/vial, 3g/vial, 20g/vial,*
30g/vial

**Sepsis, respiratory tract, skin and soft tissue,
intra-abdominal, genitourinary infx:** 3-4g IV
q4-6h; **CH** > 40kg: see adults, <40kg:
200-300mg/kg/d IV div q4-6h; DARF: ini 3g, then
GFR (ml/min): 30-60: 2g IV q4h; 10-30: 2g IV q8h;
<10: 2g IV q12h

7 A.2.5   Penicillin + β-Lactamase Inhibitor

AE (amoxicillin + clavulanate): headache, rash, N/V, diarrhea
AE (ampicillin + sulbactam): rash, N/V, pseudomembranous colitis, liver enzymes ↑
AE (piperacillin + tazobactam): rash, diarrhea, headache, N/V
AE (ticarcillin + clavulanate): hypersensitivity reactions, headache, seizures, pseudomembranous colitis, thrombophlebitis
CI (amoxicillin + clavulanate, ampicillin + sulbactam, piperacillin + tazobactam): hypersensitivity to penicillins + product ingredients

Amoxicillin + Clavulanate

PRC B, Lact +

Augmentin *Tab 250mg + 125mg, 500mg + 125mg, 875mg + 125mg, Tab (chew) 125mg + 31.25mg, 200mg + 28.5mg, 250mg + 62.5mg, 400mg + 57mg, Susp 125mg/5ml + 31.25mg/5ml, 200mg/5ml + 28.5mg/5ml, 250mg/5ml + 62.5mg/5ml, 400mg/5ml + 57mg/5ml*

UTI, respiratory tract, skin infx, sinusitis →416, **otitis media** →421: 250 +125mg PO or 500–875 +125mg bid; **CH** 20–45mg/kg/d amoxicillin component PO div bid or tid; DARF: GFR (ml/min): 10–30: 250–500 + 125mg q12h; <10: 250–500 + 125mg PO q24h

Ampicillin + Sulbactam

PRC B, Lact +

Unasyn *Inj 1g/vial + 0.5g/vial, 2g/vial + 1g/vial, 10g/vial + 5g/vial*

UTI, respiratory tract, intra-abdominal, skin and soft tissue infx: 1+0.5g = 2+1g IM/IV q6h; **CH** 50 200mg/kg/d ampicillin component iV div q6h; DARF: GFR (ml/min): > 30: q6-8h; 15-29: q12h; 5-14: q24h

Piperacillin + Tazobactam

PRC B, Lact +

Zosyn *Inj 2g/vial + 0.25g/vial, 3g/vial + 0.375g/vial, 4g/vial + 0.5g/vial, 36g/vial + 4.5g/vial, Inj 40mg/ml + 5mg/ml, 60mg/ml + 7.5mg/ml, 4g/100ml + 500mg/100ml*

Intra-abdominal, skin infx, community-acquired pneumonia →100, **febrile neutropenia**: 3 + 0.375g IV q6h; **nosocomial pneumonia** →109: 3 + 0.375g IV q4h in combination with aminoglycoside; DARF: GFR (ml/min): 20-40: 2 + 0.25g IV q6h; <20: 2 + 0.25g IV q8h

Ticarcillin + Clavulanate

PRC B, Lact +

Timentin *Inj 3g/vial + 0.1g/vial, 3g/vial + 0.2g/vial, 30g/vial + 1g/vial, Inj 3g/100ml + 100mg/100ml*

Systemic infx, UTI: 3 + 0.1g IV q4-6h; **CH** 300mg/kg/d ticarcillin component IV div q6h; DARF: ini 3.1g, then GFR (ml/min): 30-60: 2g IV q4h; 10-30: 2g IV q8h; <10: 2g IV q12h; <10 with hepatic dysfunction: 2g IV q24h

7 A.3   Cephalosporins

7 A.3.1   Cephalosporins – 1st Generation

S: act as penicillin G substitutes, but resistant to staphylococcal penicillinase; also activity against Proteus mirabilis, E. coli + Klebsiella pneumoniae; cefazolin-group: Staphylo-, Strepto-, Pneumococcus, N. meningitis, E. coli, Klebsiella, Prot. mirabilis, H. influenza
R (cefazolin-group): Enterococcus, Pseudomonas, Acinetobact., Listeria, Chlamydia, Mycoplasma, gram-neg. ß-lactamase-producing bacteria
AE (cephalosporins): allergic skin reactions, Lyell-syndrome, anaphylaxis, N/V, diarrhea, transaminases ↑, cholestasis, interstitial pneumonia, complete blood count changes, hemolytic anemia, creatinine ↑, interstitial nephritis, superinfection by bacteria or yeasts
CI (cephalosporins): hypersensitivity to cephalosporins

Cefazolin

Ancef *Inj 10mg/ml, 20mg/ml,*
500mg/vial, 1g/vial, 5g/vial, 10g/vial
Kefzol *Inj 250mg/vial, 500mg/vial,*
1g/vial, 10g/vial, 20g/vial
Generics *250mg/vial, 500mg/vial, Inj 1g/vial,*
5g/vial, 10g/vial, 20g/vial

EHL 1.5-2.5h, PRC B, Lact +

Pneumonia →106: 500mg IV/IM q12h, **mild infx**:
250-500mg IV/IM q8h, **endocarditis** →65,
septicemia: 1-1.5g IV/IM q6h, **UTI**: 1g IV/IM q12h,
surgical PRO: 1g IM/IV 30-60min preop, 0.5-1g
during surgery >2h, 0.5-1g q6-8h for 24h postop;
CH >1mo: 25-50mg/kg/d IM/IV div q6-8h;
100mg/kg/d for severe infx; DARF: GFR (ml/min):
>55: 100%, 35-54: 100% at least q8h, 11-34: 50%
q12h, 0-10: 50% q18-24h

Cephalothin

Keflin *Inj 1g/vial, 2g/vial, 4g/vial,*
20g/vial
Generics *Inj 1g/vial, 2g/vial, 4g/vial*

EHL 0.5-1h, PRC B, Lact +

Pneumonia →106, **skin infx, UTI**: 500mg IV q6h,
max 2g q4h; **surgical PRO**: 1-2g 30min preop,
during surgery, q6h postop; **CH** 100mg/kg/d div q6h;
DARF: ini 1-2g IV,
GFR (ml/min) 50-80: up to 2g q6h, 25-50: up to 1.5g
q6h, 10-25: up to 1g q6h, 2-10: up to 500mg q6h,
<2: 500mg q8h

7 A.3.2 Cephalosporins – 1st Generation – Oral Cephalosporins

S: similar spectrum to cefazolin-group, highly effective against gram-positive bacteria, low effectiveness
against gram-negative bacteria
R: Pseudomonas, Enterococcus, Prot. vulgaris, Morganella, Citrobacter, Serratia, enteric bacteria,
Acinetobact., B. fragilis, Listeria, Chlamydia, Mycoplasma
AE/CI: see Cephalosporins – 1st Generation →191

Cefadroxil

Duricef *Tab 1g, Cap 500mg, Susp 125mg/5ml,*
250mg/5ml, 500mg/5ml
Generics *Tab 1g, Cap 500mg*

EHL 1.2-1.7h , PRC B, Lact +

UTI: 1-2g/d PO qd or div bid; **skin and soft tissue
infx, pharyngitis** →418, **tonsillitis** →418: 1g/d PO
qd or div bid for 10d; **CH** 30mg/kg/d PO div bid;
DARF: ini 1g, then: GFR (ml/min): 26-50: 0.5g q12h;
10-25: 0.5g q24h; 0-10: 0.5g q36h

Cephalexin

Keflet *Tab 250mg, 500mg, 1g*
Keflex *Cap 250mg, 500mg, Susp 100mg/5ml,*
125mg/5ml, 250mg/5ml
KefTab *Tab 500mg*
Generics *Tab 250mg, 500mg, Cap 250mg, 500mg,*
Susp 100mg/5ml, 125mg/5ml, 250mg/5ml

EHL 0.9h, PRC B, Lact +

Pneumonia →106, **skin infx, UTI**: 250-500mg PO
qid, max 4g/d; **CH** 25-50mg/kg/d PO div bid-qid,
max 4g/d; DARF: GFR (ml/min) >50: 100%, <50:
250-500mg q12h

7 A.3.3   Cephalosporins – 2nd Generation

S (cephalosporins - 2nd generation): greater activity against three additional gram-negative organisms, H. influenzae, some Enterbacter aerogenes and some Neisseria species, whereas activity against gram-positive organisms is weaker; cefuroxim group: see Cephalosporins - 1st Generation →191, higher effectiveness against E. coli, Klebsiella, Prot. mirabilis, H. influenza, ß-lactamase producing bacteria; cephamycins/cefoxitin group (S/R): highly effective against ß-lactamase-producing anaerobic bacteria (for example Bacteroides)
R (cefuroxime-group): Enterococcus, Pseudomonas, Acinetobact., Listeria, Chlamydia, Mycoplasma
AE/CI: see Cephalosporins - 1st Generation →191

Cefamandol	EHL 1h, PRC B, Lact +
Mandol *Inj 1g/vial, 2g/vial, 10g/vial*	**Pneumonia →106, urinary tract, bone and joint infx**: 0.5-1g IV/IM q4-8h, max 12g/d; **CH** 50-100mg/kg/d div q4-8h; DARF: GFR (ml/min): 50-80: 0.75-2g q6h; 25-50: 0.75-2g q8h; 10-25: 1-1.25g q8h; 2-10: 0.5-1g q12h; <2: 0.25-0.75g q12h
Cefmetazole	EHL 1.2-1.8h, PRC B, Lact ?
Zefazone *Inj 1g/vial*	**Pneumonia →106, urinary tract, skin, soft tissue, intra-abdominal, surgical PRO**: 1-8g/d IV div q6-12h; DARF: GFR (ml/min): 50-90: 1-2g q12h; 30-49: 1-2g q16h; 10-29: 1-2g q24h; <10: 1-2g q48h
Cefonicid	EHL 4.5h, PRC B, Lact +
Monocid *Inj 500mg/vial, 1g/vial, 10g/vial*	**Pneumonia →106, UTI, gynecologic, skin, bone, joint infx, surgical PRO**: 1-2g IV/IM q24h; **CH** 50mg IM q24h; DARF: see Prod Info
Cefotetan	EHL 2.8-4.6h, PRC B, Lact +
Cefotan *Inj 1g/vial, 2g/vial, 10g/vial, Inj 20mg/ml, 40mg/ml*	**UTI, skin, lower respiratory, abdominal infx**: 2-6g IM/IV div bid; DARF: GFR (ml/min) 10-30: 50%, <10: 25%
Cefoxitin	EHL 0.8-1h, PRC B, Lact +
Mefoxin *Inj 20mg/ml, 40mg/ml, 1g/vial, 2g/vial, 10g/vial* **Generics** *Inj 1g/vial, 2g/vial, 10g/vial*	**Pneumonia →106, genitourinary and gynecologic infx, sepsis, intra-abdominal, skin, bone and joint infx: uncomplicated**: 1g IV q6-8h; **moderate to severe**: 1g IV q4h or 2g IV q6-8h; **severe**: 2g IV q4h or 3g IV q6h; **CH** >3mo: 80-160mg/kg/d IV div in 4-6 doses, max 12g/d; DARF: ini. 1-2g IV, then GFR (ml/min) 30-50: 1-2g IV q8-12h 10-29: 1-2g IV q12-24h, 5-9: 0.5-1g IV q12-24h, <5: 0.5g IV q24-48h

Cefuroxime-Sodium

Kefurox *Inj 750mg/vial, 1.5g/vial, 7.5g/vial*
Zinacef *Inj 750mg/vial, 1.5g/vial, 7.5g/vial*
Zinacef in Plastic Container *Inj 15mg/ml, 30mg/ml*
Generics *Inj 750mg/vial, 1.5g/vial, 7.5g/vial, Inj 15mg/ml, 30mg/ml*

EHL no data, PRC B, Lact +

Bone + joint infx: 1.5g IV/IM q8h **meningitis**: 1.5g IV q6h; **pneumonia** →106: 750-1500mg q8h; **gonorrhea** →232: 1.5g IM as single dose together with 1g Probenecid PO; **skin and soft tissue infx, UTI**: 750-1500mg IV/IM for 5-10d; **CH** >3mo: 50-100mg/kg/d div tid; DARF: GFR (ml/min): >20: 750-1500mg q8h; 10-20: 750mg q12h; <20: 750mg q24h

7 A.3.4 Cephalosporins – 2nd Generation – Oral Cephalosporins

S/R (oral cephalosporins 2nd generation): see cefuroxime-group →193
AE/CI: see Cephalosporins - 1st Generation →191

Cefaclor

Ceclor *Cap 250mg, 500mg, Susp 125mg/5ml, 187mg/5ml, 250mg/5ml, 375mg/5ml*
Ceclor cd *Tab ext.rel. 375mg, 500mg*
Generics *Cap 250mg, 500mg, Susp 125mg/5ml, 187mg/5ml, 250mg/5ml, 375mg/5ml*

EHL 30-60min, PRC B, Lact +

Respiratory tract infx, otitis media →421, **UTI, skin infx, bone and joint infx**: 250-500mg PO tid; **CH** 20-40mg/kg/d PO, max 1g/d div bid-tid; DARF: GFR (ml/min): 10-50: 100%, <10: 50%

Cefprozil

Cefzil *Tab 250mg, 500mg*
Susp 125mg/5ml, 250mg/5ml

EHL 1-2h, PRC B, Lact +

Pharyngitis →418, **tonsillitis** →418: 500mg PO qd for 10d; **sinusitis** →416: 250-500mg PO bid; **acute or exacerbation of chronic bronchitis** →105: 500mg PO bid; **skin infx**: 250-500mg PO bid; **CH** 6mo-12y: 7.5-15mg/kg PO bid; DARF: GFR (ml/min) <30: 50%

Cefuroxime-Axetil

Ceftin *Tab 125mg, 250mg, 500mg, Susp 125mg/5ml, 250mg/5ml*
Veftin *Tab 125mg, 250mg, 500mg, Susp 125mg/5ml, 250mg/5ml*

EHL 1.1-1.3h , PRC B, Lact +

Early lyme disease →227: 500mg PO bid for 20d; **bronchitis, pharyngitis** →418, **sinusitis** →416: 250mg PO bid for 7-10d; **cystic fibrosis** →114: 250-500mg PO bid; **UTI**: 125-250mg PO bid for 7-10d; **CH** >3mo: Tab: 125-250mg PO bid; Susp: 20-30mg/kg/d div bid

Loracarbef

Lorabid *Cap 200mg, 400mg*
Susp 100mg/5ml, 200mg/5ml

EHL 1h, PRC B, Lact ?

Exacerbation of chronic bronchitis →105, **pneumonia** →106, **sinusitis** →416, **uncomplicated pyelonephritis**: 400mg PO bid, **pharyngitis** →418, **skin infx, uncomplicated cystitis**: 200mg PO bid **CH** 15-30mg/kg/d PO div bid; DARF: GFR (ml/min): >50: 100%, 10-49: 50%, <10: 100% q3-5d

7 A.3.5   Cephalosporins – 3rd Generation

S (cephalosporins - 3rd generation): inferior to first generation cephalosporins against gram-positive cocci, but enhanced activity against gram-negative bacilli (see 2nd generation cephalosporins →193 plus most other enteric organisms) and Serratia marcescens. (ceftriaxone or cefotaxime: agents of choice in Tx of meningitis; ceftazidime: activity against Ps. aeruginosa); cefotaxime sodium-group: higher bactericidal effect against gram-negative germs (i.e. Klebsiella, H. influenza)
R: cefotaxime sodium-group: Enterococcus, Legionella, Chlamydia, Mycoplasma, Listeria, Clostridium diff.
AE/CI: see Cephalosporins - 1st Generation →191
AE (cefoperazone): disulfiram-like reaction with alcohol intake, phlebitis at injection site

Cefoperazone	EHL 1.6-2.4h, PRC B, Lact +
Cefobid *Inj 1g/vial, 2g/vial, 10g/vial,* *Inj 20mg/ml, 40mg/ml*	**Peritonitis, sepsis, pneumonia** →106, **skin infx, gynecologic infx**: 2-4g/d IV div bid, max 12g/d div q6-12h; **DARF**: not req
Cefotaxime	EHL 0.8-1.4h, PRC B, Lact +
Claforan *Inj 500mg/vial, 1g/vial, 2g/vial, 10g/vial* **Generics** *Inj 500mg/vial, 1g/vial, 2g/vial, 10g/vial, 20g/vial*	**Pneumonia** →106, **UTI, gynecologic, skin, intra-abdominal, bone, joint, CNS infx: uncomplicated**: 1g IM/IV q12h; **moderate/severe**: 1-2g IM/IV q8h; **severe**: 2g IV q6-8h. **life-threatening**: 2g IV q4h, max 12g/d; **neonates 1-4 wk**: 50mg/kg IV q8h, **CH** 1mo-12y: 50-180mg/kg/d IM/IV div q4-6h; DARF: GFR (ml/min): <20: 50%
Ceftazidime	EHL 1.6-2h, PRC B, Lact +
Ceptaz *Inj 1g/vial, 2g/vial, 10g/vial* **Fortaz** *Inj 500mg/vial, 1g/vial, 2g/vial, 6g/vial, Inj 20mg/ml, 40mg/ml* **Tazicef** *Inj 500mg/vial, 1g/vial, 2g/vial, 6g/vial* **Tazidime** *Inj 500mg/vial, 1g/vial, 2g/vial* **Generics** *Inj 10mg/ml, 20mg/ml, 40mg/ml*	**Complic. UTI**: 0.5g IM/IV q8-12h; **serious gynecologic, intra-abdominal, bone/joint, life-threatening infx, meningitis, febrile neutropenia**: 2g IV q8h; **pseudomonas pulmonary infx**: 30-50mg/kg IV q8h, max 6g/d, **CH** 1mo-12y: 30-50mg/kg IV q8h, max 6g/d; **cystic fibrosis with pseudomonas infx** →114: 50-75mg/kg IV q8h; DARF: GFR (ml/min): 31-50: 1g IV q12h, 16-30: 1g IV q24h; 6-15: 500mg IV q24h, <5: 500mg IV q48h
Ceftizoxime	EHL 1.1-2.3h, PRC B, Lact +
Cefizox *Inj 1g/vial, 2g/vial, 10g/vial*	**Pneumonia** →106, **sepsis, intra-abdominal, skin, bone and joint, UTI**: 1-2g IM/IV q8-12h, **life-threatening infx**: 3-4g IV q8h, **CH** >6mo: 50mg/kg IV q6-8h, max 200mg/kg/; DARF: ini 0.5-1g IV/IM, GFR (ml/min). 50-79: 0.5-1.5g q8h; 5-49: 250mg-1g q12h; 0-4: 250-500mg q24h
Ceftriaxone	EHL 5-9h, PRC B, Lact +
Rocephin *Inj 250mg/vial, 500mg/vial, 1g/vial, 2g/vial, 10g/vial, Inj 20mg/ml, 40mg/ml*	**UTI, respiratory tract, intra-abdominal infx, endocarditis** →63, **sepsis, meningitis, lyme disease** →227: 1-2g IM/IV q24h, max 4g/d; **CH** 50-75mg/kg/d IM/IV div q12-24h, max 2g/d; **meningitis**: 100mg/kg/d IV, max 4g/d; DARF: not req

7 A.3.6   Cephalosporins – 3rd Generation – Oral Cephalosporins

S/R (oral cephalosporins 3rd gen.): more effective and broader spectrum then 2nd gen. cephalosporins against gram-neg. bacteria; less effective against gram-positive bacteria
AE/CI: see Cephalosporins – 1st Generation →191

Cefdinir — EHL 1.7 (+/-0.6)h, PRC B, Lact +

Omnicef *Cap 300mg, Susp 125mg/5ml* — **Pharyngitis** →418, **tonsillitis** →418, **sinusitis** →416, **skin infx**: 300mg PO bid or 600mg qd; **CH** 7mg/kg PO bid or 14mg/kg qd; DARF: GFR (ml/min) <30: 300mg PO q24h

Cefditoren — EHL 1.6 (+/-0.4)h, PRC B, Lact +

Spectracef *Tab 200mg* — **Acute exacerbation of chronic bronchitis** →105: 400mg PO bid for 10d; **pharyngitis** →418, **tonsillitis** →418, **skin infx**: 200mg PO bid for 10d; DARF: GFR (ml/min) >50: 100%; 30-50: 200mg bid; <30: 200mg qd

Cefixime — EHL 3-4h, PRC B, Lact ?

Suprax *Tab 200mg, 400mg, Susp 100mg/5ml* — **Respir. infx , UTI, tonsillitis** →418, **pharyngitis** →418: 400mg PO qd or div bid; **gonorrhea** →232: 400-800mg PO as single dose; **CH** >6mo: 8mg/kg/d qd or div bid; DARF: GFR (ml/min): >60: 100%, 21-60: 75%, <20: 50%

Cefpodoxime — EHL 2-3h, PRC B, Lact ?

Vantin *Tab 100mg, 200mg, Susp 50mg/5ml, 100mg/5ml* — **Pneumonia** →106, **acute exacerbation of chronic bronchitis** →105: 200mg PO bid for 10-14d; **pharyngitis** →418: 100mg PO bid for 5-10d; **skin infx**: 400mg PO bid for 7-14d; **UTI**: 100mg PO bid for 7d; **gonorrhea** →232: 200mg PO as single dose; **CH** 2mo-12y: 10mg/kg/d PO div bid; DARF: GFR (ml/min): <30: q24h

Ceftibuten — EHL 1.53-2.5h, PRC B, Lact ?

Cedax *Cap 400mg, Susp 90mg/5ml, 180mg/5ml* — **Acute exacerbation of chronic bronchitis, pharyngitis** →418, **tonsillitis** →418, **otitis media** →421: 400mg PO qd for 10d; **CH** 9mg/kg PO qd; DARF: GFR (ml/min): >50: 100%, 30-49: 50%; 5-29: 25%

7 A.3.7 Cephalosporins – 4th Generation

S: wide antibacterial spectrum, Strepto- and Staphylococci (only methicillin susceptible ones); also aerobic gram-negatives like Enterobacter, E. coli, Klebsiella pneumoniae, Proteus mirabilis and Ps. aeruginosa
AE/CI: see Cephalosporins - 1st Generation →191

Cefepime	EHL 2h, PRC B, Lact ?
Maxipime *Inj 500mg/vial, 1g/vial, 2g/vial*	**Severe UTI, intra-abdominal, skin infx:** 2g IV q12h; **pneumonia** →106: 1-2g IV q12h; **febrile neutropenia:** 2g IV q8h; **CH** 2mo-16y: 50mg/kg IV q12h; DARF: GFR (ml/min): <10: 0.5-1g q24h, 11-30: 1-2g q24h

7 A.4 Carbapenems

S: almost all gram-positive and gram-negative bacteria
R: Mycoplasma, Chlamydia, Legionella, Ps. cepacia, Xanthonomas maltophilia, E. faecium
AE: N/V, diarrhea, liver enz.↑, allergic reactions, complete blood count changes, CNS DO
CI: children < 3mo, hypersensitivity to product ingredients, penicillins, cephalosporins, and other beta lactams

Ertapenem	EHL 4h, PRC B, Lact ?
Invanz *Inj 1g/vial*	**UTI, respiratory tract, intra-abdominal, gynecologic, skin infx:** 1g IV/IM qd; DARF: GFR (ml/min) >30: 100%, <30: 500mg qd
Imipenem–Cilastatin	EHL 1h, PRC C, Lact ?
Primaxin *Inj 250mg/vial, 500mg/vial, 750mg/vial*	**UTI, respiratory tract, intra-abdominal, gynecologic, bone/joint, skin infx, sepsis, endocarditis, polymicrobic:** >70kg: 250-1000mg IV q6, max 4g/d, **CH** >3mo: 15-25mg/kg IV q6h; DARF: see Prod Info
Meropenem	EHL 1h, PRC B, Lact ?
Merrem IV *Inj 500mg/vial, 1g/vial*	**Febrile neutropenia, intra-abdominal infx:** 1g IV q8h; **meningitis:** 2g IV q8h; **soft tissue/UTI:** 0.5g IV q8-12h, **CH** 3-12y: 20-40mg/kg tid; DARF: GFR (ml/min) >50: 100%; 26-50: 1g q12h; 10-25: 0.5g q12h; <10: 0.5g q24h

7 A.5 Monobactams

S: primarily against enterobacteria
R: gram-positive organisms and anaerobes
AE (aztreonam): (thrombo)phlebits, rash, abnormal liver tests, N/V, anaphylaxis, fever
CI (aztreonam): hypersensitivity to aztreonam products; precautions: RF, combination w/aminoglycosides in high doses or prolonged duration), impaired hepatic function, hypersensitivity to penicillins + cephalosporins, neonates with congenital or acquired arginase deficiency, infants with extremely low birth weight

Aztreonam   EHL 1.6h, PRC B, Lact +

Azactam *Inj 500mg/vial, 1g/vial, 2g/vial*   **Gram negative infx, moderate**: 1-2g IM/IV q8-12h; **severe**: 2g IV q6-8h; **UTI**: 0.5-1g IV/IM q12h; **CH** 30mg/kg IV/IM q6-8h, max 120mg/kg/d; DARF: ini 1-2g IV, then GFR (ml/min): 10-30: 50%; <10: 25%

7 A.6   Glycopeptides

S: aerobic and anaerobic gram-positive bacteria, methicillin resistant S. aureus (MRSA)
R: all gram-negative Bacteria, Mycoplasma, Chlamydia
AE: allergic reactions, thrombophlebitis, ototoxicity, nephrotoxicity, complete blood count changes, red man/neck syndrome, N/V
CI: hypersensitivity to product ingredients

Vancomycin   EHL 4-6h, PRC C, Lact + serum-lev. (µg/ml): peak 30-40; trough 5-10

Vancocin HCT *Cap 125mg, 250mg, Sol (oral) 250mg/5ml, 500mg/6ml, Inj 500mg/vial, 1g/vial, 2g/vial*
Vancoled *Sol (oral) 250mg/5ml, Inj 0.5g/vial, 1g/vial, 2g/vial, 5g/vial, 10g/vial*
Generics *Inj 500mg/vial, 1g/vial, 5g/vial, 10g/vial, Inj 500mg/100ml*
  MRSA infx, other staphylococcal or streptococcal infx, endocarditis →63: 1g IV q12h or 30mg/kg/d IV div q12; **clostridium difficile diarrhea** →230: 125mg PO qid for 7-10d; **CH** >1mo: 40mg/kg/d IV div q6h; DARF: GFR (ml/min): >50: 500mg IV q12h, 10-50: 500mg IV q24-48h, <10: 500mg IV q48-96h

7 A.7   Tetracyclines

S: many gram-pos. + gram-neg. bacteria, e.g. Chlamydia, Mycoplasma, Rickettsia, Yersinia, Borrelia, Leptospira, Treponema, Actinomyces
R: P. aeruginosa, Providencia, Serratia, Proteus, Morganella
AE: allergic skin reactions, phototoxic reactions, N/V/D, dizziness, reversible irregularities in bone growth (children < 8y), irreversible tooth staining + crown deformation (ch < 8y), intracranial pressure↑, complete blood count changes, superinfection by bacteria or yeasts
CI: hypersensitivity to tetracyclines, severe hepatic dysfunction, RF, children < 8y

Doxycycline   EHL 12-24h, PRC D, Lact ?

Doryx *Cap 100mg*
Monodox *Cap 50mg, 100mg*
Periostat *Tab 20mg, Cap 20mg*
Vibramycin *Cap 50mg, 100mg, Susp 50mg/5ml, Inj 100mg/vial, 200mg/vial*
Generics *Tab 50, 100mg, Cap 50mg, 100mg*
  Infx general: first day 100mg PO bid, then 100mg qd; **chlamydial infx**: 100mg PO bid for 7d; **lyme disease** →227: 100-200mg PO bid for 14-21d; **CH** >8y, <45kg: 1st d 2mg/kg PO bid, then 2.2mg/kg qd >45kg: see adults; DARF: not req

Minocycline   EHL 11-22h, PRC D, Lact +

Dynacin *Cap 50mg, 75mg, 100mg*
Minocin *Cap 50mg, 100mg, Susp 50mg/5ml, Inj 100mg/vial*
Vectrin *Cap 50mg, 75mg, 100mg*
Generics *Cap 50mg, 75mg, 100mg*
  Infx general: first day 200mg IV/PO, then 100mg q12h; **CH** >8y: first day 4mg/kg IV/PO, then 2mg/kg bid

Tetracycline	EHL 8-10h, PRC D, Lact +
Achromycin *Cap 250mg, 500mg,* *Susp 125mg/5ml* **Bristacycline** *Cap 250mg, 500mg* **Panmycin** *Cap 250mg* **Robitet** *Cap 250mg, 500mg* **Sumycin** *Tab 250mg, 500mg, Cap 250mg, 500mg,* *Susp 125mg/5ml* **Generics** *Cap 100mg, 250mg, 500mg*	**Infx general**: 250-500mg PO qid; **CH** >8y: 25-50mg/kg/d PO div bid-qid; DARF: GFR (ml/min) >50: q8-12h, 10-50: q12-24h, <10: q24h

7 A.8 Macrolides

S: Streptococcus, Pneumoccous, Chlamydia, Legionella, Mycoplasma pneumoniae, Listeria, Actinomyces, Campylobacter, H. pylori, M. avium intracellulare (MAC)
R: Brucella, enteric bacteria, Nocardia, Mycoplasma hominis, B. fragilis, Fusobacteria, Pseudomonas
AE: allergic skin reactions, N/V/D, abdominal pain, cholestasis, headache
CI: hypersensitivity to product, liver disease (erythromycin, estolate salt)

Azithromycin	EHL 11-57h, PRC B, Lact ?
Zithromax *Tab 250mg, 600mg,* *Cap 250mg,* *Susp 100mg/5ml, 200mg/5ml, 1g/pkt,* *Inj 500mg/vial*	**Community-acquired pneumonia** →106: 500mg IV qd for 2d, then 500mg PO qd for 7-10d total; **pelvic inflamm. disease**: 500mg IV for 1-2d, then 500mg PO qd for 7-10d total; **acute exacerbation of chronic bronchitis** →105, **pharyngitis** →418, **skin infx**: 1st d 500mg PO, then 250mg PO qd for 5d total; **chlamydial infx**: 1g PO as single dose; **PRO of M. avium complex**: 1.2g PO qwk; **CH otitis media**: 1st d 10mg/kg, max 500mg PO, then 5mg/kg, max 250mg PO qd for 5d total; **pharyngitis**: 12mg/kg, max 500mg PO for 5d; DARF: not req

Clarithromycin	EHL 3-7h, PRC C, Lact ?
Biaxin *Tab 250mg, 500mg,* *Tab ext.rel. 500mg,* *Susp 125mg/5ml, 187mg/5ml,* *250mg/5ml*	**Exacerbation of chronic bronchitis** →105: 250-500mg PO bid for 7-14d; **pharyngitis** →418: 250mg PO bid for 10d; **sinusitis** →416: 500mg PO bid for 14d; **community aquired pneumonia** →106: 500mg PO bid for 10d; **PRO/Tx of mycobacterium avium complex**: 500mg PO bid in combination with **antimyco-bacterial drugs; h. pylori triple Tx**: 500mg PO bid with omeprazole 20mg bid and amoxicillin 1g bid for 10d; **CH** >6mo: 7.5mg/kg PO bid; DARF: GFR (ml/min) <30: 50%

Dirithromycin	EHL 44h, PRC C, Lact ?
Dynabac *Tab ext.rel. 250mg*	**Community aquired pneumonia** →106: 500mg PO qd for 14d; **exacerb. chron. bronchitis, skin infx**: 500mg PO qd for 5-7d; DARF: not req

Erythromycin Base

E-Base *Tab ext.rel. 333mg, 500mg*
E-mycin *Tab ext.rel. 250mg, 333mg*
Eryc *Cap ext.rel. 250mg*
Ery-tab *Tab ext.rel. 250mg, 333mg, 500mg*
Ilotycin *Tab ext.rel. 250mg*
PCE *Tab 333mg, 500mg*
Generics *Tab 250mg, 500mg,*
Cap ext.rel. 250mg

EHL no data, PRC B

Respiratory, campylobacter jejuni, chlamydia, mycoplasma pneumoniae infx, nongonococcal urethritis, legionnaire's disease: 250mg PO q6h or 500mg bid, max 4g/d; **CH** 30-50mg/kg/d div q6-8h; DARF: GFR (ml/min): <10: 50-75%, max 2g/d

Erythromycin Estolate

Ilosone *Tab 500mg, Tab (chew) 125mg, 250mg, Cap 125mg, 250mg, Susp 125mg/5ml, 250mg/5ml, Susp/ Drops 100mg/ml*
Generics *Cap 250mg, Susp 125mg/5ml, 250mg/5ml*

EHL no data, PRC B, Lact +

250mg PO q6h or 500mg bid, max 4g/d, **CH** 30-50mg/kg/d div q6-8h; DARF: GFR (ml/min): <10: 50-75%, max 2g/d

Erythromycin Ethylsuccinate

E.E.S. *Tab 400mg, Tab (chew) 200mg, Gran (oral) 200mg/5ml, Susp 200mg/5ml, 400mg/ 5ml*
Eryped *Tab (chew) 200mg, Gran (oral) 200mg/5ml, 400mg/5ml,*
Pediamycin *Susp 200mg/5ml, 400mg/5ml*
Generics *Tab 400mg, Gran (oral) 200mg/5ml, Susp 200mg/5ml, 400mg/5ml*

EHL no data, PRC B, Lact +

400mg PO q6h, max 4g/d, **CH** 30-50mg/kg/d PO div q6-8h; DARF: GFR (ml/min): <10: 50-75%, max 2g/d

Erythromycin Ethylsuccinate + Sulfisoxazole

Eryzole *Gran (oral) 200 + 600mg/5ml*
Pediazole *Gran (oral) 200 + 600mg/5ml*

PRC C, Lact ?

CH otitis media: 50mg/kg/d erythromycin + 150mg/kg/d sulfisoxazole div q6h for 10d

Erythromycin Lactobionate

Erythrocin *Inj 500mg/vial, 1g/vial*
Generics *Inj 500mg/vial, 1g/vial*

EHL no data, PRC B, Lact +

15-20mg/kg/d IV div q6h, max 4g/d, **CH** 30-50mg/kg/d IV, max 4g/d; DARF: GFR (ml/min): <10: 50-75%, max. 2g/d

7 A.9 Aminoglycosides

S: enteric bacteria, Pseudomonas, Staphylococcus, Serratia, Yersinia, Pasteurella, Brucella
R: Enterococcus, Anaerobic bacteria, Streptococcus, Pneumococcus
AE: nephrotoxicity, ototoxicity, neurotoxicity, neuromuscular blockage, paresthesia, renal damage, complete blood count changes, allergic reactions, N/V/D, diziness
CI: damage of the vestibulocochlear nerve, terminal renal insufficiency, hypersensitivity to product ingredients

Amikacin

Amikin *Inj 50mg/ml, 250mg/ml*
Generics *Inj 50mg/ml, 62.5mg/ml, 250mg/ml, 500mg/ml*

EHL no data, PRC D, Lact +
serum-lev. (µg/ml): peak: 30; trough: 5-10

Gram-negative infx: 15mg/kg/d IV/IM div bid-tid, max 1.5g/d; **neonates:** ini 10mg/kg, then 7.5mg/kg IM/IV q12h; DARF: GFR (ml/min) >50: 60-90% q12h, 10-50: 30-70% q12-18h, <10: 20-30% q24-48h

Gentamicin

EHL 2h, PRC C, Lact ?
serum-level (µg/ml). peak 5-10; trough <2

Garamycin *Inj 1mg/ml, 40mg/ml*
U-gencin *Inj 10mg/ml, 40mg/ml*
Generics *Inj 0.8mg/ml, 1.2mg/ml, 1.4mg/ml,
1.6mg/ml, 1.8mg/ml, 2mg/ml, 2.4mg/ml, 10mg/ml,
40mg/ml, 40mg/100ml, 60mg/100ml, 70mg/100ml,
80mg/100ml, 90mg/100ml, 100mg/100ml,
120mg/100ml*

Gram-negative infx: 3-5mg/kg/d IV/IM div tid,
neonates: 2.5mg/kg IV/IM q8h, **CH** 2-2.5mg/kg IV/IM
q8h; DARF: GFR (ml/min) >50: 60-90% q12h,
10-50: 30-70% q12-18h, <10: 20-30% q24-48h

Paromomycin

EHL no data,

Humatin *Cap 250mg*
Generics *Cap 250mg*

Intestinal amebiasis: 25-35mg/kg/d PO div tid for
5-10d; **hepatic coma** →136: 4g/d PO in divided
doses for 5-6d; DARF: not req

Spectinomycin

EHL 1.7h, PRC B, Lact ?

Trobicin *Inj 2g/vial, 4g/vial*

Gonorrhea →232: 2g IM as a single dose
disseminated gonorrhea →232: 2g IM q12h;
CH patients <45kg: 40mg/kg IM; DARF: not req

Streptomycin

EHL 2.5h, PRC D, Lact ?

Generics *Inj 1g/2.5ml, 1g/vial, 5g/vial*

Bacterial endocarditis →63: 1g IM bid for 1wk,
then 0.5g bid for 1wk; patients >60y: 0.5g IM bid for
2wk; **TB** →235: 15mg/kg IM qd, max 1g/d or
25-30mg/kg IM max 1.5g/d 2-3 times weekly; **CH**
TB: 20-40mg/kg IM qd, max 1g/d; DARF: GFR (ml/
min) >50: 100% q24h, 10-50: 100% q24-72h, <10:
100% q72-96h

Tobramycin

EHL 2h, PRC D, Lact +
serum-level (µg/ml): peak 5-10; trough <2.

Nebcin *Inj 10mg/ml, 40mg/ml, 1.2g/vial*
Generics *Inj 10mg/ml, 40mg/ml,
Inj 1.2mg/ml, 1.6mg/ml, 80mg/100ml*

3-5mg/kg/d IV/IM div tid; **cystic fibrosis** →114:
3mg/kg IV q8h; **nebulization**: 300mg bid for 28d,
then 28d off, neonates: 4mg/kg/d IV div bid;
CH 6-7.5mg/kg/d IV/IM div tid-qid; **cystic fibrosis**:
see adults; DARF: GFR (ml/min): >50: 60-90% q8-
12h; 10-50: 30-70% q12h, <10: 20-30% q24-48h

7 A.10 Lincosamides

S: Pneumo-, Staphylo-, Streptococcus, C. diphtheria, anaerobics, B. fragilis, Cl. perfringens
R: Enteric bacteria, P. aeruginosa, Entero-, Gono-, Meningococcus, H. influenza, Mycoplasma, Listeria
AE: N/V, diarrhea, pseudomembranous enterokolitis, allergic skin reactions, LFT↑, erythema exsudativum,
thrombophlebitis (when used iv)
CI: caution with Myasthenia gravis, hypersensitivity to product ingredients

Clindamycin

EHL 1.5-5h, PRC B, Lact ?

Cleocin *Cap 75mg, 150mg, 300mg,
Sol (oral) 75mg/5ml; Inj 150mg/ml*
Generics *Cap 75mg, 150mg, 300mg,
Inj 150mg/ml*

Anaerobic and other infx: 600-1200mg/d IV div tid
or 150-450mg PO qid; **CH** 20-40mg/kg/d IV div
q6-8h or 8-20mg/kg/d PO div tid-qid; DARF: not req

7 A.11 Chloramphenicol

S: wide range of gram-positive and gram-negative organisms (note: because of its toxicity limited clinical use)
AE: N/V, irreversible aplastic anemia, rash, myelosuppression, gray baby syndrom
CI: hypersensitivity to chloramphenicol products

Chloramphenicol	EHL 1.6-3.3h, PRC C, Lact -
Chloromycetin *Inj 1g/vial*	50mg/kg/d IV div q6h, max 100mg/kg/d; DARF: not req

7 A.12 Quinolones
7 A.12.1 Nonfluorinated Quinolone

S: only enteric bacteria; **AE:** allergic skin reactions, photosensitivity, muscle weakness, muscle pain, tachycardia, BP↓ ,headache, malaise, visual DO, cholestasis, hepatitis, N/V;
CI: children in growth period, hypersensitivity to nalidixic acid, history of convulsive DO

Nalidixic Acid	EHL 60-90min, PRC B, Lact ?
Neggram *Tab 250mg, 500mg, 1g, Susp 250mg/5ml* **Generics** *Tab 250mg, 500mg, 1g*	**UTI:** 1g PO qid for 7-14d; **CH** 55-60mg/kg/d PO div qid

7 A.12.2 Fluoroquinolones 1st Group

Group I: indicated almost exclusively for UTI; **S:** enteric bacteria, Campylobacter, Salmonella, Shigella, Gonococcus; **R:** Anaerobic bacteria, Chlamydia, Mycoplasma, E. faecium, Ureaplasma; **AE** (quinolones): allergic skin reactions, phototoxicity, muscle weakness, muscle pain, tachycardia, BP↓, CNS disturbances, cholestasis, hepatitis, cristalluria; **AE** (norfloxacin): dizziness, nausea, headache, abdominal cramping; **CI** (quinolones): children < 18y/during growth period;
CI (norfloxacin): hypersensitivity to norfloxacin or other fluoroquinolones

Norfloxacin	EHL 2-4h, PRC C, Lact ?
Noroxin *Tab 400mg*	**Simple UTI**: 400mg PO bid for 3d; **complicated UTI**: 400mg PO bid for 10-21d; **traveler's diarrhea**: 400mg PO bid for 3d; **gonorrhea** →232: 800mg PO as single dose; DARF: GFR (ml/min) <30: 400mg PO qd

7 A.12.3 Fluoroquinolones – 2nd Group

S: high activity vs. gram-negatives like enterobacteria + H. influenzae, different activity vs. pseudomonas, low activity vs. Staphylo-, Pneumo-, Enterococcus, Mycoplasma, Chlamydia
AE/CI (quinolones): see Fluoroquinolones - 1st Group →202;
AE (ciprofloxacin): dizziness, headache, diarrhea; **AE** (enoxacin): headache, N/V, gastric pain, skin eruption; **AE** (lomefloxacin): phototoxicity, headache, dizziness, hypersensitivity; **AE** (ofloxacin): nausea, insomnia, headache, dizziness, diarrhea; **CI** (ciproflox., lomeflox, oflox.): hypersensitivity to product ingredients/quinolones; **CI** (enoxacin): hypersensitivity to enoxacin/quinolones, history of tendon rupture

Ciprofloxacin	EHL 3-6h, PRC C, Lact -
Cipro *Tab 100mg, 250mg, 500mg, 750mg, Susp 250mg/5ml, 500mg/5ml, Inj 200mg/20ml, 400mg/40ml*	**Simple UTI**: 100mg PO bid for 3d; **UTI, bone and joint infx**: 250-500mg PO bid or 200-400mg IV bid; **chronic bacterial prostatitis**: 500mg PO bid for 28d; **traveler's diarrhea**: 500mg PO bid for 5-7d; **typhoid fever**: 500mg PO bid for 10d; **gonorrhea** →232: 250mg PO as single dose; DARF: GFR (ml/min) 30-50: 250-500mg PO q12h; 5-29: 250-500mg PO q18h or 200-400mg IV q18-24h
Enoxacin	EHL 4.3-6.4h, PRC C, Lact ?
Penetrex *Tab 200mg, 400mg*	**Simple UTI**: 200mg PO bid for 7d; **complicated UTI**: 400mg PO bid for 14d; **gonorrhea** →232: 400mg PO as single dose; DARF: GFR (ml/min) <30: 50%
Lomefloxacin	EHL 6.35-8.19h, PRC C, Lact ?
Maxaquin *Tab 400mg*	**Exacerbation of chronic bronchitis (not due to S. pneumoniae)** →105, **simple UTI**: 400mg PO qd for 10d DARF: ini 400mg, then GFR (ml/min) 10-40: 200mg PO qd
Ofloxacin	EHL 5-7.5h, PRC C, Lact -
Floxin *Tab 200mg, 300mg, 400mg Inj 20mg/ml, 40mg/ml, Inj (floxin in dextrose 5% in plastic container) 4mg/ml, 400mg/100ml*	**UTI**: 200mg PO/IV bid for 3-10d; **exacerbation of chronic bronchitis** →105: 400mg bid for 10d; **gonorrhea** →232: 400mg PO as single dose; **prostatitis** →435: 300mg PO bid for 6wk; **Chlamydia trachomatis infx**: 300mg bid for 7d; **severe infectious diarrhea**: 300mg PO bid for 3d; DARF: GFR (ml/min): 20-50: 100% q24h, <20: 50% q24h

7 A.12.4 Fluoroquinolones – 3rd Group

S: additional activity Staphylo-, Pneumo-, Streptococcus, Chlamydia, Mycoplasma
AE, CI (quinolones): see Fluoroquinolones - 1st Group →202
AE (levofloxacin): N/V, diarrhea, headache
AE (sparfloxacin): diarrhea, photosensitivity, headache, dyspepsia, N/V
CI (levofloxacin): hypersensitivity to levofloxacin products/quinolones
CI (sparfloxacin): hypersensitivity to sparfloxacin/quinolones, class Ia or class III anti-arrhythmic agents, patients with a known QTc prolongation, unprotected sun exposure

Levofloxacin	EHL 6-8h, PRC C, Lact -
Levaquin *Tab 250mg, 500mg, 750mg, Inj 5mg/ml, 25mg/ml*	**UTI**: 250mg PO/IV for 3d (simple), 10d (complicated); **chronic bronchitis**: 500mg PO/IV qd for 7d; **community-acquired pneumonia** →106: 500mg IV/PO qd for 7-14d; **skin infx**: 500mg qd for 7-10d; DARF: ini 250- 500mg PO/IV, then GFR (ml/min): 20-49: 250mg q24h; 10-19: 250mg q48h; <10, dialysis: 250mg q48h
Sparfloxacin	EHL 16-30h
Zagam *Tab 200mg*	**Community-acquired pneumonia** →106, **exacerbation of chronic bronchitis** →105, **acute sinusitis** →416: 400mg PO 1std, then 200mg PO qd for 10d total; DARF: ini 400mg PO then GFR (ml/min): <50: 200mg q48h

7 A.12.5 Fluoroquinolones – 4th Group

S: additional activity against anaerobic bacteria
AE, CI (quinolones): see Fluoroquinolones - 1st Group →202
AE (gatifloxacin, moxifloxacin): nausea, diarrhea, headache, dizziness
AE (trovafloxacin): dizziness, headache, N/V/D, liver disease including liver failure
CI (gatifloxacin, moxifloxacin): hypersensitivity to product ingredients/quinolones
CI (trovafloxacin): hypersensitivity to trovafloxacin/alatrofloxacin products, hypersensitivity to quinolone antibiotics

Gatifloxacin	EHL 7-14h, PRC C
Tequin *Tab 200mg, 400mg, Inj 200mg/vial, 400mg/vial*	**Exacerbation of chronic bronchitis** →105, **complicated UTI, acute sinusitis** →416: 400mg IV/PO qd for 7-10d; **community-acquired pneumonia** →106: 400mg IV/PO qd for 7-14d; **gonorrhea** →232, **simple UTI**: 400mg PO/IV as single dose; DARF: ini 400mg PO then GFR (ml/min): <40: 200mg qd
Gemifloxacin	EHL no data, PRC C
Factive *Tab 320mg*	**Community-acquired pneumonia** →106: 320mg PO qd for 7d; **exacerbation of chronic bronchitis** →105: 320mg PO qd for 5d; DARF: GFR (ml/min): <40: 160mg qd
Moxifloxacin	EHL 9-16h, PRC C
Avelox *Tab 400mg, Inj. 400mg/vial*	**Community-acquired pneumonia** →106, **acute sinusitis** →416: 400mg PO/IV qd for 10d; **exacerbation of chronic bronchitis** →105: 400mg PO/IV qd for 5-10d; DARF: not req
Trovafloxacin	EHL 9-13h, PRC C, Lact ?
Trovan *Tab 100mg, 200mg Inj (alatrofloxacin mesylate) 200mg/vial, 300mg/vial*	**Community-acquired pneumonia** →106: 200mg IV/PO qd for 7-14d; **nosocomial pneumonia** →109: ini 300mg IV qd, then 200mg PO qd for 10-14d total; **intra-abdominal infx**: ini 300mg IV qd, then 200mg PO qd for 7-14d total; DARF: not req; only for Tx of serious or life-threatening infx

7 A.13 Urinary Tract Antiseptics

AE (methenamine): N/V, diarrhea, cramping
AF (nitrofurantoin): pulmonary hypersensitivity, hemolytic anemia, peripheral neuropathy, N/V/D
CI (methenamine): glaucoma, urinary bladder neck obstruction, pyloric or duodenal obstruction, cardiospasm, hypersensitivity to methenamine
CI (nitrofurantoin): anuria, pregnant patients (38-42wk gestation), neonates, hypersensitivity to nitrofurantoin

Methenamine Hippurate	EHL 4.3h, PRC C, Lact +
Hiprex *Tab 1g* **Urex** *Tab 1g*	**Tx/PRO of recurrent or chronic UTI**: 1g PO bid; **CH** 6-12y: 25-50mg/kg/d div bid; DARF: GFR (ml/min): >50: 100%; <50: not rated
Methenamine Mandelate	EHL 4.3h, PRC C, Lact +
Mandelamine *Tab 0.5g, 1g*	**Tx/PRO of recurrent or chronic UTI**: 1g PO qid; **CH** 6-12y: 50-75mg/kg/d div qid; DARF: GFR (ml/min): >50: 100%; <50: not rated
Nitrofurantoin	EHL 20min-1h, PRC B, Lact
Furadantin *Tab 50mg, 100mg* *Susp 25mg/5ml* **Macrobid** *Cap 25mg, 75mg* **Macrodantin** *Cap 25mg, 50mg, 100mg* **Generics** *Tab 50mg, 100mg*	**UTI**: 50-100mg PO qid for 7d or at least 3d after sterile urine; **CH** >1mo: 5-7mg/kg/d PO div qid for 7d or at least 3d after sterile urine; DARF: GFR (ml/min): >50: 100%; <50: not rated

7 A.14 Folate Antagonists

7 A.14.1 Sulfonamides

S (sulfonamids, including co-trimoxazole): active against selected enterobacteria, chlamydia, Pneumocystis, nocardia
S (sulfadiazin/in combination with pyrimethamine): Toxoplasma
AE (sulfonamids): N/V, allergic reactions, erythema exudativum multiforme, photosensitivity, renal damage, complete blood count changes; **AE** (sulfadiazine): crystalluria, RF; **AE** (sulfamethoxazole): crystalluria, blood dyscrasias
AE (sulfisoxazole): N/V, diarrhea, blood dyscrasias
CI: hypersensitivity to sulfonamides, previous erythema exudativum, severe hepatic + renal dysfunction, newborns, infants < 2mo, patients receiving methenamine

Sulfadiazine	EHL 7 and 16.8h, PRC C, Lact -
Generics *Tab 500mg*	**UTI**: ini 2-4g PO, then 2-4 g/d div in 3-6 doses; **rheumatic fever PRO** →64: 1g PO qd; **toxoplasmosis** →243: 1-2g PO qid in combination with pyrimethamine (25-100mg), **CH** >2mo: ini 75mg/kg PO, then 150mg/kg/d, max 6g/d div q4-6h; **toxoplasmosis** →243: 25-50mg/kg PO qid; **rheumatic fever PRO**: <30kg: 500mg PO qd; >30kg: 1g PO qd;
Sulfamethoxazole	EHL 10h, PRC C, Lact ?
Gantanol *Tab 500mg*	**UTI**: ini 2g, then 1g PO bid-tid; **CH** > 2mo: ini 50-60mg/kg, then 25-30mg/kg PO bid, max 75mg/kg/d

Sulfisoxazole　　　　　　　　　　　EHL 7h, PRC C, Lact ?

Gantrisin *Susp 500mg/5ml,*　　　**UTI**: ini 2-4g, then 4-8g/d PO div q4-6h; **CH** >2mo:
Syr 500mg/5ml　　　　　　　　　ini 75mg/kg, then 150mg/kg/d PO div q4-6h;
Sosol *Tab 500mg*　　　　　　　DARF: GFR (ml/min): >50: q6h; 10-49: q8-12h;
Generics *Tab 500mg*　　　　　<10: q12-24h

7 A.14.2 Trimethoprim

AE: rash, pruritus, effects of folate deficiency (megaloblastic anemia, leukopenia, granulozytopenia)
CI: hypersensitivity to trimethoprim products, megaloblastic anemia (folate deficiency)

Trimethoprim　　　　　　　　　EHL 5-17h, PRC C, Lact +

Primsol *Sol (oral) 25mg/5ml, 50mg/5ml*　　**Uncomplicated UTI**: 100mg PO q12h or 200mg PO
Proloprim *Tab 100mg, 200mg*　　　q24h; DARF: GFR (ml/min): 15-30: 50mg PO q12h;
　　　　　　　　　　　　　　　　<15: not rated

7 A.14.3 Co-trimoxazole

S: almost all aerobic bacteria, Pneumocystis carinii; **R:** P. aeruginosa, Treponema, Clostridium, Leptospiria, Rickettsia, Chlamydia psittaci, Mycoplasma
AE: exanthema, photodermatosis, Lyell-Syndrome, complete blood count changes, hemolytic anemia, N/V, rash, urticaria
CI: hypersensitivity to sulfonamides or trimethoprim, glucose-6-phosphat-dehydrogenase deficiency, severe complete blood count change, severe renal insufficiency, infants < 2mo

Sulfamethoxazole + Trimethoprim (Co-trimoxazole) PRC C, Lact ?

Bactrim *Inj 80+16mg/ml*　　　　　**UTI**: 800mg + 160mg PO q12h for 3-7d;
Bactrim DS *Tab 800+160mg*　　　**exacerbation of chronic bronchitis** →105: 800mg
Bactrim Pediatric *Susp 200+40mg/5ml*　+ 160mg PO q12h for 14d;
Cotrim *Tab 400+80mg, 800+160mg*　**travelers' diarrhea**: 800mg + 160mg PO q12h for
Septra *Tab 400+80mg, 800+160mg, Susp*　5d;
200+40mg/5ml, Inj 80+16mg/ml　　**pneumocystis Tx** →242: 15-20 (TMP) + 75-100
Sulfamethoprim *Tab 400+80mg, 800+160mg*　(SMZ) mg/kg/d IV div q6-8h or PO div q6h for
Sulfatrim Pediatric *Susp 200+40mg/5ml*　14-21d;
Trimeth/Sulfa *Susp 200+40mg/5ml*　**pneumocystis PRO** →243: 800mg + 160mg PO qd;
Generics *Tab 400+80mg, 800+160mg, Susp*　**CH** 40-100mg/kg + 8-20mg/kg PO/IV; DARF: GFR
200+40mg/5ml, Inj 80+16mg/ml　　(ml/min): > 30: 100%;
　　　　　　　　　　　　　　　　15-30: 50%, <30: not rated

7 A.15 Nitroimidazoles

S: obligate anaerobic bacteria (i.e. Bacteroides, Clostridium), Campylobacter, H. pylori, Gardnerella vaginalis, Trichomonas vaginalis, Giardia lamblia, Entamoeba histolytica
R: all aerobic and facultative anaerobic bacteria, Actinomyces, Propionibacteria
AE: GI disturbances, bitter/metallic taste, CNS-disturbances, seizures, allergic skin reactions, alcohol intolerance; **CI:** hypersensitivity to metronidazole

Metronidazole	EHL 6-11h, PRC B, Lact ?
Flagyl *Tab ext.rel. 750mg, Tab 250mg, 500mg, Cap 375mg, Inj 500mg/vial, 500mg/100ml* **Metro** *Inj 500mg/100ml* **Protostat** *Tab 250mg, 500mg* **Generics** *Tab 250mg, 500mg, Inj 500mg/100ml*	**Anaerobic bacterial infx**: ini 1g or 15mg/kg IV, then 500mg or 7.5mg/kg IV/PO q6h; **pseudomembranous colitis** →230: 500mg PO tid; **CH anaerobic bacterial infx:** ini 15mg/kg IV, then 7.5mg/kg IV bid or 30mg/kg/d PO div qid; DARF: GFR (ml/min) >10: 100%, <10: 50%

7 A.16 Streptogramines

S: all gram-positive cocci, incl. MRSA, E. faecium, penicillin-G-resistent Pneumococcus, Mor. catarrhalis, Legionella, Mycoplasma pneumoniae, Chlamydia, Prevotella, Fusobacteria, Peptostreptococcus, Clostridia;
R: H. influenza, E. faecalis, B. fragilis
AE: vein irritation, pruritus, erythema and burning on the face and upper body, N/V, arthralgia, myalgia, transaminases↑, bilirubin↑, alkaline phosphatase↑
CI: severe hepatic insufficiency, combination with drugs that prolong QT interval, hypersensitivity to dalfopristin/quinupristin/streptogramins

Dalfopristin + Quinupristin	PRC B, Lact ?
Synercid *Inj 350mg/vial + 150mg/vial, 420mg/vial + 180mg/vial*	**Vancomycin-resistant F. faecium infx:** 7.5mg/kg IV q0h, **complicated staphyl. skin infx:** 7.5mg/kg IV q12h; DARF: not req

7 A.17 Oxazolidinones

S: E. faecalis, E. faecium, S. aureus, MRSA, koagulaseneg. Staphylococci
S. agalactiae, S. pneumoniae, S. pyogenes, C- u. D-Streptococci, C. perfringens, Pasteurella multocida
R: H. influenzae, M. catarrhalis, Enterobacteriaceae, Neisseria, Pseudomonas
AE (linezolid): diarrhea, headache, nausea

Linezolid	EHL 5h, PRC N, Lact ?
Zyvox *Tab 400mg, 600mg, Susp 100mg/5ml, Inj 200mg/100ml*	**Vancomycin-resistant E. faecium infx:** 600mg IV/PO q12h for 14-28 d; **compli-cated skin infx, pneumonia** →106: 600mg IV/PO q12h for 10-14d; **uncomplicated skin infx:** 400mg PO q12h for 10-14d; DARF: not req

7 A.18 Other Antimicrobials

AE (fosfomycin): diarrhea, headache, N/V
AE (furazolidone): discolored urine, N/V, abdominal distress, headache, rash
CI (fosfomycin, linezolid): hypersensitivity to product ingredients
CI (furazolidone): hypersensitivity to furazolidone, children < 1mo, ethanol ingestion

Fosfomycin	EHL 5.7 (+/- 2.8)h, PRC B, Lact ?
Monurol *Susp 3g/pkt*	**UTI:** 3g PO as single dose
Furazolidone	EHL no data, PRC C, Lact -
Furoxone *Tab 100mg, Susp 50mg/15ml*	**Giardiasis:** 100mg PO qid for 7-10d; **bacterial diarrhea, cholera** →239: 100mg PO for 5-7d; **CH** 1.25-2mg/kg/d PO div qid

7 A.19 Antimycobacterials
7 A.19.1 Antituberculosis Drugs – Single Ingredient Drugs

S (ethambutol): M. tuberculosis, M. kansasii, M. avium-intracellulare
S (isoniazid): M. tuberculosis, M. kansasii
S (pyrazinamide): M. tuberculosis
S (rifampin): M. tuberculosis, gram-positive cocci, Legionella, Chlamydia, M. lepra, Meningococcus, Gonococcus, H. influenza, Bacteroides
S (streptomycin): M.tuberculosis, Brucella, Yersinia pestis, Francisella tularensis
AE (ethambutol): optic neuritis, transaminases↑, allergic reactions
AE (isoniazid): peripheral neuropathy, transaminases↑, hepatotoxicity, acne, leukopenia, microhematuria
AE (pyrazinamide): hyperuricemia, vomiting, transaminases↑, liver toxicity, disturbances of hematopoiesis, mild nausea + anorexia, arthralgia
AE (rifampin): transaminases↑, cholestasis, red discoloration of the urine, neutropenia, thrombopenia, RF
AE (streptomycin): nephrotoxicity, neurotoxicity, hypersensitivity, ototoxicity
CI (ethambutol): optic neuritis, hypersensitivity to ethambutol products
CI (isoniazid): acute liver disease, previous isoniazid-associated hepatitis, peripheral neuropathy
CI (pyrazinamide): severe hepatic dysfunction, hypersensitivity to pyrazinamide products, acute gout
CI (rifampin): severe hepatic dysfunction
CI (streptomycin): severe renal insufficiency, inner ear damage, hypersensitivity to streptomycin/ aminoglycosides

Ethambutol	EHL 2.5-4h, PRC B, Lact +
Myambutol *Tab 100mg, 400mg* **Generics** *Tab 100mg, 400mg*	**TB** →235: 15-25mg/kg qd **mycobacterium avium complex** →244: 15mg/kg qd, **CH** see adults; DARF: GFR (ml/min) 10-50: q24-36h, <10: q48h
Ethionamide	EHL 1.85-3h, PRC C, Lact ?
Trecator-SC *Tab 250mg*	**TB** →235: 15-20mg/kg/d PO, max 1g/d div bid; DARF: GFR (ml/min) >10: 100%, <10: 50%
Isoniazid	EHL 0.7-4h, PRC C, Lact +
Laniazid *Tab 50mg, 100mg, 300mg* **Nydrazid** *Inj 100mg/ml* **Generics** *Tab 100mg, 300mg,* *Syr 50mg/5ml*	**TB Tx** →235: 5mg/kg PO/IM qd, max 300mg/d PO or 15mg/kg, max 900mg biw, **CH** 10-20mg/kg/d PO, max 300mg; **TB PRO**: 300mg PO qd, **CH** 10mg/kg/d PO, max 300mg; DARF: GFR (ml/min) >10: 100%, <10: 50%
Pyrazinamide	EHL 9-23h, PRC C, Lact ?
Generics *Tab 500mg*	**TB Tx** →235: 15-30mg/kg PO qd, max 2g/d or 50-70mg/dose, max 4g/dose biw; **CH** see adults; DARF: endstage RF: 12-20mg/kg/d
Rifampin	EHL no data, PRC C, Lact +
Rifadin *Cap 150mg, 300mg,* *Inj 600mg/vial* **Rimactane** *Cap 300mg* **Generics** *Cap 150mg, 300mg, Inj 600mg/vial*	**TB** →235: 10mg/kg PO/IV qd, max 600mg/d, **meningococcal PRO**: 600mg PO bid for 2d, **CH TB**: 10-20mg/kg PO/IV qd, max 600mg/d; **CH meningococcal PRO**: 10mg/kg PO bid for 2d
Rifapentine	EHL 14-17h, PRC C, Lact ?
Priftin *Tab 150mg*	**TB** →235: 600mg PO biw for 2mo, then 1x/wk for 4mo, **CH** >12y: >45kg: see adults; <45kg: 450mg PO biw

7 A.19.2 Antituberculosis Drugs – Combinations

Isoniazid + Rifampin

Rifamate *Cap 150mg + 300mg* — **TB** →235: 2 Cap PO qd

Isoniazid + Pyrazinamide + Rifampin

Rifater *Tab 50mg + 300mg + 120mg* — **TB** →235: > 55kg: 6 Tab PO qd; 45-54kg: 5 Tab PO qd, < 44kg: 4 Tab PO qd

7 A.19.3 Other Antimycobacterials

S (dapsone): M. tuberculosis, M. leprae, Pneumocystis carinii
S (rifabutin): M. tuberculosis, M. marinum, M. kansasii, M. leprae, M. avium-intracellulare, gram-positive cocci, Legionella, Chlamydia, Gonococcus
AE (dapsone): dose-related hemolysis, methemoglobinemia, peripheral neuropathy, N/V
AE (rifabutin): red-orange discoloration of urine, N/V, liver enzymes↑, jaundice, anemia, leukopenia, eosinophilia, neutropenia, thrombopenia, fever, skin discoloration, reversible uveitis, rash
CI (dapsone): hypersensitivity to dapsone products
CI (rifabutin): hypersensitivity to other rifamycins, obstructive jaundice, acute hepatitis

Dapsone — EHL 10-50h, PRC C, Lact

Generics *Tab 25mg, 100mg* — **Leprosy:** 100mg PO qd with other anti-leprosy drugs; **CH** 1-2mg/kg/d PO, max 100mg/d; **pneumocystis PRO** →242: 100mg PO qd; **pneumocystis Tx** →242: 100mg PO qd; **CH** 2mg/kg/d PO, max 100mg/d

Rifabutin — FHL 45h, PRC B, Lact ?

Mycobutin *Cap 150mg* — **Mycobacterium avium PRO** →244: 300mg PO qd or 150mg PO bid; **mycobacterium avium Tx**: 300mg PO qd in combination with a macrolide

7 A.20 Antivirals
7 A.20.1 Anti-CMV Drugs

MA/Ind (cidofovir): nucleoside analogue, inhibition of the DNA-Polymerase; CMV retinitis
MA/Ind (foscarnet): inhibition of viral polymerases; CMV + herpes simplex infx
MA/Ind (ganciclovir, valgancicl.): nucleoside analogue, inhibition of DNA synthesis of CMV
AE (cidofovir): proteinuria, creatinine↑, neutropenia, fever, dyspnea, nausea, diarrhea, alopecia, skin rashes;
AE (foscarnet): anemia, fever, headache, N/V, nephrotoxicity
AE (ganciclovir): neutropenia, thrombocytopenia, fever, headache, nausea
AE (valganciclovir): diarrhea, neutropenia, thrombocytopenia, anemia, fever, headache, nausea, abdominal pain, insomnia, peripheral neuropathy
CI (cidofovir): creatinine > 1.5mg/dl or CrCl < 55ml/min., proteinuria > 100mg/dl
CI (foscarnet): hypersensitivity to foscarnet
CI (ganciclovir): severe leuko- or thrombopenia, children and adolescents < 18
CI (valganciclovir): hypersensitivity to valganciclovir or ganciclovir

Cidofovir	EHL , PRC C, Lact ?
Vistide *Inj 75mg/ml*	**CMV retinitis in AIDS** →244: 5mg/kg IV qwk for 2 wk, maint 5mg/kg every other wk; give probenecid 2g PO 3h before and 1g 2h and 8h after cidofovir-administration; CI if serum creatinine >1.5mg/dl or GFR < 55ml/min, or urine protein >100mg/dl; reduce to 3mg/kg if serum creatinine incr. by 0.3–0.4mg/dl from baseline
Foscarnet	EHL 3 - 6h, PRC C, Lact ?
Foscavir *Inj 2.4g/100ml*	**CMV retinitis in AIDS** →244: ini. 60mg/kg IV (over 1 h) q8h or 90mg/kg IV (over 1.5-2 h) q12h for 2-3 wk, maint 90-120mg/kg IV (over 2h) qd; **acyclovir-resistant HSV infx in immunocompromised patients**: 40mg/kg IV (over 1 h) q8-12h for 2-3 wk or until healed; DARF: see Prod Info
Ganciclovir	EHL 2.5-5h, PRC C, Lact ?
Cytovene *Cap 250mg, 500mg, Inj 500mg/vial* **Vitrasert** *implantation 4.5mg*	**CMV retinitis** →240, →244: 5mg/kg IV bid for 14-21 d, then 5mg/kg IV qd or 1g PO tid; **CMV PRO in AIDS**: 1g PO tid; DARF: see Prod Info
Valganciclovir	EHL 4h, PRC C, Lact -
Valcyte *Tab 450mg*	**CMV retinitis** →240, →244: ini 900mg PO bid for 21d, then 900mg qd; DARF: GFR (ml/min): >60: 100%; 40-59: ini 450mg bid, then 450mg qd; 25-39: ini 450mg qd, then 450mg qod; 10-24: ini 450mg qod, then 450mg biw

7 A.20.2 Anti-Herpetic Drugs

MA/Ind (acyclovir): inhibition of the viral DNA-polymerase; herpes simplex, varicella zoster
MA/Ind (famciclovir): inhibition of the DNA-Polymerase; herpes genitalis, varicella zoster
MA/Ind (valacyclovir): better resorption than acyclovir, varicella zoster infx
AE (acyclovir): renal dysfunction, exanthema, complete blood count changes, N/V
headache, rash, phlebitis; **AE** (famciclovir): headache, dizziness, diarrhea;
AE (valacyclovir): headache, N/V
CI (famciclovir): hypersensitivity to famciclovir or penciclovir; **CI** (acyclovir): hypersensitivity to acyclovir **CI**
(valacyclovir): hypersensitivity to valacyclovir or acyclovir

Acyclovir	EHL 3h, PRC B, Lact ?
Zovirax *Cap 200mg, Tab 400mg, 800mg, Susp 200mg/5ml, Inj 500mg/vial, 1g/vial* **Generics** *Tab 400mg, 800mg, Cap 200mg, Susp 200mg/5ml, Inj 50mg/vial, 500mg/vial, 1gm/vial*	**CMV infx** →240, →244: 500mg/square meter IV q8h; **herpes simplex encephalitis**: 10mg/kg IV q8h for 10d; **mucocutaneous herpes**: 5-10mg/kg IV q8h for 5-7d; **varicella zoster in immunocompromised patients**: 10-12mg/kg IV q8h for 7-14d; **varicella zoster in immunocompetent patients**: 5mg/kg IV q8h for 5-7d or 800mg PO q4h for7-10d; **ini herpes genitalis**: 200mg PO 5 x/d for 7-10d; **recurrent herpes genitalis**: 400mg PO bid for up to 12 mo; **chickenpox**: 800mg PO qid for 5d; DARF: GFR (ml/min): >50: 100% q8h (IV), 25-50: 100% q12h (IV), 10-25: 100% q24h (IV), 0-10: 50% q24h (IV)

Famciclovir	EHL 2-2.3h, PRC B, Lact ?
Famvir *Tab 125mg, 250mg, 500mg*	**Herpes simplex in AIDS**: 500mg PO bid for 7d; **recurrent genital herpes**: 125mg PO bid for 5d; **herpes PRO**: 250mg PO bid; **zoster**: 500mg PO q8h for7d; DARF: see Prod Info

Valacyclovir	EHL 2.5-3.6h, PRC B, Lact -
Valtrex *Tab 500mg*	**Herpes zoster**: 1g PO tid for 7 d; **ini. genital herpes**: 1g PO bid for 10 d; **recurrent genital herpes**: 500mg PO bid for 5d; **herpes PRO**: 500-1000mg PO qd; DARF: see Prod Info

7 A.20.3 Anti-Influenza Drugs

MA/Ind (amantadine): prevents uncoating and maturation of influenza viruses
MA/Ind (zanamivir): inhibition of the viral neuraminidase, inhibition of the release of newly built influenza
A + B viruses
AE (amantadine): nausea, dizziness, insomnia; **AE** (oseltamivir): N/V, bronchitis, insomnia, vertigo
AE (rimantadine): nausea, dizziness; **AE** (zanamivir): respiratory symptoms, thrombotic thrombocytopenic
purpura, hemolytic uremic syndrome
CI (amantadine, oseltamivir, rimantadine, zanamivir): hypersensitivity to product ingredients

Amantadine	EHL 10-14h, PRC C, Lact -
Symmetrel *Tab 100mg, Syr 50mg/5ml* **Generics** *Cap 100mg, Syr 50mg/5ml*	**Influenza A** →245: 100mg PO bid; **CH** 1-9 yr or <40kg: 5mg/kg/d PO, max. 150mg/d div bid, 10 yr and older: 100mg PO bid; **Parkinsonism** →315; DARF: ini 200mg, then GFR (ml/min) 30-50: 100mg qd, 15-29: 100mg qod, <15: 200mg q7d
Oseltamivir	EHL 1-3h, PRC C, Lact ?
Tamiflu *Cap 75mg, Susp 12mg/ml*	**Influenza A, B Tx** →245: 75mg PO bid for 5d; **Influenza A, B PRO**: 75mg PO qd; DARF: GFR (ml/min) <30: 75mg qd
Rimantadine	EHL 19.8-36.5h, PRC C, Lact -
Flumadine *Syr 50mg/5ml, Tab 100mg*	**Influenza A Tx and PRO** →245: 100mg PO bid; **CH** <10 yr, **Influenza A PRO**: 5mg/kg PO qd, max. 150mg/d; DARF: GFR (ml/min) <10: 100mg qd
Zanamivir	EHL 1.6-5.1h, PRC B, Lact ?
Relenza *Cap (inhal) 5mg*	**Influenza A, B Tx** →245: 2 inhal bid for 5d; **CH** >7 yr: see adults; DARF: not req

7 A.20.4 Interferons

MA/EF: antiviral, growth inhibiting and immune regulatory effects
AE: fever, sweating, chills, tiredness, joint and soft-tissue pains, complete blood count changes, cardiac arrhythmias, depression, tremors, convulsions, paresthesia, GI disturbances, hair loss, exanthema, pruritus
AE (interferon alfacon-1): flu like symptoms, depression, N/V, granulocytopenia
AE (interferon alfa-2b + Ribavirin): anemia, insomnia, irritability, depression, headache, nausea
CI: coronary diseases, CNS DO, severe hepatic dysfunction, RF, severe bone marrow damage
CI (interferon alfacon-1): hypersensitivity to alfa interferons/E. coli derived products
CI (interferon alfa-2b + Ribavirin): hypersensitivity to ribavirin or alfa interferon, autoimmune hepatitis

Interferon alfa 2a	EHL 3.7-8.5 h
Roferon A *Inj 3, 6, 9, 18, 36 M U/vial*	**Chronic hepatitis C** →134: 3 M U tiw SC/IM
Interferon alfa-2b	EHL 2-3 h
Intron A *Inj 3, 5, 10, 18, 25, 50 M U/vial, Sol 3, 5, 10,18, 25 M U/vial*	**Chronic hepatitis B** →134: 5 M U qd or 10 M U tiw SC/IM for 16 wk; **chronic hepatitis C**: 3 M U SC/IM tiw
Interferon alfacon-1	EHL 0.5-7h, PRC C, Lact ?
Infergen *Inj 9µg/vial, 15µg/vial*	**Chronic hepatitis C** →134: 9µg SC tiw for 24 wk; 15µg SC tiw for 24 wk for relapse or no response- 9µg dose
Interferon alfa-2b + Ribavirin	PRC X, Lact ?
Rebetron *Cap 200mg, Inj 3, 22.5, 22.8 M U/vial*	**Chronic hepatitis C** →134: Interferon alfa-2b: 3 M U SC tiw and ribavirin 600mg PO bid if >75kg; 400mg qam and 600 hs if <75kg

Interferon beta-1a | EHL 69 h PRC C, Lact ?
Avonex *Inj 33µg/vial*
Rebif *Syr 22µg/0.5ml, Syr 44µg/0.5ml* | **Relapsing form of multiple sclerosis** →317: Avonex: 30µg IM qwk; Rebif: ini 8.8µg SC tiw for 2wk, then 22µg tiw for 2wk, then 44µg tiw

Interferon beta-1b | EHL 4h PRC C, Lact ?
Betaseron *Inj 0.3mg/vial* | **Relapsing form of multiple sclerosis** →317: 0.25mg SC qod

Peginterferon alfa-2a | EHL 80h PRC C, Lact ?
Pegasys *Inj 180µg/vial* | **Chronic hepatitis C** →135: 180µg SC once a wk as monotherapy or in combination with ribavirin; DARF: hemodialysis 135µg/wk

Peginterferon alfa-2b | EHL 40h PRC C, Lact
Peg-Intron *Inj 100µg/ml, 160µg/ml, 240µg/ml, 300µg/ml* | **Chronic hepatitis C** →135: monotherapy: 1µg/kg/wk SC; combination with ribavirin: 1.5µg/kg/wk SC

7 A.20.5 Anti-Respiratory-Syncytial-Virus Drugs

MA/Ind (ribavirin): guanosine analogue, inhibition of the RNA polymerase of HCV
AE (palivizumab): rash, rhinitis, upper respiratory tract infx
AE (ribavirin): rash, respiratory dysfunction, conjunctivitis, hemolytic anemia, nausea
CI (palivizumab): hypersensitivity to palivizumab products
CI (ribavirin): hypersensitivity to ribavirin products, pregnancy

Palivizumab | EHL 13-27 d, PRC C, Lact ?
Synagis *Inj 50mg/vial, 100mg/vial* | **PRO of respiratory syncytial virus disease in high-risk infants**: 15mg/kg IM qmo

Ribavirin | EHL Inhal 9.5h, IV/PO 24-36h, PRC X, Lact ?
Copegus *Tab 200mg*
Rebetol *Cap 200mg*
Virazole *Sol (inhal) 6g/vial* | **Severe respiratory syncytial virus infx** →246: 20mg/ml as continous aerosol administrationfor 12-18h/d for 3d; **CH** see adults; **chronic hepatitis C** →134: <75kg: 400mg PO am, 600mg pm; >75kg: 600mg PO bid; only in combination with interferons (→212); DARF: GFR (ml/min) <50: not recomm.

7 A.20.6 Anti-HIV Drugs: Nucleoside Reverse Transcriptase Inhibitors

MA/Ind (nucleoside analogues): blockage of the transformation of RNA into DNA through chemically altered nucleosides in HIV-infx
AE (abacavir): N/V, fatigue, fever, headache, diarrhea, loss of appetite, lactic acidosis/severe hepatomegaly with steatosis, hypersensitivity reactions (some fatal)
AE (adefovir): asthenia, headache, abdominal pain, nausea, diarrhea, fever, renal failure
AE (didanosine, stavudine): polyneuropathy, pancreatitis, diarrhea, exanthema
AE (lamivudine): headache, N/V, pancreatitis, lactic acidosis/hepatomegaly, fatigue
AE (zalcitabine): polyneuropathy, dermatitis, mucositis, pancreatitis, granulocytopenia, anemia;
AE (zidovudine): anemia, leukopenia, myopathy, nausea, headache
CI (abacavir): severe hepatic dysfunction, hypersensitivity to abacavir products; **CI** (adefovir): hypersensitivity; **CI** (didanosine): acute pancreatitis, combination with rifampin, hypersensitivity to product ingredients; **CI** (lamivudine): hypersensitivity; **CI** (stavudine): hypersensitivity to product ingredients; **CI** (zalcitabine): polyneuropathy, pancreatitis, hypersensitivity to product ingredients; **CI** (zidovudine): leukopenia<750/µl, Hb<7.5g/dl, hypersensitivity

Abacavir (ABC)	EHL 1-2h, PRC C, Lact -
Ziagen *Tab 300mg, Sol (oral) 20mg/ml*	**HIV infx** →242: 300mg PO bid in combination with other antiretroviral drugs; **CH** 3 mo - 16 yr: 8mg/kg PO bid, max. 300mg PO bid; DARF: not req
Adefovir	EHL 1-2h, PRC C, Lact -
Hepsera *Tab 10mg*	**Chronic hepatitis B** →134: 10mg PO qd; DARF: GFR (ml/min) >50: 100%; 20-49: 10mg qod; 10-19: 10mg q72h; hemodial.: 10mg q7d
Didanosine (ddI)	EHL 1.3-1.5h, PRC B, Lact ?
Videx *Tab (chew) 25mg, 50mg, 100mg, 150mg, 200mg, Sol (oral) 100mg/packet, 167mg/packet, 250mg/packet, 10mg/ml* **Videx EC** *Cap ext.rel. 125mg, 200mg, 250mg, 400mg*	**HIV infx** →242: >60kg: 400mg PO qd or 200mg PO bid as Tab or 250mg PO bid buffered powder; <60kg 250mg PO qd or 125mg PO bid as Tab or 167mg PO bid buffered powder in combination with other antiretroviral drugs; **CH** 120mg/square meter PO bid DARF: see Prod Info
Lamivudine (3TC)	EHL 3-7h, PRC C Lact ?
Epivir *Tab 150mg, Sol (oral) 10mg/ml* **Epivir-HBV** *Tab 100mg, Sol (oral) 5mg/ml*	**HIV infx** →242: 150mg PO bid in combination with other antiretroviral drugs; **chronic hepatitis B** →134 100mg PO qd; **CH** 3 mo -16 yr, **HIV infx:** 4mg/kg, max. 150mg PO bid; DARF: **HIV-Tx** GFR (ml/min): >50: 150mg bid, 30-49: 150mg qd, 15-29: ini. 150mg, then 100mg qd, 5-14: ini. 150mg, then 50mg qd, <5: ini. 50mg, then 25mg qd
Stavudine (d4T)	EHL 0.9-1.6h, PRC C, Lact ?
Zerit *Cap 15mg, 20mg, 30mg, 40mg, Sol (oral) 1mg/ml*	**HIV infx** →242: >60kg: 40mg PO bid <60kg: 30mg PO bid; **CH** <30kg: 1mg/kg PO bid, >30kg: see adults; DARF: GFR (ml/min) >50: 100% q12h, 26-50: 50% q12h, 10-25: 50% q24h

Tenofovir (TDF)	EHL 0.9-1.6h, PRC B, Lact -
Viread *Tab 300mg*	**HIV infx** →242: 300mg PO qd in combination with other antiretroviral drugs; DARF: GFR (ml/min) <60: not rec
Zalcitabine (ddC)	EHL 1-3h, PRC C Lact ?
Hivid *Tab 0.375mg, 0.75mg*	**HIV infx** →242: 0.75mg PO tid in combination with other antiretroviral drugs; **CH** 0.015-0.04mg/kg PO qid; DARF: GFR (ml/min): 10-40: 100% q12h, <10: 100% q24h
Zidovudine (AZT, ZDV)	EHL 1h, PRC C, Lact ?
Retrovir *Tab 300mg,* *Cap 100mg,* *Syr 50mg/5ml,* *Inj 10mg/ml*	**HIV infx** →242: 600mg/d PO div bid or tid; 1mg/kg IV over 1h 5-6x/d in combination with other antiretroviral drugs; **PRO of maternal–fetal HIV transmission**: mother (>14 wk of pregnancy): 100mg PO 5x/d until start of labor, during labor, 2mg/kg IV over 1h, then 1mg/kg/h until delivery; newborn: 2mg/kg PO q6h within 12h of birth for 6 wk, **CH** 3 mo - 12 yr: 180mg/square meter q6h, max. 200mg q6h
Lamivudine + Zidovudine	PRC C, Lact ?
Combivir *Tab 150 + 300mg*	**HIV infx** →242: 1 Tab PO bid; DARF: not rec in RF
Abacavir + Lamivudine + Zidovudine	PRC C, Lact -
Trizivir *Tab 300 + 150 + 300mg*	**HIV infx** →242: 1 Tab PO bid; DARF: GFR (ml/min) <50: not rec

7 A.20.7 Anti-HIV Drugs: Non-Nucleoside Reverse Transcriptase Inhibitors

MA/Ind (efavirenz, nevirapine): direct binding on the reverse transcriptase
⇒ blockage of DNA-polymerase of HIV-1
AE (delavirdine): N/V, rash, headache, fatigue; **AE** (efavirenz): dizziness, drowsiness, impaired concentration, sleeplessness, exanthema, liver enzymes ↑; **AE** (nevirapine): rash, nausea, diarrhea, fever, headache, liver enzymes ↑, hypersensitivity to product ingredients
CI (delavirdine): hypersensitivity to delavirdine products, concomitant use with rifampin or rifabutin; **CI** (efavirenz): combination with astemizole, cisapride, midazolam, triazolam, fexofenadine, ergotamine derivates; children < 3 yr, hypersensitivity to product ingredients
CI (nevirapine): hypersensitivity to nevirapine products

Delavirdine (DLV)	EHL 2-11h, PRC C, Lact ?
Rescriptor *Tab 100mg*	**HIV infx** →242: 400mg PO tid combined with other antiretroviral; **CH** >16yr: see adults
Efavirenz (EFV)	EHL 52-76 h (1 dose), 40-55 h (x dose), Lact -
Sustiva *Cap 50mg, 100mg, 200mg; Tab 300, 600mg*	**HIV infx** →242: 600mg PO qd combined with other antiretroviral drugs; **CH** >3 yr: 10-15kg: 200mg PO qd, 15-20kg: 250mg PO qd, 20-25kg: 300mg PO qd, 25-32.5kg: 350mg PO qd, 33-40kg: 400mg PO qd, >40kg: 600mg qd

Nevirapine (NVP)	EHL 22-84h, PRC C, Lact ?
Viramune *Tab 200mg,* *Susp 50mg/5ml*	**HIV infx** →242: 200mg PO qd for 14d, then 200mg PO bid combined with other antiretroviral drugs; **CH** 2 mo - 8 yr: 4mg/kg PO qd for 14d, then 7mg/kg bid, >8 yr: 4 mg/kg PO qd x 2 wk, then 4 mg/kg bid, max. 400mg/d; **PRO of maternal-fetal HIV transmission**: mother 200mg PO as single dose at onset of labor; neonate 2mg/kg PO within 3d of birth

7 A.20.8 Anti-HIV Drugs: Protease Inhibitors

MA/Ind: specific inhibition of HIV protease ⇒ protein production ↓ (i.e. rev. transcriptase)
AE (amprenavir): N/V, diarrhea, rash, paresthesia
AE (atazanavir): jaundice, N/V, diarrhea, headache, abdominal pain
AE (indinavir, ritonavir): nausea, headache, diarrhea, tiredness, exanthema
AE (nelfinavir, saquinavir): diarrhea, nausea, exanthema
CI (amprenavir): concomitant interacting drugs, hypersensitivity to amprenavir products, children < 4yr, hepatic or RF, under disulfiram or metronidazole Tx
CI (atazanavir): hypersensitivity to a.; coadministration with midazolam, triazolam, cisapride, pimozide, ergot derivates; **CI** (indinavir): hypersensitivity to indinavir products
CI (nelfinavir): combination w/rifampin, fexofenadine
CI (ritonavir): severe hepatic insufficiency
CI (saquinavir): combination w/rifampin

Amprenavir (APV)	EHL 7-10h, PRC C, Lact -
Agenerase *Cap 50, 150mg,* *Sol (oral) 15mg/ml*	**HIV-1 infx** →242: 1200mg PO bid in combination with ohther antiretroviral drugs; **CH** 4-16yr, <50kg: Cap: 20mg/kg PO bid, max. 2400mg/d, Sol: 22.5mg/kg bid
Atazanavir (AZV)	EHL 7h, PRC B, Lact -
Reyataz *Cap 100mg, 150mg, 200mg*	**HIV infx** →242: 400mg PO qd in combination with other antiretroviral drugs
Indinavir (IDV)	EHL 1.5-2h, PRC C, Lact -
Crixivan *Cap 200mg, 333mg, 400mg*	**HIV infx** →242: 800mg PO tid in combination with other antiretroviral drugs; DARF: not req
Nelfinavir (NFV)	EHL 3.5-5h, PRC B, Lact ?
Viracept *Tab 250mg,* *Susp 50mg/scoopful*	**HIV infx** →242: 750mg PO tid or 1250mg PO bid in combination with other antiretroviral drugs; **CH** 2-13 yr: 20-30mg/kg tid
Ritonavir (RTV)	EHL 3-3.5h, PRC B, Lact ?
Norvir *Cap 100mg, Sol; oral 80mg/ml*	**HIV infx** →242: ini. 300mg PO bid, incr. at 2-3d intervalls by 100mg bid to 600mg bid in combination with other antiretroviral drugs; **CH** ini 250mg/m^2 PO bid, incr. at 2-3d intervalls by 50mg/m^2/dose to 400mg/m^2 PO bid, max. 600mg PO bid

Saquinavir (SQV)

EHL 13h, PRC B Lact?

Fortovase *Cap 200mg*
Invirase *Cap 200mg*

HIV infx →242: Fortovase: 1200mg PO tid
Invirase: 600mg PO tid in combination with other
antiretroviral drugs

7 A.20.9 Anti-HIV Drugs: Fusion Inhibitors

MA: interferes wit the entry of HIV-1 into cells by inhibiting fusion of viral and cellular membranes
AE (enfuvirtide): injection site reactions, diarrhea, nausea, fatigue, pancreatitis, pneumonia
CI (enfuvirtide): hypersensitivity to enf.

Enfuvirtide (T20)

EHL 3.8h, PRC B, Lact -

Fuzeon *Inj 90mg/1ml*

HIV-1 infx →242: 90mg SC bid; **CH** 6-16 yr: 2mg/kg
SC bid, max 90mg bid

7 A.21 Antifungals

7 A.21.1 Drugs for Subcutaneous and Systemic Mycoses

Ind (amphotericin B): Candida-species, Aspergillus, Histoplasma, Sporothrix, Blastomyces, Cryptococcus, Coccidoides; **Ind** (fluconazole): Candida-species (except C. krusei, C. glabrata), Cryptococcus, Histoplasma, Trichosporon, Dermatophytes, Blastomyces
Ind (flucytosine): Candida, Cryptococcus, Aspergillus
AE (amphotericin B): fever, chills, N/V, diarrhea, generalized pains, anemia, renal dysfunction, hypokalemia, thrombocytopenia; **AE** (caspofungin): neutropenia, anemia, headache, hypokalemia, fever, phlebitis, increased liver enzymes; **AE** (fluconazole): nausea, stomachache, diarrhea, exanthema, headache, peripheral neuropathy, LFT↑, itching; **AE** (flucytosine): complete blood count changes, liver enzymes↑, dizziness, **AE** (itraconazole): N/V, hypokalemia, LFT↑, rash; **AE** (ketoconazole): hepatitis, N/V, adrenal insufficiency
CI (amphotericin B): severe hepatic, kidney dysfunction, hypersensitivity to amphotericin B
CI (caspofungin): hypersensitivity to caspofungin; **CI** (fluconazole): severe hepatic dysfunction, great caution with children, hypersensitivity to fluconazole; **CI** (flucytosine): great caution with RF, hepatic damage, bone marrow depression, hypersensitivity to product ingredients; **CI** (itraconazole): hypersensitivity to itraconazole, concurrent use with astemizole, fexofenadine, triazolam, cisapride, oral midazolam, pimozide, quinidine
CI (ketoconazole): hypersensitivity to ketoconazole products, concurrent use with astemizole, fexofenadine, cisapride, oral triazolam

Amphotericin B

EHL 15 d, PRC B Lact ?

Fungizone *Susp 100mg/ml,*
Inj 50mg/vial
Generics *Inj 50mg/vial*

Severe fungal infx →251: test dose 1mg slow IV, if
tolerated start 0.25 mg/kg IV qd, incr. to 0.5-1.5 mg/
kg/d, max. 1.5 mg/kg/d, administration time. 2-6h;
DARF: GFR (ml/min) >50: 100% q24h, 10-50: 100%
q24h, <10: 100% q24-36h

Amphotercin B lipid complex

EHL 170h, PRC B, Lact ?

Abelcet *Inj lipid complex 5mg/ml*
Amphotec *Inj lipid complex 50mg/vial, 100mg/vial*

Severe fungal infx →251: 5 mg/kg IV qd
administration time: 2.5mg/kg/h

Amphotercin B liposome

EHL 7-153h, PRC B, Lact ?

Ambisome *Inj liposomal 50mg/vial*

Severe fungal infx →251: 3-5 mg/kg IV qd
administration time: 2h; **CH** 1mo - 16 yr:
3mg/kg IV qd

Caspofungin	EHL 9-11h, PRC C, Lact ?
Cancidas *Inj 50mg/vial, 70mg/vial*	**Invasive aspergillosis** →251: d1 70mg IV over 1h, then 50mg IV qd; DARF: not req
Fluconazole	EHL 30 h
Diflucan *Tab 50mg,100mg, 150mg, 200mg, Susp 200mg/5ml, 50mg/5ml, Inj 200mg/100ml*	**Oropharyngeal/esophageal candidiasis**: first day 200mg PO/IV qd, then 100mg qd; **vaginal cand**: 150mg PO as single dose; **systemic cand**: 400mg PO/IV qd; **CH oropharyngeal/esophageal cand**: first day 6mg/kg PO/IV qd, then 3mg/kg qd; **systemic cand** →251: 6-12 mg/kg PO/IV qd; DARF: GFR (ml/min) >50: 100%, <50: 50%
Flucytosine	EHL 3-8h, PRC C, Lact ?
Ancobon *Cap 250mg, 500mg*	**Candidiasis, cryptococcosis** →251: 50-150mg/kg/d PO div qid; DARF: GFR (ml/min): >50: q6h, 10-50: q12-24h, <10: q24-48h
Itraconazole	EHL 64h (x dose)/24h (1x), IV35h, PRC C, Lact ?
Sporanox *Cap 100mg, Inj 10mg/ml, Sol (oral) 10mg/ml*	**Aspergillosis**: →251 200mg IV bid x 2d, then 200mg IV qd; 200-400mg/d PO for 3 mo; **blastomycosis**: 200mg IV bid x 2d, then 200mg IV qd; 200-400mg/d PO; **esophageal, oropharngeal cand**: 100-200mg PO swish and swallow; **onychomycosis, toenails**: 200mg PO qd for 12 wk; DARF: GFR (ml/min) > 30: 100%, <30: IV not rated
Ketoconazole	EHL 2-12h, PRC C, Lact ?
Nizoral *Tab 200mg* **Generics** *Tab 200mg*	**Various fungal infx**: 200-400mg PO qd; **CH >2 yr**: 3.3-6.6mg/kg PO qd; DARF: not req
Terbinafine	EHL 22-26h, PRC B, Lact -
Lamisil *Tab 250mg*	**Onychomycosis, fingernails**: 250mg PO qd for 6 wk; **onychomycosis, toenails**: 250mg PO qd for 12 wk; **superficial mycoses**: 250mg PO qd for 1-4 wk; **systemic mycoses**: 250-500mg PO qd for 1-16 mo; DARF: GFR (ml/min) <50: 50%
Voriconazole	EHL 6h, PRC D , Lact -
Vfend *Tab 50mg, Tab 200mg; Inj 200mg*	**Invasive aspergillosis, scedosporium-, fusarium infx**: ini 6mg/kg IV q12h, after 2doses 4mg/kg q12h; 200mg PO bid, may incr. to 300mg PO bid; <40kg: 100mg PO bid, may incr. to 150mg bid;

7 A.21.2 Drugs for Superficial Mycoses

Ind (clotrimazole): cutaneous, oral, vaginal candidiasis, dermatomycosis; **Ind** (griseofulvin microsize/microcrystalline, ultramicrosize/ultra-microcrystalline): dermal fungal-, ringworm infx; **Ind** (nystatin): Candida, Blastomyces, Coccidioides, Histoplasma, Aspergillus
Ind (terbinafine): dermal fungal infx, onychomycosis
AE (clotrimazole): N/V, transient elevations in LFT, contact dermatitis; **AE** (griseofulvin microsize/microcrystalline, ultramicrosize/ultra-microcrystalline): N/V, headache, rash, photosensitivity; **AE** (nystatin): in high doses: diarrhea, vaginal irritation/pain, N/V, rash
AE (terbinafine): local irritation, N/V, LFT ↑
CI (clotrimazole): hypersensitivity to clotrimazole; **CI** (griseofulvin microsize/microcrystalline, ultramicrosize/ultra-microcrystalline): hypersensitivity to griseofulvin products, porphyria, hepatocellular failure; **CI** (nystatin): hypersensitivity to nystatin products; **CI** (terbinafine): hypersensitivity to terbinafine products

Clotrimazole	EHL 3.5-5h, PRC B, Lact ?
Mycelex *troche/lozenge; oral;10mg*	**Oropharyngeal candidiasis**: 1 troche dissolved slowly in the mouth 5x/d for 14d; **PRO**: 1 troche dissolved slowly in mouth tid; **CH** >3 yr: see adults
Griseofulvin microsize	EHL no data, PRC N, Lact ?
Gris-peg *Tab 125mg, 250mg* **Ultragris** *Tab 165mg, 330mg* **Grifulvin V** *Tab 125mg, 250mg, 500mg,* *Susp (or) 125mg/5ml*	**Tinea** →364: 500mg PO qd, max. 1g; **CH** 10-20mg/kg/d PO qd
Griseofulvin ultramicrosize	EHL no data, PRC N, Lact ?
Gris-PEG *Tab 125mg, 250mg* **Grisactin** *Cap 250mg, Tab 500mg* **Grisactin ultra** *Tab 125mg, 165mg, 250mg,* *330mg* **Fulvicin-u/f** *Tab 250mg, 500mg* **Fulvicin p/g** *Tab 125mg, 165mg, 250mg, 330mg*	**Tinea** →364: 330 or 375mg PO qd, max. 750mg; **CH** 5-10mg/kg/d PO qd
Nystatin	EHL no data, PRC C, Lact +
Korostatin *Tab vag 100,000 U* **Mycostatin** *Tab 200,000 U, 500,000 U, Susp* *100,000 U/ml* **Nilstat** *Powder (oral) 100%, Tab 500,000 U, Tab* *(vag) 100,000 U, Susp 100,000 U/ml* **Nystex** *Susp 100,000 U/ml* **Generics** *Tab 500,000 U, Tab (vag) 100,000 U,* *Powder (oral) 100%, Susp 100,000 U/ml*	**Oral candidiasis**: 400000-600000 U PO qid **GI candidiasis**: 0.5-1 M U PO tid; **infants**: 200000 U PO qid; **CH** see adults

7 A.22 Antiparasitics

AE (albendazole): leukopenia, hepatic abnormalities, headache; **AE** (atovaquone): fever, rash, N/V, diarrhea; **AE** (iodoquinol): optic neuritis/atrophy, peripheral neuropathy; **AE** (ivermectin): headache, pruritus; **AE** (mebendazole): abdominal pain, diarrhea, rash; **AE** (metronidazole): seizures, N/V, metallic taste; **AE** (nitazoxanide): abdominal pain, diarrhea, vomiting, headache, **AE** (pentamidine): leukopenia, thrombocytopenia, hypotension, chest pain, rash; **AE** (praziquantel): malaise, headache; **AE** (pyrantel): N/V, headache; **AE** (pyrimethamine): Steven's-Johnson syndrome, megaloblastic anemia, leukopenia; **AE** (thiabendazole): N/V, psychotic reactions;
CI (albendazole): hypersensitivity to albendazole or benzimidazoles; **CI** (atovaquone, ivermectin, mebendazole, metronidazole): hypersensitivity to product; **CI** (iodoquinol): hepatic damage, hypersensitivity to iodine + 8-hydroxyquinolones, **CI** (nitoxanide): hypersensitivity to n.; **CI** (pentamidine): hypersensitivity to pentamidine; **CI** (praziquantel): hypersensitivity to praziquantel, ocular cysticercosis; **CI** (pyrantel): liver disease, myasthenia gravis; **CI** (pyrimethamine): hypersensitivity to pyrimethamine products, megaloblastic anemia (folate deficiency); **CI** (thiabendazole): hypersensitivity to thiabendazole, Pro of pinworm infestation

Albendazole	EHL 8-12h, PRC C, Lact ?
Albenza *Tab 200mg*	**Hydatid disease**: > 60kg: 400mg PO bid, < 60kg: 15mg/kg/d PO, max. 800mg/d div bid for 28d followed by a 14d drug-free intervall, for a total of 3 cycles; **neurocysticercosis**: > 60kg: 400mg PO bid, < 60kg: 15mg/kg/d PO, max. 800mg/d for 8-30d; **hookworm, pinworm, roundworm, whipworm**: 400mg (**CH** >2 yr: 200mg) PO as a single dose, **strongyloidiasis**: 400mg PO qd for 3d **cutaneous larva migrans**: 200mg PO bid for 3d; DARF: not req
Atovaquone	EHL 50-84h, PRC C, Lact ?
Mepron *Tab 250mg, Susp 750mg/5ml*	**Pneumocystis carinii Tx** →242: 750mg PO bid for 21d; **pneumocystis carinii PRO** →243: 1500mg PO qd **toxoplasmosis** →243: 750mg PO qid; **CH** 13-16 yr: see adults
Iodoquinol	EHL no data, PRC C, Lact ?
Yodoxin, Diiodohydroxyquin *Tab 210mg, 650mg, Powder 25g*	**Intestinal amebiasis**: 630-650mg PO tid for 20d; **CH** 40mg/kg/d PO div tid for 20d; max. 1.95g/d
Ivermectin	EHL 16-35 h
Stromectol *Tab 3mg 6mg*	**Strongyloidiasis**: 200µg/kg PO as single dose; **onchocerciasis**: 150µg/kg PO q3-12 mo; **cutaneous larva migrans**: 12mg PO as single dose; **CH** >15 kg **onchocerciasis**: 150µg/kg PO as single dose
Mebendazole	EHL 1.5-5.5h, PRC C, Lact ?
Vermox *Tab (chew) 100mg*	**Roundworm, whipworm, hookworm**: 100mg PO bid for 3d; **pinworm**: 100mg PO as single dose; **CH** >2 yr: see adults; DARF: not req

Metronidazole — EHL 6-11h, PRC B, Lact ?

Flagyl *Tab ext.rel. 750mg, Cap 375mg, Inj 500mg/vial, 500mg/100ml*
Metro *Inj 500mg/100ml*
Protostat *Tab 250mg, 500mg*
Generics *Inj 500mg/100ml, Tab 250mg, 500mg*

Amebic dysentery: 750mg PO tid for 5-10d **amebic liver abscess**: 500-750mg PO tid for 5-10d; **giardiasis**: 250mg PO tid for 5d; **trichomoniasis**: 250mg PO tid for 7d; **CH** **amebic dysentery**: 35-50mg/kg/d PO, max. 750mg/dose, div tid for 10 d; **amebic liver abscess**: 50mg/kg/d PO div tid, max. 2.4g/d, for 7d; **giardiasis**: 15mg/kg/d PO div tid for 7-10d; **trichomoniasis**: 15mg/kg/d PO div tid for 7d; DARF: GFR (ml/min) >10: 100%, <10: 50%

Nitazoxanide — PRC B, Lact ?

Alinia *Susp 100mg/5ml*

Diarrhea by Cryptosporidium parvum, Giardia lamblia: CH 1-4yr: 100mg PO bid for 3d; 4-11yr: 200mg PO bid for 3d

Pentamidine — EHL 6.4 h-9h, PRC C, Lact -

Nebupent *Sol (inhal) 300mg, 600mg/vial*
Pentam *Inj 300mg/vial*
Generics *Inj 300mg/vial*

Pneumocystis carinii Tx →242: 4mg/kg IM/IV qd for 14-21d; **pneumocystis carinii PRO** →243: 300mg nebulized 1x q4 wk or 4mg/kg IV 1x q4 wk; **CH** >5 yr: see adults; DARF: not req

Praziquantel — EHL 0.8-3h, PRC B

Biltricide *Tab 600mg*

Schistosomiasis: 60mg/kg PO div tid for 1d **liver flukes**: 75mg/kg PO div tid for 1d **neurocysticercosis**: 50mg/kg/d PO div tid for 15d; **cestodiasis**: 10mg/kg PO as single dose; **CH** >4 yr: **schistosomiasis**: 60mg/kg PO div tid for 1d; DARF: not req

Pyrantel — EHL no data, PRC C, Lact ?

Combantrin *Tab 125 mg, Susp 50mg/ml*
Pin-X *Inj 50mg/ml*

Pinworm, roundworm: 11 mg/kg PO, max. 1g as single dose

Pyrimethamine — EHL 80-96h, PRC C, Lact +

Daraprim *Tab 25mg*

Toxoplasmosis →243, **immunocompetent patients**: 50-75mg PO qd for 1-3 wk, then 50% of first dose for 4-5 wk; **toxoplasmosis in AIDS**: ini. 200mg PO, then 50-100mg qd; **secondary PRO of toxoplasmosis in AIDS**: 50mg PO qd, give with folinic acid (10-15 mg qd) and sulfadiazine or clindamycin; **CH toxoplasmosis**: 1mg/kg/d PO div bid for 2-4 d, then 50% of 1st dose for 1 mo; DARF: not req

Thiabendazole — EHL no data, PRC C Lact ?

Mintezol *Susp 500mg/5ml, Tab (chew) 500mg*

Strongyloidiasis, cutaneous larva migrans: 22mg/kg PO bid for 2d; **trichinosis**: 22mg/kg PO bid for 2-4d

7 A.23 Antimalarials
7 A.23.1 Antimalarials – Single Ingredient Drugs

AE (chloroquine): corneal clouding, pigmented retinopathy, methemoglobinemia, ECG changes, exanthema, muscle weakness; **AE** (doxycycline): photosensitivity, epigastric distress; **AE** (mefloquine): GI/CNS DO, psychoses, dysrhythmias, leuko-/thrombopenia, sinus bradycardia, seizures, liver transaminases ↑ ; **AE** (primaquine): anemia, leukocytosis, abdominal pain; **AE** (quinine): thrombocytopenia, convulsions, urticaria, hypoglycemia, hemolytic uremic syndrome; **CI** (chloroquine): retinopathy, G6PD deficiency, hypersensitivity to product, retinal/visual field changes; **CI** (doxycycline): hypersensitivity to doxycycline/tetracycline, children < 8yr; **CI** (mefloquine): psychoses, cardiomyopathy, epilepsy; **CI** (primaquine): concomitant medications which cause bone marrow suppression, rheumatoid arthritis, lupus erythematosus; **CI** (quinine): hypersensitivity to quinine, glucose–6–phosphate dehydrogenase deficiency, myasthenia gravis

Chloroquine Phosphate	EHL 6-60 d, PRC C, Lact +
Aralen *Tab 300mg, Inj 40mg/ml* **Generics** *Tab 150mg, 300mg*	**Malaria PRO** →248: 500mg PO 1x/wk from 2 wk before exposure to 6 wk after **malaria Tx** →249: d1: 1g PO, then 500mg PO after 6h, then 500mg PO qd on d2 and 3; **extraintestinal amebiasis**: 1g PO qd for 2d, then 500mg PO qd for 2-3 wk; **CH malaria PRO**: 5mg/kg PO 1x/wk from 2 wk before exposure to 6 wk after **malaria Tx**: 10mg/kg PO, max. 600mg, then 5mg/kg, max. 300mg after 6, 18 and 24h; DARF: GFR (ml/min) <10: 50%
Doxycycline	EHL 12-24h, PRC D, Lact ?
Doryx *Cap 100mg* **Monodox** *Cap 50mg, 100mg* **Vibramycin** *Cap 50mg, 100mg; Susp 50mg/5ml* **Generics** *Cap 50mg, 100mg*	**Malaria PRO** →248: 100mg PO qd from 2d before exposure to 4 wk after **malaria Tx** →249: 200mg PO qd for 7 d with quinine; DARF: not req
Mefloquine	EHL 13-30 d, PRC C, Lact ?
Lariam *Tab 250mg*	**Malaria PRO** →248: 250mg PO 1x/wk from 1wk before exposure to 4 wk after **malaria Tx** →249: 1250mg PO single dose; **CH malaria PRO**: 1x/wk, 15-19kg: ¼ Tab PO, 20-30kg: ½ Tab PO, 31-45kg: ¾ Tab PO, >45kg: 1 Tab PO; **malaria Tx** <45 kg: 15mg/kg PO, then 10mg/kg given 6-8h after first dose
Primaquine Phosphate	EHL 4-7h, PRC C, Lact ?
Primaquine *Tab 15mg*	**PRO of p. vivax and p. ovale relapse** →248: 15mg PO qd for 14d; **CH** 0.3mg/kg PO for 14d
Quinidine Gluconate	EHL no data, PRC ? Lact ?
Quinaglute *Tab ext.rel. 324mg* **Generics** *Inj 80mg/ml, Tab ext.rel. 324mg*	**Severe p. falcip. malaria** →249: ini. 10mg/kg IV over 1-2h, then 0.02 mg/kg/min for 72 h or until parasitemia <1%, or PO meds tolerated
Quinine Sulfate	EHL no data, PRC X, Lact ?
Generics	**Malaria Tx** →249: 650mg PO tid for 3-7 d with doxycycline or pyrimethamine/sulfadoxine

7 A.23.2 Antimalarials – Combinations

AE (a. + p.): fever, headache, myalgia; AE (p. + s): blood dyscrasias, Stevens-Johnson syndrome, myelosuppression, toxic nephrosis; CI (a. + p.): hypersensitivity to atovaquone, hypersensitivity to proguanil; CI (p. + s.): hypersensitivity to pyrimethamine or sulfonamides, infants, severe liver or renal disease, blood dyscrasias

Atovaquone + Proquanil	PRC C, Lact ?
Malarone *Tab 250 + 100mg* **Malarone pediatric** *Tab 62.5 + 25mg*	**Malaria PRO** →248: 1 Tab PO qd from 2d before to 7d after exposure; **malaria Tx** →249: 4 Tab PO qd for 3d; **CH malaria PRO**: from 2d before to 7d after exposure, 11–20kg: 1 ped Tab PO qd, 21–30kg: 2 ped Tab PO qd, 31–40kg: 3 ped Tab PO qd, >40kg: 1 adult Tab PO qd; **malaria Tx**: for 3 d, 11–20kg: 1 adult Tab PO qd, 21–30kg: 2 adult Tab PO qd, 31–40kg; 3 adult Tab PO qd, >40kg: 4 adult Tab PO qd
Pyrimethamine + Sulfadoxine	PRC C, Lact +
Fansidar *Tab 25 + 500mg*	**Malaria PRO** →248: 1 Tab PO 1x/wk from 2d before to 4–6 wk after exposure; **malaria Tx** →249: 2–3 Tab PO as single dose; **CH malaria PRO**: 1x/wk from 2d before to 4–6 wk after exposure; 2 mo–4 yr: 1/4 Tab PO, 4–8 yr: 1/2 Tab PO, 9–14 yr: 3/4 Tab PO; **CH malaria Tx**: single dose, 2 mo–4 yr: 1/2 Tab PO, 4–8 yr: 1 Tab PO, 9–14 yr: 2 Tab PO

7 B. Infections – Therapies

Helmut Albrecht, MD
Division of Infectious Diseases
Emory University, Atlanta, GA

7 B.1 Empiric Antimicrobial Therapy

Cardiovascular System
- Infective endocarditis →63
- Endocarditis prophylaxis →65

Respiratory System
- Chronic bronchitis, acute exacerbations →105
- Community-acquired pneumonia (CAP) →106
- Hospital-acquired pneumonia →109
- Pleural infections →111
- Infections in cystic fibrosis →115

Rheumatolgy
- Reactive arthritis/Reiter's syndrome
  (enteropathic form) →278

Gastroenterology
- Infectious esophagitis →130
- PUD, Helicobacter →131
- Diverticular disease →132
- Biliary/necrotizing pancreatitis →134
- Viral hepatitis →134

Nephrology, Urology
- Urinary tract infection (UTI) →428
- Pyelonephritis →428
- Urosepsis →429
- Acute post-streptococcal glomerulonephritis
  →429
- Urethritis →434
- Prostatitis →435
- Epididymitis →436

Neurology
- Meningitis →310
- Encephalitis →310

Ophthalmology
- Hordeolum, chalazion →386
- Blepharitis →386
- Infections of the eyelids →388
- Dacryoadenitis, dacryocystitis →388
- Conjunctivitis →390
- Keratitis →392

ENT
- Rhinosinusiitis →416
- Furuncles of the nose →417
- Tonsillitis →418
- Pharyngitis →418
- Bacterial laryngitis, epiglottitis →419
- Perichondritis, external otitis →419
- Herpes zoster oticus →421
- Otitis media →421
- Mastoiditis →422
- Sialadenitis →422

Dermatology
- Abscess →361
- Acne vulgaris →361
- Lyme borreliosis →370
- Condyloma acuminata →363
- Eczema →366
- Scabies, pediculosis →370
- Erysipelas, erythrasma →367
- Folliculitis →367
- HSV infection →368
- Impetigo →369
- Tinea, tinea versicolor →374
- Rosacea →373
- Sexually transmitted diseases →373
- Pityriasis rosea →372

7 B.2   Specific Antibacterial Therapy
7 B.2.1   Organism – Antibiotic

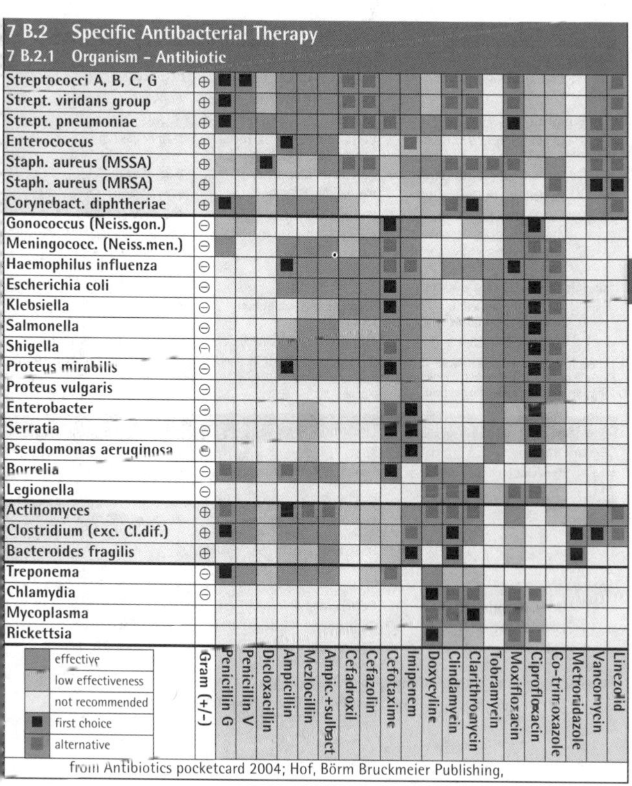

from Antibiotics pocketcard 2004; Hof, Börm Bruckmeier Publishing,

7 B.2.2   Acinetobacter Species

Empiric therapy

	Carbapenem →197	**Imipenem–Cilastim** (Primaxin)	*0.5g IV q6h*
		Meropenem (Merrem)	*1g IV q8h*

Alternatives

	Cephalosporin 3rd Gen. →195	**Ceftazidime** (Ceptaz, Fortaz, Tazicef, Tazidime, Gens)	*1–2g IV q8-12h*
or	**Cephalosporin 4th Gen.** →197	**Cefepime** (Maxipime)	*1–2g IV q12h*
or	**Penicillin 4th Gen.** →190	**Piperacillin** (Pipril)	*3–4g IV/IM q4-6h*
PLUS	**Fluoroquinolone** →203	**Ciprofloxacin** (Cipro)	*400mg IV q8-12h*
or	**Aminoglycoside** →200 (often most sensitive to amikacin)	**Amikacin** (Amikin, Gens)	*15mg/kg IV qd (check level in prolonged Tx)*

Carbapenem-resistant isolates

	Acylaminopenicillin + lactamase inhibitor →191	**Ampicillin + Sulbactam** (Unasyn)	*3g IV q6h*
or	**Polymxyin** →413	**Colistin** (Coly-Mycin M)	*5mg/kg qd (div bid-qid)*

If hospital-acquired often multi-drug resistant, adjust empiric Tx according to local susceptibility pattern. Double coverage for serious infection until susceptibility tests available. Duration of Tx dependant on location and severity of infection.

7 B.2.3   Actinomyces Species

Empiric therapy

wk1 – wk4 (wk6)	**Benzylpenicillin** →187	**Penicillin G** (Pfizerpen, Gens)	*10–20 M IU IV qd (div qid or cont Inf), for 4–6wk*
then		**Penicillin V** (Beepen VK, Betapen VK, Ledercillin VK, Pen-vee K, Uticillin VK, V-cillin VK, Veetids, Gens)	*0.5–1g qid PO for 2–6mo*

Alternatives

or	**Cephalosporin 3rd Gen.** →195	**Ceftriaxone** (Rocephin)	*1–2g IV qd*
or	**Lincosamide** →201	**Clindamycin** (Cleocin, Gens)	*300–600mg IV tid-qid*
or	**Chloramphenicol** →202	**Chloramphenicol** (Chloromycetin)	*12.5–15mg/kg IV q6h*

In Penicillin allergic patients or Penicillin-resistant isolates

	Tetracycline →198	**Doxycycline** (Doryx, Monodox, Periostat, Vibramycin, Gens)	*0.1g IV/PO bid*

7 B.2.4   Alcaligenes xylosoxidans

	Carbapenem →197	Imipenem-Cilastin (Primaxin)	0.5g q6h
		Meropenem (Merrem)	1g q8h
or	Folate antagonist + p-Aminobenzoic acid antagonist →206	Sulfamethoxazole + Trimethoprim (Cotrimoxazole) (Bactrim, Cotrim, Septra, Sulfamethoprim, Sulfatrim, Gens)	8-10mg trimethoprim equivalent/kg IV (div bid-qid) or 800+160mg PO bid

Alcaligenes xylosoxidans are usually resistant to penicillins, cephalosporins (some sensitive to ceftazidime), FQ, aztreonam. Duration of Tx dependant on location and severity of infection.

7 B.2.5   Bacillus anthracis (Anthrax)

	Fluoroquinolone →203	Ciprofloxacin (Cipro)	500-750mg PO bid, or 400mg IV bid, max 400mg IV tid for 100d
or	Tetracycline →198	Doxycycline (Doryx, Monodox, Periostat, Vibramycin, Gens)	d1: 200mg PO/IV qd, then 100mg PO/IV qd

Note: Severe infections (pulmonary, bacteremia, meningitis) usually require multi-drug and intensive supportive Tx. Immediately notify local/federal authorities.

7 B.2.6   Bacteroides fragilis

Infection below diaphragm

	Antiprotozoal →206 (nitroimidazole)	Metronidazole (Flagyl, Metro, Metryl, Protostat, Gens)	250-500mg PO bid-qid, 500mg IV bid-qid

Infection above diaphragm

	Lincosamide →201	Clindamycin (Cleocin, Gens)	150-450mg PO bid-tid, 200-600mg IV tid-qid

Also effective: carpapenems, moxifloxacin, beta-lactams/beta-lactamase inhibitor combinations, chloramphenicol. Duration of Tx depends on location/severity of infection

7 B.2.7   Bordetella pertussis

1st choice

	Macrolide →199	Clarithromycin (Biaxin)	250mg PO bid for 2wk

In intolerance

	Folate antagonist + p-Aminobenzoic acid antagonist →206	Sulfamethoxazole + Trimethoprim (Cotrimoxazole) (Bactrim, Cotrim, Septra, Sulfamethoprim, Sulfatrim, Gens)	8-10mg trimethoprim equivalent/kg IV (div bid-qid for 14d), 800+160mg PO bid

7 B.2.8   Borrelia burgdorferi

1st choice

	Tetracycline →198	Doxycycline (Doryx, Monodox, Periostat, Vibramycin, Gens)	d1: 200mg PO/IV qd, then 100mg PO/IV qd

In children

	Benzylpenicillin →187	**Penicillin V** (Beepen VK, Betapen VK, Ledercillin VK, Pen-vee K, Uticillin VK, V-cillin VK, Veetids, Gens)	*0.6-1.5 M IU PO tid for 21d*

In neuroborreliosis

	Cephalosporin 3rd Gen. →195	**Ceftriaxone** (Rocephin)	*1-2g IV qd for 2-4wk*

7 B.2.9   Borrelia recurrentis

1st choice	**Tetracycline** →198	**Doxycycline** (Doryx, Monodox, Periostat, Vibramycin, Gens)	*0.2g IV once*
or	**Benzylpenicillin** →187	**Penicillin G** (Pfizerpen, Gens)	*0.5-10 M IU IV qid-6x/d*

7 B.2.10 Brucella abortus, melitensis, suis, canis

1st choice

	Tetracycline →198	**Doxycycline** (Doryx, Monodox, Periostat, Vibramycin, Gens)	*200mg PO qd for 6wk*
Plus	**Antimycobacterial** →208	**Rifampin** (Rifadin, Rimactane, Generic)	*10mg/kg PO qd for 6wk*
or	**Aminoglycoside** →200	**Gentamicin** (Garamycin, U-gencin, Gens)	*2-5mg/kg IV/IM qd (monitor drug level)*

CH < 8 years

	Folate antagonist + p-Aminobenzoic acid antagonist →206	**Sulfamethoxazole + Trimethoprim** (Cotrimoxazole) (Bactrim, Cotrim, Septra, Sulfamethoprim, Sulfatrim, Gens)	*800+160mg PO/IV bid*
Plus	**Antimycobacterial** →208	**Rifampin** (Rifadin, Rimactane, Generic)	*10mg/kg PO qd*
or	**Aminoglycoside** →200	**Gentamicin** (Garamycin, U-gencin, Generic)	*2-5mg/kg IV/IM qd (monitor drug level)*

Endocarditis, meningoencephalitis, relapses

	Tetracycline →198	**Doxycycline** (Doryx, Monodox, Periostat, Vibramycin, Gens)	*500mg PO qd-tid*
plus	**Aminoglycoside** →200	**Gentamicin** (Garamycin, U-gencin, Gens)	*2-5mg/kg IV/IM qd (monitor drug level)*
plus	**Antimycobacterial** →208	**Rifampin** (Rifadin, Rimactane, Generic)	*10mg/kg PO qd*

Chronic disease, osteomyelitis

1st choice	**Aminoglycoside** →200	**Gentamicin** (Garamycin, U-gencin, Gens)	*2-5mg/kg IV/IM qd (monitor drug level)*
plus	**Antimycobacterial** →208	**Rifampin** (Rifadin, Rimactane, Generic)	*10mg/kg PO qd*

plus	**Tetracycline** →198	**Doxycycline** (Doryx, Monodox, Periostat, Vibramycin, Gens)	*500mg PO qd-tid for 5mo*
OR	**Antimycobacterial** →208	**Rifampin** (Rifadin, Rimactane, Generic)	*10mg/kg PO qd*
plus	**Folate antagonist + p-Aminobenzoic acid antagonist** →206	**Sulfamethoxazole + Trimethoprim** (Cotrimoxazole) (Bactrim, Cotrim, Septra, Sulfamethoprim, Sulfatrim, Gens)	*800+160mg PO/IV bid*

B.2.11 Campylobacter

Enteritis (Campylobacter jejuni)

	Macrolide →199	**Clarithromycin** (Biaxin)	*250mg PO bid for 3d*
or	**Fluoroquinolone** →203	**Ciprofloxacin** (Cipro)	*250-750mg PO bid for 3d*

Note: resistance to fluoroquinolones rising

Sepsis (Campylobacter fetus)

	Fluoroquinolone →203	**Ciprofloxacin** (Cipro)	*400mg IV bid*
plus	**Aminoglycoside** →200	**Gentamicin** (Garamycin, U-gencin, Gens)	*2-5mg/kg IV/IM qd (monitor drug level)*

B.2.12 Chlamydia

Psittacosis (Chlamydia psittaci)

	Tetracycline →198	**Doxycycline** (Doryx, Monodox, Periostat, Vibramycin, Gens)	*200mg PO/IV bid*
or	**Macrolide** →199	**Azithromycin** (Zithromax)	*500mg PO qd*
		Clarithromycin (Biaxin)	*500mg PO bid*

Urethritis (Chlamydia trachomatis)

	Macrolide →199	**Azithromycin** (Zithromax)	*500mg PO qd (once)*
or	**Tetracycline** →198	**Doxycycline** (Doryx, Monodox, Periostat, Vibramycin, Gens)	*100mg PO bid for 7-20d*

Lymphogranuloma venereum (Chlamydia trachomatis)

	Tetracycline →198	**Doxycycline** (Doryx, Monodox, Periostat, Vibramycin, Gens)	*200mg PO/IV qd for 3wk*
or	**Macrolide** →199	**Clarithromycin** (Biaxin)	*250mg PO bid*

B.2.13 Clostridium perfringens (Gas Gangrene)

Primary Tx: surgical debridement

plus	**Benzylpenicillin** →187	**Penicillin G** (Pfizerpen, Gens)	*24 M IU IV qd (div qid-6x/d)*
plus	**Lincosamide** →201	**Clindamycin** (Cleocin, Gens)	*900mg IV tid*

In penicillin allergy

	Macrolide →199	**Erythromycin** (Erythrocin, Gens)	*1g IV q6h*
or	**Tetracycline** →198	**Doxycycline** (Vibramycin, Gens)	*200mg IV bid*

7 B.2.14 Clostridium botulinum (Botulism)

	Specific antidote (toxin binding ⇒ toxin effects ↓)	**Botulinin Antitoxin (ABE)** (CDC)	*1-2 vials IV q4h for 4-5 doses, duration depends on response; not indicated in infants*

Comment: Consider use as bioweapon if no reasonable exposure history. Prolonged supportive therapy (irreversible binding of toxin)

7 B.2.15 Clostridium tetani (Tetanus)

Antibiotic

	Benzylpenicillin →187	**Penicillin G** (Pfizerpen, Gens)	*12-24 M IU IV qd (div qid-6x/d) for >30d*
or	**Tetracycline** →198	**Doxycycline** (Vibramycin, Gens)	*200mg IV bid for >30d*

Symptomatic

	Benzodiazepine →330 (sedation)	**Diazepam** (Diastat, Diazepam Intensol, Valium, Gens)	*5-15mg IV/PR*
plus	**Non–depolarisizing muscle relaxant** →284 (compet. ACH-antagonism)	**Pancuronium bromide** (Pavulon)	*Ini 0.008-0.01mg/kg IV, then 0.02-0.04mg/kg IV*
plus	**Beta–1–selective blocker** →23 (CO↓, neg. chronotropic, neg. inotropic, central sympathetic activity↓)	**Metoprolol** (Lopressor, Toprol-xl, Gens)	*50-100mg PO qd-bid; 5-10mg slowly IV qd, max 15mg IV*
plus	**Immunoglobulin serum** →258 (toxin neutralization)	**Tetanus Immune Globulin** (BayTet)	*6000 IU IM*

7 B.2.16 Clostridium difficile (Pseudomembranous Colitis)

	Antiprotozoal →206 (nitroimidazole)	**Metronidazole** (Flagyl, Protostat, Gens)	*500mg PO tid for 10-14d*
or	**Glycopeptide** →198	**Vancomycin** (Vancocin, Vancoled, Gens)	*250mg PO qid for 10d*

7 B.2.17 Corynebacterium diphtheriae

	Immunoglobulin serum (toxin neutralisation)	**Diphtheria antitoxin**	*30,000-50,000 IU IV Inf over 1h, up to 120.000 IU*
plus	**Macrolide** →199	**Clarithromycin** (Biaxin)	*250mg PO bid for 10d*

7 B.2.18 Coxiella burnetti

Acute Q fever

	Tetracyclin →198	**Doxycycline** (Doryx, Monodox, Periostat, Vibramycin, Gens)	*d1: 200mg PO/IV qd, then 100mg PO/IV qd for 10-12d or 3d after defervescence*
or	**Macrolide** →199	**Clarithromycin** (Biaxin)	*250-500mg PO bid*

Endocarditis, chronic disease

	Tetracycline →198	**Doxycycline** (Doryx, Monodox, Periostat, Vibramycin, Gens)	*d1: 200mg PO/IV qd, then 100mg PO/IV qd (>12mo)*
plus	**Antimycobacterial** →208	**Rifampin** (Rifadin, Rimactane, Gens)	*10mg/kg PO/IV qd, max 750mg*
Or	**Fluoroquinolone** →203	**Ciprofloxacin** (Cipro)	*500-750mg PO bid, or 200-400mg IV bid*
plus	**Antimycobacterial** →208	**Rifampin** (Rifadin, Rimactane, Gens)	*10mg/kg PO/IV qd, max 750mg*

7 B.2.19 Enterobacter

If hospital acquired, often beta-lactamase producers

	Carbapenem →197	**Imipenem–Cilastim** (Primaxin)	*0.5g IV q6h*
		Meropenem (Merrem)	*1g IV q8h*
or	**Fluoroquinolone** →203	**Ciprofloxacin** (Cipro)	*400mg IV bid*

7 B.2.20 Enterococci

Ampicillin-sensitive isolates

	Aminopenicillin →189	**Ampicillin** (Omnipen, Principen, Totacillin, Gens)	*2g IV qid-6x/d*
plus	**Aminoglycoside** →200	**Gentamicin** (Garamycin, U-gencin, Gens)	*1-1.5mg/kg IV/IM q8h (monitor drug level)*

In Penicillin allergy or resistance

	Glycopeptide →198	**Vancomycin** (Vancocin, Vancoled, Gens)	*1g IV bid as short Inf (monitor drug level)*
plus	**Aminoglycoside** →200	**Gentamicin** (Garamycin, U-gencin, Gens)	*1-1.5mg/kg IV/IM q8h (monitor drug level)*

Vancomycin-resistant F. faecium

	Oxazolidinone →207	**Linezolid** (Zyvox)	*600mg IV bid*
or	**Streptogramine** →207	**Dalfopristin + Quinupristin** (Synercid)	*7.5mg/kg IV q8h*

7 B.2.21 Escherichia coli

Community acquired

	Fluoroquinolone →203	Ciprofloxacin (Cipro)	*250-750mg PO bid*

Hospital acquired

Hospital acquired strains may become multi-drug resistant and require alternative antibiotics. Choice based on local susceptability pattern.

7 B.2.22 Francisella tularensis (Tularemia)

	Aminoglycoside →200	Gentamicin (Garamycin, U-gencin, Gens)	*1-1.5mg/kg IV/IM q8h for 7-14d (monitor drug level)*

7 B.2.23 Gonococci

Note: always treat patient and partner for Gonococci and Chlamydia!

Urethritis, cervicitis, proctitis (uncomplicated)

	Cephalosporin 3rd Gen. →195	Ceftriaxone (Rocephin)	*0.125g IV qd (once)*
or	Fluoroquinolone →203	Ciprofloxacin (Cipro)	*500mg PO qd (once)*
Plus	Tetracycline →198	Doxycycline (Doryx, Monodox, Periostat, Vibramycin, Gens)	*200mg PO qd for 7d*
or	Macrolide →199	Azithromycin (Zithromax)	*1g PO once*

Complicated (salpingitis, endometritis, epididymitis, ...)

	Cephalosporin 3rd Gen. →195	Ceftriaxone (Rocephin)	*1g IV qd for 10d*
Plus	Tetracycline →198	Doxycycline (Doryx, Monodox, Periostat, Vibramycin, Gens)	*200mg PO/IV qd for 7d*
or	Macrolide →199	Azithromycin (Zithromax)	*1g PO once*

Sepsis, arthritis, meningitis, endocarditis

	Cephalosporin 3rd Gen. →195	Ceftriaxone (Rocephin)	*1g IV qd for 2-4wk*

Generalized disease in newborns

After amniotic fliud infection and gonorrhea of the mother

	Cephalosporin 2nd Gen. →193	Cefuroxime (Kefurox, Zinacef, Gens)	*100mg/kg IV qd*

7 B.2.24 Haemophilus ducreyi (soft chancre)

In general

	Cephalosporin 3rd Gen. →195	Ceftriaxone (Rocephin)	*0.25g IV qd (once)*
or	Fluoroquinolone →203	Ciprofloxacin (Cipro)	*1g PO qd for 3d*

7 B.2.25 Haemophilus influenza

Sepsis

	Cephalosporin 3rd Gen. →195	**Ceftriaxone** (Rocephin)	*1-2g IV qd*
or	**Fluoroquinolone** →203	**Ciprofloxacin** (Cipro)	*200-400mg IV bid*

Epiglottitis in children

	Cephalosporin 2nd Gen. →193	**Cefuroxime** (Kefurox, Zinacef, Gens)	*0.75-1.5g IV tid for 1wk*

Pneumonia

	Cephalosporin 3rd Gen. →195	**Ceftriaxone** (Rocephin)	*1g IV q12h for 10–14d*

Meningitis

	Cephalosporin 3rd Gen. →195	**Ceftriaxone** (Rocephin)	*2g IV q12h for 10–14d*

In children additionally to prevent hearing damage

	Glucocorticoid →148 (anti-inflammatory)	**Dexamethasone** (Decadron, Hexadrol, Mymethasone, Gens)	*0.15mg/kg IV q6h for 4d*

Prophylaxis following exposure to patient with meningitis

	Antimycobacterial →208	**Rifampin** (Rifadin, Rimactane, Generic)	*10mg/kg PO bid for 4d*

7 B.2.26 Klebsiella

	Cephalosporin 3. Gen. →195	**Ceftriaxone** (Rocephin)	*1g IV q12h*
plus	**Fluoroquinolone** →203	**Ciprofloxacin** (Cipro)	*250-750mg PO bid, 100-200mg IV bid*

In severe infection

plus	**Aminoglycoside** →200	**Gentamicin** (Garamycin, U-gencin, Gens)	*2-5mg/kg IV/IM qd (monitor drug level)*

Duration depending on location and severity. Hospital acquired strains may become multi-drug resistant + require modified Tx depending on local susceptibility patterns.

7 B.2.27 Legionella

	Fluoroquinolone →203	**Ciprofloxacin** (Cipro)	*400mg IV bid*
or	**Macrolide** →199	**Azithromycin** (Zithromax)	*500mg IV qd*

In severe infection

plus	**Antimycobacterial** →208	**Rifampin** (Rifadin, Rimactane, Generic)	*0.6g IV qd;* **Ped** *6-10mg/kg IV qd*

Following defervescence

	Macrolide →199	**Clarithromycin** (Biaxin)	*250-500mg PO bid for 1-3wk*

7 B.2.28 Leptospira

In mild infection

Tetracycline →198	**Doxycycline** (Doryx, Monodox, Periostat, Vibramycin, Gens)	*200mg PO qd for 7d*

In severe infection

	Benzylpenicillin →187	**Penicillin G** (Pfizerpen, Gens)	*1.5 M IU IV qid for 7d*
or	Aminopenicillin →189	**Ampicillin** (Omnipen, Principen, Totacillin, Gens)	*0.5–2g IV qid*

7 B.2.29 Listeria

Sepsis, endocarditis, meningoencephalitis

	Aminopenicillin →189	**Ampicillin** (Omnipen, Principen, Totacillin, Gens)	*2g IV q4h,* **Ped** *400mg/kg IV qd for >4–6wk*
poss. plus	Aminoglycoside →200	**Gentamicin** (Garamycin, U-gencin, Gens)	*2–5mg/kg IV/IM qd (monitor drug level)*

Comment: Ampicillin plus Sulfamethoxazole + Trimethoprim may become preferred Tx for patients with meningitis

Penicillin allergy

	Folate antagonist + p-Aminobenzoic acid antagonist →206	**Sulfamethoxazole + Trimethoprim** (Cotrimoxazole) (Bactrim, Cotrim, Septra, Sulfamethoprim, Sulfatrim, Gens)	*800+160mg IV bid*
poss. plus	Aminoglycoside →200	**Gentamicin** (Garamycin, U-gencin, Gens)	*2–5mg/kg IV/IM qd (monitor drug level)*

7 B.2.30 Meningococci – Meningitis, Sepsis

1st choice	**Benzylpenicillin** →187	**Penicillin G** (Pfizerpen, Gens)	*0.1–4 M IU IV qid-6x/d (until 7–10d after defervescence)*
or	**Cephalosporin 3rd Gen.** →195	**Ceftriaxone** (Rocephin)	*4g IV qd,* **Ped** *50–80mg/kg IV qd*

Cephalosporin in Penicillin allergy

7 B.2.31 Meningococci – Prophylaxis after Exposure to Meningococcal Carrier

1st choice	**Antimycobacterial** →208	**Rifampin** (Rifadin, Rimactane, Generic)	*0.6g PO bid,* **Ped** *10mg/kg PO bid for 2d*
or	**Fluoroquinolone** →203	**Ciprofloxacin** (Cipro)	*500mg Tab qd (once)*
Or	**Cephalosporin 3rd Gen.** →195	**Ceftriaxone** (Rocephin)	*1g IV qd (once)*

Cephalosporin in pregnancy

7 B.2.32 Mycobacterium tuberculosis

Treatment of latent tuberculosis (prophylaxis)

	Antimycobacterial →208	Isoniazid (Laniazid, Gens)	5mg/kg PO qd (max 300mg); **Ped** 10mg/kg PO qd for 6-9mo
plus	Vitamin →145 (for prevention of INH-associated neuropathy)	Vitamin B6 = Pyridoxine (Gens)	25-50mg PO qd for 6-9mo

Pulmonary tuberculosis

	Antimycobacterial →208	Rifampin (Rifadin, Rimactane, Generic)	10mg/kg PO qd for 6mo
plus	Antimycobacterial →208	Isoniazid (Laniazid, Gens)	5mg/kg PO qd for 6mo
plus	Vitamin →145 (for prevention of INH-associated neuropathy)	Vitamin B6 = Pyridoxine (Gens)	25-50mg PO qd for 6mo
plus	Antimycobacterial →208	Ethambutol (Myambutol, Gens)	15mg/kg PO qd for 2mo
plus	Antimycobacterial →208	Pyrazinamide (Gens)	25-30mg/kg qd for 2mo

Extrapulmonary tuberculosis

	Antimycobacterial →208	Rifampin (Rifadin, Rimactane, Generic)	10mg/kg PO qd for 1-2yr
plus	Antimycobacterial →208	Isoniazid (Laniazid, Gens)	5mg/kg PO qd for 1-2yr
plus	Vitamin →145 (for prevention of INH-associated neuropathy)	Vitamin B6 = Pyridoxine (Gens)	25-50mg PO qd for 1-2yr
plus	Antimycobacterial →208	Ethambutol (Myambutol, Gens)	15mg/kg PO qd for 2mo
plus	Antimycobacterial →208	Pyrazinamide (Gens)	25-30mg/kg qd for 2mo

Miliary tuberculosis, TB meningitis, and TB suppurative pleuritis

	Glucocorticoid →148 (anti-inflammatory, sensitivity of β-recept. ↑)	Prednisone (Deltasone, Meticorten, Prednisone Intensol, Gens)	Ini 30-50mg PO qd, taper to 10-20mg PO qd for 1-4wk

Some experts recommend addition of glucocorticoids for miliary tuberculosis, TB meningitis, and TB suppurative pleuritis

7 B.2.33 Mycoplasma

	Macrolide →100	Clarithromycin (Biaxin)	250mg PO bid
or	Tetracycline →198	Doxycycline (Doryx, Monodox, Periostat, Vibramycin, Gens)	d1: 200mg PO/IV, then 100mg PO qd

7 B.2.34 Nocardia

1st choice

	Folate antagonist + p-Aminobenzoic acid antagonist →206	**Sulfamethoxazole + Trimethoprim** (Cotrimoxazole) (Bactrim, Cotrim, Septra, Sulfamethoprim, Sulfatrim, Gens)	*800+160mg PO/IV bid for 6mo (longer in CNS disease or immuno-compromised)*
or	**Tetracycline** →198	**Minocycline** (Dynacin, Minocin, Vectrin, Gens)	*200mg PO/IV bid for 6mo*

In severe cases, until stabilization

	Carbapenem →197	**Imipenem–Cilastatin** (Primaxin)	*0.5-1g IV tid-qid, max 50mg/kg/ d or 4g/d*
plus	**Cephalosporin 3. Gen.** →195	**Cefotaxime** (Claforan, Gens)	*1g IV tid*
then	After stabilization: Cotrimoxazole or Tetracycline (see 1st choice)		

7 B.2.35 Pneumococci - Pneumonia (usually lobar-/segmental pneumonia)

1st choice

	Benzylpenicillin →187	**Penicillin G** (Pfizerpen, Gens)	*0.5-10 M IU IV qid-6x/d for 8-10d*
or	**Cephalosporin 3rd Gen.** →195	**Ceftriaxone** (Rocephin)	*1g IV qd,* **Ped** *50mg/kg qd for 8-10d*

In penicillin or cephalosporin allergy

	Macrolide →199	**Clarithromycin** (Biaxin)	*250mg PO bid*

In areas or patients with increased risk of penicillin resistance

	Fluoroquinolone →203	**Moxifloxacin** (Avelox)	*400mg IV/PO qd*
		Levofloxacin (Levaquin)	*500mg IV/PO qd*
		Gatifloxacin (Tequin)	*400mg IV/PO qd*

7 B.2.36 Pneumococci - Meningitis

	Glycopeptide →198	**Vancomycin** (Vancocin, Vancoled, Gens)	*1g IV bid as short Inf,* **Ped** *50mg/kg IV qd for 10-14d*
Plus	**Benzylpenicillin** →187	**Penicillin G** (Pfizerpen, Gens)	*1-2 M IU IV qid,* **Ped** *0.5 M IU/kg qd for 10-14d*
or	**Cephalosporin 3rd Gen.** →195	**Ceftriaxone** (Rocephin)	*2g IV bid,* **Ped** *50mg/kg IV bid for 10-14d*

7 B.2.37 Proteus mirabilis (especially UTI)

	Aminopenicillin →189	**Ampicillin** (Omnipen, Principen, Totacillin, Gens)	*1g PO tid-qid; 0.5-2g IV tid-qid, max 5g IV tid*

7 B.2.38 Proteus vulgaris

	Cephalosporin 3. Gen. →195	**Cefotaxime** (Claforan, Gens)	*1-2g IV bid*

7 B.2.39 Pseudomonas aeruginosa

Sepsis, pneumonia

	Carbapenem →197	**Imipenem–Cilastatin** (Primaxin)	*1g IV tid-qid, max 50mg/kg/d or 4g/d*
or	**Cephalosporin 3rd Gen.** →195	**Ceftazidime** (Ceptaz, Fortaz, Tazicef, Tazidime, Gens)	*2g IV tid, **Ped** 100-200mg/kg IV qd*
or	**Acylaminopenicillin** →189	**Piperacillin** (Pipracil)	*4g IV tid*
Plus	**Fluoroquinolone** →203	**Ciprofloxacin** (Cipro)	*400mg IV q8h*
or	**Aminoglycoside** →200	**Gentamicin** (Garamycin, U-gencin, Gens)	*2-5mg/kg IV/IM qd (monitor drug level)*

UTI

	Fluoroquinolone →203	**Ciprofloxacin** (Cipro)	*250-750mg PO bid*

7 B.2.40 Rickettsia

Tetracycline →198	**Doxycycline** (Doryx, Monodox, Periostat, Vibramycin, Gens)	*200mg IV/PO qd (until 6d after defervescence)*

Rickettsia prowazeki (typhus), R. rickettsii (Rocky Mountain spotted fever), R. tsutsugamushi (scrub typhus)

7 B.2.41 Salmonella

	Fluoroquinolone →203	**Ciprofloxacin** (Cipro)	*500-750mg PO bid for 2wk*
or	**Cephalosporin 3rd Gen.** →195	**Ceftriaxone** (Rocephin)	*1-2 g IV qd, **Ped** 50mg/kg IV qd for 2wk*

Chronic Carriers

	Fluoroquinolone →203	**Ciprofloxacin** (Cipro)	*500mg PO bid for 4wk*

7 B.2.42 Serratia

	Aminoglycoside →200	**Amikacin** (Amikin, Gens)	*10-15mg/kg/d IV/IM qd*
Plus	**Cephalosporin 3rd Gen.** →195	**Ceftazidime** (Ceptaz, Fortaz, Tazicef, Tazidime, Gens)	*2g IV tid*
or	**Fluoroquinolone** →203	**Ciprofloxacin** (Cipro)	*100-750mg PO/IV bid*
or	**Carbapenem** →145	**Imipenem–Cilastatin** (Primaxin)	*0.5-1g IV tid-qid, max 50mg/kg/d or 4g/d*

7 B.2.43 Shigella

Adults

Fluoroquinolone →203	**Ciprofloxacin** (Cipro)	*500mg PO bid for 1-3d*

Children

Folate antagonist + p-Aminobenzoic acid antagonist →206	**Sulfamethoxazole + Trimethoprim** (Cotrimoxazole) (Bactrim, Cotrim, Septra, Sulfamethoprim, Sulfatrim, Gens)	*10-15mg TMP eyuivalent/kg PO/IV bid for 5-7d*

7 B.2.44 Staphylococcus, Methicillin-sensitive (MSSA)

Naphthylpenicillin →188	**Nafcillin** (Nallpen, Unipen, Gens)	*2g IV tid-6x/d*

In Penicillin-allergy

Cephalosporin 1st Gen. →191	**Cefazolin** (Ancef, Kefzol, Gens)	*0.5-2g IV bid-tid (until defervescence)*

7 B.2.45 Staphylococcus aureus, Methicillin-resistant (MRSA) and Coagulase-negative Staphylococcus species

	Glycopeptide →198	**Vancomycin** (Vancocin, Vancoled, Gens)	*1g IV bid as short Inf for 7-28 d;* **Ped** *50mg/kg IV qd*
or	**Oxazolidinone** →207	**Linezolid** (Zyvox)	*600mg IV bid for 7-28d*

143. Stevens DL, Herr D, Lampiris H, Hunt JL, Batts DH, Hafkin B. Linezolid versus Vancomycin for the Treatment of Methicillin-Resistant Staphylococcus aureus Infections. Clin Infect Dis 2002; 34: 1481-90

Sepsis, endocarditis

add	**Aminoglycoside** →200	**Gentamicin** (Garamycin, U-gencin, Gens)	*1-1.5mg/kg IV/IM tid for 3d*

In infection involving bones or prosthetic material

add	**Antimycobacterial** →208	**Rifampin** (Rifadin, Rimactane, Generic)	*10mg/kg PO qd*

7 B.2.46 Streptococci, Group A

Strep throat, scarlet fever

Benzylpenicillin →187	**Penicillin V** (Beepen VK, Betapen VK, Ledercillin VK, Pen-vee K, Uticillin VK, V-cillin VK, Veetids, Gens)	*0.6-1.5 M IU PO tid for 2wk*

In penicillin allergy

Macrolide →199	**Clarithromycin** (Biaxin)	*250mg PO bid,* **Ped** *12mg/kg qd*

Sepsis			
	Benzylpenicillin →187	**Penicillin G** (Pfizerpen, Gens)	*10-20 M IU IV qd for 1-2wk*
then		**Penicillin V** (Beepen VK, Betapen VK, Ledercillin VK, Pen-vee K, Uticillin VK, V-cillin VK, Veetids, Gens)	*1.5-3 M IU PO qd for 2wk*

In penicillin allergy			
	Cephalosporin 1st Gen. →191	**Cefazolin** (Ancef, Kefzol, Gens)	*0.5-2g IV bid-tid*

7 B.2.47 Streptococci, Beta-hemolytic

Subacute bacterial endocarditis			
	Benzylpenicillin →187	**Penicillin G** (Pfizerpen, Gens)	*20-30 M IU IV qd (div in 2-3 short Inf) for 3wk*
plus	**Aminoglycoside** →200	**Gentamicin** (Garamycin, U-gencin, Gens)	*1-1.5mg/kg IV/IM tid (monitor drug level)*

In penicillin allergy			
	Cephalosporin 1st Gen. →191	**Cefazolin** (Ancef, Kefzol, Gens)	*0.5-2g IV bid-tid for 3wk*
plus	**Aminoglycoside** →200	**Gentamicin** (Garamycin, U-gencin, Gens)	*2-5mg/kg IV/IM qd (monitor drug level)*

7 B.2.48 Treponema pallidum, Aquired Syphilis

Primary/secondary syphilis			
	Depot Benzylpenicillin →187	**Procaine Penicillin** (Pfizerpen-as, Wycillin, Gens)	*1.2 M IU IM once*

Late latent syphilis			
	Depot Benzylpenicillin →187	**Procaine Penicillin** (Pfizerpen-as, Wycillin, Gens)	*1.2 M IU IM qwk for 3wk*

Tertiary syphilis, neurosyphilis			
	Benzylpenicillin →187	**Penicillin G** (Pfizerpen, Gens)	*10-20 M IU IV Inf qd (div qid-6x/d or cont Inf) for 14d*

In penicillin allergy			
	Cephalosporin 3rd Gen. →195	**Ceftriaxone** (Rocephin)	*1g IV qd for 14d*
or	**Tetracycline** →198	**Doxycycline** (Vibramycin, Gens)	*200mg IV qd for 3wk*

7 B.2.49 Vibrio cholerae (Cholera)

Antibiotic Therapy			
	Folate antagonist + p-Aminobenzoic acid antagonist →206	**Sulfamethoxazole + Trimethoprim** (Bactrim, Cotrim, Septra, Sulfamethoprim, Sulfatrim, Gens)	*800+160mg PO/IV bid for 3d*

or	**Tetracycline** →198	**Doxycycline** (Doryx, Monodox, Periostat, Vibramycin, Gens)	*300mg PO/IV qd once*
or	**Fluoroquinolone** →203	**Ciprofloxacin** (Cipro)	*500mg PO bid for 3d*
Adjuvant Therapy			
poss.	**Glucose electrolyte solution** (volume substitution)	**WHO „Oral rehydration formula"** (Glucose, Na^+Cl^-, $Na^+HCO_3^-$, K^+Cl^-)	*20g Glucose + 3.5g Na^+Cl^- + 2.5g $NaHCO_3^-$ + 1.5g K^+Cl^- in 1 l H_2O PO prn*
poss.	**Glucose solution** (nutrition substitution)	**Glucose 20%**	*Ca. 2000 kcal qd prn*
poss.	**Isotonic saline solution** (volume + electrolyte substitution)	**Saline 0.9%**	*IV after CVP and elecrolytes prn*
poss.	**Cristalloid plasma expander** (volume + electrolyte substitution)	**Ringer's solution**	*prn*

7 B.2.50 Vibrio parahaemolyticus

poss.	**Folate antagonist + p–Aminobenzoic acid antagonist** →206	**Sulfamethoxazole + Trimethoprim** (Cotrimoxazole) (Bactrim, Cotrim, Septra, Sulfamethoprim, Sulfatrim, Gens)	*800+160mg PO/IV bid for 5-7d*
or	**Tetracycline** →198	**Doxycycline** (Doryx, Monodox, Periostat, Vibramycin, Gens)	*200mg PO/IV qd for 5-7d*

7 B.2.51 Yersinia

	Folate antagonist + p–Aminobenzoic acid antagonist →206	**Sulfamethoxazole + Trimethoprim** (Cotrimoxazole) (Bactrim, Cotrim, Septra, Sulfamethoprim, Sulfatrim, Gens)	*800+160mg PO/IV bid*
or	**Fluoroquinolone** →203	**Ciprofloxacin** (Cipro)	*500mg PO bid*

7 B.3 Specific Antiviral Therapy
7 B.3.1 Cytomegalovirus

In retinitis, pneumonia in Non–HIV

	Virostatic →209 (purine antagonist, inhibits DNA polymerase)	**Ganciclovir** (Cytovene)	*5-10mg/kg IV over 1h qd for 2-4wk*
or	**Virostatic** →209 (pyrophasphate analogue, then polymerase inhibitor)	**Foscarnet** (Foscavir)	*wk1-3: 90mg/kg IV bid, then 90-120mg/kg IV qd for 2-4wk*

Prevention in transplant recipients

Virostatic →209 (purine antagonist, inhibits DNA polymerase)	**Ganciclovir** (Cytovene, Valcyte)	*500-1000 mg PO tid (up to 120d after transplantation)*

7 B.3.2 Ebstein-Barr Virus (Inf. Mononucleosis)

General measures

poss.	**Aniline derivative** →269 (analgesic, antipyretic)	**Acetaminophen** (Acephen, Neopap, Tylenol, Gens)	*500-1000mg PO/PR tid-qid prn*

In Severe infection

Virostatic →211 (purine antagonist, DNA polymerase inhibitor)	**Acyclovir** (Zovirax, Gens)	*10mg/kg IV tid or 800mg 5x/d PO for 2-3 wk*

7 B.3.3 Herpes Simplex Virus

Meningoencephalitis, systemic infection

Virostatic →211 (purine antagonist, inhibits DNA polymerase)	**Acyclovir** (Zovirax, Gens)	*10mg/kg IV tid for 2-3 wk*

Primary genital infection

Virostatic →211 (purine antagonist, inhibits DNA polymerase)	**Valacyclovir** (Valtrex)	*400mg PO tid*

Recurring genital infection

Virostatic →211 (purine antagonist, inhibits DNA polymerase)	**Acyclovir** (Zovirax, Gens)	*Ini 400mg PO tid, then 200mg PO bid*

Keratitis

Virostatic →378 (pyrimidine antagonist ⇒ transcription errors)	**Trifluridine solution (oph)** (Viroptic)	*Admin q4h*

Herpes labialis

Virostatic →211, →352 (purine antagonist, inhibits DNA polymerase)	**Acyclovir 0.5%** (Zovirax)	*Admin q4h for ca. 5d*

7 B.3.4　Human Immunodeficiency Virus, Anti–HIV Therapy

Note: HIV expertise required

Combination of 2 nucleoside/nucleotide reverse transcriptase inhibitors (NRTIs)

	NRTI →214 (nucleoside reverse transcriptase inhibitor ⇒ virostatic)	**Zidovudine (AZT)** (Retrovir)	*250-300mg PO bid* *(not azt + d4T)*
		Zalcitabine (ddC) (Hivid)	*0.75mg PO tid* *(not ddI + ddC)*
		Didanosine (ddI) (Videx, Videx EC)	*<60kg: 250mg PO qd,* *>60kg: 400mg PO qd* *(not ddI + ddC)*
		Lamivudine (3TC) (Epivir, Epivir-HBV)	*150mg PO bid*
		Stavudine (d4T) (Zerit)	*<60kg: 30mg PO bid,* *>60kg: 40mg PO bid* *(not azt + d4T)*
		Abacavir (ABC) (Ziagen)	*300mg PO bid (Caution: hypersensitivity)*
	NRTI (nucleotide RTI ⇒ virostatic)	**Tenofovir Disoproxil Fumarate (TDF)** (Viread)	*300mg PO qd*

With either a protease inhibitor

Plus	**Protease inhibitor** →216 (production of immature, non-infectous viral hulls, virostatic)	**Amprenavir (APV)** (Agenerase)	*1200mg PO bid*
		Indinavir (IDV) (Crixivan)	*800mg PO tid or 800mg PO bid in combination with ritonavir*
		Nelfinavir (NFV) (Viracept)	*1250mg PO bid*
		Ritonavir (RTV) (Norvir)	*600mg PO bid*
		Ritonavir (RTV) + Lopinavir (LPV) (Kaletra)	*400/100mg PO bid*
		Saquinavir (SQV) (Fortovase, Invirase)	*600mg PO tid or 400mg PO bid in combination with ritonavir*

Or a non-nucleoside reverse transcriptase inhibitor (NNRTIs)

or	**NNRTI** →215 (non-nucleoside reverse-transcriptse inhibitor ⇒ virostatic)	**Delavirdine (DLV)** (Rescriptor)	*400mg PO tid*
		Efavirenz (EFV) (Sustiva)	*600mg PO qd*
		Nevirapine (NVP) (Viramune)	*200mg PO qd for 14d, then 200mg PO bid*

7 B.3.5　HIV, Opportunistic Infections

Pneumocystis carinii, 1st choice

Folate antagonist + p–Aminobenzoic acid antagonist →206	**Sulfamethoxazole + Trimethoprim** (Cotrimoxazole) (Bactrim, Cotrim, Septra, Sulfamethoprim, Sulfatrim, Gens)	*5mg TMP equivalent/kg IV tid for 21d*

Pneumocystis carinii, in moderate/severe pneumonia (pO$_2$ <70 mm Hg)

plus	**Glucocorticoid** →148 (anti-inflammatory, sensitivity of β-recept. ↑)	**Prednisone** (Deltasone, Meticorten, Prednisone Intensol, Gens)	*40mg bid for 5d, then 40mg qd for 5d, then 20mg qd for 11d*

Pneumocystis carinii, in Cotrimoxazole failure/intolerance

	Antiparasitic →220 (diamidine derivative)	**Pentamidine** (Pentam, Gens)	*4mg/kg IV qd for 14-21d*
or	**Hydroxy-naphthochinone** →220	**Atovaquone** (Mepron)	*1500mg PO qd for 21d*
or	**Lincosamide** →201	**Clindamycin** (Cleocin, Gens)	*600mg PO/IV tid*
plus	**Anti-malarial** →222	**Primaquine** (Gens)	*30mg base PO qd*

Pneumocystis carinii, primary prophylaxis

	Folate antagonist + p-Aminobenzoic acid antagonist →206	**Sulfamethoxazole + Trimethoprim** (Cotrimoxazole) (Bactrim, Septra, Gens)	*800+160mg IV tiw*
or	**Hydroxy-naphthochinone** →220	**Atovaquone** (Mepron)	*1500mg PO qd*
or	**Antimycobacterial** →208	**Dapsone** (Gens)	*100mg PO qd*

Toxoplasma gondii, 1st choice →250

	Dihydrofolate reductase inhibitor →220	**Pyrimethamine** (Daraprim, Gens)	*100-200 mg PO qd for 3d, then 50-75 mg (until >3wk after resolution)*
plus	**Sulfonamide** →205 (folate antagonist)	**Sulfadiazine** (Gens)	*4-8g PO qd*
plus	**Folic acid derivative** (thrombocytopenia Pro)	**Folinic acid** (Leucovorin, Gens)	*15mg PO qd*

Toxoplasma gondii, alternative →250

	Dihydrofolate reductase inhibitor →220	**Pyrimethamine** (Daraprim, Gens)	*100-200 mg PO qd for 3d then 50-75 mg (until 3wk after resolution)*
plus	**Lincosamide** →201	**Clindamycin** (Cleocin, Gens)	*600mg PO/IV qid*
plus	**Folic acid derivative** (thrombocytopenia Pro)	**Folinic acid** (Leucovorin, Gens)	*15mg PO qd*

Toxoplasma gondii, primary prophylaxis →250

	Folate antagonist + p-Aminobenzoic acid antagonist →206	**Sulfamethoxazole + Trimethoprim** (Cotrimoxazole) (Bactrim, Cotrim, Septra, Sulfamethoprim, Sulfatrim, Gens)	*800+160mg PO qd*
or	**Hydroxy-naphthochinone** →220	**Atovaquone** (Mepron)	*1500-2250mg PO qd*

or	Sulfone derivative →209	Dapsone (Gens)	*0.1g PO qd*
Plus	Dihydrofolate reductase inhibitor →220	Pyrimethamine (Daraprim, Gens)	*25mg PO biw*
Plus	Folic acid derivative (thrombocytopenia Pro)	Folinic acid (Leucovorin, Gens)	*15mg PO biw*

Mycobacterium tuberculosis →235

	Antimycobacterial →208	Rifampin (Rifadin, Rimactane, Generic)	*10mg/kg PO qd for 6mo*
plus	Antimycobacterial →208	Isoniazid (Laniazid, Gens)	*5mg/kg PO qd for 6mo*
plus	Vitamin →145 (prevention of INH-associated neuropathy)	Vitamin B6 = Pyridoxine (Gens)	*25-50mg PO qd for 6mo*
plus	Antimycobacterial →208	Ethambutol (Myambutol, Gens)	*15mg/kg PO qd for 2mo*
plus	Antimycobacterial →208	Pyrazinamide (Gens)	*25-30mg/kg qd for 2mo*

Mycobacterium avium

	Macrolide →199	Clarithromycin (Biaxin)	*500mg PO bid*
plus	Antimycobacterial →208	Ethambutol (Myambutol, Gens)	*15mg/kg PO qd*
poss. plus	Antimycobacterial →208	Rifabutin (Mycobutin)	*300-450mg PO qd*

Varizella–Zoster virus →246

1sr choice	Virostatic →211 (purine antagonist, DNA polymerase inhibitor)	Acyclovir (Zovirax, Gens)	*10mg/kg IV tid*

Cytomegalovirus (CMV: retinitis, colitis, →240)

	Virostatic →209 (purine antagonist, DNA polymerase inhibitor)	Ganciclovir (Cytovene, Valcyte)	*5mg/kg IV bid for 14-21d, then 5mg/kg IV qd (5-7d/wk) or 1g PO tid*
or	Virostatic →209 (pyrophosphate analogue, DNA polymerase inhibitor)	Foscarnet (Foscavir)	*90mg/kg IV bid over >1h for 14-21d, then 90-120mg/kg qd over >2h*

Cryptococcus neoformans →252

	Antifungal – polyene →217 (antimycotic, membrane deposition)	Amphotericin B (Fungizone, Gens)	*Test dose 1mg slow IV, if tolerated: 0.7mg/kg IV qd over 2-6h*
plus	Antimetabolite →217 (antimycotic)	Flucytosine (Ancobon)	*25mg/kg PO qid*
Or in mild cases	Antifungal – azole →217	Fluconazole (Diflucan)	*400mg IV qd*

Cryptosporidium

No established effective therapy! Symptomatic control of diarrhea and amelioration of immune deficiency mainstay of therapy!

oss.	**Antiparasitic** →220 (benzimidazole derivative)	**Albendazole** (Albenza)	*400mg PO bid*
oss.	**Aminoglycoside** →200	**Paromomycin** (Humatin)	*500mg PO tid for 2–4wk*
oss.	**Macrolide** →199	**Azithromycin** (Zithromax)	*1200mg PO qd for 4wk*

Microsporida

	Antiparasitic →220 (benzimidazole derivative)	**Albendazole** (Albenza)	*400mg PO bid*

Candidiasis, mucosal →251

	Antifungal – azole →217	**Fluconazole** (Diflucan)	*100–200mg PO qd*

Candidiasis, severe →251

	Imidazole derivative →217 (antimycotic)	**Fluconazole** (Diflucan)	*Up to 800mg IV qd*
r	**Antifungal – polyene** →217 (antimycotic, membrane deposition)	**Amphotericin B** (Fungizone, Gens)	*Test dose 1mg slow IV, if tolerated: 0.3–0.6mg/kg IV qd over 2–6h (Caution: toxicity)*
oss. lus	**Antimetabolite** →217 (antimycotic)	**Flucytosine** (Ancobon)	*25–30mg/kg IV tid*

B.3.6   Influenza Virus

Uncomplicated

oss.	**Opioid** →270 (antitussive) x	**Codeine** (Gens)	*30–50mg PO bid, max 150mg qd prn*
oss.	**Aniline derivative** →269 (analgesic, antipyretic)	**Acetaminophen** (Acephen, Infants' feverall, Neopap, Tylenol, Gens)	*500–1000mg PO/PR tid-qid prn*

Severe

	Virostatic →211 (neuroaminidase inhibitor)	**Zanamivir** (Relenza)	*Inhal 10mg bid for 5d*
r		**Oseltamivir** (Tamiflu)	*75mg PO bid for 5d*

Also effective in influenza A

	Virostatic →211	**Amantadine** (Symmetrel)	*100mg PO bid (qd if >65yr) for 3–7d*
r		**Rimantadine** (Flumadine)	*100mg PO bid (qd if >65yr) for 3–7d*

B.3.7   Measles Virus

oss.	**Aniline derivative** →269 (analgesic, antipyretic)	**Acetaminophen** (Acephen, Infants' feverall, Neopap, Tylenol, Gens)	*10–15mg/kg PO/PR q4-6h prn, max 5 doses/d*

7 B.3.8 Mumps Virus

poss.	**Aniline derivative** →269 (analgesic, antipyretic)	**Acetaminophen** (Acephen, Infants' feverall, Neopap, Tylenol, Gens)	*10-15mg/kg PO/PR q4-6h prn, max 5 doses/d*

7 B.3.9 Respiratory Syncytial Virus (RVS)

	Virostatic →213 (purine antagonist)	**Ribavirin** (Rebetol, Virazole)	*Dissolve 6g in 300ml, as aeroso over 12-18h for 3-7d*

7 B.3.10 Varicella–Zoster Virus

Varicella (in immunosuppressed patient or pneumonia)

	Virostatic →211 (purine antagonist, inhibits DNA polymerase)	**Acyclovir** (Zovirax, Gens)	*10mg/kg IV tid for 10d*

Shingles

	Virostatic →211 (purine antagonist, inhibits DNA polymerase)	**Valacyclovir** (Valtrex)	*500-1000mg PO tid*

7 B.4 Specific Antiparasitic Therapy

7 B.4.1 Ascaris lumbricoides (roundworm)

	Anthelmintic →220 (tubulin binding, glucose uptake ↓)	**Mebendazole** (Vermox)	*100mg PO bid x 6 doses or 500mg PO once*
poss.	**Anthelmintic** →220 (benzimidazole)	**Albendazole** (Albenza)	*400mg PO (once)*
or	**Anthelmintic** →220 (inhibits choline esterase)	**Pyrantel** (Combantrin, Pin-X)	*10mg/kg PO to max 1g (once)*

7 B.4.2 Echinococci

	Antiparasitic →220 (benzimidazole)	**Albendazole** (Albenza)	*400mg PO bid for 28d*

Effective in E. granulosus = dog tapeworm infection, E. multilocularis = fox tapeworm infection usually requires surgical intervention

7 B.4.3 Entamoeba histolytica

Hepatic abscess, enteritis

	Antiprotozoal →206 (nitroimidazole)	**Metronidazole** (Flagyl, Metro, Metryl, Protostat, Gens)	*750mg PO/IV tid for 10d*
then	**Aminoglycoside** →200	**Paromomycin** (Humatin)	*500mg PO tid for 7d*

7 B.4.4   Enterobius vermicularis (pinworm, oxyuriasis)

	Anthelmintic →220 (inhiblts choline esterase)	**Pyrantel** (Combantrin, Pin-X)	*10mg/kg PO once, rep after 14d*
or	**Anthelmintic** →220 (benzimidazole)	**Albendazole** (Albenza)	*400mg PO once, rep after 14d*
or	**Anthelmintic** →220 (tubulin binding, glucose uptake ↓)	**Mebendazole** (Vermox)	*100mg PO once, rep after 14d*

7 B.4.5   Lamblia intestinalis (Giardiasis)

	Antiprotozoal →206 (Nitroimidazole)	**Metronidazole** (Flagyl, Protostat, Gens)	*250mg PO tid for 5d*
or	**Nitroimidazole** →206 (antiprotozoal)	**Tinidazole** (Fasigyn)	*2g PO qd (once)*
or	**Antiparasitic** →220 (benzimidazole)	**Albendazole** (Albenza)	*400mg PO qd for 5d*

7 B.4.6   Leishmaniasis

1st choice

	Antiprotozoal (pentavalent organic antimon connection)	**Stibogluconate** (Pentostam)	*20mg/kg IV/IM qd for 3-4wk*

In resistance

	Diamidine derivative →220	**Pentamidine** (Pentam, Gens)	*2-4mg/kg IV qd for 14d*
or	**Antifungal - polyene** →217 (antimycotic, membrane deposition)	**Amphotericin B** (Fungizone, Gens)	*Test dose 1mg slow IV, if tolerated: 1mg/kg IV qd over 2-6h for 20d or 0.5 mg/kg IV qod for 8wk (Caution: toxicity)*
or	**Antifungal** →217 (polyene derivative, membrane deposition)	**Liposomal Amphotericin B** (Ambisome)	*3-5mg/kg IV qd on d1-5, d14*

7 B.4.7   Plasmodium (Malaria), Prophylaxis

Individualized decision based on risk and travel destination recommended!
1st prophylaxis: protection from mosquito bites!

Zone A = no chloroquine resistance

Antimalarial →222 (DNA intercalation, Hb utilization disturbance; schizonticide)	**Chloroquine** (Aralen, Gens)	*300mg base qwk (1wk before until 4wk after trip)*

Zone B = moderate chloroquine resistance
Zone C = multiresistance areas

	Antimalarial →222 (DNA intercalation, Hb utilization disturbance; schizonticide)	**Mefloquine** (Lariam)	*1 Tab qwk (1wk before until 4wk after trip)*
or	**Tetracycline** →198	**Doxycycline** (Doryx, Monodox, Periostat, Vibramycin, Gens)	*100 mg PO qd*

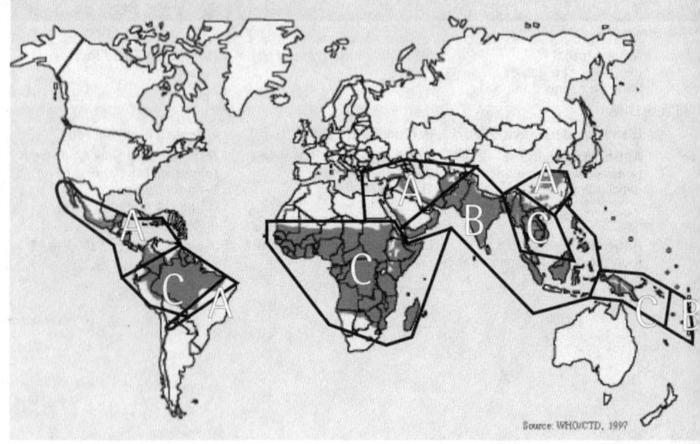

7 B.4.8   Plasmodium, Therapy

P. malariae, P. ovale, chloroquine sensitive P. vivax and P. falciparum

	Antimalarial →222 (DNA intercalation, Hb utilization disturbance; schizonticide)	**Chloroquine** (Aralen, Gens)	*Ini 600mg base PO, then 300mg base after 6, 24, and 48h*

Additionally for P. vivax and P. ovale (relapse prophylaxis)

	Antimalarial →222	**Primaquine** (Gens)	*15mg base PO qd for 14d*

Chloroquine-resistant P. falciparum or P. vivax

	Antimalarial →222	**Quinine** (Gens)	*Ini 20mg/kg IV over 4h, then 10mg/kg IV tid for 3-7d*
plus	**Tetracycline** →198	**Doxycycline** (Doryx, Monodox, Periostat, Vibramycin, Gens)	*100mg PO bid for 7d*
Or	**Antimalarial** →222	**Quinine** (Gens)	*Ini 20mg/kg IV over 4h, then 10mg/kg IV tid for 3-7d*
plus	**Antimalarial combination** →223	**Pyrimethamine + Sulfadoxine** (Fansidar)	*3 Tab qd, once on last day of quinine admin*
Or	**Antimalarial** →222	**Mefloquine** (Lariam)	*Ini 750mg base, at 6h 500mg, at 12h: 250mg*
Or	**Antimalarial** →222	**Halofantrine** (Halfan)	*500mg q6h x 3 doses, rep after 1wk*
Or	**Antimalarial** →222	**Artesunate** (experimental drug)	*Ini 20mg/kg over 4h, then 10mg/kg IV tid*
plus	**Antimalarial** →222	**Mefloquine** (Lariam)	*Ini 750mg base, at 6h 500mg*
Or	**Antimalarial combination** →223	**Atovaquone + Proguanil** (Malorone)	*4 Tabs qd PO with food for 3d*

Additionally for P. vivax (relapse prophylaxis)

	Antimalarial →222	**Primaquine** (Gens)	*15mg base PO qd for 14d*

7 B.4.9   Schistosoma

S. haematobium, S. mansoni, S. mekongi, S. japonicum

	Anthelmintic →220 (tetanic contracture, worm paralysis)	**Praziquantel** (Biltricide)	*20mg/kg PO bid (4-6h apart) for 1d*

7 B.4.10 Taenia (tapeworm)

Anthelmintic →220 (tetanic contracture, worm paralysis)	**Praziquantel** (Biltricide)	*10mg/kg PO once*

T. saginata = cattle tapeworm, T. solium = pork tapeworm

7 B.4.11 Toxoplasma gondii, Pregnancy Toxoplasmosis

Before 16th week of pregnancy

Macrolide →199	**Spiramycin** (available from FDA)	*1g PO tid*

After 16th week of pregnancy

	Dihydrofolate reductase inhibitor →220	**Pyrimethamine** (Daraprim, Gens)	*25mg PO qd*
plus	**Sulfonamide** →205 (folate antagonist)	**Sulfadiazine** (Gens)	*1g PO qid*
plus	**Folic acid derivative** (thrombocytopenia Pro)	**Folinic acid** (Leucovorin, Gens)	*10mg PO qd*

7 B.4.12 Toxoplasma gondii, Chorioretinitis

	Dihydrofolate reductase inhibitor →220	**Pyrimethamine** (Daraprim, Gens)	*25mg PO qd (until >1-2wk after resolution)*
plus	**Sulfonamide** →205 (folate antagonist)	**Sulfadiazine** (Gens)	*1g PO qid (until >1-2wk after resolution)*
plus	**Folic acid derivative** (thrombocytopenia Pro)	**Folinic acid** (Leucovorin, Gens)	*10-15mg PO qd*

In congenital toxoplasmosis, sight-threatening chorioretinitis, and meningitis in adults

plus	**Glucocorticoid** →148 (anti-inflammatory, sensitivity of β-recept. ↑)	**Prednisone** (Deltasone, Meticorten, Prednisone Intensol, Gens)	*0.5 mg/kg PO bid until CSF protein lower or inflammatory activity controlled*

7 B.4.13 Trichomonas vaginalis

Antiprotozoal →206 (nitroimidazole)	**Metronidazole** (Flagyl, Protostat, Gens)	*500mg PO bid for 7d or 2g PO once*

7 B.5   Specific Antifungal Therapy
7 B.5.1   Aspergillus

Antifungal – polyene →217 (antimycotic, membrane deposition)	**Amphotericin B** (Fungizone, Generic)	*Test dose 1mg slow IV, if tolerated: 1mg/kg IV qd over 2-6h for 10-21d (Caution: toxicity)*

In mild cases or following initial Amphotericin Tx

Antifungal – azole →217	**Itraconazole** (Sporanox)	*200mg IV PO qd-tid (for up to 2-5mo)*

7 B.5.2   Candida

Candidemia

Antifungal – azole →217	**Fluconazole** (Diflucan)	*1.d: 400-800 mg IV/PO, then 200-400mg IV/PO qd*

Endocarditis, unstable patient

	Antifungal – polyene →217 (antimycotic, membrane deposition)	**Amphotericin B** (Fungizone, Gens)	*Test dose 1mg slow IV, if tolerated: 1mg/kg IV qd over 2-6h (Caution: toxicity)*
plus	**Antimetabolite** →217 (antimycotic)	**Flucytosine** (Ancobon)	*25-37.5mg/kg PO qid*

UTI

Antifungal – azole →217	**Fluconazole** (Diflucan)	*100-200mg PO qd for 1-5d*

Dermal infection

or	**Antifungal – azole** →217	**Clotrimazole cream** (Lotrimin, Mycelex, Gens)	*Admin bid*

90% C. albicans

7 B.5.3   Coccidioides immitis

	Antifungal – azole →217	**Itraconazole** (Sporanox)	*200-400mg PO qd-bid for 3-12mo*
or	**Antifungal – polyene** →217 (antimycotic, membrane deposition)	**Amphotericin B** (Fungizone, Gens)	*Test dose 1mg slow IV, if tolerated: 0.0-1mg/kg IV qd over 2-6h (until 2-3g total dose, followed by prolonged itra/fluco Tx)*

Meningitis

Antifungal – azole →217	**Fluconazole** (Diflucan)	*400-800mg IV/PO qd (indefinitely)*

7 B.5.4 Cryptococcus neoformans

Mild cases

	Antifungal – azole →217	**Fluconazole** (Diflucan)	*d1: 400mg IV/PO then 200-400mg PO qd for 8wk-6mo*

Severe cases

	Antifungal – polyene →217 (antimycotic, membrane deposition)	**Amphotericin B** (Fungizone, Gens)	*Test dose 1mg slow IV, if tolerated: 0.5–1mg/kg IV qd over 2-6h for 3wk, followed by prolonged fluconazole (see above)*
plus	**Antimetabolite** →217 (antimycotic)	**Flucytosine** (Ancobon)	*25mg/kg PO qid for 3wk*

7 B.5.5 Dermatophytes

Onychomycosis (usually dermatophytes, also mixed infections)

	Antifungal – azole →217	**Itraconazole** (Sporanox)	*100-200mg PO qd (up to 3-6mo; as cure: admin for 1wk, 3wk pause, 3-6 cycles)*
or	**Antifungal – allylamine** →217	**Terbinafine** (Lamisil)	*250mg PO qd for 6wk*

Tinea

	Antifungal – azole →217	**Clotrimazole cream** (Lotrimin, Mycelex, Gens)	*Admin bid*

In refractory tinea capitis (ringworm)

	Antifungal – allylamine →217	**Terbinafine** (Lamisil)	*250 mg PO qd for 4-8wk*

7 B.5.6 Histoplasma capsulatum

Moderate disease

	Antifungal – azole →217	**Itraconazole** (Sporanox)	*200mg PO qd for 9mo*

Severe disease

d1-d10 (d20)	**Antifungal – polyene** →217 (antimycotic, membrane deposition)	**Amphotericin B** (Fungizone, Gens)	*Test dose 1mg slow IV, if tolerated: 1mg/kg IV qd over 2-6h for 10-20d, then Itraconazole*
then	**Antifungal – azole** →217	**Itraconazole** (Sporanox)	*100-200mg PO qd (long term)*

Meningitis

d1-d10 (d20)	**Antifungal – polyene** →217 (antimycotic, membrane deposition)	**Amphotericin B** (Fungizone, Gens)	*Test dose 1mg slow IV, if tolerated: 1mg/kg IV qd over 2-6h for 10-20d, then Fluconazole*
then	**Antifungal – azole** →217	**Fluconazole** (Diflucan)	*400-800mg IV/PO qd indefinitely*

7 B.5.7   Mucor

	Antifungal - polyene →217 (antimycotic, membrane deposition)	**Amphotericin B** (Fungizone, Gens)	*Test dose 1mg slow IV, if tolerated: 0.8–1.5 mg/kg IV qd over 2–6h (total dose 2.5–3g)*

7 B.5.8   Pityriasis versicolor

	Antifungal - azole →217	**Ketoconazole** (Nizoral)	*2% cream/shampoo apply to affected areas qd for 2wk*
or	**Selenium sulfate** →360	**Selenium sulfate** (Selsun, several "dandruff shampoos")	*Apply to affected areas qd for 2wk*
or	**Antifungal - azole** →217	**Ketoconazole** (Nizoral)	*400mg PO once*

8 A. Immunology – Drugs

8 A.1 Vaccines

8 A.1.1 Combinations

AE (Diphtheria + Tetanus + Pertussis vaccine): injection site reaction, fever, irritability, drowsiness
AE (Diphtheria + Tetanus + Pertussis + Hep. B + Polio vaccine): hypersensitivity reactions, injection site reaction, drowsiness, restlessness, fever, fussiness, decreased appetite
AE (Haemophilus B + N. meningitidis + Hepatitis B Vaccine): see Prod Info
CI (Diphtheria + Tetanus + acellular Pertussis vaccine): hypersensitivity to the vaccine or thimerosal, adults and children > 7y, active infection, febrile illness, history encephalopathy secondary to DPT vaccine
CI (Diphtheria + Tetanus + Pertussis + Hep. B + Polio vaccine): infants of HbsAG-positive mothers, patients older than 7y, immunosuppressed patients, patients hypersensitive to yeast, neomycin, or polymyxin B
CI (Haemophilus B + N. meningitidis + Hepatitis B Vaccine): hypersensitivity to product ingredients, see Prod Info

Diphtheria + Tetanus + acellular Pertussis Vaccine EHL no data, PRC C, Lact -	
Daptacel *Inj 0.5ml single dose* **Infanrix** *Inj 0.5ml single dose* **Tripedia** *Inj 0.5ml single dose; Inj 7.5ml multidose*	**Diphtheria, tetanus, pertussis immunization:** 0.5ml IM at 2, 4, 6 and 15-18mo of age; booster dose at 4-6y
Diphtheria + Tetanus + acelllular Pertussis + Hepatitis B + Polio Vaccine PRC C	
Pediarix *Inj 0.5ml single dose*	**Diphtheria, tetanus, pertussis, Hepatitis B, Polio immunization: CH** 6wk-7y: 3 doses of 0.5ml IM at 6-8wk intervals
Diphtheria + Tetanus Toxoid	EHL no data
Generics *Inj 2LF U + 5 LF U/0.5ml*	**Tetanus, diphtheria immunization** →230: >7y: 0.5ml IM, rep after 4-8wk and after 6-12mo; 0.5ml booster dose q10y
Haemophilus B + Neisseria meningitidis OMPC + Hepatitis B Vaccine PRC C, Lact ?	
Comvax *Inj 7.5µg (haemophilus B PRB) + 125µg (neisseria meningitidis OMPC) + 5µg (HBsAg)/0.5ml*	**H. influenzae B and Hepatitis B vaccination:** 0.5ml IM at 2, 4, and 12-15mo of age

8 A.1.2 Toxoids (Bacteria)

AE (tetanus toxoid): injection site pain, fever
CI (tetanus toxoid): hypersensitivity to tetanus tox. products, infx, poliomyelitis outbreak

Tetanus Toxoid	EHL no data, PRC C, Lact ?
Generics *Inj 5 LF U/0.5ml*	**Tetanus immunization** →230: 0.5ml IM, rep after 4-8wk and after 6-12mo; give 0.5ml booster dose q10y; **CH** <1y: 0.5ml IM, rep after 4 and 8wk and after 6-12mo; > 1y: see adults

8 A.1.3   Polysaccharid-Vaccines (Bacteria)

AE (pneumococcal vaccine): injection site pain, anaphylaxis; **AE** (meningococcal vaccine): see Prod Info; **CI** (pneumococcal vaccine): hypersensitivity to pneumococcal vaccine products, Hodgkin's disease within 10d of or during Tx; **CI** (meningococcal vaccine): any acute illness, sensitivity to thimerosal or any other component of the vaccine

Meningococcal Polysaccharide Vaccine	EHL no data, PRC C
Menomune-A/C/Y/W-135 *Inj 50µg of "isolated product" from each of Groups A, C, Y and W-135/0.5ml*	**Meningococcal infx PRO:** 0.5ml SC; **CH** 3-18mo: 0.5ml SC, rep after 3mo; > 2y: see adults
Pneumococcal Vaccine	EHL no data
Pneumovax 23 Merck *Inj 25µg of each polysaccharide type/0.5ml* **Pnu-Imune** *Inj 25µg of each of the 23 purified polysaccharide types/0.5ml*	**Pneumococcal infx PRO:** 0.5ml IM/SC

8 A.1.4   Inactivated Vaccines (Bacteria)

AE (cholera vaccine): fever, malaise, headache
CI (cholera vaccine): illness, hypersensitivity to cholera vaccine

Cholera Vaccine	EHL no data, PRC C, Lact ?
Cholera vaccine USP *Inj 1.5ml + 20ml vials (8U of each serotype antigen (Ogawa and Inaba)/ ml)*	**Cholera immunization:** 0.5ml SC/IM, rep after 1-4wk; **CH** >10y: see adults, **CH** 5-10y: 0.3ml SC/IM, rep after 1-4wk; **CH** 6mo-4y: 0.2ml SC/IM, rep after 1-4wk

8 A.1.5   Live Attenuated Vaccines (Bacteria)

AE: flu-like syndrome, hematuria, urinary frequency, dysuria
CI: positive tuberculin tests, burns, AIDS, immunocompromised status, fever unknown origin, UTI (intravesical BCG), hypersensitivity to BCG vaccine

BCG Vaccine	EHL no data
Tice BCG *Inj 50mg/vial*	Different BCG vaccine products are available for TD immunization; route of immunization and dose depends on product; see Prod Info; **TB immunization:** 0.2-0.3ml percutanous; **CH** >1mo: see adults, **CH** <1mo: 50%

8 A.1.6 Inactivated Vaccines (Viruses)

AE (hepatitis A vaccine): fever, injection site pain/soreness, headache
AE (hepatitis B vaccine): fever, injection site soreness/erythema
AE (influenza vaccine): fever, pain, redness at injection site, malaise
AE (japanese encephalitis vaccine): fever, headache, injection site pain
AE (poliovirus vaccine): fever, injection site reaction, fussiness and crying in children
AE (rabies vaccine): dizziness, malaise, injection site reaction, myalgias, nausea
CI (hepatitis A vaccine): hypersensitivity to hepatitis A vaccine
CI (hepatitis B vaccine): hypersensitivity to hepatitis B vaccine/yeast
CI (influenza vaccine): allergy to chicken feathers/dander/eggs, hypersensitivity to vaccine/ thimerosol, active acute respiratory disease/infections
CI (japanese encephalitis vaccine): hypersensitivity to japanese encephalitis vaccine
CI (poliovirus vaccine): hypersensitivity to streptomycin, neomycin, polymixin B, hypersensitivity to polio vaccine products
CI (rabies vaccine): hypersensitivity to rabies vaccine products, fever

Hepatitis A Vaccine	EHL no data, PRC C, Lact ?
Havrix *Inj 360U/ml, 720U/ml, 1440U/ml* **Vaqta** *Inj 25U/ml, 50U/ml*	**Hep. A immunization:** Havrix: 1440 U IM, rep after 6-12mo; Vaqta: 50 U IM, rep after 6mo; **CH** 2-17y: Havrix: 720 U IM, rep after 6-12mo; Vaqta: 25 U IM, rep after 6-18mo
Hepatitis B Vaccine	EHL no data, PRC C, Lact ?
Engerix–B *Inj 10µg/0.5ml (pediatric), Inj 20µg/ml (adult)* **Recombivax HB** *Inj 5µg/0.5ml (pediatric), Inj 10µg/ml (adult)*	**Hep. B immunization: Engerix–B:** 20µg IM, rep after 1 + 6mo **Recombivax HB:** 10µg IM, rep after 1 + 6mo; **CH Engerix–B:** 10µg IM within 7d of birth, rep after 1 + 6mo; **Recombivax HB:** 5µg IM within 7d of birth, rep after 1 + 6mo
Hepatitis A + B Vaccine	EHL no data, PRC C, Lact ?
Twinrix *Inj 720U + 20µg/ml*	**Hep. A+B immunization:** 720 + 20µg IM, rep after 1 + 6mo
Influenza Vaccine	EHL no data, PRC C, Lact +
Fluzone *Inj 45µg/0.5ml* **Fluogen** *Inj 45µg/0.5ml*	**Influenza virus PRO:** 0.5ml IM once yearly; **CH** 6-35mo: 0.25ml IM, rep after 4wk; 3-8y: 0.5ml IM, rep after 4wk; 9-12y: see adults
Japanese Encephalitis Vaccine	EHL no data
JE-Vax *Inj single dose vial, 10 dose vial*	**Japanese encephalitis immunization:** 1ml SC on d 0, 7, 30; 1ml booster dose may be given after 2y; **CH** 1-3y: 0.5ml SC on d 0, 7, 30; > 3y: see adults
Poliovirus Vaccine	EHL no data
Ipol *Inj 40 D antigen U of Type1 + 8 D antigen U of Type2 + 32 D antigen U of Type 3 poliovirus/0.5ml*	**Poliomyelitis immunization:** IPOL: 0.5ml SC, rep after 1 and 6-12mo

Rabies Vaccine 9	EHL no data, PRC C, Lact ?
Imovax *Inj: 1ml is equal to or greater than 2.5 U of rabies antigen* **RabAvert** *Inj: the potency of 1.0ml RabAvert is at least 2.5 U of rabies antigen*	**Rabies immunization, pre exposure:** 1ml IM on d 0, 7, 21 or 28; **post exposure:** 1ml IM on d 0, 3, 7, 14, 28, 90 with a concommitant dose of 20 U/kg rabies IG on d 0; **CH** see adults

8 A.1.7 Live Attenuated Vaccines (Viruses)

AE (varicella vaccine): fever, N/V, injection site pain/swelling
AE (yellow fever vaccine): fever, malaise, headache
CI (varicella vaccine): hypersensitivity to varicella vaccine products, blood dyscrasias, immunodeficiency, active TB
CI (yellow fever vaccine): hypersensitivity to yellow virus vaccine products/eggs, child younger than 4mo of age, blood transfusion or IG therapy within 8wk

Varicella Vaccine	EHL no data, PRC C, Lact ?
Varivax *Inj 1350 PFU (plaque forming U) of Oka/ Merck varicella virus/0.5ml*	**Varicella immunization:** 0.5ml SC, rep after 4–8wk; **CH** > 12y: see adults; 1–12y: 0.5ml SC as single dose

Yellow Fever Vaccine	EHL no data, PRC C, Lact +
YF–Vax *5.04 Log $_{10}$ Plaque Forming Units (PFU)/ 0.5ml*	**Yellow fever immunization:** 0.5ml SC as single dose; **CH** > 9mo: see adults

8 A.1.8 Other Vaccines

AE (lyme disease vaccine): injection site reaction, flu like symptoms; AE (plague vaccine): see Prod Info
AE (typhoid vaccine): fever, rash, N/V, myalgia, diarrhea
CI (lyme disease vaccine): hypersensitivity to vaccine or its components; CI (plague vaccine): see Prod Info
CI (typhoid vaccine): hypersensitivity to typhoid vaccine products, immunodeficiency, persistent diarrhea, GI illness

Lyme Disease Vaccine	EHL no data, PRC C, Lact ?
LYMErix *Inj 30µg/0.5ml*	**Lyme disease immunization:** 30µg IM, rep after 1 and 12mo; **CH** >15y: see adults

Plague Vaccine	EHL no data
Plague Vaccine USP 20 *Inj 2000 million inactivated Yersinia pestis (strain 195/P)/ml*	**Plague immunization:** 1ml IM, then 0.2ml IM after 1–3mo, then 0.2ml IM after 5–6mo

Typhoid Vaccine	EHL no data
Typhim Vi *Inj 25 µg of purified Vi polysaccharide/ 0.5ml* **Typhoid Vaccine USP** *Inj 8 U/ml* **Vivotif Berna** *Cap 2-6 × 10^9 colony-forming U of viable S. typhi Ty21a/5-50 × 10^9 bact. cells of non-viable S. typhi Ty21a*	**Typhoid fever immunization:** **Typhim Vi:** 0.5ml IM as single dose; **Typhoid Vaccine USP:** 0.5ml SC, rep after 4wk; **CH** >10y: see adults; **CH** <10y: 0.25ml SC, rep after 4wk; **Vivotif Berna:** 1 Cap PO 1h ac on d 1, 3, 5, 7; **CH** >6y: see adults

8 A.2   Immunoglobulins

AE (hepatitis B IG): rash, pain at injection site, joint pain; **AE** (IG): flushing of face, hypotension, tachycardia, chest tightness, rash; **AE** (rabies IG human): fever, pain at injection site, hypersensitivity reaction; **AE** (RSV IG): fluid overload, O_2 saturation ↓, exacerbation of respiratory distress, fever; **AE** (tetanus IG): fever, redness, pain at injection site, myalgia; **AE** (varicella-zoster IG): injection site reaction **CI** (hepatitis B IG): hypersensitivity to IG products; **CI** (IG): hypersensitivity to IG, blood products, IgA deficiency; **CI** (rabies IG human): hypersensitivity to rabies IG/thimerosal
CI (RSV IG): hypersensitivity to RSVIG or other human IG, selective IgA deficiency
CI (tetanus IG): hypersensitivity to tetanus IG products, patients with IgA deficiency
CI (varicella-zoster IG): IgA deficiency, hypersensitivity to IG products/neomycin, immunodeficiency, blood dyscrasias, fever/respiratory, illness/active TB

Hepatitis B Immune Globulin	EHL 17.5d/25d, PRC C, Lact ?
BayHep *Inj 0.5ml syringe, 1ml vial, 5ml vial* **H-BIG** *0.5ml syringe, 1ml vial, 4ml vial, 5ml vial*	**Post-exposure PRO:** 0.06ml/kg IM, repeat in 1mo for persons, who are not given hepatitis B vaccine. Initiate hepatitis B vaccine series **PRO of infants born to HBsAG (+) mothers:** 0.5ml IM within 12h of birth. Initiate hepatitis B vaccine series

Immune Globulin	EHL 3-5wk, PRC C, Lact no data
BayGam *Inj (IM form) 2ml, 10ml single dose vials* **Gamimune N 5%** *Inj 0.5g, 2.5g, 5.0g, 10.0g, 12.5g protein* **Gamimune N 10%** *Inj 1g, 5g, 10g, 20g protein* **Sandoglobulin** *Inj 1g, 3g, 6g, 12g size vials*	**Hep. A post-exposure PRO** (i.e. household or institutional contacts): 0.02ml/kg IM; **Hep. A pre-exposure PRO:** < 3mo length of stay = 0.02ml/kg IM;> 3mo length of stay = 0.06ml/kg IM and rep. q4-6mo; **measles:** 0.2-0.25ml/kg IM within 6d of exposure, max 15ml; **CH pediatric HIV:** 400mg/kg IV inf q28d; **measles:** 0.2-0.25ml/kg IM within 6d of exposure, max 15ml

Rabies Immune Globulin	EHL 21d, PRC C, Lact ?
BayRab, Imogam *Inj 150 U/ml*	**Post-exposure PRO:** 20IU/kg (0.133ml/kg), infiltrated in the area around the wound and the rest given IM

RSV Immune Globulin	EHL 22-28d, PRC, Lact no data
RespiGam *Inj 20ml, 50ml single use vial*	**RSV PRO in CH** <24mo. 1.5ml/kg/h x 15min; incr rate as clinical condition permits to 3ml/kg/h x 15min, then to a max rate of 6ml/kg/h; max total dose/mo 750mg/kg
Tetanus Immune Globulin	EHL 3-5wk, PRC B/C, Lact no data
BayTet *Inj 250U/vial*	**Tetanus PRO** →230: 250U IM at time of injury; higher doses in severe injuries, severely contaminated wounds, or wounds >24h old, see Prod Info ; **tetanus Tx** →230: dose adjusted to severitiy of infx/clinical situation; usually TIG 3000-6000 U IM; **CH >7y:** see adults; **smaller CH, CH <7y:** 4 U/kg IM
Varicella-Zoster Immune Globulin	EHL 3wk, PRC C, Lact ?
VZIG *Inj 1.25ml vial, 6.25ml vial*	**Passive immunization to varicella:** **IM (gluteal):** </= 10kg: 125U at one site; 10.1-20kg: 250U at a single site, 20.1-30kg: 375U with no > 2.5ml at a single site, 30.1-40kg: 500 U with no > 2.5ml at a single site, > 40kg: 625U with no > 2.5ml at a single site; spezialized dosing for post-exposure PRO in immundeficient patients

8 A.3 Immunosuppressives

AE (azathioprine): N/V, diarrhea, pancytopenia, fever, risk of infection↑, cholestasis, pancreatitis, alopecia; **AE** (cyclosporine): renal damage, hepatic DO, cardiotoxic, tremors, hirsutism, gingival hypertrophy, edema; **AE** (daclizumab): N/V, headache, dizziness, tremor; **AE** (mycophenolate mofetil): myelosuppression, HTN, tremor, diarrhea, N/V; **AE** (sirolimus): thrombocyto-, leukopenia, hyperlipidemia, headache, periph. edema; **AE** (tacrolimus): HTN, N/V, diarrhea, headache/tremor, infx; **CI** (azathioprine): hypersens. to 6-mercaptopurine, severe renal/hepatic/bone marrow damage, severe infx; **CI** (cyclosporine): renal dysfunction, uncontrollable HTN, uncontrollable infx, tumors, severe hepatic diseases; **CI** (daclizumab, sirolimus, tacrolimus): hypersens. to product; **CI** (mycophenolate mofetil): hypersens. to mycophenolate mofetil/mycophenolic acid, hypersens. to IV formulation

Azathioprine	EHL 3h, PRC D, Lact -
Imuran *Tab 50mg, Inj. 100mg/vial* **Generics** *Tab 50mg, Inj. 100mg/vial*	**Renal transplant:** ini 3-5mg/kg PO/IV qd, maint 1-3mg/kg; **rheumatoid arthritis** →276: ini 1mg/kg/d PO, maint 1-2.5mg/kg/d
Basiliximab	EHL 7.2 +/- 3.2d, PRC B, Lact ?
Simulect *Inj 20mg/vial*	**Renal transplant:** 20mg IV 2h prior to transpl., rep after 4d; **CH** 2-15y: 12mg/m^2 2h prior to transpl., rep after 4d
Cyclosporine	EHL 19h, PRC C, Lact -
Neoral *Cap 25mg, 100mg, Sol (oral) 100mg/ml* **Sandimmune** *Cap 25mg, 50mg, 100mg, Sol (oral) 100mg/ml, Inj 50mg/ml* **Generics** *Cap 25mg, 50mg, 100mg*	**Organ transplant:** ini 15mg/kg/d PO for 7-14d, then decrease 5%/wk, maint 5-10mg/kg/d; IV: 1/3 of PO dose; **rheum. arthritis** →276: ini 2.5mg/kg/d PO div bid, incr prn after 8-12wk by 0.5-0.75mg/kg/d, max 4mg/kg/d
Daclizumab	EHL 44-360h, PRC C, Lact ?
Zenapax *Inj 25mg/5ml*	**Renal transplant:** 1mg/kg IV 24h prior to transpl., rep q14d for a total of 5 doses
Mycophenolate Mofetil	EHL 16-18h, PRC C, Lact ?
Cellcept *Tab 500mg, Cap 250mg, Susp 200mg/ml, Inj 500mg/vial*	**Renal transplant:** 1g IV/PO bid; **heart transplant:** 1.5g IV/PO bid; **liver transplant:** 1.5g PO bid; 1g IV bid
Sirolimus	EHL 57-63h, PRC C, Lact ?
Rapamune *Sol (oral) 1mg/ml*	**Renal transplant:** **ini** 6mg for 1d, maint 2mg PO qd; DARF: not req
Tacrolimus	EHL 8.7-11.3h, PRC C, Lact -
Prograf *Cap 0.5mg, 1mg, 5mg, Inj 5mg/ml*	**Liver/renal transplant:** ini 0.03-0.05mg/kg/d IV cont. inf, maint 0.1-0.2mg/kg PO div bid

8 A.4 Recommended Childhood Immunization Schedule

Vaccine	Months									Years		
	Birth	1	2	4	6	12	15	18	24	4–6	11–12	14–18
Hepatitis B	Hep B #1		Hep B #2		Hep B #3						Hep B	
Diphtheria, Tetanus, Pertussis			DTaP	DTaP	DTaP		DTaP			DTaP	Td	
H. influenzae type b			Hib	Hib	Hib	Hib						
Inactivated Polio			IPV	IPV	IPV					IPV		
Pneumococcal Conjugate			PCV	PCV	PCV	PCV						
Measles, Mumps, Rubella						MMR				MMR	MMR	
Varicella						Var					Var	
Hepatitis A									Hep A – in selected areas			

Range of acceptable ages for vaccination

Vaccines to be given if previously recommended doses were missed of given earlier than recommended minimum age

Approved by the Advisory Committee on Immunization Practices (ACIP), the American Academy of Pediatrics (AAP), and the American Academy of Family Physicians (AAFP), United States, January–December 2001

9 A. Rheumatology – Drugs

9 A.1   Antirheumatics
9 A.1.1   Gold

MA: inhibition of leukocyte migration into synovial membrane
EF: influence on rheumatoid process
AE: hair loss, dermatitis, stomatitis, pancytopenia, renal damage
AE (auranofin): rash, abdominal cramps, N/V, pruritus, proteinuria, diarrhea, anemia
AE (aurothioglucose): stomatitis, proteinuria, blood dyscrasias, pruritus/dermatitis
AE (gold sodium thiomalate): pruritus/rash, mucous membrane reactions, nephrotic syndrome, hematologic toxicity
CI: renal insufficiency, complete blood count changes, hepatic damage
CI (auranofin): hypersensitivity to gold salts, severe colitis, pulmonary fibrosis, exfoliative dermatitis, bone marrow aplasia, hematological DO
CI (aurothioglucose): SLE, untreat. CHF/DM, blood DO, severe HTN, urticaria, eczema, colitis
CI (gold sodium thiomalate): toxicity to gold/heavy metals, SLE, severe debilitation

Auranofin	EHL 15-31d, PRC C, Lact ?
Ridaura *Cap 3mg*	**Rheumatoid arthritis** →276: 3mg PO bid or 6mg PO qd; max 9mg/d; **CH** 0.1-0.15mg/kg/d PO; max 0.2mg/kg/d
Aurothioglucose	EHL 3-27d, PRC C, Lact ?
Solganal *Inj 50mg/ml*	**Rheumatoid arthritis** →276: 1st wk: 10mg IM, 2nd wk: 25mg IM; maint 25-50mg IM q2-4wk; **CH** 1st wk: 0.25mg/kg IM, incr 0.25mg/kg/wk to maint 1mg/kg qwk to total of 20 doses; max 50mg/wk; DARF: contraind. in renal DO
Gold Sodium Thiomalate	EHL 5d, PRC C, Lact ?
Myochrysine *Inj 25mg/ml, 50mg/ml*	**Rheumatoid arthritis** →276: 1st wk: 10mg IM, 2nd wk: 25mg, then 25-50mg/wk until cumulative dose of 0.8-1g; maint 25-50mg q other wk for 2-20wk; **CH** test dose 10mg IM, then 1mg/kg/wk until cumulative dose of 0.8-1g; max 50mg/dose maint 1mg/kg q2-4wk; DARF: GFR (ml/min) >50: 100% <50: not rec

9 A.1.2   Hydroxychloroquine

AE: agranulocytosis, ocular toxicity, skin/mucosal pigmentation, N/V; **CI**: retinal or visual field changes from prior use, hypersens. to hydroxychloroquine, long-term use in children

Hydroxychloroquine Sulfate	EHL 40d, PRC C, Lact ?
Plaquenil *Tab 200mg* **Generics** *Tab 200mg*	**Rheumatoid arthritis** →276: 400-600mg PO qd maint.: 200-400mg PO qd; **LE**: 400mg PO qd-bid maint 200-400mg PO qd; **CH** 3-5mg/kg/d PO, max 400mg/d or max 7mg/kg/d

9 A.1.3 Sulfasalazine

MA: prostaglandin synthesis ↓ ⇒ influence on rheumatoid process
AE: headache, N/V, GI distress, reversible oligospermia
CI: hypersensitivity to sulfasalazine/sulfa drugs/salicylates

Sulfasalazine	EHL 7.6h, PRC B, Lact ?
Azulfidine *Tab 500mg, Susp 250mg/5ml* **Azulfidine en-tabs** *Tab (coated) 500mg* **Generics** *Tab 500mg*	**Rheumatoid arthritis** →276: ini 500mg PO qd-bid; maint 1g bid; **CH** ini 10mg/kg/d PO; maint 30-50mg/kg/d div bid, max 2g/d

9 A.1.4 Immunosuppressants

MA (methotrexate): immunosuppressive, synthesis of cytokines ↓
EF: influence on rheumatoid process
AE (methotrexate): exanthema, hair loss, GI ulcers, N/V, hematopoietic DO, lung fibrosis
CI (methotrexate): acute infx, severe bone marrow depression, hepatic DO, GI ulcers, RF

see Azathioprine →260

Methotrexate (MTX)	EHL no data, PRC X, Lact -
Folex *Inj 25, 50, 100, 250mg/vial* **Rheumatrex** *Tab 2.5mg* **Generics** *Tab 2.5mg* *Inj 2.5mg/ml, 25mg/ml*	**Rheumatoid arthritis** →276: 7.5-15mg/wk PO/IM; DARF: GFR (ml/min) >50: 100%, 10-50: 50%

9 A.1.5 Disease-Modifiying Antirheumatics

MA (adalimumab): recombinant monoclonal antibody binding to TNF
MA (anakinra): recombinant interleukin-1 receptor antagonist
MA (etanercept): genetically engineered fusion protein composed of TNF receptors ⇒ binds 2 molecules of TNF and prevents them from binding to cellular receptors
MA (infliximab): monoclonal antibody specifically binding to TNF
MA (leflunomide): inhibition of dihydroorotate dehydrogenase ⇒ inhibition of pyrimidine synthesis ⇒ lymphocyte proliferation ↓ ⇒ influence on rheumatoid process
AE (adalimumab): serious to fatal infections incl. tuberculosis, fungal infections, allergic reaction, malignancies, CNS demyelinating disease, arrhythmias, pancytopenia, leukopenia, formation of autoantibodies, lupus-like-syndrome; **AE** (anakinra): neutropenia, infections, headache, injection site reactions; **AE** (etanercept): injection site reaction, headache, rhinitis; **AE** (infliximab): dyspnea, urticaria, flushing, headache, infections, recurrent malignancies; **AE** (leflunomide): diarrhea, HTN, transaminases↑, exanthema, hair loss, bone marrow depression, susceptibility to infx↑; **CI** (adalimumab): hypersensitivity to a., active infection, concurrent life-vaccination; **CI** (anakinra): hypersensitivity to E. coli-derived products; **CI** (etanercept): hypersensitivity to etanercept products, **CI** (infliximab): heart failure NYHA III-IV, hypersensitivity to murine proteins; **CI** (leflunomide): severe immunodeficiencies, restricted hematopoiesis, severe infections, hepatic dysfunction, moderate and severe RF, children and adolescents < 18

Adalimumab	EHL 10-20d, PRC B, Lact ?
Humira *Inj 40mg/syringe*	**Rheumatoid arthritis** →276: 40mg SC q2wk, may incr to 40mg qwk if not on MTX

Anakinra	EHL 4-6h, PRC B, Lact ?
Kineret *Inj 100mg/vial*	**Rheumatoid arthritis** →276: 100mg SC qd

Etanercept	EHL 90-300h, PRC B, Lact ?
Enbrel *Inj 25mg/vial*	**Rheumatoid arthritis** →276, **psoriatic arthritis** →279: 25mg SC biw; **CH** 4-17y: 0.4mg/kg SC biw; max 25mg/dose; DARF: not req
Infliximab	EHL 8-9.5d, PRC B, Lact ?
Remicade *Inj 100mg/vial*	**Rheumatoid arthritis** →276: 3mg/kg IV, rep after 2 and 6wk, thereafter q8wk, in combination with methotrexate
Leflunomide	EHL 4-28d, PRC X, Lact -
Arava *Tab 10mg, 20mg, 100mg*	**Rheumatoid arthritis** →276: 100mg PO qd for 3d; maint 10-20mg PO qd; DARF: not req

9 A.2   Nonsteroidal Anti-Inflammatory Drugs
9 A.2.1   NSAID - Salicylates

MA/EF: inhibition of cyclooxygenase ⇒ synthesis of prostaglandins ↓ ⇒ analgesic, antiinflammatory, antipyretic; inhibition of blood platelet aggregation (aspirin)
Note: salicylate-containing products are not recommended for use in children and teenagers with chicken pox, influenza or flu symptoms
AE: allergic skin reactions, dizziness, nausea, tinnitus, GI ulcerations, bronchospasm, hematopoietic DO, renal dysfunctions, abscess formation after IM administration
AE (aspirin): pancytopenia, acid-base balance DO, bleeding time ↑; **AE (diflunisal):** GI distress, rash
AE (trilisate): tinnitus and GI complaints (most frequent AE), hearing impairment, headache, lightheadedness, dizziness, drowsiness, lethargy (less frequent AE)
CI (acid NSAIDs): GI ulcerations, hematopoietic DO; **CI (aspirin):** restricted use in children and adolescents with febrile diseases (danger of Reye's syndrome); **CI (diflunisal):** hypersensitivity to diflunisal, asthma, allergic reactions to ASA or other anti-inflammatories; **CI (trilisate):** hypersensitivity to non-acetylated salicylates, renal insufficiency, hepatic DO, gastritis/peptic ulcer disease, precaution with pulmonal diseases

Aspirin (Acetylsalicylic Acid)	EHL 4.7-9h, PRC D, Lact ?
Aspergum *Chewing Gum 227mg* **Bayer Aspirin** *Tab 81mg, 163mg, 325mg, 500mg, 650mg, 975mg, Tab (chew) 81mg* **Easprin** *Tab 975mg* **Ecotrin** *Tab 81mg, 325mg, 500mg* **Genacote** *Tab 325mg, 500mg* **Halfprin** *Tab 81mg, 162mg* **Sureprin** *Tab 81mg, 162mg* **Zorprin** *Tab (ext.rel.) 800mg* **Generics** *Tab 81mg, 325mg, 500mg, 650mg, 975mg, Tab (chew) 81mg,* *Supp 60mg, 120mg, 200mg, 300mg, 325mg, 600mg, 650mg*	**Pain** →302, **fever:** 325-650mg PO/PR q4h prn, max 3.9g/d; **rheumatoid arthritis** →276: 3.2-6g/d in div doses; **rheumatic fever** →63: 1g q3-6h; **CH** 2-14y: **fever:** 10-15mg/kg PO q4h, max 60-80mg/kg/d; DARF GFR < 10ml/h: not rated
Choline-magnesium-trisalicylate	EHL 2-12h, PRC C, Lact -
Trilisate *Tab 500mg, 750mg, 1g* *Susp. 500mg/5ml*	**Rheumatoid arthritis** →276, **osteoarthritis** →275: 1.5g PO bid; **pain** →302, **fever:** 1000-1500mg PO bid

Diflunisal — EHL 8-12h, PRC C, Lact ?

Dolobid *Tab 250mg, 500mg*
Generics *Tab 250mg, 500mg*

Pain →302: ini 1g PO, maint 250-500mg q8-12h; **rheumatoid arthritis** →276, **osteoarthritis** →275: 500mg-1g PO div bid, max 1.5g/d; DARF: GFR (ml/min) > 50: 100%, <50: 50%

Salsalate — EHL 1h, PRC C, Lact ?

Disalcid *Cap 500mg*
Salflex *Tab 750mg*

Rheumatoid arthritis →276, **osteoarthritis** →275: 3g PO div bid-tid, max 1.5g/d; DARF: GFR (ml/min) > 50: 100%, <50: 50%

9 A.2.2 NSAID – Propionic Acid Derivates

MA/EF: see NSAID, Aspirin + other salicylates →264
AE (fenoprofen): headache, somnolence, dizziness, dyspepsia, tinnitus; **AE** (flurbiprofen): headache, GI distress, ocular burning/stinging, rash, ulcers; **AE** (ibuprofen): nausea, heartburn, ulcers, rash;
AE (ketoprofen): malaise, dizziness, GI distress, rash, tinnitus; **AE** (ketorolac): GI distress, ulcers, headache/dizziness; **AE** (naproxen): GI upset, headache, edema, dizziness; **AE** (oxaprozin): GI distress, rash
CI (fenoprofen, ibuprofen, ketoprofen, naproxen): hypersensitivity to product ingredients, asthma, allergic reactions to ASA, other anti-inflammatories
CI (flurbiprofen): hypersensitivity to flurbiprofen products, asthma, allergic reaction to ASA/other anti-inflammatories, ocular epithelial herpes simplex keratitis
CI (ketorolac, oxaprozin): hypersensitivity to product ingredients, allergy to ASA or other inflammatories, syndrome of nasal polyps and angioedema

---

Fenoprofen — EHL 3h, PRC D, Lact +

Nalfon *Tab 600mg, Cap 200mg, 300mg*
Generics *Tab 600mg, Cap 200mg, 300mg*

Pain →302: 200mg PO q4-6h prn; **rheumatoid arthritis** →276, **osteoarthritis** →275: 300-600mg PO tid-qid; DARF: not req

---

Flurbiprofen — EHL 5.7h, PRC B, Lact ?

Ansaid *Tab 50mg, 100mg*
Generics *Tab 50mg, 100mg*

Rheumatoid arthritis →276, **osteoarthritis** →275: 200-300mg/d PO div bid-qid

---

Ibuprofen — EHL 1.8-2.0h, PRC D, Lact +

Advil *Tab 200mg, Cap 200mg, Susp 100mg/5ml*
Children's advil *Susp 100mg/5ml*
Ibu *Tab 400mg, 600mg, 800mg*
Ibu-Tab *Tab 400mg, 600mg*
Motrin *Tab 100mg, 300mg, 400mg, 600mg, 800mg, Tab (chew) 50mg, 100mg, Drops 40mg/ml, Susp 100mg/5ml, 40mg/ml*
Generics *Tab 300mg, 400mg, 600mg, 800mg, Susp 100mg/5ml*

Rheumatoid arthritis →276, **osteoarthritis** →275: 1200-3200mg/d PO div tid-qid;
pain, dysmenorrhea: 400mg PO q4-6h;
CH juv. rheumatoid arthritis: 30-50mg/kg/d PO div tid-qid, max 2.4g/d;
CH fever, pain: 5-10mg/kg PO q6-8h prn, max 40mg/kg/d; DARF: not req

---

Ketoprofen — EHL 2-4h, PRC B, Lact ?

Orudis *Cap 25mg, 50mg, 75mg*
Oruvail *Cap ext.rel. 100mg, 150mg, 200mg*
Generics *Cap 25mg, 50mg, 75mg, Cap ext.rel. 100mg, 150mg, 200mg*

Rheumatoid arthritis →276, **osteoarthritis** →275: 100-300mg/d PO div tid-qid; **pain** →302, **dysmenorrhea:** 25-50mg PO q6-8h
CH juv. rheumatoid arthritis: 25-50mg bid; DARF: see Prod Info

Ketorolac   EHL 5.3h, PRC C, Lact ?

Acular PF *Tab 10mg, Inj 15mg/ml, 30mg/ml*
Toradol *Tab 10mg, Inj 15mg/ml, 30mg/ml, 60mg/ 2ml*
Generics *Tab 10mg, Inj 15mg/ml, 30mg/ml, 60mg/ 2ml*

Pain: ini 30–60mg IM or 15–30mg IV or 15–30mg IV/ IM q6h; max IV/IM, 120mg/d; 10mg PO q4–6h prn; max PO 40mg/d; DARF: see Prod Info

Naproxen   EHL 12–15h

Anaprox *Tab 250mg*
EC-Naprosyn *Tab ext.rel. 375mg, 500mg*
Naprelan *Tab ext.rel. 375mg, 500mg, 750mg*
Naprosyn *Susp 25mg/ml*
Generics *Tab 250mg, 375mg, 500mg, Tab ext.rel. 375mg, 500mg, Susp 25mg/ml*

Rheumatoid arthritis →276, **osteoarthritis** →275, **ankylosing spondylitis** →277: 250–500mg PO bid; **pain** →302, **dysmenorrhea**: ini 500mg, maint 250mg q6–8h prn; **CH** (rheumatoid arthritis): 10mg/kg/d div bid; DARF: not req

Oxaprozin   EHL 24–69h, PRC C, Lact ?

Daypro *Tab 600mg*
Generics *Tab 600mg*

Rheumatoid arthritis →276, **osteoarthritis** →275: 1200mg PO qd, max 1800mg/d; DARF: severe renal impairment: 600mg PO qd

9 A.2.3   NSAID – Acetic Acid Derivates

MA/EF: see NSAID, Aspirin + other salicylates →264
AE (diclofenac): nausea/diarrhea, constipation, headache, burning/stinging, ulcers; **AE** (diclofenac + misoprostol): abdominal pain, nausea, diarrhea; **AE** (etodolac): GI distress, malaise, dizziness
AE (indomethacin): headache, GI distress; **AE** (nabumetone): headache/dizziness, edema, GI distress
AE (sulindac): headache, dizziness, rash/pruritus, GI distress, edema; **AE** (tolmetin): edema, dizziness, GI distress, BP ↑; **CI** (diclofenac + misoprostol): hypersensitivity to diclofenac or misoprostol, asthma or allergic reactions with aspirin or NSAIDS; **CI** (diclofenac, etodolac, nabumetone, sulindac, tolmetin): hypersensitivity to product ingredients, allergic reactions to ASA or other anti-inflammatories, asthma
CI (indomethacin, in addition): history of recent rectal bleeding or proctitis

Diclofenac   EHL 2h, PRC B, Lact ?

Voltaren *Tab del.rel. 25mg, 50mg, 75mg*
Voltaren-xr *Tab ext.rel. 100mg*
Generics *Tab ext.rel. 25mg, 50mg, 75mg, Tab del. rel 100mg*

Osteoarthritis →275, **rheumatoid arthritis** →276: 50mg PO bid-tid or 75mg bid or 100mg qd; **ankylosing spondylitis** →277: 25mg PO qid, **pain** →302, **dysmenorrhea**: 50mg PO tid

Diclofenac + Misoprostol

Arthrotec *Tab ext. rel. 50mg + 200µg, 75mg + 200µg*

Osteoarthritis →275: 50mg/200µg PO bid-tid or 75mg/200µg bid; **rheumatoid arthritis** →276: 50mg/200µg PO bid-qid or 75mg/200µg bid ; DARF: GFR < 30ml/min: contraind.

Etodolac   EHL 6–7h, PRC C, Lact ?

Lodine *Cap 200mg, 300mg*
Lodine xl *Tab ext.rel. 400mg, 500mg, 600mg*
Generics *Tab 400mg, 500mg, Tab ext.rel. 400mg, 500mg, 600mg, Cap 200mg, 300mg*

Pain →302: 200–400mg PO q6–8h; max 1000mg/d; max in patients weighing < 60kg is 20mg/kg/d; **rheumatoid arthritis** →276, **osteoarthritis** →275: ini 400–500mg PO bid or 300mg bid-tid; maint 400–1000mg/d

Indomethacin
EHL 4.5h, PRC D, Lact +

Indocin *Cap ext.rel. 25mg, 50mg, Susp 25mg/5ml, Supp 50mg*
Indocin SR *Cap ext.rel. 75mg*
Indo-lemmon *Cap ext.rel. 25mg, 50mg*
Indomethagan *Supp 50mg*
Generics *Cap ext.rel. 25mg, 50mg, 75mg, Susp 25mg/5ml*

Rheumatoid arthritis →276, **osteoarthritis** →275: 25mg PO bid-tid, max 200mg/d
bursitis, tendinitis: 75-150mg/d PO/PR div tid-qid; DARF: not req

---

Ketorolac
EHL 5.3h, PRC C, Lact ?

Acular PF *Tab 10mg, Inj 15mg/ml, 30mg/ml*
Toradol *Tab 10mg, Inj 15mg/ml, 30mg/ml, 60mg/2ml*
Generics *Tab 10mg, Inj 15mg/ml, 30mg/ml, 60mg/2ml*

Pain →302: ini 30-60mg IM or 15-30mg IV or 15-30mg IV/IM q6h; max IV/IM 120mg/d; 10mg PO q4-6h prn; max PO 40mg/d; DARF: see Prod Info

---

Nabumetone
EHL unknown, PRC C, Lact ?

Relafen *Tab 500mg, 750mg*
Generics *Tab 500mg, 750mg*

Rheumatoid arthritis →276, **osteoarthritis** →275: 500mg PO bid, maint 1-2g/d; DARF not req

---

Sulindac
EHL 7.8h, PRC D, Lact -

Clinoril *Tab 150mg, 200mg*
Generics *Tab 150mg, 200mg*

Rheumatoid arthritis →276, **osteoarthritis** →275, **ankylosing spondylitis** →277: 150mg PO bid, **bursitis, tendinitis, gout** →171: 200mg PO bid; max 400mg/d; **CH** limited data, 4mg/kg/d PO div bid has been used; DARF: not req

---

Tolmetin
EHL 5h, PRC C, Lact -

Tolectin DS *Cap 400mg*
Tolectin *Tab 200mg, 600mg*
Generics *Tab 200mg, 600mg, Cap 400mg*

Rheumatoid arthritis →276, **osteoarthritis** →275: 200-600mg PO tid, max 1800mg/d, **CH** >2y: ini 20mg/kg/d PO div tid-qid, maint 15-30mg/kg/d div tid-qid; DARF: not req

9 A.2.4 NSAID - Anthranilic Acid

MA/EF: see NSAID, Aspirin + other salicylates →264
AE (meclofenamate): diarrhea, GI distress, rash, dizziness, headache
CI (meclofenamate): hypersensitivity to meclofenamate products, asthma allergic reactions to ASA or other anti-inflammatories

Meclofenamate
EHL 0.8-5.3h, PRC D, Lact ?

Meclomen *Cap 50mg, 100mg*
Generics *Cap 50mg, 100mg*

Pain →302: 50mg PO q4-6h prn, max 400mg/d, **dysmenorrhea**: 100mg PO tid for 6 d, **rheumatoid arthritis** →276, **osteoarthritis** →275: 200-400mg/d PO div tid-qid

9 A.2.5   NSAID – Cyclooxygenase-2-Inhibitors

MA/EF (celecoxib, rofecoxib, valdecoxib): high selectivity for cyclooxygenase-2; inhibition of cyclooxygenase $\Rightarrow$ synthesis of prostaglandins ↓
AE (celecoxib): dyspepsia, abdominal pain, GI effects
AE (rofecoxib): heartburn, N/V, HTN, edema
AE (valdecoxib): dyspepsia, headache, abdominal pain, nausea, diarrhea, edema
CI (celecoxib): hypersensitivity to celecoxib products, hypersensitivity to ASA or other anti-inflammatory drugs, hypersensitivity to sulfonamides
CI (rofecoxib): hypersensitivity to rofecoxib, allergic or asthma reaction to ASA/NSAIDs
CI (valdecoxib): hypersensitivity to valdecoxib, allergic or asthma reaction to ASA/NSAIDs

Celecoxib	EHL 11h , PRC C, Lact ?
Celebrex *Cap 100mg, 200mg*	**Osteoarthritis** →275: 100mg PO bid or 200mg qd; **rheumatoid arthritis** →276: 100-200mg PO bid
Rofecoxib	EHL 17h, PRC C, Lact ?
Vioxx *Tab 12.5mg, 25mg, 50mg* *Susp 12.5mg/5ml, 25mg/5ml*	**Osteoarthritis** →275: 12.5-25mg PO qd **pain** →302; **dysmenorrhea**: 50mg PO qd
Valdecoxib	EHL 8-11h, PRC C, Lact ?
Bextra *Tab 10mg, 20mg*	**Osteoarthritis** →275: 10mg PO qd; **dysmenorrhea**: 20mg PO bid; DARF: not rec in advanced RF

9 A.2.6   Other NSAIDs

MA/EF: see NSAID, Aspirin + other salicylates →264
AE (meloxicam): dyspepsia, flatulence, abdominal pain, diarrhea
AE (piroxicam) GI distress, rash, dizziness, ulcers, edema
CI (meloxicam): hypersensitiviy to meloxicam, allergic reactions to aspirin/NSAIDS
CI (piroxicam): hypersensitivity to piroxicam products, asthma, allergic reactions to ASA or other anti-inflammatories

Meloxicam	EHL 15-20h, PRC N, Lact ?
Mobic *Tab 7.5mg*	**Osteoarthritis** →275: 7.5mg PO qd, max 15mg/d; DARF: see Prod Info
Piroxicam	EHL 50h, PRC C, Lact +
Feldene *Cap 10mg, 20mg* **Generics** *Cap 10mg, 20mg*	**Rheumatoid arthritis** →276, **osteoarthritis** →275: 20mg PO qd or div bid; DARF: not req

9 A.3   Other Non-Opiod Analgesics
9 A.3.1   Aniline Derivates

MA: inhibition of cyclooxygenase ⇒ synthesis of prostaglandins ↓
EF: anti-inflammatory, analgesic, only mildly antiphlogistic
AE: allergic skin reactions, headache, bronchospasm, renal damage (tubular and papillary necrosis, interstitial nephritis), hepatic damage
CI: restricted use in presence of hepatic DO, Meulengracht's syndrome, renal DO

Acetaminophen (Paracetamol)   EHL no data, PRC B, Lact +

Acephen *Supp 120mg, 325mg, 650mg*
Infants' feverall *Supp 80mg*
Neopap *Supp 120mg*
Tylenol *Tab ext.rel. 650mg*
Generics *Tab 325mg, 500mg, 650mg, Tab (chew) 80mg, Tab ext.rel. 650mg, Cap 325mg, 500mg, Drops 80mg/0.8ml, Supp 120mg, 325mg, 650mg*

Pain →302, **fever**: 325-1000mg PO/PR q4-6h, max 4g/d; **CH** 10-15mg/kg/dose PO/PR q4-6h, max 5 doses/d; DARF: GFR (ml/min) >50: q4h, 10-50: q6h, <10: q8h

9 A.3.2   Non-Opioid Analgesic Combinations

Acetaminophen + Butalbital + Caffeine   PRC C, Lact ?

Anoquan *Cap 325 + 50 + 40mg*
Fioricet *Tab 325 + 50 + 40mg*
Generics *Tab 325 + 50 + 40mg, Cap 325 + 50 + 40mg*

Tension headache: 1-2 Tab PO q4h, max. 6 Tab/d

Aspirin + Butalbital + Caffeine   PRC D, Lact ?

Butal Compound *Tab 325 + 50 + 40mg*
Fiorinal *Tab 325 + 50 + 40mg, Cap 325 + 50 + 40mg*
Ianorinal *Tab 325 + 50 + 40mg*
Generics *Tab 325 + 50 + 40mg*

Tension headache: 1-2 Tab/Cap PO q4h

Aspirin + Caffeine + Orphenadrine   PRC D, Lact ?

Invagesic *Tab 385 + 30 + 25mg*
Invagesic forte *Tab 770 + 60 + 50mg*
Norgesic *Tab 385 + 30 + 25mg*
Norgesic forte *Tab 770 + 60 + 50mg*
Orphengesic *Tab 385 + 30 + 25mg*
Orphengesic forte *Tab 770+60+50mg*
Generics *Tab 385 + 30 + 25mg, Tab 770 + 60 + 50mg*

Musculoskeletal pain →304: 1-2 Tab PO tid-qid; forte: 1/2-1 Tab PO tid-qid

Aspirin + Methocarbamol   PRC D, Lact ?

Robaxisal *Tab 325 + 400mg*
Generics *Tab 325 + 400mg*

Acute painful musculoskeletal conditions →304: 2 Tab PO qid

9 A.4   Opioids
9 A.4.1   Opioid Agonists

MA/EF: stimulation of central opiate receptors ⇒ analgesic, sedative, respiratory depression, antitussive, emetic and antiemetic (see AE); **AE**: respiratory depression, sedation, bradycardia, hypotensive circulation DO, pruritus, bronchospasm, transpiration, spasms of pancreatic and bile ducts, constipation, seizures, miosis, tolerance development, urinary retention; **CI**: restricted use for children < 1, addiction to opiates, pancreatitis, respiratory DO; **Note**: all are PRC D if used for prolonged periods or in high doses at term

Codeine Phosphate
EHL 2.5-3.5h, PRC C, Lact +

Generics *Tab 30mg, Sol (oral) 15mg/5ml, Inj 15mg/ml, 30mg/ml*

Pain →302: 15-60mg PO/IM//SC q4-6h; **cough**: 10-20mg PO/SC q4-6h prn; **CH pain**: > 2y: 0.5-1mg/kg/dose PO/SC/IM q4-6h, **cough**: 2-6y: 1mg/kg/d PO div qid, max 30mg/24h; 6-12y: 5-10mg PO q4-6h prn; max 60mg/24h; DARF: GFR (ml/min) > 50: 100%, 10-50: 75%, <10: 50%

Fentanyl
EHL no data, PRC C, Lact ?

Actiq *Buccal/lozenge (oral) 0.2mg, 0.4mg, 0.6mg, 0.8mg, 1.2mg,1.6mg*
Duragesic *Film (ext.rel, TD) 0.6mg/24h, 1.2mg/24h, 1.8mg/24h, 2.4mg/24h*
Fentanyl Oralet *Buccal/lozenge (oral) 0.1mg, 0.2mg, 0.3mg, 0.4mg*
Sublimaze *Inj 0.05mg/ml*
Generics *Inj 0.05mg/ml*

Chronic pain →302: 25-100µg/h patch q72h **breakthrough CA pain**: ini 200µg PO (oral transmucosal), titrate dose

Hydromorphone
EHL 2.5h, PRC C, Lact ?

Dilaudid *Tab 2mg, 4mg, 8mg, Liquid (oral) 1mg/ml, Supp 3mg, Inj 1mg/ml, 2mg/ml, 4mg/ml*
Dilaudid-HP *Inj 10mg/ml*
Generics *Tab 8mg, Sol (oral) 5mg/5ml, Inj 10mg/ml*

Pain →302: 2-4mg PO q4-6h; 1-2mg IM/SC/IV q4-6h prn; 3mg PR q6-8h

Levorphanol
EHL 11h, PRC C, Lact ?

Levo-Dromoran *Tab 2mg, Inj 2mg/ml*
Generics *Tab 2mg*

Pain →302: 2-3mg PO/SC q6-8h prn; 2-4mg IM q6-8h prn; 1-2mg IV q6-8h prn

Meperidine
EHL 3.2-3.7h, PRC B, Lact +

Demerol *Tab 50mg, 100mg, Syr 50mg/5ml, Inj 25mg/ml, 50mg/ml, 75mg/ml, 100mg/ml*
Generics *Tab 50mg, 100mg, Inj 10mg/ml, 25mg/ml, 50mg/ml, 75mg/ml, 100mg/ml*

Pain →302: 50-150mg IV/IM/SC/PO q3-4h prn, **CH** 1-2mg/kg q3-4h IM/SC/PO; DARF: GFR (ml/min) > 50: 100%, 10-50: 75%, <10: 50%

Methadone
EHL 23h, PRCB, Lact ?

Dolophine HCT *Tab 5mg, 10mg, Syr 10mg/30ml, Inj 10mg/ml*
Methadose *Tab 5mg, 10mg, Tab (dispersible) 40mg, Sol (oral) 10mg/ml*
Generics *Tab 5mg, 10mg, Tab disp. 40mg, Sol (oral) 5mg/5ml, 10mg/ml, 10mg/5ml, Powder (comp) 50g/ bot, 100g/bot, 500g/bot*

Pain →302: 2.5-10mg PO/SC/IM q3-4h prn; **narcotic addiction**: 40-180mg PO qd, taper dose as appropriate to avoid withdrawal symptoms; **CH pain**: .0.1-0.2mg/kg PO q6h; DARF: GFR (ml/min) > 50: q6h, 10-50: q8h, <10: q8-12h

Morphine Sulfate	EHL no data, PRC C, Lact ?
Astramorph pf *Inj 0.5mg/ml, 1mg/ml* **Avinza** *Cap ext.rel. 30mg, 60mg, 90mg, 120mg* **Duramorph pf** *Inj 0.5mg/ml, 1mg/ml* **Infumorph** *Inj 10mg/ml, 25mg/ml* **Kadian** *Cap ext.rel. 20mg, 50mg, 100mg* **MS contin** *Cap ext.rel. 15mg, 30mg, 60mg, 100mg, 200mg* **MSIR Oral Solution** *Sol (oral) 10mg/5ml, 20mg/5ml* **Numorphan** *Supp 5mg* **Oramorph SR** *Tab ext.rel. 15mg, 30mg, 60mg, 100mg* **Roxanol** *Sol (oral) 20mg/ml, 100mg/5ml* **Generics** *Tab ext. rel 15mg, 30mg, 60mg, 100mg, 200mg; Inj 0.5mg/ml, 1mg/ml, 2mg/ml, 15mg/ml; Supp 10mg*	**Pain** →302: 5-30mg PO q4h; ext.rel.: 15-200mg PO qd-bid; 10mg IM/SC q4h; 2-10mg IV q4h; 10-20mg PR q4h; **CH** 0.1-0.2mg/kg IM/SC/IV q2-4h, max 15mg/dose; DARF: GFR (ml/min) > 50: 100%, 10-50: 75%, <10: 50%
Oxycodone	EHL 3.2-8h, PRC C, Lact ?
Oxycontin *Tab ext.rel. 10mg, 20mg, 40mg, 80mg, 160mg* **Roxicodone** *Tab 15mg, 30mg*	**Pain** →302: 10-30mg PO q6h prn; ext.rel.; 10mg PO q12h
Oxymorphone	EHL no data, PRC B/D, Lact ?
Numorphan *Supp 5mg* *Inj 1mg/ml, 1.5mg/ml*	**Pain** →302: 1-1.5mg SC/IM q4-6h prn; 0.5mg IV q4-6h prn; 5mg PR q4-6h prn
Propoxyphene	EHL 6-12h, PRC D, Lact ?
Darvon-N *Tab 100mg, Susp 50mg/5ml* **Darvon** *Cap 32mg, 65mg* **Dolene** *Cap 65mg* **Kesso-gesic** *Cap 65mg* **Generics** *Cap 32mg, 65mg*	**Pain** →302: 65mg PO q4h prn, max 390mg/d; DARF: GFR (ml/min) > 50: 100%, 10-50: 100%, <10: not rec

9 A.4.2 Opioid Agonist–Antagonists and Combinations

AE (bupren.): N/V, hypotension, sedation; **AE** (butorphanol): sedation, drowsiness, N/V, diplopia
AE (dezocine): N/V, sedation, headache, dizziness; **AE** (nalbuphine): sedation, sweatiness, N/V, dizziness, resp. depression; **AE** (pentaz.): physical dependence, resp. depression, hallucinations, confusion, N/V
CI (bupren.): hypersens. to buprenorphine; **CI** (butorphanol): hypersens. to butorphanol, benzethonium
CI (dezocine): hypersens. to dezocine, concomitant CNS depressants; **CI** (nalbuphine): hypersens. to nalbuphine, oxymorphone, naloxone; **CI** (pentaz.): hypersens. to pentazocine, naloxone (PO)

Buprenorphine	EHL 37h, PRC C, Lact ?
Buprenex *Inj. 0.3mg/ml* **Generics** *Inj 0.3mg/ml*	**Moderate to severe pain** →302: 0.3-0.6mg IM/IV q6-8h prn, max single dose 0.6mg
Buprenorphine + Naloxone	EHL 37h, PRC C, Lact -
Suboxone *Tab 2 + 0.5mg, 8 + 2mg*	**Opioid dependence** →302: see Prod Info

Butorphanol	EHL 4-7h, PRC C, Lact +
Stadol *MDI (nasal) 1mg/puff* *Inj 1mg/ml, 2mg/ml* **Generics** *Inj 1mg/ml, 2mg/ml*	**Postop pain, pain** →302: 0.5-2mg IV q3-4h prn; 1-4mg IM q3-4h prn, 1mg intranasally q3-4h prn; DARF: GFR (ml/min) > 50: 100%, 10-50: 75%, < 10: 50%
Dezocine	EHL 2.6-2.8h, PRC C, Lact ?
Dalgan *Inj 10mg/vial*	**Pain** →302: 5-20mg IM q3-6h prn, max 20mg/d; 2.5-10mg IV q2-4h prn; DARF: see Prod Info
Nalbuphine	EHL 2.2 + 2.6h, PRC B, Lact ?
Nubain *Inj 10mg/ml, 20mg/ml* **Generics** *Inj 1.5mg/ml, 10mg/ml, 20mg/ml*	**Pain** →302: 10-20mg SC/IM/IV q3-6h prn; **anesth**: 0.3-3mg/kg IV, then 0.25-0.5mg/kg prn
Pentazocine	EHL 2-3.6h, PRC C, Lact ?
Talwin *Inj 30mg/ml* **Talwin NX** *Tab 50mg pentazocine + 0.5mg naloxone*	**Pain** →302: 30mg IV/IM/SC q3-4h prn; max 360mg/d; 50-100mg PO q3-4h; max 600mg/d; DARF: GFR (ml/min) > 50: 100%, 10-50: 75%, <10: 50%

9 A.4.3 Opioid Antagonists

MA: competitive blockage of opiate receptors; **AE**: withdrawal syndrome in opiate addicts, allergic reactions; **AE (nalmefene)**: N/V, headache, dizziness, tachycardia; **AE (naloxone)**: opiate withdrawal symptoms; **CI**: hypersensitivity to product ingredients

Nalmefene	EHL 8.5-10.8h, PRC B, Lact ?
Revex *Inj 0.1mg/ml, 1mg/ml*	**Opioid overdose** →483: 0.5-1mg IV; **postop respiratory depression**: 0.25 µg/kg IV, rep. after 2-5min prn
Naloxone	EHL 30-81min, PRC B, Lact ?
Narcan *Inj 0.02mg/ml, 0.4mg/ml, 1mg/ml* **Generics** *Inj 0.02mg/ml, 0.4mg/ml, 1mg/ml*	**Opioid overdose** →483: 0.4-2mg IV/IM/SC, rep. prn q2-3min; **postop respiratory depression**: 0.1-0.2mg IV rep. prn q2-3min; **CH opiod overdose < 20kg**: 0.1mg/kg IV, **> 20kg**: 2mg IV, rep. prn q2-3min; **postop respiratory depression**: 10µg/kg IV/IM/SC rep. prn q2-3min; DARF: not req

9 A.5 Opioid Analgesic Combinations

Codeine + Acetaminophen	PRC C, Lact ?
Capital and Codeine *Susp 12mg + 120mg/5ml* **Tylenol with Codeine** *Sol (oral) 12mg + 120mg/5ml* **Generics** *Sol (oral) 12mg + 120mg/5ml*	**Pain** →302: 15ml PO q4h prn; **CH 3-6y**: 5ml PO q4-6h prn, 7-12y: 10ml PO q4-6h prn
Codeine + Acetaminophen + Butalbital + Caffeine	PRC C, Lact -
Fioricet with Codeine *Cap 30 + 325 + 50 + 40mg* **Generics** *Cap 30 + 325 + 50 + 40mg*	**Pain** →302: 1-2 Cap PO q4h prn, max 6 Cap/d

Codeine + Aspirin + Butalbital + Caffeine — PRC C, Lact -

Fiorinal with Codeine No 3 *Cap 30 + 325 + 50 + 40mg*
Generics *Cap 30 + 325 + 50 + 40mg*

Pain →302: 1-2 Cap PO q4h prn, max 6 Cap/d

Codeine + Carisoprodol + Aspirin — PRC N, Lact -

Soma Compound with Codeine *Tab 16 + 200 + 325mg*
Generics Tab 16 + 200 + 325mg

Musculoskeletal pain →304: 1-2 Tab PO qid prn

Hydrocodone + Acetaminophen — PRC C, Lact ?

Allay *Cap 5 + 500mg*
Anexsia *Tab 5 + 500mg, 7.5 + 650mg, 10 + 660mg*
Co-gesic *Tab 5 + 500mg*
Hydrocet *Cap 5 + 500mg*
Hy-phen *Tab 5 + 500mg*
Lorcet-hd *Cap 5 + 500mg*
Norco *Tab 10 + 325mg*
Vicodin *Tab 5 + 500mg, 10 + 660mg, 7.5 + 750mg*
Generics *Tab 2.5 + 500mg, 5 + 500mg, 7.5 + 500mg, 10 + 500mg, 7.5 + 650mg, 10 + 650mg, Cap 5 + 500mg*

Pain →302: 1 Tab PO q4-6h prn, max 4g acetaminophen/d

Hydrocodone + Ibuprofen — PRC C, Lact ?

Vicoprofen *Tab 7.5 + 200mg*

Pain →302: 1 Tab PO q4-6h prn

Oxycodone + Acetaminophen — PRC C, Lact -

Oxycet *Tab 5 + 325mg*
Percocet *Tab 2.5 + 325mg, 5 + 325mg, 7.5 + 500mg, 10 + 650mg*
Roxilox *Cap 5 + 500mg*
Roxicet *Tab 5 + 325mg, 5 + 500mg, Sol (oral) 5 + 325mg/5ml*
Tylox *Cap 5 + 500mg*
Generics *Tab 5 + 325mg, 7.5 + 500mg, 10 + 650mg, Cap 5 + 500mg*

Pain →302: 1 Tab PO q6h prn; max 4g acetaminophen/d

Oxycodonehydrochloride + Oxycodoneterephthalate + Aspirin — PRC D, Lact ?

Percodan-demi *Tab 2.25 + 0.19 + 325mg*
Percodan *Tab 4.5 + 0.38 + 325mg;*
Roxiprin *Tab 4.5 + 0.38 + 325mg*
Generics *Tab 4.5 + 0.38 + 325mg*

Pain →302: 1 Tab PO q6h prn

Pentazocine + Acetaminophen — PRC C, Lact ?

Talacen *Tab 25 + 650mg*
Generics *Tab 25 + 650mg*

Pain →302: 1 Tab PO q4h prn

Propoxyphene + Acetaminophen — PRC D, Lact +

Darvocet *Tab 50 + 325mg, 100 + 650mg*
Generics *Tab 50 + 325mg, 65 + 650mg, 100 + 650mg*

Pain →302: 1 Tab (100 + 650mg) or 2 Tab (50 + 325mg) PO q4h prn

Propoxyphene + Aspirin + Caffeine	PRC D, Lact ?
Darvon compound 65 *Cap 65 + 389 +32.4mg* **Propoxyphene compound 65** *Cap 65 + 389 + 32.4mg*	**Pain** →302: 1 Cap PO q4h prn
Tramadol + Acetaminophen	PRC D, Lact ?
Ultracet *Tab 37.5 + 325mg*	**Pain** →302: 2 Tab PO q4-6h prn, max 8 Tab/d; DARF: GFR (ml/min) <30: max. 2 Tab q12h

9 A.6 Other Analgesics

AE (tramadol): drowsiness, dizziness, constipation, headache, N/V
CI (tramadol): hypersensitivity to tramadol, intoxication with alcohol or CNS depressants

Tramadol	EHL 6.3-6.4h, PRC C, Lact -
Ultram *Tab 50mg*	**Pain** →302: 50-100mg PO q4-6h prn, max 400mg/d; **CH** > 1y: 1-2mg/kg/dose PO q4-6h; DARF: GFR (ml/min) <30: q12h

9 B. Rheumatology – Therapies

Gary Gilkeson, MD
Division of Rheumatology and Immunology, Department of Medicine
Medical University of South Carolina, Charleston, SC

9 B.1   Raynaud Syndrome

	Calcium antagonist →28 (vasodilation)	Nifedipine (Adalat, Adalat cc, Procardia, Procardia XL, Gens)	*5mg PO tid, up to max. 180mg/d; Caution: cimetidine/ grape fruit juice increase levels, toxicity of vincristine↑, digoxin level ↑*
		Any calcium channel blocker	
poss	**Isosorbide dinitrate** →36 (vasodilation)	Isosorbide dinitrate cream	*Admin cream 1% for acute episodes*
poss	**Antiplatelet drugs** →74 (phosphodiesterase/platelet aggregation-adhesion inhibition)	Aspirin - ASA (Ascriptin, Asprimox, Bayer Aspirin, Bufferin, Easprin, Ecotrin, Empirin, Genprin, Halfprin, St. Joseph Pain Reliever, Zorprin, Gens)	*81mg PO qd*
		Dipyridamole (Persantine, Gens)	*75mg qid*

9 B.2   Fibromyalgia

poss	**Tricyclic Antidepressant** →321 (distancing from pain, sleep inducing)	Amitriptyline (Clavil, Elavil, Endep, Gens)	*25mg PO qd qpm, incr dose prn until sleep achieved; Caution: with digitalis increased danger of arrhythmias*
		Other tricyclics	
plus	physical Tx + psychosomatic care + endurance sports!		

9 B.3   Osteoarthritis

9 B.3.1   In Activated Arthrosis

poss	**Analgesic – aniline derivative** →269 (inhibits cyclooxygenase → prostaglandins ↓)	Acetaminophen (Tylenol, Gens)	*1000mg PO qid*
poss	**NSAID** →265, →266 (inhibits cyclooxygenase ⇒ prostaglandins ↓ ⇒ anti-inflammatory, analgesic)	Diclofenac (Voltaren, Voltaren-XR, Gens)	*50mg qd-tid (max. 150mg/d)*
		Ibuprofen (Advil, Children's advil, Motrin, Gens)	*800-1600mg/d PO div tid-qid; well tolerated*
		Indomethacin (Indocin SR, Indocin, Gens)	*25mg PO bid-tid, max 200mg/d; Note: strongest analgesic EF, highest rate of AE*

NSAID ⇒ methotrexate levels ↑ ⇒ liver toxicity↑; interaction with warfarin!

poss	**Local anesthetic** →285 (muscle relaxation in tenseness)	Bupivacaine 0.25% (Marcaine HCT, Sensorcaine, Gens)	*2-5ml Inj IM*
poss	**Glucocorticoid** →148, →285 (anti-inflammatory, immunosuppressive)	Triamcinolone acetonide (Aristocort, Kenalog) + Lidocaine (Gens)	*Intraarticular Inj: large joint: 10-20mg, middle size joint: 5-10mg, small joint: 2-5mg; max. 4 Inj/y, at least 3-4wk apart*
poss	**Viscous compounds** (structure modifying)	Hyaluronic acid (Hyalgan, Synvisc)	*Intraarticular Inj qwk for 3-4wk*
		Glucosamine sulfate (Gens)	*500mg PO tid*

9 B.4   Rheumatoid Arthritis
9 B.4.1   Symptomatic Therapy (Acute Episode)

In General

	NSAID →265, →266 (inhibits cyclooxygenase ⇒ prostaglandins ↓ ⇒ anti-inflammatory, analgesic, antipyretic)	Naproxen (Anaprox, Naprelan, Naprosyn, Gens)	*500mg PO bid*
		Indomethacin (Indocin SR, Indocin, Gens)	*25-50mg PO bid-tid, 75mg (SR) PO qd-bid, 50-100mg PR qd-bid prn*
		Diclofenac (Voltaren, Voltaren-XR, Gens)	*50mg PO qd-tid (max 150mg)*
		Ibuprofen (Advil, Children's advil, Motrin, Gens)	*1-2 SR Tab PO bid-qid, max. 1600mg/d; note: well tolerated*

NSAID ⇒ methotrexate levels ↑ ⇒ liver toxicity ↑; interaction with warfarin!

In ventricular/duodenal ulcers

	NSAID – Cyclooxygenase-2-Inhibitor →268 (inhibits cyclooxygenase-2 ⇒ prostaglandins ↓ ⇒ anti-inflammatory, analgesic)	Rofecoxib (Vioxx)	*12.5-25mg PO qd, max. 25mg/d*
		Celecoxib (Celebrex)	*100-200mg PO bid, max. 400mg/d*
		Valdecoxib (Bextra)	*10-20mg PO qd*
poss	**Glucocorticoid** →148 (anti-inflammatory, immunosuppressive)	Prednisolone (Onapred, Pediapred, Prelone, Gens)	*40mg PO qd; ini dose depending on symptoms*
or	**Opioid** →274 (analgesia)	Tramadol (Ultram)	*Up to 50-100mg PO qid Caution: IA with other psychotropic drugs; with MAOIs severe CNS-AEs*

Intraarticular injections

poss	**Glucocorticoid** →148, →285 (anti-inflammatory, immunosuppressive)	Triamcinolone acetonide (Aristocort, Kenalog) + Lidocaine (Gens)	*Intraarticular Inj: large joint: 10-20mg, middle size joint: 5-10mg, small joint: 2-5mg (max. 2 Inj/y, 3-4wk apart)*

9 B.4.2   Basal Therapy in Mild Courses

Antirheumatic →262 (stabilization of lysosome membrane, influence on BG-metabolism)	Hydroxychloroquine (Plaquenil, Gens)	*Long-term Tx: 200-400mg PO qd (at least 3mo, if successful maint.Tx)*

9 B.4.3   Basal Therapy in Moderately Severe Courses

Antirheumatic – acetic acid derivative →263 (prostaglandin synthesis ↓)	Sulfasalazine (Azulfidine, Azulfidine en-tabs, Gens)	*Wk 1: 500mg PO qd, wk 2: 500mg PO bid, wk 3: 500mg PO tid, wk 4: 500mg PO qid; at least 3mo, if successful, maint.Tx; IA: EF of warfarin, antidiabetics↑, iron absorption↓*
Antibiotic →198 (tetracycline)	Minocycline (Dynacin, Minocin, Vectrin, Gens)	*100mg IV/PO qd*

9 B.4.4   Basal Therapy in Severe Courses

	Immunosuppressant →263 (cytokine synthesis ↓)	Methotrexate (Folex, Rheumatrex, Gens)	*7.5-20mg/wk PO, incr up to 25mg/wk prn as SC Inj*
In intolerance plus			
	Vitamin →147	Folic acid (Folicet, Gens)	*1mg PO qd*
In CI against methotrexate and failure with other basal therapeutics			
1st choice	**Disease-modifiying antirheumatic** →263 (inhibition of T-cell pyrimidine biosynthesis ⇒ immunomodulation)	Leflunomide (Arava)	*d1-3: 100mg, from d4 10-20mg qd (at least 4-6wk until results, then maint Tx); no simultan. live vaccination*
2nd choice	(monoclonal Ab against TNFα)	Infliximab (Remicade)	*3mg/kg IV over 2h, poss rep at 2wk, 6wk, then q8wk*
or	(soluble TNFα-Receptor)	Etanercept (Enbrel)	*25mg SC biw*
or	(IL1 Receptor antagonist)	Anakinra (Kineret)	*100mg SC qd*

9 B.5   Ankylosing Spondylitis

9 B.5.1   Symptomatic Therapy (Acute Episode)

NSAID →266 (inhibits cyclooxygenase → prostaglandins ↓ ⇒ anti-inflammatory, analgesic, antipyretic)	Indomethacin (Indocin SR, Indocin, Gens) **Other NSAIDs**	*25-50mg PO bid-tid, 75mg (SR) PO qd-bid, 50-100mg PR qd-bid*

9 B.5.2   Peripheral Joint Involvement

poss	**Antirheumatic – acetic acid derivative** →263 (prostaglandin synthesis ↓)	Sulfasalazine (Azulfidine, Azulfidine en-tabs, Gens)	*Wk 1: 500mg PO qd, wk 2: 500mg PO bid, wk 3: 500mg PO tid, wk 4: 500mg PO qid*
poss	**Glucocorticoid** →148 (anti-inflammatory, immunosuppressive)	Prednisone (Deltasone, Meticorten, Gens)	*40mg PO qd (ini dose depending on symptoms)*
poss	**Immunosuppressant** →263 (cytokine synthesis ↓)	Methotrexate (Folex, Rheumatrex, Gens)	*7.5-20mg/wk PO*

In intolerance plus

	Vitamin →147	Folic acid (Gens)	*1mg qd*

9 B.5.3   Involvement of the Axial Skeleton

Clinical studies

	Disease-modifiying antirheumatic →263 (monoclonal Ab against TNFα)	Infliximab (Remicade)	*3-5mg/kg IV over 2h, rep at 2wk, 6wk and then q8wk*
	Disease-modifiying antirheumatic →263 (soluble TNFα-Receptor)	Etanercept (Enbrel)	*25mg SC biw*

9 B.6   Reactive Arthritis, Reiter's Syndrome

9 B.6.1   Symptomatic Therapy (acute episode)

	NSAID →266 (inhibits cyclooxygenase ⇒ prostaglandins ↓ ⇒ anti-inflammatory, analgesic, antipyretic)	Indomethacin (Indocin SR, Indocin, Indo-lemmon, Indomethagan, Gens) **Other NSAIDs**	*25-50mg PO bid-tid, 75mg (SR) PO qd-bid, 50-100mg PR qd-bid*
poss	**Glucocorticoid** →148 (anti-inflammatory, immunosuppressive)	Prednisone (Deltasone, Meticorten, Gens)	*40mg PO qd (ini dose depending on symptoms)*

9 B.6.2   Chronic Course

poss	**Antirheumatic – acetic acid derivative** →263 (prostaglandin synthesis ↓)	Sulfasalazine (Azulfidine, Azulfidine en-tabs, Gens)	*Wk 1: 500mg PO qd, wk 2: 500mg bid, wk 3: 500mg tid, wk 4: 500mg qid (at least 3mo)*
poss	**Immunosuppressant** →263 (cytokine synthesis ↓)	Methotrexate (Folex, Rheumatrex, Gens)	*7.5-20mg/wk PO*

In intolerance plus

	Vitamin →147	Folic acid (Gens)	*1mg qd PO qd*

9 B.6.3 Enteropathic Form

Chlamydia, Mykoplasma

Tetracycline →198 (antibiosis)	Doxycycline (Doryx, Vibramycin, Gens)	*100mg PO qd; IA: milk + antacid resorbtion↓, safety of contracept.↓, EF of digoxin ↑*

Yersinia

Fluoroquinolone →203 (antibiosis)	Ciprofloxacin (Cipro)	*250-750mg PO bid*
IA with NSAIDs: spasmophilia ↑, half-life of diazepam ↑		

9 B.7 Psoriatic Arthritis
9 B.7.1 Symptomatic

NSAID →266 (inhibits cyclooxygenase ⇒ prostaglandins ↓ ⇒ anti-inflammatory, analgesic, antipyretic)	Indomethacin (Indocin SR, Indocin, Gens)	*25-50mg PO bid-tid, 75mg (SR) PO qd-bid, 50-100mg PR qd-bid*

9 B.7.2 Basal Therapy

poss	**Antirheumatic – acetic acid derivative** →263 (prostaglandin synthesis ↓)	Sulfasalazine (Azulfidine, Azulfidine en-tabs, Gens)	*Wk 1: 500mg PO qd, wk 2: 500mg bid, wk 3: 500mg tid, wk 4: 500mg qid (at least 3mo)*
or poss	**Immunosuppressan** →263t (cytokine synthesis ↓)	Methotrexate (Folex, Rheumatrex, Gens)	*7.5-20mg/wk PO*

In intolerance plus

Vitamin →147	Folic acid (Gens)	*1mg PO qd*

9 B.8 Systemic Lupus Erythematosus
9 B.8.1 In Skin Involvement

poss	**NSAID** →266 (inhibits cyclooxygenase ⇒ prostaglandins ↓ ⇒ anti-inflammatory, analgesic)	Diclofenac (Voltaren, Voltaren-XR, Gens)	*50mg PO/PR qd-tid, 100mg (SR) PO qd or 75mg IM qd*
		Any NSAID	
poss	**Antirheumatic** →262 (stabilization of lysosome membrane)	Hydroxychloroquine (Plaquenil, Gens)	*200mg PO bid*
poss	**Glucocorticoid** (anti-inflamm., immunosupp.)	Prednisone (Deltasone, Meticorten, Gens)	*1mg/kg PO qd (ini dose depending on symptoms)*

9 B.8.2 Slight Visceral Involvement (Pleuritis, Pericarditis)

poss	**NSAID** →266 (inhibits cyclooxygenase ⇒ prostaglandins ↓ ⇒ anti-inflammatory, analgesic)	Diclofenac (Voltaren, Voltaren-XR, Gens)	*50mg PO bid-tid or 100mg PO qd*

poss	**Glucocorticoid** →148 (anti-inflammatory, immunosuppressive)	Prednisolone (Onapred, Pediapred, Prelone, Gens)	*1mg/kg PO qd (ini dose depending on symptoms, red slowly)*
poss	**Antirheumatic** →262 (stabilization of lysosome membrane)	Hydroxychloroquine (Plaquenil, Gens)	*Long-term Tx: 200mg PO bid*

9 B.8.3　Severe Visceral Involvement (Lupus Nephritis, Myocarditis)

Tx of choice	**Alkylating agent** (immunosuppression)	Cyclophosphamide (Cytoxan, Neosar)	*0.5-1g/m² q4wk IV, or 2-4mg/kg PO qd*
plus	**Acrolein neutralisation** (reacts with urotoxic metabolites of cyclophosphamide ⇒ cystitis PRO)	Mesna (Uromitexan, Mesnex)	*200-400mg IV before, 4h after + 8h after cyclophosphamide Inf (prn, in most patients not needed)*
poss	**Glucocorticoid** →148 (anti-inflamm., immunosup.)	Prednisone (Deltasone, Meticorten, Gens)	*1mg/kg, red slowly*
poss	**Immunosuppressant** →260 (cytokine synthesis ↓)	Cyclosporine (Neoral, Sandimmune, Gens)	*1-3mg/kg/d PO (not in combination with cyclophosphamide)*

9 B.9　Progressive Systemic Sclerosis
9 B.9.1　In Skin Involvement

poss	**Immunosuppressant**, →263 (cytokine synthesis ↓)	Methotrexate (Folex, Rheumatrex, Gens)	*7.5-20mg/wk PO/IM*
poss		Cyclosporine (Neoral, Sandimmune, Gens)	*3mg/kg/d PO div bid*

No proven effective Tx! No influence on organic changes.

9 B.9.2　In Pulmonary Involvement

	Alkylating agent (immunosuppression)	Cyclophosphamide (Cytoxan, Neosar)	*2-4mg/kg qd or 500-1000mg/ m² IV q4wk*

9 B.9.3　In Pulmonary Hypertension

	Direct vasodilator →31 (prostaglandin-I2- analogue)	Epoprostenol (Flolan)	*2ng/kg/min constant IV Inf with initial ICU monitoring*
	Endothelin-1 receptor antagonist →32	Bosentan (Tracleer)	*62.5mg PO bid for 4wk, then 125mg bid*

Do right coronary catheter to test effectiveness before administration

9 B.10　Temporal Arteritis

	Glucocorticoid →148 (anti-inflammatory, immunosuppressive)	Prednisone (Deltasone, Meticorten, Gens)	*Ini 60mg PO qd until results, then taper over 2-3mo until < 10mg/d, then red by 1mg/d q4-8wk; in loss of vision pulse Tx: 1g IV for 3d (maint. for 6-12 mo)*

9 B.11 Polymyalgia Rheumatica

	Glucocorticoid →148 (anti-inflammatory, immunosuppressive)	Prednisone (Deltasone, Meticorten, Gens)	*Ini 10-20mg qd, then taper slowly over 8-12mo*

9 B.12 Panarteritis Nodosa
9 B.12.1 Slight

poss	**Glucocorticoid** →148 (anti-inflammatory, immunosuppressive)	Prednisone (Deltasone, Meticorten, Gens)	*Ini 40mg PO qd, red by 10mg q5d to 20mg qd, then red by 5mg q3-4wk*

9 B.12.2 Severe (Systemic Involvement)

	Glucocorticoid →148 (anti-inflammatory, immunosuppressive)	Prednisolone (Onapred, Pediapred, Prelone, Gens)	*1mg/kg PO qd (ini dose depending on symptoms, red slowly)*
	Alkylating agent (immunosuppression)	Cyclophosphamide (Cytoxan, Neosar)	*0.5g/m^{2}q 3-4wk IV or 2-4mg/kg qd PO*
plus	**Acrolein neutralisation** (reacts with urotoxic metab. of cyclophos. ⇒ cystitis PRO)	Mesna (Uromitexan, Mesnex)	*200-400mg IV before, 4h after + 8h after cycloph. Inf (prn)*

9 B.13 Wegener's Granulomatosis
9 B.13.1 Localized Initial Stage

poss rarely ind	**Antibiotic** →206 (folate antagonist + p-aminobenzoic acid antagonist)	Sulfamethoxazole + Trimethoprim (Bactrim, Septra, Sulfamethoprim, Sulfatrim, Gens)	*160+800mg PO bid; IA: EF of anticoagulants, antidiabetics, phenytoin, MTX, thiazides↑ ; risk of thrombopenia↑*

9 B.13.2 Generalized Stage

	Glucocorticoid →148 (anti-inflammatory, immunosuppressive)	Prednisolone (Onapred, Pediapred, Prelone, Gens)	*1-2mg/kg PO qd q1-2wk red by 10mg to 20mg qd, then red by 5mg q2-3wk; poss pulse Tx: 500-1000mg for 3d IV*
	Alkylating agent (immunosuppression)	Cyclophosphamide (Cytoxan, Neosar)	*0.5-1g/m^2/3-4wk IV or 2-4mg/kg PO qd*
plus	**Acrolein neutralisation** (reacts with urotoxic metabolites of cycloph. ⇒ cystitis PRO)	Mesna (Uromitexan, Mesnex)	*200-400mg IV before, 4h after + 8h after cycloph. Inf (prn, in most patients not needed)*

9 B.14 Sjögren's Syndrome

	Film builder (artificial tears)	Hypromellose 5% (Ocucoat)	*Apply prn*
	Epithelializing agent (corneal protection/care)	Dexpanthenol (Bepanthen, Panthenol)	*Apply bid-qid*
	Salivary stimulant	Cevimeline (Evoxac)	*30mg tid*

10 A. Anesthetics – Drugs

10 A.1 Intravenous Anesthetics and Sedatives

10 A.1.1 Barbiturates

MA (methohexital): short-acting barbiturate, hypnotic, no analgesia
MA (thiopental): barbiturate, hypnotic, anticonvulsive, decrease of intracranial pressure
AE (methohexital): BP↓, resp. depression, bronchospasm, excitation, confusion, lethargy
AE (thiopental): BP↓↓, resp. depression, bronchospasm, hemolytic anemia, vasodilation, intracranial pressure changes, hepatotoxicity, erythema
CI (methohexital): patients with contraindications to general anesthesia, porphyria, hypersensitivity to barbiturates
CI (thiopental): shock, status asthmaticus, intoxications, porphyria, severe CVS disease, hypersensitivity to thiopental products/barbiturate

Methohexital	EHL 3.9 +/- 2.1h, PRC B, Lact ?
Brevital Sodium *Inj 500mg/vial, 2.5g/vial, 5g/vial*	**Anesthesia induction**: 1-1.5mg/kg IV, maint 20-40mg q4-7min prn

Thiopental	EHL 3-18h, PRC
Pentothal *Inj (Sol) 250mg, 400mg, 500mg, Inj (Powder) 500mg/vial, 1g/vial, 5g/vial*	**Anesthesia induction**: 3-5mg/kg IV convulsive state: 75-125mg IV; **CH** 1-12y: **anesthesia induction**: 5-6mg/kg IV; DARF: GFR (ml/min) >10: 100%, <10: 75%

10 A.1.2 Benzodiazepines

MA/EF: opening of chloride channels ⇒ inhibiting function of GABA neurons↑, especially in the limbic system ⇒ sedative, sleep inducing, anxiolytic, muscle relaxing; **AE** (midazolam): amnesia, N/V, respiratory depression; **CI** (midazolam): acute narrow angle glaucoma, hypersensitivity to midazolam products

Midazolam	EHL 2-5h, PRC D, Lact ?
Versed *Inj 1mg/ml, 5mg/ml* **Generics** *Inj 1mg/ml, 5mg/ml*	**Anesthesia induction**: 0.15-0.35mg/kg IV; **sedation**: 0.05-0.1mg/kg IV, maint. 0.02-0.1mg/kg/h; **CH** 0.5-5y: **sedation**: 0.05-0.1mg/kg IV; **CH** 6-12y: **sedation**: 0.025-0.05mg/kg IV; DARF: GFR (ml/min): >10: 100%, <10: 50%

10 A.1.3 Opioids

MA/EF: stimulation of central opiate receptors ⇒ analgesic, sedative
AE (alfentanil): muscle rigidity, arrhythmias, dizziness, N/V, apnea
AE (fentanyl): respiratory depression, muscle rigidity, N/V, urinary retention, sedation
AE (remifentanil): hypotension, bradycardia, N/V
AE (sufentanil): respiratory depression, N/V, skeletal muscle rigidity, HTN, drowsiness, urinary retention
CI (alfentanil, fentanyl, remifentanil, sufentanil): hypersensitivity to product ingredients/opioid agonists

Alfentanil	EHL 90-111min, PRC C, Lact ?
Alfenta *Inj 0.5mg/ml* **Generics** *Inj 0.5mg/ml*	**Anesthesia**: individualized according to type and duration of surgical procedure/anesthesia; 8-75µg/kg IV, maint 0.5-3µg/kg/min according to duration of surgical procedure

Fentanyl — EHL 2-7h, PRC C, Lact ?
Sublimaze *Inj 0.05mg/ml*
Generics *Inj 0.05mg/ml*
Pain →302: 50-100µg IV/IM q1-2h prn; **anesthesia adjunct**: 2-50µg/kg IV

Remifentanil — EHL 3-10min, PRC C, Lact ?
Ultiva *Inj 1mg/vial, 2mg/vial, 5mg/vial*
Anesthesia induction: 0.5-1µg/kg/min IV, maint 0.05-2µg/kg/min; DARF not req

Sufentanil — EHL 158-164min, PRC C, Lact ?
Sufenta *Inj 0.05mg/ml*
Generics *Inj 0.05mg/ml*
Analgesic adjunct: 1-8µg/kg IV; **anesthesia**: 8-30µg/kg IV, then 10-50µg prn; **CH** < 12y: **anesthesia**: 10-25µg/kg IV, then 25-50µg prn

10 A.1.4 Etomidate

EF: hypnotic for induction of anesthesia, no analgesia
AE: resp. depression, myoclonia, N/V, emergence psychoses, injection site pain
CI: children < 6y, hypersensitivity to etomidate products

Etomidate — EHL 2.6-3.5h, PRC C, Lact ?
Amidate *Inj 2mg/ml*
Anesthesia: ini 0.3mg/kg IV, maint 10-20µg/kg/min

10 A.1.5 Ketamine

EF: analgesic, hypnotic without considerable respiratory depression
AE: BP ↑, tachycardia, intracranial pressure ↑, hypersalivation, unpleasant/vivid dreams, muscle hyperactivity, N/V
CI: severe HTN, pre-eclampsia, intracranial pressure ↑ without adequate artificial respiration, hypersensitivity to ketamine products, conditions where HTN is hazardous

Ketamine — EHL 2-3h, PRC D, Lact -
Ketalar *Inj 10mg/ml, 50mg/ml, 100mg/ml*
Generics *Inj 50mg/ml, 100mg/ml*
Anesthesia: 1-2mg/kg IV; 5-10mg/kg IM; maint. 0.1-0.5mg/min IV; **sedation, analgesia**: 0.2-0.75mg/kg IV, maint 5-20µg/kg/min, **CH anesthesia**: 1-2mg/kg IV; 5-10mg/kg IM; maint 0.01-0.03mg/kg/min IV; **CH sedation, analgesia**: 0.2-1mg/kg IV maint 5-20µg/kg/min

10 A.1.6 Propofol

MA/EF: hypnotic for induction and maintenance of anesthesia, no analgesia
AE: BP ↑, respiratory depression, bradycardia, seizures, adrenal suppression, apnea, injection site pain, cardiac arrest
CI: decompensated cardiac insufficiency, ch < 3y, hypersensitivity to propofol products

Propofol — EHL 40-200min, PRC B, Lact ?
Diprivan *Inj 10mg/ml*
Generics *Inj 10mg/ml*
Anesthesia induction: 1-2.5mg/kg IV, maint 100-200µg/kg/min IV; **ICU sedation**: 5-50µg/kg/min; **CH > 3y: anesthesia induction**: 2.5-3.5mg/kg IV, maint 125-300µg/kg/min; **sedation**: 1-2mg/kg IV, maint 75-100µg/kg/min; DARF: not req

10 A.2 Neuromuscular Blockers

10 A.2.1 Depolarising Muscle Relaxants

MA/EF: permanent depolarization of the motor endplate, prevention of the immediate repolarization
AE: allergic skin reactions, fasciculations, muscle pain, coronary dysrythmias, bradycardia, hyperkalemia, malignant hyperthermia, IOP ↑
CI: impossibility of artificial respiration, anamnestic malignant hyperthermia, susceptibility to hyperkalemia ↑, acute phase of major trauma/major burns, hypersensitivity to succinylcholine

Succinylcholine	EHL < 1min, PRC C, Lact ?
Anectine *Inj 20mg/ml, 0.5g/vial, 1g/vial* **Quelicin** *Inj 20mg/ml, 50mg/ml, 100mg/ml* **Generics** *Inj 20mg/ml*	**General anesthesia**: ini 0.6mg/kg IV, maint 0.5–10mg/min; **CH general anesthesia**: ini 1–2mg/kg IV; DARF: not req

10 A.2.2 Non-Depolarising Muscle Relaxants

MA/EF: competitive displacement of acetylcholine at the nicotinergic receptors of the motor endplate ⇒ prevention of depolarization; **AE:** bronchospasm, tachycardia, urticaria, hypotension
AE (cisatracurium): bradycardia, flushing; **AE (mivacurium):** flushing; **AE (pancuronium):** HTN, salivation; **AE (rapacuronium):** bradycardia/tachycardia; **AE (rocuronium):** severe pain on injection, HTN; **AE (vecuronium):** brady-/tachycardia, allergic reactions, hypotension; **CI:** impossibility of artificial respiration; caution with myasthenia gravis and Eaton-Lambert-Syndrome; **CI (cisatracurium, mivacurium):** hypersensitivity to cisatracurium/benzylisoquinoliniums; **CI (pancuronium):** hypersensitivity to pancuronium or bromide products; **CI (rapacuronium, rocuronium, vecuronium):** hypersensitivity to product ingredients

Cisatracurium	EHL 22-31min, PRC B, Lact ?
Nimbex *Inj 2mg/ml* **Nimbex preservative free** *Inj 2mg/ml, 10mg/ml*	**General anesthesia**: ini 0.15mg/kg IV maint. 1–2µg/kg/min IV; **ICU long-term use**: 3µg/kg/min IV; **CH 2-12y**: **general anesthesia**: ini 0.1mg/kg IV

Mivacurium	EHL 1.8-2min, PRC C, Lact ?
Mivacron *Inj 2mg/ml* **Mivacron in Dextrose 5%** *Inj 0.5mg/ml*	**General anesthesia**: ini 0.15–0.25mg/kg IV, maint 0.1mg/kg q15min or 4µg/kg/min; **CH 2-12y**: **general anesthesia**: ini 0.2mg/kg IV, maint 0.1mg/kg q10-15min or 10-15µg/kg/min

Pancuronium	EHL 89-140min, PRC C, Lact ?
Pancuronium *Inj 1mg/ml, 2mg/ml* **Pavulon** *Inj 1mg/ml, 2mg/ml* **Generics** *Inj 1mg/ml, 2mg/ml*	**General anesthesia**: 0.06–0.1mg/kg IV, maint 0.01–0.06mg/kg q80-150min; DARF: GFR (ml/min) >10: 100%, <10: not rated

Rapacuronium	EHL 72-175min, PRC C, Lact ?
Raplon *Inj 100mg/vial, 200mg/vial*	**General anesthesia**: ini 1.5mg/kg IV, maint 0.5mg/kg IV prn; **CH 1mo –12y**: **general anesthesia**: ini 2mg/kg IV

Rocuronium	EHL 84-131min, PRC B, Lact ?
Zemuron *Inj 10mg/ml* **Zemuron (p/f)** *Inj 10mg/ml*	**General anesthesia**: ini 600µg/kg IV, maint 75-225µg/kg prn

Vecuronium — EHL 65-80min, PRC C, Lact ?

Norcuron *Inj 10mg/vial, 20mg/vial*
Generics *Inj 10mg/vial; 20mg/vial*

General anesthesia: 0.075-0.1mg/kg IV, maint 0.01-0.015mg/kg, rep q15-40min prn

10 A.3 Local Anesthetics

MA/EF: membrane permeability for cations ↓, especially Na^+ ⇒ excitability of nerve fibers ↓
AE: dizziness, vomiting, drowsiness, convulsions, bradycardia, dysrhythmias, shock
AE (bupivacaine): arterial hypotension, ventricular arrhythmias, CNS excitation
AE (etidocaine): cardiac/respiratory arrest, autonomic deficits, seizures, pain on injection
AE (lidocaine): seizures, drowsiness, tremors, hypotension
AE (mepivacaine): fetal bradycardia, respiratory arrest, seizures, allergic reaction, porphyria
CI (topical anesthetics): severe conduction disturbances, acute decompensated coronary insufficiency, shock, infections around injection site, known allergy
CI (bupivacaine): regional IV anesthesia, paracervical block, shock or myasthenia gravis, hypersensitivity to bupivacaine products
CI (etidocaine): hypersensitivity to etidocaine
CI (lidocaine, mepivacaine): hypersensitivity to product ingredients/amide-type anesthetics

Bupivacaine — EHL no data

Marcaine HCT *Inj 0.25%, 0.5%, 0.75%, Inj (spinal) 0.75%*
Sensorcaine *Inj 0.25%, 0.5%, 0.75%, Inj (spinal) 0.75%*
Generics *Inj 0.25%, 0.5%, 0.75%, Inj (spinal) 0.75%*

Local infiltration: 175mg (0.25% sol.);
complete motor blockade, epidural: 75-150mg (0.5-0.75% sol.);
dental anesthesia: 9-18mg (0.5% sol.)

Etidocaine — EHL 2.5h, PRC B, Lact ?

Duranest *Inj 1%; Inj (with 0.005mg/ml epinephrine Bitartrate) 1%, 1.5%*

Epidural block: 100-300mg (1% sol.)
dental anesthesia: 15-75mg (1.5% sol.)
peripheral nerve block: 50-400mg (1% sol.)

Lidocaine — EHL 1.5-2h, PRC B, Lact +

Otocaine *Inj (with epinephrine) 2%*
Xylocaine *Inj 0.5%, 1%, 1.5%, 2,0%*
Xylocaine (with epinephrine) *Inj 0.5%, 1%, 1.5%, 2,0%*
Generics *Inj 0.5%, 1%, 1.5%, 2,0%, Inj (with epinephrine) 0.5%, 1%, 1.5%, 2,0%*

Caudal anesthesia: 200-300mg (1% sol.)
epidural anesthesia: 250-300mg (1-2% sol.);
arrhythmias →62

Mepivacaine — EHL 1.9-3.2h, PRC C, Lact ?

Carbocaine *Inj 1%, 1.5%, 2%, 3%*
Isocaine HCT *Inj 3%*
Polocaine MPF *Inj 1%, 1.5%, 2%*
Polocaine *Inj 1%, 2%, 3%*
Scandonest plain *Inj 3%*
Generics *Inj 1%, 2%, 3%*

Brachial nerve block: 50-400mg (1-2% sol);
epidural nerve block: 150-300mg (1-2% sol);
local infiltration: up to 400mg (0.5-1% sol.)

11 A. Neurology – Drugs

11 A.1 Anticonvulsants

MA (carbamazepine): repeated stimulation of afferences ⇒ stimulus answer ↓
MA (benzodiazepines; clonazepam, diazepam, lorazepam): opening of chloride channels ⇒ inhibiting function of GABA neurons ↑, especially in the limbic system
MA (fosphenytoin, phenytoin): ion permeability ↓ ⇒ membrane stabilization
MA (lamotrigine): blockage of presynaptic Na^+ channels ⇒ release of excitatory amino acids ↓
MA (phenobarbital): reinforcement of inhibitory effect of GABA in the CNS
MA (oxcarbazepine, topiramate): membrane stabilization by blockage of Na- channels, antagonization of the excitatory effect of glutamate, reinforcement of the inhibitory effect caused by GABA
MA (tiagabine): reuptake of GABA in neurons ↓
MA (valproic acid, vigabatrin): enzymatic breakdown of GABA ↓
EF (benzodiazepines; diazepam, phenobarbital): sedative, sleep inducing, anxiolytic, anti-aggressive, anti-convulsive, muscle relaxing
AE (carbamazepine): headache, dizziness, ataxia, dysopias, cholestatic hepatitis, disturbances of haematopoiesis, bradycardic cardiac arrhythmias, allergic reactions
AE (benzodiazepines; clonazepam, diazepam, lorazepam): tiredness, sleepiness, drowsiness, confusion, paradox reactions, anterograde amnesia, respiratory depression, psychic and physical addiction
AE (fosphenytoin, phenytoin): gingival hyperplasia, hypertrichosis, dizziness, ataxia, complete blood count changes
AE (oxcarbazepine): tiredness, dizziness, headache, nausea, diplopia, hyponatremia, acne, alopecia, exanthema
AE (phenobarbital): tiredness, dizziness, anterograde amnesia, dizziness, ataxia, dysopias, porphyria, N/V, hepatic dysfunction, bradycardia, respiratory depression, skin reactions, complete blood count changes, enzyme ind., addiction
AE (valproic acid): tiredness, tremors, hair loss, hepatic damage, coagul. DO
CI (carbamazepine): AV block, severe hepatic dysfunction, combination with MAO-inhib.
CI (benzos; clonazepam, diazepam, lorazepam): myasthenia gravis, severe hepatic damage, respiratory insufficiency, ataxia
CI (fosphenytoin, phenytoin): AV block II° - III°, sick sinus, cardiac insufficiency
CI (phenobarbital): porphyria, severe hepatic and renal dysfunction, status asthmaticus, respiratory insufficiency
CI (valproic acid): liver diseases in family history, see also: sedatives/barbiturates →330 and sedatives/benzodiazepines →330

Carbamazepine

EHL 12-17h (mult. dose), 25-65h (1x dose), PRC D, Lact +, serum-level (µg/ml): 4-12

Carbatrol *Cap, ext.rel. 100mg, 200mg, 300mg*
Epitol *Tab (chew) 100mg, Tab 200mg*
Mazepine *Tab (chew) 100mg, 200mg, Susp 100mg/ 5ml*
Tegretol *Tab (chew) 100mg, Tab 200mg, Susp 100mg/5ml*
Tegretol-XR *Tab (chew) 100mg, 200mg, 400mg*
Generics *Tab (chew) 100mg, Tab 200mg, Susp 100mg/5ml*

Mania →343: 200mg PO qd-bid, incr by 200mg/d q2-4d, maint 600-1600mg/d, max 2,000-3,000mg/d; **epilepsy** →313: ini 200mg PO bid, incr by 200mg/d qwk div tid-qid or bid (ext.rel.); maint 800-1,200mg/d, max 1,200mg/d, max 1,600mg/d; **CH** >12 y: ini 200mg PO bid, or 100mg PO qid (susp), incr by 200mg/d qwk div tid-qid or bid (ext.rel.), max 1,000mg/d (age 12-15 y), max 1,200mg/d (age >15 y); **CH** 6-12 y: 100mg PO bid or 50mg PO qid (susp), incr by 100mg/d qwk div tid-qid or bid (ext.rel.), 15-30mg/kg/d PO div bid-qid, maint 400-800mg/d, max 1,000mg/d; **CH** <6 y: 10-20mg/kg/d PO div bid-qid, max 35 mg/kg/d; **trigeminal neuralgia** →307: ini 100mg PO bid or 200mg PO qd (ext. rel.) or 50mg PO qid (susp), incr by 200mg/d prn, maint 400-800mg/d, max 1,200mg/d; **migraine PRO** →307: 600mg/d, 10-20mg/kg/d PO div bid; DARF: not req

Clonazepam

EHL 30-40h, PRC C, Lact ?
serum-level (ng/ml): 25-30

Klonopin rapidly disintegrating *Tab (orally disint) 0.125mg, 0.25mg, 0.5mg, 1mg, 2mg*
Klonopin *Tab 0.125mg, 0.25mg, 0.5mg, 1mg, 2mg*
Generics *Tab 0.5mg, 1mg, 2mg*

Epilepsy →312: ini 0.5mg PO tid, incr by 0.5-1mg q3d, max 20mg/d; **CH** <10 y or <30kg: ini 0.01-0.03mg/kg/d (max 0.05mg/kg/d) PO div bid-tid, incr by 0.25- 0.5mg q3d up to 0.1-0.2mg/kg/d div tid, **neuralgias**: 2-4mg/d PO; **anxiety** →345, **panic DO** →345: →330

Diazepam

EHL 22-54h, PRC D, Lact ?

Diastat *Gel (rectal) 2.5mg/0.5ml, 5mg/ml, 10mg/ 2ml, 15mg/3ml, 20mg/4ml*
Diazepam Intensol *Conc (oral) 5mg/ml*
Valium *Tab 2mg, 5mg, 10mg; Inj 5mg/ml*
Generics *Tab 2mg, 5mg, 10mg, Sol (oral) 5mg/5ml; Inj 5mg/ml*

Status epilepticus →311: 5-10mg IV, rep in 10-15min, max 30mg; **CH** 1 mo-5 y: 0.2-0.5mg/kg IV slowly q2-5min to max 5mg, >5 y: 1mg IV slowly q2-5min to max 10mg, rep q2-4h prn; **epilepsy, adj Tx** →312: 2-10mg PO bid-qid; **CH** >6 mo: 1-2.5mg PO tid-qid, <5 y: max 5mg/d, >5 y: max 10mg; **seizure activity** ↑ : 0.2-0.5 mg/kg PR or 14-27kg: 5mg, 28-50kg: 10mg, 51-75kg: 15mg, 76-111kg: 20mg, rep prn in 4-12h, max 20mg/d or **CH** 2-5 y: 0.5 mg/kg PR, 6-11 y: 0.3 mg/kg PR, <12 y: 0.2 mg/kg PR; **alcohol withdrawal** →339: ini 10mg PO tid-qid x 24h, then red to 5mg tid-qid prn; DARF: not req; **muscle spasm** →298, **sedation** →338, **anxiety** →345: →330

Ethosuximide

PRC C, Lact ? serum-level (µg/ml): 40-100

Zarontin *Cap 250mg, Syr 250mg/5ml*
Generics *Syr 250mg/5ml*

Epilepsy →312: 500mg PO qd or div bid, incr by 250mg/d q4-7d, maint 20-30mg/kg/d div qd-bid, max 1.5 g/d; **CH** 3-6 y: 250mg PO qd, incr by 250mg/d q4-7d, maint 20-30mg/kg/d, >6 y: 500mg PO qd, incr by 250mg/d q4-7d, maint 20-30mg/kg/d, max 1.5g/d

Felbamate	EHL 20-23h, PRC C, Lact ? serum-level (μg/ml): 18-83
Felbatol *Tab 400mg, 600mg,* *Susp 600mg/5ml*	**Epilepsy** →312: ini 400mg PO tid, incr by 600mg/d q2wk, max 3,600mg/d; **Lennox-Gastaut syndrome, CH** 2-14 y: ini 15mg/kg/d PO div tid-qid, incr by 15mg/kg/d qwk, max 45mg/kg/d; DARF: sometimes req (no exact data)
Fosphenytoin	EHL (Phenytoin): 12-29h, PRC D, Lact ? serum-level (μg/ml): 10-20
Cerebryx *Inj 50mg mg PE/ml* *(PE = phenytoin equivalents)*	**Status epilepticus** →311: 15-20mg PE/kg IV, max IV rate 100-150mg PE/min; **CH** 15-20mg PE/kg IV at rate <2mg PE/kg/min; **seizure PRO:** 10-20mg PE/kg IM; maint 4-6mg PE/kg/d
Gabapentin	EHL 5-7h, PRC C, Lact ?
Neurontin *Tab 600mg, 800mg,* *Cap 100mg, 300mg, 400mg*	**Epilepsy (adj Tx)** →313: ini 300mg PO tid, incr by 300mg/d q3-5d, maint 300-600mg PO tid, max 3,600mg/d; **CH** >12 y: adult dose; **neuropathic pain:** 300mg PO tid, max 3,600mg/d; **restless leg syndrome:** 300-2,700mg/d PO; **mania** →343: ini 300mg PO hs, titrate to 900-2,400mg/d in div doses; DARF: CrCl(ml/min) 30-60: 300mg PO bid, 15-30: 300mg PO qd, <15: 300mg PO qod
Lamotrigine	EHL 25-30h, PRC C, Lact ?
Lamictal CD *Tab (chew) 5mg, 25mg, 100mg* **Lamictal** *Tab 25mg, 100mg, 150mg, 200mg*	**Epilepsy (adj Tx with valproic acid)** →312: ini 25mg PO qod x 2wk, then 25mg PO qd x 2wk, incr by 25-50mg/d q1-2wk, maint 100-400mg/d div qd-bid, maint with valproic acid alone: 100-200mg/d div qd-bid; **epilepsy (adj Tx with enzyme-inducing antiepileptic drugs):** ini 50mg PO qd x 2wk, then 50mg PO bid x 2wk, incr by 100mg/d q1-2wk, maint 150-250mg PO bid; **Lennox-Gastaut (adj Tx with valproic acid) CH** 2-12 y: ini 0.15mg/kg/d PO div qd-bid x 2wk, then 0.3mg/kg/d PO div qd-bid x 2wk, incr q1-2wk, maint 1-5mg/kg/d, max 200mg/d; **Lennox-Gastaut (adj Tx with enzyme-inducing antiepileptic drugs) CH** 2-12 y: ini 0.6mg/kg/d PO div bid x 2wk, then 1.2mg/kg/d PO div bid x 2wk, incr q1-2wk, maint 5-15mg/kg/d, max 400mg/d; **bipolar depression:** ini 25-50mg PO qd, incr to 100-500mg/d div bid; DARF: reduce maint dose
Levetiracetam	EHL 6-8h, PRC C, Lact ?
Keppra *Tab 250mg, 500mg, 750mg*	**Epilepsy (adj Tx)** →313: ini 500mg PO bid, incr by 1,000mg/d q2wk, max 3,000mg/d; DARF: CrCl (ml/min), 50-80: 500-1,000mg PO bid, 30-50: 250-750mg PO bid, <30: 250-500mg PO bid, endstage RF: 500-1,000mg PO qd

Lorazepam

EHL 10-20h, PRC D, Lact ?

Ativan *Tab 0.5mg, 1mg, 2mg*
Inj 2mg/ml, 4mg/ml
Lorazepam Intensol
Conc (oral) 2mg/ml
Generics *Tab 0.5mg, 1mg, 2mg,*
Sol (oral) 0.5mg/5ml;
Inj 1mg/0.5ml, 2mg/ml, 4mg/ml

Status epilepticus →311: 0.05-0.1mg/kg IV x 2-5min or 4mg IV, rep prn 0.05mg/kg in 5-15min, max single dose 4mg/kg, max 8mg/12h; **anxiety** →345: 0.05mg/kg IV, max IV dose 4mg, max 2mg (preop), ini 1-2mg PO bid-tid, maint 2-6mg/d, max 10mg/d; **insomnia:** 2-4mg PO hs; DA in mild and moderate RF: use lowest effective dose in severe RF: contraind.

Oxcarbazepine

EHL 1-2.5h, metabolites 8-11h, PRC C, Lact ?

Trileptal *Tab 150mg, 300mg, 600mg*

Epilepsy →313, **monotherapy:** ini 300mg PO bid, incr by 300mg/d q3d, maint 1,200mg/d, max 2,400mg/d; **epilepsy, adj:** ini 300mg PO bid, incr by 600mg/d qwk, maint 1,200mg/d, max 2,400mg/d; **CH** 4-16 y: ini 8-10mg/kg/d div bid, max loading dose 600mg/d, maint 900mg/d (20-29kg), 1,200mg/d (29.1-39kg), 1,800mg/d (>39kg); DARF: CrCl (ml/min) <30: reduce ini dose by 50%, titrate carefully

Phenobarbital

EHL 1.5-4.0d, PRC D, Lact -
serum-level(µg/ml): 15-40

Barbita *Tab 16mg*
Eskabarb *Cap 65mg, 97mg*
Hypnette *Tab 16.2mg*
Luminal Sodium *Inj 60, 130mg/ml*
Generics *Tab 15mg, 16.2mg, 30mg, 32.4mg, 60mg, 64.8mg, 97.2mg, 100mg,*
Elixir 20mg/5ml, 30mg/7.5ml,
Inj 65mg/ml, 130mg/ml

Epilepsy →311: 60-250mg/d PO qd or 2-3mg/kg/d; **CH** 1-5 y: 6-8mg/kg/d PO/IV, 6-12 y: 4-6mg/kg/d PO/IV, >12 y: 1-3mg/kg/d IV/PO; **status epilepticus** →311: 15-20mg/kg IV, max IV rate 60mg/min, max 20mg/kg; **sedation** →338: 30-120mg PO qd/bid/tid, max 400mg/d; DARF: not req in mild/moderate RF, reduce in severe RF, no long term use

Phenytoin

EHL 22h, PRC D, Lact +
serum-level (µg/ml): 10-20

Dilantin *Tab (chew) 50mg,*
Cap 30mg, 100mg, Susp 125mg/5ml,
Inj 50mg/ml
Phenytoin Sodium *Cap ext.rel. 100mg*
Inj 50mg/ml
Phenytoin Sodium Prompt *Cap 100mg*
Generics *Cap 100mg, Susp 125mg/5ml,*
Inj 50mg/ml

Epilepsy →311: ini 400mg PO, then 300mg in 2h and 4h, after 1d maint 300mg PO qd (ext.rel.)/div tid; **CH** >6 y: 5mg/kg/d PO div bid-tid, maint 4-8mg/kg/d, max 300mg/d; **status epilepticus** →311: 10-15mg/kg IV, max rate 50mg/min, then 100mg IV/PO q6-8h; **CH** >6 y: 10-20mg/kg IV, max 1-3mg/kg/min, DARF: no loading dose

Primidone

EHL 3.3-7h, metabol. 29-150h, PRC D, Lact ?
serum-level(µg/ml): 5-12

Myidone *Tab 250mg*
Mysoline *Tab 250mg, 50mg*
Susp 250mg/5ml
Generics *Tab 250mg*

Epilepsy →313: 125mg PO qhs, incr x 10d, maint
250mg PO tid-qid, max 2g/d;
CH <8 y: ini 50mg PO qhs x 3d, incr to 50mg PO bid
x 3d, incr to 100mg PO bid x 3d, then incr to maint
125-250mg PO tid or 10-25 mg/kg/d div tid-qid,
CH >8 y: ini 100-125mg PO qhs x 3d, incr to
100-125mg PO bid x 3d, incr to 100-125mg PO x 3d,
incr to maint 250mg tid-qid or 750-1,000mg/kg/d
div tid-qid; **essential tremor:** incr to 250mg PO tid
DARF: GFR (ml/min) >50: dosing q8h, 10-50: dosing
q8-12h, <10: dosing q12-24h

Tiagabine

EHL 7-9h, PRC C, Lact ?

Gabitril *Tab 2mg, 4mg, 12mg, 16mg, 20mg*

Epilepsy, adj Tx →313: 4mg PO qd, incr by 4-8mg
q1wk, max 56mg/d div bid-qid; **CH** 12-18 y: 4mg PO
qd, incr by 4mg q1-2wk, max 32mg/d div bid-qid

Topiramate

EHL 18-24h, PRC C, Lact ?

Topamax Sprinkle *Cap 15mg, 25mg*
Topamax *Tab 25mg, 100mg, 200mg*

Epilepsy, adj Tx →313: ini 50mg PO qhs, incr by
5mg/d qwk, maint 200mg PO bid, max 1,600mg/d;
CH 2-16 y: ini 1-3mg/kg/d (or 25mg/d) PO qhs, incr
by 1-3mg/kg/d q1-2wk up to 5-9mg/kg/d div bid;
DARF: CrCl (ml/min) <70: 50%

Valproic Acid

EHL 6-17h, PRC D, Lact + serum-level
(µg/ml): 50-100 (epilepsy), 25-125 (mania)

Depacon *Inj 100mg/ml*
Depakene *Cap 250mg, Syr 250mg/5ml*
Myproic Acid *Syr 250mg/5ml*
Generics *Cap 250mg, Sol 250mg/5ml,*
Syr 250mg/5ml

Seizures →312: 10-15mg/kg/d PO or IV inf x 60min,
max 20mg/min, incr by 5-10mg/kg/d qwk, max
60mg/kg/d, div doses >250mg/d into bid-qid;
CH >10 y: 10-15mg/kg/d PO or IV inf x 60min, max
20mg/min, incr by 5-10mg/kg/d qwk, max
60mg/kg/d, div doses >250mg/d into bid-qid;
absence seizures →312: 10-24.9kg: 250mg/d,
25-39.9kg: 500mg/d, 40-59.9kg: 750mg/d, 60-
74.9kg: 1,000mg/d, 75-89.9kg: 1,250mg/d, div doses
<250mg/d into bid-qid; **migraine:** →292;
mania: →325

Zonisamide

EHL 63h, PRC C, Lact -
serum-level (µg/ml): 15-40

Zonegran *Cap 100mg*

Epilepsy, adj →313: ini 100mg PO qd x 2wk, then
incr to 200mg PO div bid, then prn q2wk by 100mg
to 300 resp 400mg/d div bid, max 600mg/d;
DARF: slower dosage titration req

11 A.2　Migraine Therapy
11 A.2.1　5-HT$_1$ Agonists

MA/EF: serotonin agonism (5-HT$_1$D-Rec) $\Rightarrow$ vasoconstriction; Tx of migraine attack
AE: heaviness, feeling of pressure, tiredness, dizziness, flush;
CI: hypersensitivity to sumatriptane, ischemic coronary diseases, heart attack, vasospastic angina, M. Raynaud, HTN, not with (dihydro-)ergotamine

Almotriptan	EHL 3-4h, PRC C, Lact ?
Axert *Tab 6.25mg, 12.5mg*	**Migraine Tx** →306: 6.25-12.5 mg PO, rep prn after 2h, max 2 doses/24h; DARF: ini 6.25mg, max 12.5mg/24h
Eletriptan	EHL 4h, PRC C, Lact ?
Relpax *Tab 20mg, 40mg*	**Migraine Tx** →306: 20-40mg PO, rep prn in 2h, max 80mg/24h
Frovatriptan	EHL 26h
Frova *Tab 2.5mg*	**Migraine Tx** →306: 2.5 mg PO, rep prn q2h, max 7.5mg/24h; DARF: not req
Naratriptan	EHL 5-8h, PRC C, Lact ?
Amerge *Tab 1mg, 2.5mg*	**Migraine Tx** →306: 1-2.5mg PO, rep prn in 4h, max 5mg/24h; >4 Tx/mo not established; DARF: CrCl (ml/min) <15: contraind., mild RF: max 2.5mg/d, reduce ini dose
Rizatriptan	EHL 2-3h, PRC C, Lact ?
Maxalt *Tab 5mg, 10mg* **Maxalt-MLT** *Tab (orally disint) 5mg, 10mg*	**Migraine Tx** →306: 5-10mg PO, rep prn in 2h, max 30mg/24h, >4 Tx/mo not established, under propranolol Tx max 5mg PO tid
Sumatriptan	EHL 2h, PRC C, Lact -
Imitrex *Tab 25mg, 50mg, Spray (nasal) 5mg/Spray, 10mg/Spray, 20mg/Spray* *Inj 6mg/0.5ml*	**Migraine Tx** →306: 6mg SC, rep prn in 1h, max 12mg/d or 25mg PO, rep q2h 25-100mg, max 200mg (if 1st dose was SC), max 300mg/d (if 1st dose was PO) or 5-20mg intranasally, rep prn q2h, max 4mg/d, >4 Tx/mo not established; **cluster headache** →306: 6mg SC, rep. prn in 1h, max 12mg/d
Zolmitriptan	EHL 2.5-3h, PRC C, Lact ?
Zomig *Tab 2.5mg 5mg* **Zomig ZMT** *Tab (orally disint) 2.5mg*	**Migraine Tx** →306: 1.25-2.5 mg PO, rep prn q2h, max 10mg/24h; DARF: not req

11 A.2.2　Ergot Derivates

MA/EF (dihydroergotamine): stimulation of serotonin rec. $\Rightarrow$ constriction of venous capacity vessels; interval Tx; **MA/EF (ergotamine):** mostly α-receptor agonism $\Rightarrow$ vasoconstriction; migraine attack Tx; **AE (dihydro-, ergotamine):** N/V, peripherally inadequate circulation; **CI (dihydro-, ergotamine):** hypersensitivity to seca alkaloids, severe coronary insufficiency, vascular diseases, severe hepatic dysfunction

Caffeine, Ergotamine	EHL 3-6 (C.), 1.5-2.5h (E.), PRC X, Lact -
Cafergot *Supp 100mg+2mg* **Ercatab** *Tab 100mg+1mg* **Wigraine** *Tab 100mg+1mg*	**Migraine** →306, **cluster headache** →306: ini 2 tab PO, then 1 tab q30min prn, max 6 tab/attack, max 10 tab/wk or max 2 supp/attack, max 5 supp/wk; DARF: contraind.
Dihydroergotamine	EHL 7-9h, PRC X, Lact -
D.H.E. 45 *Inj 1mg/ml* **Migranal** *Spray (nasal) 0.5mg/inh*	**Migraine** →306: 1mg IV/IM/SC, rep prn q1h, max 2mg(IV) or 3mg(IM/SC)/24h or 1 spray (0.5mg) in each nostril, rep in 15min, max 4 sprays (2mg)/24h or 8 sprays (4mg)/wk; DARF: contraind. in severe RF
Methysergide	EHL 45-62min, PRC X, Lact -
Sansert *Tab 2mg*	**Migraine** →306/**cluster headache PRO** →306: ini 2mg PO qd, titrate to 4-8mg/d PO div bid-qid with meals, taper dose x 2-3 wk prior to discontinuation, 3-4 wk of drug-free interval after 6-mo Tx; DARF: contraind.

11 A.2.3 Migraine Therapy – Other Drugs

MA/EF (divalproex, valproic acid): potassium conductance ↑ ⇒ neuronal activity ↓
AE, CI (divalproex, valproic acid) →286

Isometheptene, Dichloralphenazone, Acetaminophen PRC ?, Lact ?	
Midrin *Cap 65mg+100mg+325mg*	**Tension and vascular headache:** 1-2 cap PO q4h, max 8 cap/ d; **migraine** →306: ini 2 cap PO, then 1 cap q1h, max 5 cap/12h; DARF: contraind. in severe RF
Acetaminophen, Aspirin, Caffeine	PRC D, Lact -
Excedrin Extra Strength (Migraine) *Tab 250mg + 250mg + 65mg*	**Migraine** →306: 2 tab PO prn q6h, max 8 tab/d
Divalproex Sodium	EHL 6-17h, PRC D, Lact + serum-level(µg/ml): 70-120
Depakote *Cap (ext.rel) 125mg VAE,* *Tab (ext.rel) 125, 250, 500mg VAE* *(VAE = valproic acid equivalents)*	**Migraine PRO** →306: 250mg PO bid, titrate to max 1,000mg/d; DARF: not req
Valproic Acid	EHL 6-17h, PRC D, Lact + serum-level(µg/ml): 70-120
Depakene *Cap 250mg, Syr 250mg/5ml* **Myproic Acid** *Syr 250mg/5ml* **Generics** *Cap 250mg, Syr 250mg/5ml*	**Migraine PRO** →306: 250mg PO bid, titrate to max 1,000mg/d; DARF: not req; **epilepsy** →312; **mania:** →325

11 A.3 Alzheimer's - Cholinesterase Inhibitors

MA/EF: reversible and noncompetitive inhibition of centrally-active acetylcholinesterase ⇒ concentration of acetylcholine ↑ ⇒ synaptic transmission ↑ ⇒ cognitive function ↑
AE (donepezil, rivastigmine): N/V, diarrhea, anorexia, muscle cramps, insomnia, fatigue, urinary incontinence, psychiatric disturbances, hypotension;
AE (tacrine): LFT ↑, ataxia, dizziness, confusion, insomnia
CI: hypersensitivity to one of the substances or other cholinesterase inhibitors, GI disease, concurrent use of NSAIDs, asthma, obstructive pulmonary disease, sick sinus syndrome, SV cardiac conduction conditions, history of seizures, major surgery
CI (rivastigmine): DM, CVS/pulmonary disease, urogenital tract obstruction, Parkinson's disease (exacerbation), renal/hepatic insufficiency,
CI (tacrine): history of or current liver disease

Donepezil	EHL 70h, PRC C, Lact ?
Aricept *Tab 5mg, 10mg*	**Alzheimer's dementia** →340: ini 5mg PO qhs, incr prn to 10mg PO qhs after 4-6wk, max 10mg/d; DARF: limited data
Galantamine	EHL 7-8h, PRC B, Lact -
Reminyl *Tab 4mg, 8mg, 12mg; Sol (oral) 4mg/ml*	**Alzheimer's dementia** →340: ini 4mg PO bid, incr prn by 4mg q4wk to 8-12mg PO bid, max 32mg/d; DARF: moderate RF: max 16mg/d; severe RF: not rec
Rivastigmine	PRC B, Lact ?
Exelon *Cap 1.5mg, 3mg, 4.5mg, 6mg, Sol (oral) 2mg/ml*	**Alzheimer's dementia** →340: ini 1.5mg PO bid, incr to 3mg PO bid >2wk, prn incr to 4.5mg PO bid up to 6mg PO bid q2wk, max 12mg/d; DARF: not req
Tacrine	EHL 2-4h, PRC C, Lact ?
Cognex *Cap 10mg, 20mg, 30mg, 40mg*	**Alzheimer's dementia** →340: ini 10mg PO qid for 4 wk, incr to 20mg qid, incr by 40mg/d q4wk prn, max 160mg/d; DARF: not req

11 A.4 Parkinsonian Drugs

11 A.4.1 Anticholinergic Parkinsonian Drugs

MA/EF: inhibition of central cholinergic neurons ⇒ plus symptoms rigor and tremor ↓
AE: confusion to psychosis, mydriasis, accommodation disturbances, glaucoma, oral dryness, micturition disturbances, fatigue, tachycardia, thermostatic dysregulation
CI: glaucoma, micturition disturbances, tachyarrhythmia, cognitive impairment; use in patients over 65 only if strictly indicated

Benztropine Mesylate	PRC C, Lact ?
Cogentin *Tab 0.5mg, 1mg, 2mg* *Inj 1mg/ml* **Generics** *Tab 0.5mg, 1mg, 2mg*	**Parkinsonism** →315: ini 0.5-2mg/qhs PO/IM/IV, incr by 0.5mg qwk, max 6mg/d, div qd-qid; **drug-induced extrapyramidal DOm:** 1-4mg PO/IM/IV qd bid, **CH** >3 y: 1-2mg/d IM/IV div qd-bid

Biperiden	EHL 18.4-24.3h, PRC C, Lact ?
Akineton *Tab 2mg*	**Parkinsonism** →315: 2mg PO bid-tid, incr prn to max 16mg/d; **(drug-induced) extrapyramidal DO** →344: 2mg PO qd-tid or 2mg IM/IV q30min prn, max 8mg/24h; **CH** 0.04mg/kg/dose IM, rep prn q30min, max 4 doses/d
Trihexyphenidyl	EHL 3.7h, PRC C, Lact ?
Artane *Tab 2mg, 5mg, Elixir 2mg/5ml* **Tremin** *Tab 2mg, 5mg* **Trihexane** *Tab 2mg, 5mg* **Generics** *Tab 2mg, 5mg, Elixir 2mg/5ml*	**Parkinsonism** →315: ini 1mg PO qd, incr by 2mg/d q3-5d, max 6-10mg/d div tid with meals, postencephalic max 15mg/d div qid with meals; **drug-induced extrapyramidal DO** →344: ini 1mg PO qd, titrate prn in 4-8h to 5-15mg PO/d div qd-qid; DARF: not req

11 A.4.2 COMT Inhibitors

MA/EF: inhibition of catechol-O-methyltransferase (COMT) ⇒ levodopa plasma levels↑ (in combination with levodopa only) ⇒ favorable on all Parkinson symptoms, particularly akinesia and psychic disturbances

Entacapone	EHL 2.4h, PRC C, Lact ?
Comtan *Tab 200mg*	**Parkinsonism, adj** →315: ini 200mg PO with each levodopa/carbidopa dose, max 1,600mg/d (div 8 times/d); DARF: not req
Tolcapone	EHL 1.6-3h, PRC C, Lact ?
Tasmar *Tab 100mg, 200mg*	**Parkinsonism, adj** →315: ini 100mg PO tid, incr prn to 200mg PO tid, max 600mg/d, withdraw drug if no benefits after 3 wk; DARF: caution in severe RF

11 A.4.3 MAO-B-Inhibitors

MA/EF: irreversible inhibition of monoamino oxidase (MAO) with greater affinity for type B; dopamine-catabolism↓; **AE:** nausea, dizziness, abdominal pain, confusion, halluzinations, dyskinesias, dry mouth; **CI:** combination with meperidine

Selegiline	EHL 2h, PRC C, Lact ?
Eldepryl *Cap 5mg* **Generics** *Cap 5mg, Tab 5mg*	**Parkinsonism** →315: 5mg PO bid in combination with levodopa

11 A.4.4 Glutamate Receptor Antagonists (Dopaminergic)

MA: blockage of striatal glutamate receptors → acetylcholine release ↓
EF: influences mainly akinesia and rigor (see also: antiviral drugs)
AE: GI disturbances, nausea, hypersensibility, paranoid psychosis with optical hallucinations; **CI:** states of confusion, epilepsy, severe hepatic dysfunction, RF

Amantadine	EHL 10-14h, PRC C, Lact -
Symmetrel *Tab 100mg, Syr 50mg/5ml* **Generics** *Tab 100mg, Cap 100mg,* *Sol 50mg/5ml, Syr 50mg/5ml*	**Parkinsonism** →315: 100mg PO bid, max 400mg/d; **drug-incuded extrapyramidal DO** →344: 100mg PO bid, max 300mg/d; **PRO and Tx of influenza A infx:** →245; DARF: GFR (ml/min) >50: normal dose q12-24h, 10-50: normal dose q48-72h, <10: normal dose q168h

11 A.4.5 Levodopa (Dopaminergic)

MA/EF: Levodopa (L-Dopa) crosses blood-brain-barrier, is taken up by dopaminergic cells and decarboxylated into dopamine; has a favorable effect on all Parkinson symptoms, particularly akinesia and psychic disturbances. Decarboxylase inhibitors (carbidopa, benserazide, DDI = dopamine decarboxylase inhibitors) do not cross the blood-brain-barrier preventing L-Dopa from being decarboxylated peripherally.
AE: nausea, anorexia, arrhythmias, postural hypotension, nervousness, anxiety, insomnia; in course of treatment hallucinations and paranoia.
Long-term AE: biphasic dystonia ("on-off" phenomenon) with a sudden onset of akinesia ("off", painful muscular cramps) followed by a sudden rebound of drug effect ("on", possibly with so-called peak-of-dose hyperkinesia)
CI: glaucoma, severe psychosis

Levodopa + Carbidopa	EHL 15min (metabol. 15h), PRC C, Lact ? ser.-lev. (µg/ml): 0.3-1.6 (mild), 4-7 (sev. DO)
Sinemet *Tab 100mg+10mg,* *100mg+ 25mg, 250mg+25mg* **Sinemet CR** *Tab ext.rel. 100mg+25mg,* *200mg+50mg* **Generics** *Tab 100mg+10mg, 100mg+25mg,* *250mg+25mg, Tab ext.rel. 100mg+25mg,* *200mg+50mg*	**Parkinsonism** →315: ini 1 Tab (100+25) PO tid, incr by 1 Tab/d q1-2d prn, max 8 Tab/d (800+200mg) or ini 1 Tab (100+10) PO tid-qid, incr by 1 Tab/d q1-2d prn, max 8 Tab/d (800+80mg); higher levodopa doses: 1 Tab (250+25) PO tid-qid, incr by ½-1 Tab q1-2d, max 8 Tab/d (2g+200mg); ext.rel: ini 1 Tab (200+50) PO bid, separate doses >6h, incr prn q3d; max 2g+200mg/d; DARF: not req

11 A.4.6 Dopamine Receptor Agonists (Dopaminergic)

MA/EF: direct dopaminergic agonist; has a favorable effect on all Parkinson symptoms, particularly akinesia and psychic disturbances
AE: CV complications, confusion, paranoid psychosis with optical hallucinations
CI: HTN, coronary heart disease, psychic disturbances, GI ulcer or bleeding

Bromocriptine	EHL 50h, PRC C, Lact -
Parlodel *Cap 2.5mg, 5mg*	**Parkinsonism** →315: 1.25mg PO bid, incr by 2.5mg/d q14-28d, maint 10-40mg/d max 100mg/d; **neuroleptic malignant syndr.:** 2.5- 15mg PO tid; **lactation suppression, acromegaly** →183, **hyperprolactinemia** →183: →158; DARF: not req

Pergolide	EHL 27h, PRC B, Lact ?
Permax *Tab 0.05mg, 0.25mg, 1mg*	**Parkinsonism** →315: 0.05mg PO qd x 2d, incr by 0.1- 0.15mg/d q3d x 12d, then incr by 0.25mg/d q3d, maint 3.5mg/d div tid (plus levodopa 650-1,000mg/d), max 5mg/d; **acromegaly** →183: ini 0.05mg/d PO qd, incr qwk by 0.1mg up to 0.1-1.5mg/d; **hyperprolactinemia** →183: 0.025-0.6 mg/d PO qd
Pramipexole	EHL 8-14h, PRC C, Lact ?
Mirapex *Tab 0.125mg, 0.25mg, 0.5mg, 1mg, 1.5mg*	**Parkinsonism** →315: ini 0.125mg PO tid, incr by 0.125mg/dose qwk, maint 0.5-1.5mg PO tid; DARF: CrCl (ml/min) <15: contraind.
Ropinirole	EHL 6h, PRC C, Lact ?
Requip *Tab 0.25mg, 0.5mg, 1mg, 2mg, 3mg, 4mg, 5mg*	**Parkinsonism** →315: 0.25mg PO tid, incr by 0.25mg PO tid qwk up to 1mg PO tid, prn incr by 0.5mg PO tid qwk up to 3mg PO tid, prn incr by 1mg PO tid qwk, max 24mg/d (8mg tid); DARF:CrCl (ml/min) 30-50: not req

11 A.5 Mannitol

MA: osmotic binding of water in the tubule lumen of the kidney
EF: water excretion ↑ with only a small increase in electrolyte elimination
AE: exsiccation, hypernatremia, volume load; **CI:** cardiac insufficiency, pulmonary edema

Mannitol	EHL 71-100min, PRC C, Lact ?
Osmitrol 5% in water *Inj 5g/100ml* **Osmitrol 10% in water** *Inj 10g/100ml* **Osmitrol 15% in water** *Inj 15g/100ml* **Osmitrol 20% in water** *Inj 20g/100ml* **Resectisol in PICont** *Sol (irrigation) 5g/100ml* **Generics** *Mannitol 5% Inj 5g/100ml* *Mannitol 10% Inj 10g/100ml* *Mannitol 15% Inj 15g/100ml* *Mannitol 20% Inj 20g/100ml* *Mannitol 25% Inj 12.5g/50ml*	**Intracranial HTN:** 0.25g/kg IV x 30-60min, rep q6-8h; **ICP↑, head trauma:** 0.25-1g/kg IV x 20min, rep q4-6h prn; **ICP↑/cerebral edema:** 0.25-1 g/kg/dose IV x 20-30min, then 0.25-0.5 g/kg/dose IV q4-6h prn; **CH** >12 y: 0.25g/kg/dose IV, rep q5min prn, incr dose slowly to 1g/kg/dose prn, max 2g/kg/dose; **acute RF (Tx)** →432: 100g/24h IV as 15%-20% sol; **acute RF (PRO):** 50-100g; **intraoc. pressure:** 1.5-g/kg IV x 30-60min as 15%-20% sol; DARF: contraind. in severe RF

11 A.6 Myasthenia Gravis Drugs – Cholinergics

MA/EF: inhibition (pyridostigmine, neostigmine), binding (edrophonium) of choline esterase ⇒ acetylcholine ↑
AE: muscle spasms, abdominal/urinary cramps, salivation, diarrhea, nausea, bradycardia, miosis
CI: bronchial asthma, iritis, mechanical intestinal/urinary/biliar obstruction, intestinal/urinary/biliar spasms, Parkinsonism, myotonia

Edrophonium
EHL 1.3-2.4h, PRC C, Lact +

Enlon *Inj 10mg/ml*
Reversol *Inj 10mg/ml*
Tensilon *Inj 10mg/ml*
Tensilon preservative free *Inj 10mg/ml*
Generics *Inj 10mg/ml*

Myasthenia gravis diagnosis →319: >34kg: 2mg IV in 15-30sec (test dose), if no reaction occurs in 45sec → 8mg IV; **CH** <34 kg: 1mg IV (test dose), if no reaction occurs in 45sec → 1mg IV q30-45sec, max 5mg; >34 kg: 2mg IV (test dose), if no reaction occurs in 45sec → 1mg IV q30-45sec, max 10mg; **neuromuscular blockade antagonism:** 10mg (1ml) IV slowly x 30-45sec, rep prn, max 40mg; DARF: probably req

Neostigmine
EHL 15-90min, PRC C, Lact +

Prostigmin *Tab 15mg,*
Inj 0.25mg/ml, 0.5mg/ml, 1mg/ml
Generics *Tab 15mg,*
Inj 0.5mg/ml, 1mg/ml

Myasthenia gravis →319: 15-375mg PO qd div tid-qid, average 150mg/d or 0.5mg IM/SC prn; **neuromuscular blockade reversal:** 0.5-2mg IV single shot, rep prn; **urinary retention:** ini 0.5mg SC/IM, after the bladder is emptied, rep 0.5mg SC/IM q3h, max 5 doses

Pyridostigmine
EHL 97min (IV)-200min (oral), PRC C, Lact +

Mestinon *Tab 60mg, Tab ext.rel. 180mg,*
Syr 60mg/5ml, Inj 5mg/ml
Regonol *Inj 5mg/ml*

Myasthenia gravis →319: ini 60mg PO tid, incr slowly, maint 200mg PO tid, or 180mg PO qd/bid (ext.rel.) or 2mg IM/IV q2-3h, max 1,500mg/d; neonates: 5mg PO q4-6h or 0.05-0.15mg/kg IM q4-6h, reduce gradually; **neuromuscular blockade reversal:** 0.1-0.25mg/kg IV bolus; DARF: probably not req

11 A.7 Skeletal Muscle Relaxants

MA/EF (Baclofen): inhibits transmission at spinal level, depresses CNS ⇒ muscle spasms ↓
MA/EF (Carisoprodol, Chlorzoxazone, Cyclobenzaprine, Metaxalone, Methocarbamol): CNS depressant with sedative and skeletal muscle relaxant effect
MA/EF (Dantrolene): acts directly on skeletal muscle
MA/EF (Orphenadrine): atropine-like on cerebral mot. centers, medulla ⇒ muscle spasm ↓
MA/EF (Tizanidine): a2-adrenergic receptor agonist
AE (Baclofen): sedation, drowsiness, nausea, hypotonia
AE (Dantrolene: drowsiness, dizziness, weakness, malaise, fatigue, diarrhea, anorexia, nausea, headache, rash
AE (Carisoprolol, Diazepam): drowsiness, tiredness, sleepiness, confusion, paradox reactions, anterograde amnesia, respiratory depression, psychic and physical addiction
AE (Chlorzoxazone, Cyclobenzaprine): dizziness, drowsiness, lightheadedness, dry mouth
AE (Metaxalone: dizziness, drowsiness, GI irritation, headache, lightheadedness, N/V, nervousness
AE (Methocarbamol): dizziness, drowsiness, lightheadedness, blurred vision, diplopia
AE (Orphenadrine): anticholinergic, dry mouth, urinary hesitancy, blurred vision, mydriasis, drowsiness, headache, weakness, intraocular pressure ↑, palpitation, tachycardia
AE (Tizanidine): drowsiness, dizziness, dry mouth, nausea, GI Disturbances, hypotension
CI (Baclofen): peptic ulcers; **CI** (Carisoprodol): porphyria, hepatic/renal function impairment;
CI (Chlorzoxazone): hepatic/renal function impairment; **CI** (Cyclobenzaprine): arrhythmias, congestive heart failure, hyperthyroidism, after MI; **CI** (Dantrolene): hepatic impairment, acute muscle spasm;
CI (Diazepam): myasthenia gravis, severe hepatic damage, respiratory insufficiency, ataxia; **CI** (Metaxalone): hemolytic anemia, hepatic/severe renal function impairment; **CI** (Methocarbamol): renal function impairment, brain damage, epilepsy; **CI** (Orphenadrine): Achalasia, bladder neck obstruction, duodenal/pyloric obstruction, glaucoma, myasthenia gravis, prostatic hypertrophy, stenosing peptic ulcer
CI (Tizanidine): severe hepatic impairment

Baclofen	EHL 3-6.8h, PRC C, Lact +
Lioresal *Tab 10mg, 20mg, Inj (intrathecal)* *0.05mg/ml, 0.5mg/ml, 2mg/ml* **Generics** *Tab 10mg, 20mg*	**Muscle spasticity** →304: 5mg PO tid; maint 40-80mg/d div tid; 300-800mg/d intrathecal; **CH** 2-7 y: 10-15mg/d PO div tid; max 40mg/d
Carisoprodol	EHL 8h, PRC C, Lact -
Soma *Tab 350mg* **Generics** *Tab 350mg*	**Musculoskeletal DO** →304: 350mg PO qid; DARF: not required
Chlorzoxazone	EHL 1.1h, PRC C, Lact ?
Parafon Forte DSC *Tab 500mg* **Strifon forte DSC** *Tab 500mg* **Generics** *Tab 250mg, 500mg*	**Musculoskeletal pain** →304: 250-750mg PO tid-qid; **CH** 125-500mg PO tid-qid
Cyclobenzaprine	EHL 1-3d, PRC B, Lact ?
Flexeril *Tab 10mg* **Generics** *Tab 10mg*	**Muscle spasm** →304: 10mg PO tid; max 60mg/d, not longer than 2-3wk
Dantrolene	EHL 8.7h, PRC C, Lact ?
Dantrium *Cap 25mg; 50mg; 100mg* *Inj 20mg/vial*	**Spasticity** →304: ini 25mg PO qd; maint 100mg bid-qid; **malignant hyperthermia** →473: 1mg/kg IV, rep.rep. until symptoms subside or to max 10mg/kg; **CH** ini 0.5mg/kg PO bid; maint 0.5-3mg/kg bid-qid

Diazepam	EHL 0.83-2.25d, PRC D, Lact ?
Diastat *Gel (rectal) 2.5mg/0.5ml, 5mg/ml, 10mg/2ml, 15mg/3ml, 20mg/4ml* **Diazepam Intensol** *Conc (or) 5mg/ml* **Valium** *Tab 2mg, 5mg, 10mg* **Generics** *Tab 2mg, 5mg, 10mg, Sol (oral) 5mg/5ml, Inj 5mg/ml*	**Muscle spasm** →304: 2-10mg PO/IM/IV tid-qid; DARF: not required; **sedation** →338, **anxiety** →345: →330; **epilepsy** →311: →286
Metaxalone	EHL 2-3h, PRC C , Lact -
Skelaxin *Tab 400mg*	**Musculoskeletal DO** →304: 800mg PO tid-qid; DARF: contraind. in RF
Methocarbamol	EHL 0.9 - 2 h, PRC C, Lact +
Robaxin *Tab 500mg, 750mg, Inj 100mg/ml* **Generics** *Tab 500mg, 750mg, Inj 100mg/ml*	**Musculoskeletal pain** →304: 750-1500mg PO qid or 1000mg IM/IV tid for 48-72h. maint 1000mg PO qid; DARF contraind. in RF
Orphenadrine	EHL 13.2 - 20.1 h, PRC C, Lact ?
Norflex *Tab ext.rel. 100mg, Inj 30mg/ml* **Generics** *Tab ext.rel. 100mg, Inj 30mg/ml*	**Musculoskeletal pain** →304: 100mg PO bid; 60mg IV/IM bid
Tizanidine	EHL 2.5 h, PRC C, Lact ?
Zanaflex *Tab 2mg, 4mg*	**Muscle spasticity** →304: ini 4mg PO tid, maint 8mg tid; max 36mg/d

11 A.8 Other Neurology Drugs

MA/EF (nimodipine): calcium channel blocker, predominantly arterial vasodilation, but different to other calcium channel blockers, effect on cerebral vessels ↑
MA (riluzole): presynaptic release of glutamic acid ↓, stabilization of inactivated voltage-dependent sodium channels, MA partially unclear
EF (riluzole): anti-convulsant, neuroprotective
AE (nimodipine): hypotension, flush, reflex tachycardia, ankle edema, headache, complete blood count changes, gingival hyperplasia
AE (riluzole): asthenia, transaminase ↑, nausea
CI (nimodipine): shock, hypotension, significant aortic stenosis; heart failure (NYHA III-IV)
CI (riluzole): history of or current neutropenia, liver/renal impairment, HTN, other CNS DO

Glatiramer	PRC B, Lact ?
Copaxone *Inj 20mg/vial*	**Multiple sclerosis** →317: 20mg SC qd
Nimodipine	EHL 8-9h, PRC C, Lact ?
Nimotop *Cap 30mg*	**Subarachnoid hemorrhage** (Hunt/Hess grades I-III): ini < 96h post hemorrhage, 60mg PO q4h x 21d prn, or 0.5µg/kg/min IV (continuous inf) x 7-10d
Riluzole	EHL 12-14h, PRC C, Lact ?
Rilutek *Tab 50mg*	**Amyotrophic lateral sclerosis:** 50mg PO bid; DARF: should be considered (Prod)

11 A.9 Glasgow Coma Scale, Dermatomes

Glasgow Coma Scale (GCS)		
Eye opening	spontaneous	4
	to verbal command	3
	to pain	2
	none	1
Best verbal response	oriented	5
	confused	4
	inappropriate words	3
	incompreh. sounds	2
	none	1
Best motor response	obeys commands	6
	localizes pain	5
	withdraws from pain	4
	flexion to pain	3
	extension to pain	2
	none	1
GCS-Score		3–15

GCS > 8 = Somnolent		
>12	mild	
12–9	moderate	
somnolence: sleepy, easy to wake		
stupor: hypnoid, hard to awake		

GCS < 8 = Unconscious		
8–7	coma grade **I**	light coma
6–5	coma grade **II**	
4	coma grade **III**	deep coma
3	coma grade **IV**	

coma grade I: directed defensive movements, normal tone, no impairment of pupillary and eye movements, vestibulo-ocular reflex (VOR) positive
II: undirected defensive movements, normal to increased tone, light response present, pupils variable
III: undirected movements, increased tone, pupils variable, mostly contracted, unequal, decreased response to light, generalized extension and flexion, unisocoria, path. VOR
IV: No reaction to pain, flabby tone, pupils dilated and fixed, VOR -, craniocaudal loss of brainstem reflexes

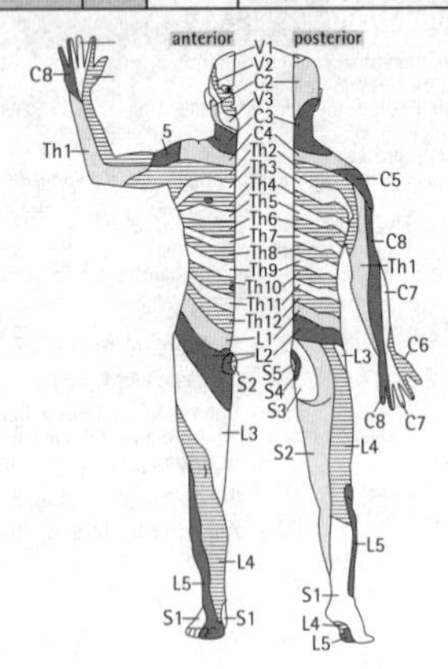

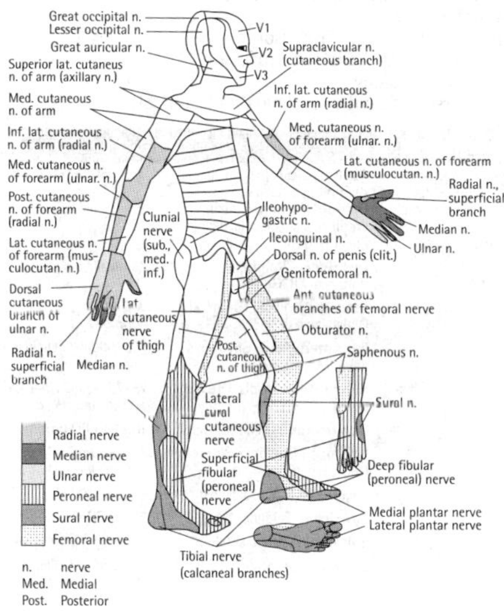
Great occipital n.
Lesser occipital n.
Great auricular n.
Superior lat. cutaneus n. of arm (axillary n.)
Med. cutaneous n. of arm
Inf. lat. cutaneous n. of arm (radial n.)
Med. cutaneous n. of forearm (ulnar. n.)
Post. cutaneous n. of forearm (radial n.)
Lat. cutaneous n. of forearm (musculocutan. n.)
Dorsal cutaneous branch of ulnar n.
Radial n. superficial branch
Median n.
Clunial nerve (sub., med. inf.)
Lat. cutaneous nerve of thigh
V1
V2
V3
Supraclavicular n. (cutaneous branch)
Inf. lat. cutaneous n. of arm (radial n.)
Med. cutaneous n. of forearm (ulnar. n.)
Lat. cutaneous n. of forearm (musculocutan. n.)
Radial n., superficial branch
Median n.
Ulnar n.
Ileohypo-gastric n.
Ileoinguinal n.
Dorsal n. of penis (clit.)
Genitofemoral n.
Ant. cutaneous branches of femoral nerve
Obturator n.
Post. cutaneous n. of thigh
Saphenous n.
Sural n.
Lateral sural cutaneous nerve
Superficial fibular (peroneal) nerve
Deep fibular (peroneal) nerve
Medial plantar nerve
Lateral plantar nerve
Tibial nerve (calcaneal branches)
Radial nerve
Median nerve
Ulnar nerve
Peroneal nerve
Sural nerve
Femoral nerve
n.   nerve
Med.   Medial
Post.   Posterior
lat.   Lateral

11 B. Neurology - Therapies

William R. Tyor, MD, Professor
Timothy D. Carter, MD, Associate Professor
Zoltan Kaliszky, MD
Paul B. Pritchard, III, MD, Professor
Aljoeson Walker, MD, Assistant Professor
Department of Neurology
Medical University of South Carolina, Charleston, SC

11 B.1   Pain Control

A.	NSAID - nonsteroidal anti-inflammatory drug →264 (exact mechanism of action unknown, inhibition of cyclooxygenase and lipoxygenase; reduction of prostaglandin synthesis)	**Aspirin - ASA** (Ascriptin, Asprimox, Bayer Aspirin, Bufferin, Easprin, Ecotrin, Empirin, Genprin, Halfprin, Zorprin, Gens)	*325-650mg PO q4-6h*
		Diclofenac (Voltaren, Voltaren-XR, Gens)	*75mg PO bid*
		Etodolac (Lodine, Lodine XL, Gens)	*200-400mgH PO bid–tid, ext.rel 400mg-1g PO qd*
		Ibuprofen (Advil, Children's advil, Motrin, Gens)	*200-800mg PO tid-qid*
		Ketoprofen (Orudis, Oruvail, Gens)	*25-75mg PO tid–qid, ext.rel 100-200mg PO qd*
		Nabumetone (Relafen, Gens)	*1000mg PO qd/bid*
		Naproxen (Anaprox, Naprelan, Naprosyn, Gens)	*250-500mg PO bid, ext.rel 750-1000mg PO qd*
		Oxaprozin (Daypro, Gens)	*1200mg PO qd*
		Piroxicam (Feldene, Gens)	*20mg PO qd*
		Salsalate (Salflex, Disalcid)	*3000mg PO qd (div q8-12h)*
		Sulindac (Clinoril, Gens)	*150-200mg PO bid*

B.	**Narcotic analgesic – Opioid agonist** →270 (act at opiate receptors)	**Codeine** (Gens)	*15-60mg PO q4-6h, short acting*
		Meperidine (Demerol, Gens)	*50-150mg q3-4h PO/IM/IV; Note: lowers seizure threshold, avoid ext. use*
		Oxycodone (Oxy Contin, Roxicodone)	*5-30mg PO q6h prn, short acting; ext.rel 10-160mg PO q12h, longer acting; note: severe abuse potential*
		Propoxyphene (Darvon, Darvon-N, Dolene, Kesso-gesic, Gens)	*65-100mg PO q4h prn*
		Fentanyl (Actiq/PO, Duragesic patch, Fentanyl Oralet/PO, Sublimaze/Inj, Gens)	*50-100µg IV/IM, typically given prior to OP; transdermal patch with 25, 50, 75 or 100µg/h, change patch q3d, good for chronic use; 1 U PO prn episode, max 4 U/d*
		Morphine sulfate (Astramorph, Avinza, Duramorph, Infumorph, Kadian, MS Contin, MSIR, Numorphan, Oramorph, Roxanol, Gens)	*10-30mg PO q4h, short acting, poor absorption; ext.rel 15-30mg PO q8-12h, longer acting, good for chronic use; 0.1-0.2mg/kg IV/IM/SC up to 15mg q4h*
		Hydromorphone (Dilaudid, Gens)	*2-4mg PO q4-6h, 1-4mg IM,/SC/IV q4-6h; Note: severe abuse potential*
		Methadone (Dolophine, Methadose, Gens)	*2.5-10mg q3-4h PO prn Pain long acting, good for chronic use*
C.	**Narcotic analgesic – Opioid agonist/antagonist** →271 (act at opiate receptors)	**Nalbuphine** (Nubain, Gens)	*10-20mg IV/IM/SC q3-6h*
		Butorphanol (Stadol nasal spray, Gens)	*1 spray q3-4h (=1mg/spray); note: frequently abused drug*

D.	**Narcotic combinations** →272 (short acting narcotic analgesics combined with non–narcotic drugs)	**Hydrocodone 5mg + Acetaminophen 500mg** (Allay, Anexsia, Co-gesic, Hydrocet, Hy-phen, Lorcet, Vicodin, Gens)	*1-2 Tab PO q4-6h prn*
		Hydrocodone 7.5mg + Ibuprofen 200mg (Vicoprofen)	*1-2 Tab PO q4-6h prn*
		Oxycodone/Acetamino–phen 5mg + 325mg (Oxycet, Percocet, Roxicet, Gens) **5mg + 500mg** (Roxilox, Roxicet, Tylox, GensGens)	*1 Tab PO q6h prn*
		Oxycodone 5mg + ASA 325mg (Percodan)	*1 Tab PO q6h prn*
		Propoxyphene 100mg + Acetaminophen 650mg (Darvocet, Gens)	*1 Tab PO q4h prn*
E.	**Tricyclic antidepressant** →320 (inhibit norepinephrine and serotonin reuptake)	**Amitriptyline** (Clavil, Elavil, Endep, Gens)	*Ini 10–25mg PO qhs, incr slowly, usual dose 50-100mg/d*
F.	**Antiepileptic** →286 (in neuropathic pain, see also seizures, →311)	**Gabapentin** (Neurontin)	*Ini 100mg PO tid, incr grad, max 3600mg/d*
		Carbamazepine (Carbatrol, Epitol, Mazepine, Tegretol/-XR, Trileptal, Gens)	*Ini 200mg PO bid, then tid, incr grad, max 1600mg/d; ext.rel 400-600mg PO bid*
		Topiramate (Topamax)	*Ini 10-25mg PO qpm, in wk2 incr to bid, then incr slowly, max 1600mg/d*
G.	**Topical agent** →37 (ionic influx ↓, depolariz. threshold ↑)	**Lidocaine** (Lidoderm)	*Patch topically, max 3 at once up to 12h/d; jelly 2.5-5%, topically as dir.*
H.	**Others** →274	**Tramadol** (Ultram)	*50-100mg PO q4-6h prn*
		Note: red in renal/hepatic impairment or elderly	

Kaliszky, 2003

11 B.2 Lower Back Pain

1.	**NSAID**	**See Pain Control,** →302	
2.	**NSAID, COX-2 inhibitor** →268 (inhibits cyclooxygenase-2 ⇒ prostaglandins ↓ ⇒ anti-inflammatory, analgesic)	**Celecoxib** (Celebrex)	*100-200mg PO qd-bid, max. 400mg/d*
		Rofecoxib (Vioxx)	*12.5-25mg PO qd, max. 25mg/d*

3. Plus	**Centrally acting muscle relaxants** →298	**Baclofen** (Lioresal, Gens)	*Ini 5mg PO tid; max dose 20mg PO qid*
		Carisoprodol (Soma, Gens)	*350mg PO tid–qid; Note: frequently abused!*
		Chlorzoxazone (Parafon Forte, Strifon Forte, Gens)	*Ini 500–750mg PO tid-qid, then decr to 250mg PO tid/qid*
		Cyclobenzaprine (Flexeril, Gens)	*Ini 10mg PO tid, max 60mg/d*
		Metaxalone (Skelaxin)	*800mg PO tid-qid*
		Methocarbamol (Robaxin, Gens)	*For acute pain: 1500mg PO qid, maint 1000mg PO qid or 750mg PO q4h*
		Orphenadrine (Norflex, Gens)	*100mg PO bid; 60mg IV/IM q12h*
		Tizanidine (Zanaflex)	*Ini 4-8mg PO q6-8h, incr according to guideline, max 36mg/d*
	Benzodiazepine →330 (Bind to benzodiazepine receptors, enhance GABA effects)	**Clonazepam** (Klonopin, Gens)	*Ini 0.5mg PO bid; incr up to 3mg PO tid*
		Diazepam (Valium, Gens)	*Ini 2mg PO tid; max 10mg PO tid- qid*
	Note: Use benzodiazepines carefully – frequently abused!		
4.	**Other analgesic** →274 (non narcotic, centrally acting analgesic, similar effect to opioids)	**Tramadol** (Ultram)	*50-100mg PO q4-6h prn; Note: red in renal/hepatic impairment or elderly*
5.	**Tricyclic antidepressant** →320 (norepinephrine and serotonin re uptake inhibition)	**Amitriptyline** (Clavil, Elavil, Endep, Gens)	*Ini 10-25mg PO qhs; grad incr by 25mg, >100mg/d rarely necessary*
	Note: Many different antidepressants are used for neuropathic pain, off-label.		

Important note: In general, avoid the use of narcotic analgesics! For acute relapses may use narcotic analgesics for short periods of time (see pain section, →302).

6.	**Local Tx**: blocks release the substance P and other neuropeptides)		
	Dermatologic agent →359	**Capsaicin** (Zostrix, Gens)	*0.025% cream: apply up to tid-qid locally*

Surgical Interventions: should be determined by an expert in pain Tx:
  Intrathecal Narcotic Pump

Kaliszky, 2003

11 B.3   Cluster Headaches
11 B.3.1   Acute Treatment

	Oxygen inhalation (blood oxygenation)	**Oxygen 100%**	*7 l/min nasal cannula (up to 15min)*
Poss	**Serotonin receptor agonist** →291 (through 5-HT$_1$-receptor ⇒ vasoconstriction)	**Sumatriptan** (Imitrex)	*6mg SC, may rep once/24h (statpak)*
or	**Ergot derivative** →291 (serotonine rec. agonism ⇒ vasoconstriction, pro-inflam. neuropeptide release↓)	**Dihydroergotamine** (D.H.E. 45, Migranal)	*1mg IV or IM qh up to 3mg/d; 2mg nasal spray (5mg both nostrils, rep at 15min)*

11 B.3.2   Prophylaxis in > 1 Attack Daily

	Glucocorticoid →148 (anti-inflammatory)	**Methylprednisolone** (Medrol, Depo-Medrol, Solu-Medrol, Gens)	*40-80mg qd for 5d, then taper quickly, disc in <3wk*
	Calcium channel blocker →29 (affects release of substance P, vasodilation)	**Verapamil** (Calan, Calan SR, Covera-HS, Isoptin, Isoptin SR, Verelan, -PM, Gens)	*80-120mg PO tid-qid, max 480mg/d*
or	**Mood stabilizer** →325 (mechanism of action unclear, alteration of electrical conductivity, arterial relaxation)	**Lithium carbonate** (Eskalith, Eskalith-CR, Lithane, Lithobid, Gens)	*600-900 mg/d PO (div bid-tid), incr to 600-1200 mg/d prn (div bid-qid), max 1800mg/d*
or	**Ergot derivative** →291 (serotonin antagonist with partial agonist activity, cerebral vessel regulation)	**Methysergide** (Sansert)	*Slowly incr to 4-10mg qd; Caution: requires drug holiday for 4 wk every 3-4mo, due to severe AE (fibrosis)*

Walker, 2003

11 B.4   Migraine
11 B.4.1   Acute Treatment

	NSAID – nonsteroidal anti-inflammatory drug →265	**Ibuprofen** (Advil, Advil Migraine, Motrin, Motrin Migraine, Gens)	*200mg PO bid*
		See Lower Back Pain section for **other NSAID**, →304	
	NSAID + Caffeine →292	**Acetaminophen 250mg, Aspirin 250mg + Caffeine 65mg** (Excedrin, Excedrin Migraine)	*2 tab PO prn q6h, max 8 tab/d*
	Isometheptene →292 (sympathomimetic ⇒ constricting dilated cerebral vessels)	**Isometheptene Mucate** (Midrin)	*Ini 2 Cap PO, then 1 Cap/h, max 10 Cap/d (1Cap=65mg)*

Ergot derivative →291 (cerebral vessel regulation)	**Dihydroergotamine** (D.H.E. 45, Migranal)	*2mg PR; 1-2mg IM/IV (Caution: vomiting); 2mg nasal spray/d*
Caution in angina pectoris, myocardial-/cerebral infarct: need 24h between administrations of dihydroergotamine!		
Serotonin receptor agonist →291 (serotonin agonism through 5-HT$_1$-receptor ⇒ vasoconstriction)	**Almotriptan** (Axert)	*6.25-12.5mg PO*
	Frovatriptan (Frova)	*2.5mg PO*
	Naratriptan (Amerge)	*1-2.5mg PO*
	Rizatriptan benzoate (Maxalt, Maxalt-MLT)	*5-10mg PO, max 30mg/d; Caution: under propranolol Tx max 5mg PO tid*
	Sumatriptan (Imitrex)	*25-100mg PO, 6mg SC, 20mg nasal spray*
	Zolmitryptan (Zomig, Zomig ZMT)	*2.5-5mg PO*

Walker, 2003

11 B.4.2 Prophylaxis in > 2 Attacks/mo

Betablocker →23 (vascular tone sympathetic)	**Propranolol** (Inderal, Inderal LA, Gens)	*Ini 60 mg PO qd (div bid, ext.rel qd), titrate prn, max 320 mg/d; long-term admin*
	Timolol (Blocadren, Gens)	*10mg PO bid-tid*
Antiepileptic →286 (GABAergic effects ↑)	**Valproic acid** (Depacon, Depakene, Depakote, Myproic Acid, Gens)	*Ini 125-250 mg/d PO, titrate prn, max 1500 mg/d*
Ergot derivative →291 (serotonin antagonist/ partial agonist ⇒ cranial and peripheral blood vessel constriction)	**Methysergide** (Sansert)	*Slowly incr to 4-10mg qd; Caution: requires drug holiday for 4 wk every 3-4mo, due to severe AE (fibrosis)*

Walker, 2003

11 B.5 Trigeminal Neuralgia

	Anticonvulsive →286 (repeated stimulation of afferences ⇒ increased response to stimuli ↓)	**Carbamazepine** (Carbatrol, Epitol, Mazepine, Tegretol/-XR, Trileptal, Gens)	*Ini 200mg PO tid, incr to max 1200mg/d PO (div 6x/d; after plasma level)*
or	**Anticonvulsive** →286 (ion permeability ↓ ⇒ membrane stabilization)	**Phenytoin** (Dilantin, Gens)	*Slowly incr to 100mg PO tid-5 times/d (after plasma level)*
		Valproic acid (Depacon, Depakene, Depakote, Myproic Acid, Gens)	*Ini 5-10mg/kg incr by 5-10mg/kg/d qwk, max 60mg/kg/d*
		Gabapentin (Neurontin)	*Ini 300mg PO, dose up by 1 Tab over 3d; then incr according to symptoms*

or	**Antipsychotic –** **D$_2$ antagonist** →328 (antagonism at central dopamine receptors)	**Pimozide** (Orap)	*Slowly incr to 4–12mg/d PO; cholinergic AE*
or	**Myotonolytic** →298 (antispastic)	**Baclofen** (Lioresal, Gens)	*10–20mg qid*

Walker, 2003

11 B.6 Cerebrovascular Disease
11 B.6.1 Acute Ischemic Stroke

Thrombolytic Tx

	Intravenous thrombolytic Tx →73 (plasminogen activation ⇒ fibrin proteolysis)	**rt-PA – Alteplase** (Activase I.V.)	*0.9mg/kg, max 90mg, over 60min IV, start with 10% of total dose as IV bolus over 1min; Only to carefully selected patients meeting all in-/ exclusion criteria*

Note: Decision must be made on an individual basis following NINDS guidelines. Patients treated with IV tPA must not receive any other anticoagulant, antiplatelet agent, or thrombolytic for 24h after initial tPA Tx.

	Intraarterial thrombolytic Tx →73 (plasminogen activation ⇒ fibrin proteolysis)	**rt-PA – Alteplase** (Activase I.V.)	

May be useful for carefully selected patients, who are not candidates for IV tPA. At centers with appropriate expertise.

Antiplatelet drug Tx

poss	**Antiplatelet drug** →74 (phosphodiesterase/platelet aggregation-adhesion inhibition)	**Aspirin – ASA** (Ascriptin, Asprimox, Bayer Aspirin, Bufferin, Easprin, Ecotrin, Empirin, Genprin, Halfprin, St. Joseph Pain Reliever, Zorprin, Gens)	*325mg PO qd started within 48h of symptom onset*

For patients who are not candidates for thrombolytic Tx. Has been associated with improved outcome.

	Antiplatelet drug →74 (inhibition of adenosine diphosphate-mediated platelet aggregation)	**Clopidogrel** (Plavix)	*75mg PO qd*
		Ticlopidine (Ticlid)	*250mg PO bid*
	Antiplatelet drug →74 (Dipyridamole: inhibition of cAMP-mediated platelet aggregation)	**Aspirin +** **Dipyridamole-ER** (Aggrenox)	*1 Cap (25+200mg ext.rel) PO bid*

Clopidogrel, Ticlopidine, Dipyridamole for patients with acute stroke who are not candidates for thrombolytic Tx and cannot take ASA

Anticoagulant Tx

poss	**Heparin, unfractionated** →70 (inhibition of thrombin and Factor Xa ⇒ conversion of fibrinogen to fibrin ↓)	**Heparin** (Gens)	*5000 U SC q8-12h, or adj dose based on PTT for IV administered heparin*
	While conclusive evidence regarding its utility is unavailable, many practitioners use dose adjusted IV heparin, especially for stroke of presumed embolic origin or secondary to large artery disease.		

General Measures

- BP monitoring (avoid even relative hypotension)
- Check ECG
- Supplemental O_2 (if hypoxic)
- Normoglycemia
- Normothermia
- Maintain fluid and electrolyte balance
- Evaluate for dysphagia/risk of aspiration
- Avoid indwelling urinary catheters if possible
- Deep venous thrombosis prophylaxis (low dose subcutaneously administered heparin or sequential compression stockings, →68)
- Rehabilitation

These measures are widely recommended and generally thought to reduce the frequency of complications and improve outcome.

11 B.6.2 Stroke Prevention

	Antiplatelet drug →74 (inhibition of platelet aggregation)	**Aspirin - ASA** (Ascriptin, Asprimox, Bayer Aspirin, Bufferin, Easprin, Ecotrin, Empirin, Genprin, Halfprin, Zorprin, Gens)	*50–1300mg PO qd*
		Clopidogrel (Plavix)	*75mg PO qd*
		Ticlopidine (Ticlid, Gens)	*250mg PO bid; Caution: need for monitoring WBC and risk for TTP*
		Aspirin + Dipyridamole-ER (Aggrenox)	*1 Cap (25+200mg ext.rel) PO bid*
	For patients **with atrial fibrillation** and **CI** to anticoagulation, ASA 325 mg qd has shown to decrease the risk of stroke.		
or	**Oral anticoagulant** →72 (inhibition of vitamin K-dependent coagulation factor synthesis)	**Warfarin** (Coumadin)	*Ini 2-5mg PO qd for 2-4d, maint 2-10mg/d PO; adj dose to maint INR 1.4 to 2.8;* **in AF** *adj dose to maint INR 2–3;*
	For patients **with prior stroke, without AF and without prosthetic heart valves** Warfarin has shown to have approximately the same efficacy as ASA. In patients **with atrial fibrillation, without CI to anticoagulation** adjusted dose warfarin has shown to substantially reduce the risk of stroke.		

For Patients with Coronary Artery Disease and Hypercholesterolemia

| **HMG Co–A Reductase Inhibitors** →42 (Statins) | **Simvastatin** (Zocor) | *Ini 10-20mg qd, titrate based on cholesterol levels* |
| | **Pravastatin** (Pravachol) | |

While specific evidence regarding efficacy of other agents in this class is not currently available, many practitioners use other statins in this setting.

For Patients with Carotid Artery Stenosis

Carotid Endarterectomy
- **Symptomatic carotid stenosis**: Patients with > 70% stenosis benefit from carotid endarterectomy compared to medical Tx alone when the surgery is done with low perioperative complication rates.
- **Asymptomatic carotid stenosis:** There is evidence that patients with > 60% asymptomatic carotid stenosis may benefit from endarterectomy when the surgery is done with low perioperative complication rates.

For All Patients

General Measures
- Hypertension control
- Smoking cessation
- Hyperlipidemia Tx (with statins)
- Avoiding heavy alcohol use
- Exercise
- Healthy dietary habits
- Control of diabetes

All of these measures have generally been shown to decr the risk of stroke. While tight control of diabetes has not been shown to decr stroke risk to date, tight control has been shown to decrease many other complications and is appropriate.

Carter, 2003

11 B.7   Meningitis, Encephalitis

*Before the initiation of the antibacterial Tx, consider consultation with an Infectious Disease specialist.

11 B.7.1 In General

Initial therapy (with no pathogen proven)

| | **Cephalosporin – 3rd gen. – nonpseudomonal** →195 (broad spectrum antibiotic – cell wall mucopeptide synthesis↓) | **Ceftriaxone** (Rocephin) | *1–2g IV q12h* |
| or | | **Cefotaxime** (Claforan, Gens) | *2g IV q6-8h (up to q4h)* |

If significant local resistance to Pneumococcus exists

| plus | **Glycopeptide** →198 | **Vancomycin** (Vancocin, Vancoled, Gens) | *1g IV q12h* |

If age > 50yr

| plus | **Aminopenicillin** →189 | **Ampicillin** (Omnipen, Principen, Totacillin, Gens) | *150-200 mg/kg/d IV (div q3-4h)* |

11 B.7.2 In the Immunocompromised

	Aminopenicillin →189	**Ampicillin** (Omnipen, Principen, Totacillin, Gens)	*150-200 mg/kg/d IV (div q3-4h)*
plus	**Cephalosporin – 3rd gen** →195 (broad spectrum antibiotic)	**Ceftazidime** (Ceptaz, Fortaz, Tazicef, Tazidime, Gens)	*2g IV q8h*

11 B.7.3 In Head Trauma, CSF Shunt, Neurosurgery

	Vancomycin →198 (inhibition of cell wall and RNA synthesis)	**Vancomycin** (Vancocin, Vancoled, Gens)	*1g IV q12h*
plus	**Cephalosporin – 3rd gen** →195 (broad spectrum antibiotic)	**Ceftazidime** (Ceptaz, Fortaz, Tazicef, Tazidime, Gens)	*2g IV q8h*

Tx must be modified according to the CSF culture, sensitivity results.

11 B.7.4 In Suspected Tuberculosis (3-Drug Therapy)

	Antimycobacterial →208 (inhibition of lipid and nucleic acid synthesis)	**Isoniazid** (Laniazid, Nydrazid, Gens)	*300mg PO qd (until ruled out)*
plus/or	**Antimycobacterial** →208 (inhibition of DNA-depend. RNA polymerase)	**Rifampin** (Rifadin, Rimactane, Gens)	*600mg PO qd (until ruled out)*
plus/or	**Antimycobacterial** →208 (inhibition of metabolite synthesis)	**Ethambutol** (Myambutol, Gens)	*10-20mg/kg/d (until ruled out)*
plus/or	**Antimycobacterial** →208 (MA unknown)	**Pyrazinamide** (Gens)	*30mg/kg/d (until ruled out)*

Any regimen must use multiple drugs to which M tuberculosis is susceptible. Therapy must be taken regularly and must continue for a period sufficient to resolve the illness.

Tyor, 2003

11 B.8 Seizures

11 B.8.1 Generalized Tonic–Clonic Status Epilepticus

	Antiepileptic, benzodiazepine →286 (GABAergic effect ↑)	**Lorazepam** (Ativan, Gens)	**Adults:** *4mg slowly IV (at 2mg/min), may rep after 10-15min, max 8mg*
plus	**Antiepileptic** →286 (ion permeability ↓, stabilizes Na⁺ channels ⇒ membrane stabilization)	**Phenytoin** (Dilantin, Gens)	**Adults:** *20mg/kg IV, max rate 50mg/min*
		Fosphenytoin (Cerebryx)	**Adults:** *15-20mg PE/kg IV, max IV rate 100-150mg PE/min*

Preferable to use phosphenytoin, a pro-drug of phenytoin (**PE** = phenytoin equivalents); can be given more quickly IV without risk of local infiltration.

11 B.8.2 Prolonged Seizures, Seizure Clusters

Antiepileptic, benzodiazepine →286 (GABAergic effect ↑)	**Diazepam** (Diastat - Gel for rectal admin)	**Adults:** *10-20mg PR qd*

11 B.8.3 Generalized Seizures: Myoclonic

Antiepileptic, benzodiazepine →286 (GABAergic effect ↑)	**Clonazepam** (Klonopin, Gens)	**Adults:** *ini < 1.5mg/d (div tid), incr by 0.5-1.0mg/d until control achieved or AE encountered*
or/plus **Antiepileptic** →286 (GABAergic effect ↑)	**Lamotrigine** (Lamictal)	**>12yr:** *ini 25mg/d, incr qwk, target 500mg/d:* *if pat. premedicated with valproate ini 25mg qod, incr qwk after first 2wk*

Ini dose depends on whether patient already takes valproic acid (VPA), which increases risk of Stevens-Johnson syndrome and toxic epidermal necrolysis.

11 B.8.4 Generalized Seizures: Absence

Antiepileptic, T-calcium channel blocker →286 (T-type Ca^{++} currents ↓)	**Ethosuximide** (Zarontin, Gens)	**>6yr:** *ini 500mg/d, incr by 250mg/d qwk, to 15-40mg/kg/d div qd-bid;* **<6yr:** *ini 10mg/kg/d, incr by 5-10mg/kg/d qwk to 15-40mg/kg/d*
or/plus **Antiepileptic** →286 (blocks Na^+ channels, GABAergic effects ↑)	**Valproic acid** (Depacon, Depakene, Depakote, Myproic Acid, Gens)	**Ped** *ini 10-15mg/kg/d (div bid), incr by 10-15mg/kg/d qwk to 30-60mg/kg/d, according to clinical response / serum levels*

Caution: Cases of fatal hepatic necrosis have been reported in use of valproic acid, with peak incidence < age 2yr; analyze risk/benefit in younger patients!

11 B.8.5 Generalized Seizures: Primarily Generalized Tonic-Clonic Seizures

adjunctive **Antiepileptic, benzodiazepine** →286 (GABAergic effect ↑)	**Clonazepam** (Klonopin, Gens)	**Adults:** *ini < 1.5mg/d (div tid), incr by 0.5-1.0mg/d until control achieved or AE encountered;* **CH <10yr or <30kg**: *ini 0.01-0.03mg/kg/d PO (div bid-tid), incr by 0.25- 0.5mg q3d up to 0.1-0.2mg/kg/d (div tid)*
last resort **Antiepileptic, glutamate modulator** →286 (inhibits NMDA subtype glutamate receptors)	**Felbamate** (Felbatol)	**Adults:** *ini 400mg PO tid, incr by 600mg/d q2wk, max 3,600mg/d;* **Ped** *ini 15mg/kg/d (div tid-qid), incr by 15mg/kg/d qwk, aiming at 45mg/kg/d (div tid-qid)*

Caution: Because of serious, potentially fatal complications of aplastic anemia and hepatotoxicity, use of Felbamate should be limited to patients with severe, uncontrolled seizures who have had an inadequate reponse to previous agents.

Antiepileptic →286 (GABAergic effect↑)	Lamotrigine (Lamictal)	**>12yr:** *ini 25mg/d, incr qwk, target 500mg/d: if pat. premedicated with valproate ini 25mg qod, incr qwk after first 2wk*

Ini dose depends on whether patient already takes valproic acid (VPA), which increases risk of Stevens-Johnson syndrome and toxic epidermal necrolysis.

Antiepileptic →286 (Na⁺ channel blocking, GABAergic effect↑)	Topiramate (Topamax)	**>17yr:** *ini 25-50mg/d. incr by 25-50mg/d qwk, target 400mg/d (div bid); smaller doses may be effective in some cases.*
Antiepileptic →286 (blocks Na⁺ channels, GABAergic effects↑)	Valproic acid (Depacon, Depakene, Depakote, Myproic Acid, Gens)	**Ped** *ini 10-15mg/kg/d (div bid), incr by 10-15mg/kg/d qwk to 30-60mg/kg/d, according to clinical response / serum* **adults:** *ini 250-500mg bid, incr to 1-3g/d, according to clinical response / serum levels*

Caution: Cases of fatal hepatic necrosis have been reported in use of valproic acid, with peak incidence < age 2yr; analyze risk/benefit in younger patients!

11 B.8.6 Partial Seizures, Secondarily Generalized Tonic-Clonic Seizures

Antiepileptic →286 (stabilizes Na⁺ channel)	Carbamazepine (Carbatrol, Epitol, Mazepine, Tegretol/-XR, Trileptal, Gens)	**Adults:** *ini 200mg bid. incr by 200mg/d qwk, target 800-1200mg/d (div tid, ext.rel div bid)*
Antiepileptic, glutamate modulator →286 (inhibits NMDA subtype glutamate receptors)	Felbamate (Felbatol)	**Adults:** *ini 400mg PO tid, incr by 600mg/d q2wk, max 3.6g/d;* **Ped** *ini 15mg/kg/d (div tid-qid), incr by 15mg/kg/d qwk, up to 45mg/kg/d (div tid-qid)*

Caution: Because of serious, potentially fatal complications of aplastic anemia and hepatotoxicity, use of Felbamate should be limited to patients with severe, uncontrolled seizures who have had an inadequate reponse to previous agents.

Antiepileptic →286 (blockade of Na⁺ channels, stabilization of hyperexcited neural membranes)	Oxcarbazepine (Trileptal)	**Adults:** *ini 300mg bid, incr by 600mg/d qwk, maint 1.2g/d, max 2.4g/d.* **Ped** *ini 8-10mg/kg/d (div bid), incr qwk by 10mg/kg/d to 20-45mg/kg/d (div bid).* **CH** *< 8yr may require higher dosage.*
Antiepileptic →286 (MA unknown)	Levetiracetam (Keppra)	**Adults:** *ini 500mg bid, incr prn by 1000mg q2wk, max 3g/d (div bid)*

Antiepileptic →286 (brain GABA concentration ↑)	**Gabapentin** (Neurontin)	**CH 3–12yr:** *ini 10-15mg/kg/d (div tid), incr q3d to 40mg/kg/d for CH 3-4yr and 25-35mg/kg/d for CH 5yr or older.* **CH >12yr, adults:** *ini 300mg tid, taper by 300-400mg/d q5d to max 1800mg; some patients may require higher doses*
Antiepileptic →286 (ion permeability ↓, stabilizes Na⁺ channels ⇒ membrane stabilization)	**Phenytoin** (Dilantin, Gens)	**Adults:** *ini 300mg/d, maint usually 3-5mg/kg/d (div tid, ext.rel. qd), lower in the elderly, use serum levels;* **Ped** *typical maint dose 4-8mg/kg/d*
Antiepileptic →286 (GABAergic effects ↑)	**Primidone** (Myidone, Mysoline, Gens)	**Adults** *ini 50-100mg qhs. grad incr to 5-20mg/kg/d (div tid-qid)* **Ped** *ini 1-2 mg/kg/d, grad incr to 5-20mg/kg/d (div bid-qid)*
Antiepileptic →286 (GABAergic effects ↑)	**Tiagabine** (Gabitril)	*Ini 4mg/d, incr qwk by 4mg, usual maint dose 32-56mg/d (div bid-qid)*
Antiepileptic →286 (Na⁺ channel blocking, GABAergic effect ↑)	**Topiramate** (Topamax)	**Adults >17yr:** *ini 25-50mg/d. incr by 25-50mg/d qwk, target 400mg/d (div bid); smaller doses may be effective in some cases.*
Antiepileptic →286 (blocks Na⁺ channels, GABAergic effects ↑)	**Valproic acid** (Depacon, Depakene, Depakote, Myproic Acid, Gens)	**Ped** *ini 10-15mg/kg/d (div bid), incr by 10-15mg/kg/d qwk to 30-60mg/kg/d, according to clinical response and serum levels;* **Adults:** *ini 250-500mg bid, incr to 1000-3000mg/d, according to clinical response + serum levels*

Caution: Cases of fatal hepatic necrosis have been reported in use of valproic acid, with peak incidence < age 2yr; analyze risk/benefit in younger patients!

Antiepileptic →286 (modulates voltage dependent ion channels)	**Zonisamide** (Zonegram)	**Adults:** *ini 100mg/d, may incr q2wk by 100mg/d (qd or div bid), max 400mg/d*

11 B.8.7 Seizures in Suspected Herpes simplex Type I Infection

Antiviral →211 (DNA polymerase inhibitor, incorporation into viral DNA)	**Acyclovir** (Zovirax)	*10mg/kg IV q8h x 10d*

Antiepileptic →286 (inhibits Na$^+$ and Ca^{++} currents, GABAergic effects↑)	**Topiramate** (Topamax)	*Adults >17yr: Ini 25-50mg/d. incr by 25-50mg/d qwk, target 400mg/d (div bid); smaller doses may be effective in some cases*
Antiepileptic →286 (blocks Na$^+$ channels, GABAergic effects↑)	**Valproic acid** (Depacon, Depakene, Depakote, Myproic Acid, Gens)	*Ini 250-500mg tid, grad incr to 1-3g qd, according to clinical response + serum levels*

Pritchard, 2003

11 B.8.8 Surgical Interventions

Surgical interventions should be determined by an expert Epileptologist.

Vagus Nerve Stimulator

For medically intractable **partial seizures**: in selected patients reduces seizure frequency. Device must be programmed to meet individual needs + tolerance.

Ablative Surgery

For medically intractable **partial seizures**: Removal of the epileptogenic zone including local topectomy, temporal lobectomy, frontal lobectomy, and even hemispherectomy.

Pritchard, 2003

11 B.9 Parkinsonism

11 B.9.1 Parkinsonism in Patients < 50yr

	MAO-B inhibitor →294 (irreversible inhibitor, dopaminergic activity↑)	**Selegiline** (Eldepryl, Gens)	*5mg PO bid; Note: admin 2nd dose at noon to avoid insomnia.*
plus/or	**Indir. dopamine agonist** →295 (glutamate receptor antagonism)	**Amantadine** (Symmetrel, Gens)	*100mg PO bid*
	Mainly if bradykinesia prominent.		
plus/or	**Centrally acting Anticholinergic** →293 (plus symptoms rigor, tremor↓)	**Trihexyphenidyl** (Artane, Tremin, Trihexane, Gens)	*1mg PO bid, max 6-10mg/d*
		Benztropine (Cogentin, Gens)	*0.5mg PO bid, max 4-6mg/d*
	If tremor is prominent.		

Amantadine and the centrally acting Anticholinergics are not commonly used any more.

11 B.9.2 Parkinsonism in Patients 50 – 59yr

1.	**Dopamine agonist** →295 (mainly D2 dopamine receptor stimulation)	**Bromocriptine** (Parlodel)	*Ini 1.25mg PO qhs, usual effective dose 10–30mg/d (div tid), max 100mg/d*
		Pergolide (Permax)	*Ini 0.05mg PO qd, usual effective dose 2–3mg/d (div tid), max 5mg/d*
		Pramipexole (Mirapex)	*Ini 0.125mg PO tid, grad incr to 0.5–1.5mg PO tid*
		Ropinirole (Requip)	*Ini 0.25mg PO tid, grad incr to 1mg PO tid, max 24mg/d*
2.	**MAO–B inhibitor** →294 (irreversible inhibitor, dopaminergic activity ↑)	**Selegiline** (Eldepryl, Gens)	*5mg PO bid; Note: admin 2nd dose at noon to avoid insomnia.*
3.	**Dopamine agonist** →295 (L–Dopa → dopamine in central dopaminerg. cells; Carbidopa inhibits periph. decarbox. of L–Dopa)	**Levodopa + Carbidopa** (Sinemet, Sinemet CR, Gens)	*Ini 25+100mg bid-tid, then incr q1–4d prn, max 200mg/d Carbidopa; ext.rel ini 25+100 – 50+200mg PO bid*
4. poss	**Indirect dopamine agonist** →295 (glutamate receptor antagonism)	**Amantadine** (Symmetrel, Gens)	*100mg PO bid*
	May add for bradykinesia and rigidity.		
5. poss	**Anticholinergic** →293	**Trihexyphenidyl** (Artane, Tremin, Trihexane, Gens)	*1mg PO bid, max 6–10mg/d*
		Benztropine (Cogentin, Gens)	*0.5mg PO bid, max 4–6mg/d*
	May add for persisting tremor.		
6. poss	**COMT Inhibitor** →294 (inhibition of catechol-O-methyltransferase COMT ⇒ levodopa ↑)	**Entacapone** (Comtan)	*200mg PO concomitantly with each Sinemet dose, max 1600mg/d (div 8x/d)*
	May also be added.		

11 B.9.3 Parkinsonism in Patients > 60yr

	Dopamine agonist →295 (L–Dopa → dopamine in central dopaminerg. cells; Carbidopa inhibits periph. decarbox. of L–Dopa)	**Levodopa + Carbidopa** (Sinemet, Sinemet CR, Gens)	*Ini 25+100mg bid-tid, then incr q1–4d prn, max 200mg/d Carbidopa; ext.rel ini 25+100 – 50+200mg PO bid*

plus/or	**Dopamine agonist** →295 (mainly D2 dopamine receptor stimulation)	**Bromocriptine** (Parlodel)	*Ini 1.25mg PO qhs, usual effective dose 10-30mg/d (div tid), max 100mg/d*
		Pergolide (Permax)	*Ini 0.05mg PO qd, usual effective dose 2-3mg/d (div tid), max 5mg/d*
		Pramipexole (Mirapex)	*Ini 0.125mg PO tid, grad incr to 0.5-1.5mg PO tid*
		Ropinirole (Requip)	*Ini 0.25mg PO tid, grad incr to 1mg PO tid, max 24mg/d*

11 B.9.4 Surgical Interventions – Deep Brain Stimulation

Deep brain stimulation should be reserved for special cases, best identified by a Parkinson's disease expert:
- **Pallidum**: For tremor, stiffness, and rigidity
- **Subthalamic nucleas**: For tremor, stiffness, and rigidity
- **Thalamus**: For tremor

Kaliszky, 2003

11 B.10 Multiple Sclerosis
11 B.10.1 Acute Episode (Relapse) Treatment

1.	**Glucocorticoid** →148 (anti-inflammatory, immuno-suppressive)	**Methylprednisolone** (Medrol, Depo-Medrol, Solu-Medrol, Gens)	*1000mg/d IV x 3-7d*
2.		**Prednisone** (Deltasone, Meticorten, Gens)	*Ini 60-80mg PO/d for 3-7d and taper over 8-12d; oral steroid taper with or without IV steroids*

11 B.10.2 Preventive Therapy for Relapsing-Remitting MS

1.	**Beta-Interferon** →212 (many immuno-modulatory effects)	**Interferon Beta-1A** (Avonex)	*30µg (6 M IU) IM qwk*
		Interferon Beta-1A (Rebif)	*44µg (12 M IU) SC tiw*
		Interferon Beta-1B (Betaseron)	*8 M IU (250µg) SC qod*
2.	**Immunomodulator** →299 (many immuno-modulatory effects)	**Glatiramer acetate** (Copaxone)	*20mg SC qd*

11 B.10.3 Preventive Therapy for Secondary Progressive MS

	Antineoplastic antibiotic (DNA-reactive, cytocidal)	**Mitoxantrone** (Novantrone)	*12mg/m² IV q3mo, max total dose 140mg; Caution: needs cardiac, hematological and liver function monitoring.*

or	**Antimetabolite, immunosuppressant** →263 (inhibits dihydrofolate reductase, lymphocyte proliferation↓, cytokine synthesis↓)	**Methotrexate sodium** (Folex, Rheumatrex, Gens)	*2.5mg PO/IM q12h for 3 doses once a week (=7.5mg/wk); based on limited trials*
plus/or	**Beta-Interferon** →212 (many immuno-modulatory effects)	**Interferon Beta-1B** (Betaseron)	*8 M IU (250µg) SC qod*
		Interferon Beta-1A (Avonex)	*30µg (6 M IU) IM qwk*

Conflicting results of trials but probably only effective for secondary progressive form of MS with continued relapses.

Tyor, 2003

11 B.11 Huntington's Chorea

Treatment for movement disorder component

1.	**Neuroleptic** →328 (central dopamine D_2 receptor antagonism)	**Haloperidol** (Haldol)	*0.5-5mg PO bid-tid; Caution: severe AE including Parkinsonism!*
or	**Atypical antipsychotic** →326 (Dopamine D_2 and serotonin 5-HT receptor antagonist)	**Quetiapine** (Seroquel)	*Ini 25mg PO bid, max 150-750mg/d; eye exam q6mo for cataracts!*
		Olanzapine (Zyprexa)	*Ini 5-10mg PO qd, maint 10-15mg/d*
plus/or	**Dopamine depleting agent** →31 (depletes central biogenic monoamine stores)	**Reserpine** (Serpalan, Gens)	*Ini 0.25mg PO bid, max 2-5mg/d; Caution: severe AE including orthostatic hypotension, depression*
plus/or	**Benzodiazepine** →330 (binds to benzodiazepine receptors; enhances GABA effects)	**Clonazepam** (Klonopin, Gens)	*Ini 0.5mg PO bid, incr up to 3mg PO tid prn*
poss	For akinetic/rigid form: - **L-dopa** (see Parkinsonism Tx, →315) - **Bromocriptine** (see Parkinsonism Tx, →315)		

Kaliszky, 2003

11 B.12 Myasthenia Gravis

	Cholinesterase inhibitor ▸297 (⇒ acetylcholine ↑)	**Pyridostigmine** (Mestinon, Gens)	*Titrate individually 30-120mg PO q3-6h; long acting, espec. effective qhs; Caution: monitor for cholinergic excess!*
or	**Glucocorticoid** →148 (anti-inflammatory, immunosuppressive)	**Prednisone** (Deltasone)	*Ini low dose 10-20mg PO qd, monitor closely; incr slowly to 1mg/kg/d*
		Methylprednisolone (Medrol, Depo-Medrol, Solu-Medrol)	*Ini low dose 10-20mg PO qd, monitor closely; incr slowly to 1-1.5mg/kg/d*
	Eventually reduce steroids to lowest possible dose, qod schedule		
or	**Immunosuppressive** →260 (purine antangonist)	**Azathioprine** (Imuran)	*Ini 50mg PO qd, incr up to 2-3mg/kg PO qd*
or	**Immunosuppressive** →260 (inhibition of interleukin-2 activation of T-lymphocytes)	**Cyclosporine** (Gengraf, Neoral, Sandimmune, SangCya, Gens)	*Ini 2.5 mg/kg bid, maint lowest effective dose*
or	**Sugical and intervenous Tx:** - **Elective thymectomy** (remove tumor thymoma) past the age of puberty; long-term clinical improvement - **Plasmapheresis** effective short-term Tx for acute exacerbations; removal of circulating antibodies including autoimmune antibodies responsible for MG; helpful to stabilize and used as prophylaxis qwk, qmo and/or bi-monthly; caution: need to evaluate for IgA deficiency		
or	**Immunotherapy** →258 (MA unknown)	**IV Gamma globulin** (Sandoglobulin IV)	

Patients with myasthenic or cholinergic crisis require intensive care monitored setting/treatment, due to their unpredictable course.

Walker, 2003

12 A. Psychiatry – Drugs

12 A.1 Antidepressants

12 A.1.1 Serotonin-Norepinephrine Reuptake Inhibitors (SNRI) – Tricyclics, Tertiary amines

MA: inhibit reuptake of serotonin and norepinephrine into presynaptic vesicles (primarily serotonine)
AE (SNRIs): oral dryness, acute glaucoma, constipation, micturition disturbances, hypotension, arrhythmia, cardiomyopathy, dizziness, headache, restlessness, insomnia, confusion
AE (amitryptiline): drowsiness, CVS effects, seizures, hypotension, anticholinergic effects
AE (clomipramine): anticholinergic effects, somnolence, tremor, weight gain
AE (doxepin): drowsiness, CVS effects, seizures, anticholinergic effects
AE (imipramine): anticholinergic effects, seizures, weight gain, confusion, CVS effects
AE (trimipramine): sedation, weight gain, anticholinergic effects, seizures
CVS effects
CI (SNRIs): glaucoma, AV block III°, combination with MAO inhibitors or Tryptophan, hypersensitivity to product ingredients/TCAs, recovery period after MI

Amitriptyline	EHL 15h (range 9-25h), PRC D/C, Lact ?
Clavil *Tab 10mg, 25mg, 50mg, 75mg, 100mg, 150mg, Inj 10mg/ml* **Elavil** *Tab 10mg, 25mg, 50mg, 75mg, 100mg, 150mg, Inj 10mg/ml* **Endep** *Conc (oral) 40mg/ml* **Generics** *Tab 10mg, 25mg, 50mg, 75mg, 100mg, 150mg*	**Depression** →341: **outpatient:** ini 75mg/d PO (in div doses), gradually incr prn to max 150mg/d; **inpatient:** ini 100mg/d PO in div doses, gradually incr prn to 200-300mg/d prn; IM: ini 80-120mg IM in 4 div doses; DARF: not req, see Prod Info
Clomipramine	EHL 19-37h (mean 32h), PRC C, Lact +
Anafranil *Cap 25mg, 50mg, 75mg* **Generics** *Cap 25mg, 50mg, 75mg*	**Obsessive compulsive DO** →346: ini 25mg/d PO, gradually incr over 2wk to 100mg/d, then gradually incr prn to max 250mg/d; **CH >10 y + OCD:** ini 25mg/d PO, gradual incr over 2wk prn to max 3mg/kg/d or 100mg/d, then incr prn to max 3mg/kg/d or 200mg/d
Doxepin	EHL 16.8h (range 8-25h), PRC C, Lact -
Sinequan *Cap 10, 25, 50, 75, 100, 150mg, Conc (oral) 10mg/ml* **Generics** *Cap 10, 25, 50, 75, 100, 150mg, Conc (oral) 10mg/ml*	**Depression** →341: individualized doses, gradually incr to 75-150mg/d (outpatients) or 150-300mg/d (inpatients); DARF: probably not req, see Prod Info
Imipramine	EHL 6-18h, PRC D, Lact ?
Tofranil *Tab 10mg, 25mg, 50mg* **Generics** *Tab 10mg, 25mg, 50mg* *Conc (oral) 25mg/ml*	**Depression** →341: inpatients: ini 100mg/d in div doses, gradually incr to 200mg/d prn, further incr prn after 2wk up to 250-300mg/d; outpatients: ini 75mg/d (qd or in div doses) incr prn to max 150-200mg/d; DARF: not req

Trimipramine	EHL 23h, PRC C, Lact ?
Surmontil *Cap 25mg, 50mg,100mg*	**Depression** →341: outpatients: ini 75mg/d PO in div doses, maint 50-150mg/d, max 200mg/d; inpatients: ini 100mg/d in div doses, prn gradually incr to 200mg/d, max 250-300mg/d; adholescents: ini 50mg/d, max 100mg/d

12 A.1.2 SNRI – Tricyclics, Secondary amines

MA: inhibit reuptake of serotonin and norepinephrine, primarily norepinephrine
Note: may cause less anticholinergic side effects than tertiary amines. Orthostatic hypotension, arrythmias. Don't use with MAOIs
AE/CI (SNRIs): see also SNRIs - tricyclics - tertiary amines →320
AE (desipramine): N/V, CVS + anticholinergic effects, sedation, seizures
AE (nortriptyline): sedation, CVS + anticholinergic effects, weight gain, seizures
AE (protriptyline): CVS + anticholinergic effects, restlessness, weight gain, seizures
CI (desipramine, nortriptyline): concomitant use of MAO inhibitors, recovery following myocardial infarction, hypersensitivity to product ingredients or TCAs
CI (protriptyline; additional): administration with cisapride

Desipramine	EHL 14.3-24.7h (average 17.1h), PRC C, Lact ?
Norpramin *Tab 10mg, 25mg, 50mg, 75mg, 100mg, 150mg* **Generics** *Tab 10mg, 25mg, 50mg, 75mg, 100mg, 150mg*	**Depression** →341: ini 25-75mg PO qam, maint 100-200mg qd or div, max. 300mg/d; adolescents: 25-100mg/d, max 150mg/d; DARF: sec Prod Info
Nortriptyline	EHL 15-39h, PRC D, Lact ?
Aventyl HCT *Cap 10mg, 25mg, Sol (oral) 10mg/5ml* **Pamelor** *Cap 10mg, 25mg, 50mg, 75mg, Sol (oral) 10mg/5ml* **Generics** *Cap 10mg, 25mg, 50mg, 75mg, Sol (oral) 10mg/5ml*	**Depression** →341: ini 25-50mg PO qhs, maint 50-150mg/d (qd or div); max 150mg/d; adolescents: 30-50mg/d; DARF: not req
Protriptyline	EHL 54-198h, PRC C, Lact ?
Vivactil *Tab 5mg, 10mg* **Generics** *Tab 5mg, 10mg*	**Depression** →341: ini 15-40mg/d PO, div tid-qid, incr prn to a max of 60mg/d

12 A.1.3 SNRI – Tricyclics/Polycyclics, 2nd Generation

MA: inhibit reuptake of serotonin and norepinephrine, primarily norepinephrine
EF: antidepressant, psychomotor sedation, anxiolytic
AE/CI: see also SNRIs - tricyclics - tertiary amines →320
AE (amoxapine): dizziness/drowsiness, anticholinergic effects, seizures, extrapyramidal effects, CVS effects
AE (maproptiline): vertigo, blurred vision, seizures, drowsiness, urinary retention
CI (amoxapine, maproptiline): hypersensitivity to product ingredients, MAO inhibitors concurrently or within 2wk of therapy, MI (during acute recovery period)

Amoxapine	EHL 8h, PRC C, Lact ?
Asendin, Generics *Tab 25mg, 50mg, 100mg, 150mg*	**Depression** →341: ini 25-50mg PO bid-tid, maint 120-300mg/d, max 400mg/d

Maprotiline | EHL 27-58h (mean 43h), PRC B, Lact ?

Ludiomil *Tab 25mg, 50mg, 75mg*
Generics *Tab 25mg, 50mg, 75mg*

Depression →341: ini 25-75mg PO qd x 2wk, (100-150mg PO qd in severe cases), incr prn by 25mg q2wk, maint 75-150mg/d, max 225mg/d; DARF: not req

12 A.1.4 SNRI - Non-Tricyclic

MA: inhibit reuptake of serotonin and norepinephrine
Note: Decrease dose in renal or hepatic impairment. Monitor for increases in BP. Don't use with MAOIs, caution with cimetidine and haloperidol
AE (venlafaxine): nausea, anorexia, sedation, dizziness
CI (venlafaxine): hypersensitivity to venlafaxine hydrochloride, concomitant use of MAOI

Venlafaxine | EHL 5h, PRC C, Lact ?

Effexor *Tab 25mg, 37.5mg, 50mg, 75mg, 100mg*
Effexor XR *Cap ext.rel. 37.5mg, 75mg, 150mg*

Depression →341: ini 75mg/d PO div bid-tid (Effexor), incr prn by 75mg/d q ≥ 4d, max 375mg/d (in div doses); ext.rel.: ini 37.5-75mg PO qd, incr by 75mg/d q ≥ 4d, max 225mg/d; **generalized anxiety DO** →345: ini 37.5-75mg PO qd (ext. rel.), incr prn by 75mg/d q ≥ 4d, max 225mg/d; DARF: GFR (ml/min) 10-70: 50-75%, <10, hemodialysis: 50%; see Prod Info

12 A.1.5 Norepinephrine-Dopamine Reuptake Inhibitors (NDRI)

MA: inhibits reuptake of norepinephrine, some dopamine
AE: N/V, seizures/tremors, agitation, insomnia, hypersensitivity reactions
CI: seizures, bulimia, anorexia, concomitant MAO inhibitors, hypersensitivity to bupropion products, concomitant use of other bupropion products

Bupropion | EHL 14h (chronic dosing: 21h), PRC B, Lact ?

Wellbutrin *Tab 75mg, 100mg*
Wellbutrin SR *Tab ext.rel. 50mg, 100mg, 150mg*
Generics *Tab 75mg, 100mg*

Depression →341: **ini** 100mg PO bid, after ≥ 3d incr to 300mg/d (div tid) prn; max 150mg/dose, 450mg/d; ext. rel.: ini 150mg PO qam, incr to 150mg bid as early as day 4; max 400mg/d div bid; DARF: is req, see Prod Info

12 A.1.6 Monoamine Oxidase Inhibitors (MAOI)

MA (tranylcypromine): irreversible inhibition of MAO type A and B ⇒ oxidative break-down ↓ ⇒ synaptic conc of epinephrine, noradrenaline, serotonin ↑
EF: antidepressant, mainly psychomotor activation
AE (MAOIs): sudden changes of BP, insomnia, restlessness, dizziness, sexual dysfunction
CI (MAOIs): combination with: other antidepressants, pethidine (= meperidine), levodopa, severe hepatic dysfunction, severe HTN, acute delirium

Isocarboxazid	EHL no data, PRC C, Lact ?
Marplan *Tab 10mg*	**Depression** →341: ini10mg/d PO bid, maint 10-40mg/d, max 60mg/d div bid-qid, caution with doses over 40mg/d
Phenelzine	EHL no data, PRC C, Lact ?
Nardil *Tab 15mg*	**Depression** →341: ini 15mg/d PO tid, usual effective dose 45-90mg/d in div doses; DARF: not req
Tranylcypromine	EHL 1.5-3.5h, PRC C, Lact ?
Parnate *Tab 10mg*	**Depression** →341: ini 10mg/d PO, incr prn by 10mg/d at 1-3wk intervals, maint 30mg/d in div doses, max 60mg/d

12 A.1.7 Selective Serotonin Reuptake Inhibitors (SSRI)

MA: selective inhibition of serotonin reuptake ⇒ serotonin levels in synaptic cleft ↑
EF: antidepressant, psychomotor activation
AE (SSRIs): sleeplessness, agitation, somnolence, headache, N/V, diarrhea, arrhythmias, ejaculation disturbances
AE (citalopram): nausea, dry mouth, sweating, somnolence, ejaculation DO
AE (fluoxetine): insomnia, asthenia, tremor, headache, GI complaints
AE (fluvoxamine): somnolence, headache, agitation, N/V, insomnia
AE (paroxetine): headache, sedation, dry mouth, insomnia, dizziness, nausea
AE (sertraline): GI complaints, tremor, headache, insomnia, male sexual dysfunction
CI (SSRIs): simultaneous treatment with MAO inhibitors, triptophan and oxitriptan; caution in children and adolescents < 18, hypersensitivity to product ingredients
CI (fluoxetine, in addition): present or recent treatment with thioridazine
CI (fluvoxamine, in addit.): coadministration of fexofenadine, astemizole or cisapride
CI (sertraline, in addition): oral concentrate with disulfiram due to alcohol content

Citalopram	EHL 33-37h, PRC C, Lact ?
Celexa *Tab 10mg, 20mg, 40mg* *Sol (oral) 10mg/5ml*	**Depression** →341: ini 20mg PO qd, incr to 40mg/d at an interval of >1wk, max 60mg/d; DARF: to be used cautiously in renal impairment; see Prod Info
Escitalopram	EHL 27-32h, PRC C, Lact ?
Lexapro *Tab 5mg,10mg, 20mg,* *Sol (oral) 5mg/5ml*	**Depression** →341: 10mg PO qd, incr prn to 20mg/d DARF: to be used cautiously in severe renal impairment; see Prod Info
Fluoxetine	EHL 4-6d (chronic); 1-3d (acute), PRC C, Lact -
Prozac *Tab 10mg, Cap 10mg, 20mg, 40mg, Cap ext rel 90mg, Sol (oral) 20mg/5ml* **Sarafem** *Cap 10mg, 20mg*	**Depression** →341/**obsessive compulsive DO** →346: ini 20mg PO qam, incr prn q several wk, max 80mg/d; ext.rel.: 90mg PO once weekly; **bulimia:** 60mg PO qam; DARF: see Prod Info

Fluvoxamine
EHL 15.6h, PRC C, Lact ?

Luvox *Tab 25mg, 50mg, 100mg*
Generics *Tab 25mg, 50mg, 100mg*

Obsessive compulsive DO →346, **depression** →341:
ini 50mg PO hs, incr prn by 50mg q4-7d
(doses above 100mg/d: div bid); max 300mg/d;
8–17y + obsessive compulsive DO: ini 25mg PO hs,
incr prn by 25mg q4-7d (doses above 50mg/d: div
bid), max: 200mg/d; DARF: low starting dosage
+ careful monitoring; see Prod Info

Paroxetine
EHL 17-22h, PRC C, Lact ?

Paxil *Tab 10mg, 20mg, 30mg, 40mg*
Susp 10mg/5ml
Paxil CR *Tab ext.rel. 12.5mg, 25mg, 37.5mg*

Depression →341: ini 20mg PO qam, incr prn by
10mg/d q ≧ 1wk, max 50mg/d; ext.rel.: ini 25mg PO
qam, incr prn by 12.5mg/d q ≧ 1wk, max 62.5mg/d;
obsessive compulsive DO →346: ini 20mg PO qam,
incr by 10mg/d q ≧ 1wk, rec dosage 40mg/d, max
60mg/d; **panic DO** →346: ini. 10mg PO qam; incr by
10mg/d, q ≧ 1wk, rec dosage 40mg/d, max 60mg/d;
social anxiety DO →345: 20mg/d PO qam; DARF: ini
10mg/d, max 40mg/d; for paroxetine ext. rel. ini
12.5mg/d, max 50mg/d

Sertraline
EHL 24h, PRC C, Lact ?

Zoloft *Tab 25mg, 50mg, 100mg,*
Conc (oral) 20mg/ml

Depression →341/**obsessive compulsive DO** →346:
ini 50mg/d PO, prn gradually incr at ≧1wk intervals,
max 200mg/d; **6–12 y/OCD:** 25mg/d PO, **13–17 y/
OCD:** 50mg/d PO; **panic** →346/**postrraumatic stress
DO:** ini 25mg/d PO, incr after 1wk to 50mg/d, prn
further incr q ≧1wk, max 200mg/d; **premenstrual
dysphoric DO:** 50-100mg/d PO; DARF: not req

12 A.1.8 Serotonin Antagonists and Reuptake Inhibitors (SARI)

MA: serotonin antagonists and reuptake inhibitors (serotonin-5-HT$_2$ antagonists); trazodone: selective
serotonin reuptake inhibitor, at low doses, trazodone appears to act as a serotonin antagonist and at higher
doses as an agonist
AE (nefazodone): dry mouth, nausea, somnolence, dizziness, blurred vision
AE (trazodone): dry mouth, dizziness, drowsiness, N/V, hypotension
CI (nefazodone): hypersensitivity to phenylpiperazine antidepressants, administration of fexofenadine/
astemizole/cisapride/MAOIs/pimozide/triazolam, caution with alprazolam, many other drug interactions
CI (trazodone): hypersensitivity to trazodone, carcinoid syndrome, initial recovery phase of myocardial
infarction

Nefazodone
EHL 1.9-5.3h, PRC C, Lact ?

Serzone *Tab 50mg, 100mg, 150mg, 200mg, 250mg*

Depression →341: ini 100mg PO bid, incr prn by
100-200mg/d, div bid, at >1wk intervals, maint
300-600mg/d div bid-tid

Trazodone
EHL 7.1h, PRC C, Lact ?

Desyrel, Generics *Tab 50mg, 100mg, 150mg,*
300mg

Depression →341: 50-150mg/d PO in div doses, incr
gradually prn by 50mg q3-4d, max 400mg/d div
(outpatients), 600mg/d div (inpatients); DARF: not
req

12 A.1.9 Norepinephrine Antagonist and Serotonin Antagonists (NASA)

MA: norepinephrine antagonist and serotonin antagonist (norepinephrine, serotonin $5\text{-}HT_2$ and $5\text{-}HT_3$)
AE (Mitrazapine): drowsiness, dizziness, constipation, appetite $\uparrow$, weight gain $\uparrow$, dry mouth, agranulozytosis (0,1%)
CI (Mitrazapine): hypersensitivity to mirtazapine. Don't use with MAOIs

Mirtazapine	EHL 20-40h, PRC C, Lact ?
Remeron *Tab 15mg, 30mg, 45mg* **Remeron Soltab** *Tab (orally disint), 15mg, 30mg, 45mg*	**Depression** →341: ini 15mg/d PO, incr prn in intervals of >1-2wk to 15-45mg/d; DARF: see Prod Info

12 A.2 Antimanic (Bimodal) Drugs

MA/EF (lithium): influence on phosphatidylinositol metabolism → Tx/PRO of manic depressive states, PRO of schizoaffective psychoses
MA (valproic acid): inhibition of the enzymatic breakdown of GABA
AE (lithium): polydipsie, polyuria, GI disturbances, tremors, goiter, hypothyroidism, renal damage
AE (valproic acid): tiredness, tremors, hair loss, hepatic damage, coagulation DO
CI (lithium): severe coronary dysfunction, M. Addison, RF
CI (valproic acid): liver diseases in family, hypersensitivity to valproic acid

Lithium	EHL 14-24h, PRC D, Lact -, serum level(mEq/l): 1-1.5 (acute), 0.6-1.2 (chronic)
Eskalith *Cap 300mg* **Eskalith CR** *Tab ext.rel. 450mg* **Lithane** *Tab 300mg* **Lithobid** *Tab ext.rel. 300mg* **Generics** *Tab 300mg, Cap 150mg, 300mg, 600mg*	**Acute mania** →343: 900-1800mg/d PO div bid-tid; **long-term use:** maint 300mg PO tid-qid; ext.rel. 600mg bid; DARF: GFR (ml/min); > 50: 100%, 10-50: 50-75%, < 10: 25-50%
Valproic Acid	EHL no data, PRC D, Lact + serum level: trough: 50-100µg/ml
Depakene *Cap 250mg, Syr 250mg/5ml* **Depakote** *Tab 125mg, 250mg, 500mg* **Myproic Acid** *Syr 250mg/5ml* **Generics** *Cap 250mg, Syr 250mg/5ml*	**Mania** →343: 250mg PO tid (Depakote), adjust dose rapidly to lowest therapeutic dose; DARF: see Prod Info; **epilepsy** →312: →286; **migraine** →306: →291
see Carbamazepine →286	

12 A.3 Antipsychotics
12 A.3.1 Atypical – Serotonin Dopamine Receptor Antagonists (SDA)

AE (aripiprazole): headache, anxiety, insomnia, lightheadedness, somnolence, akathisia, suicidal thoughts, seizures, bradycardia, nausea, vomiting, constipation, neuroleptic malignant syndrome, increased suicide risk; **AE** (clozapine): agranulocytosis, sedation, salivation, CVS effects, dizziness/vertigo, seizures; **AE** (olanzapine): somnolence, agitation, dizziness, constipation; **AE** (quetiapine): somnolence, dizziness, dry mouth, constipation; **AE** (risperidone): somnolence, dry mouth, constipation, blurred vision, extrapyramidal effects; **AE** (ziprasidone): somnolence, akathisia, weight gain, dizziness, extrapyramidal symptoms
CI (aripiprazole): hypersensitivity to arip.; **CI** (clozapine): myeloproliferative DO, clozapine induced agranulocytosis un controlled epilepsy, coma, hypersensitivity to clozapine; **CI** (olanzapine, quetiapine): hypersensitivity to product ingredients; **CI** (risperidone): hyperprolactinemia, hypersensitivity to risperidone; **CI** (ziprasidone): QT-prolongation, hypersensitivity to ziprasidone

Aripiprazole	EHL 75-94h, PRC C, Lact -
Abilify *Tab 5mg, 10mg, 15mg, 20mg, 30mg*	**Schizophrenia** →344: ini. 10-15mg PO qd, incr prn q2wk to max 30mg/d; DARF: not req
Clozapine	EHL 8-12h, PRC B, Lact -
Clozaril *Tab 25mg, 100mg* **Generics** *Tab 25mg, 100mg*	**Tx–resistent schizophrenia** →344: ini. 12.5mg PO qd-bid, incr by 25-50mg/d to 300-450mg/d (div bid-tid) by the end of 2wk, max 600-900mg/d
Olanzapine	EHL 21-54h (mean: 30h), PRC C, Lact ?
Zyprexa *Tab 2.5mg, 5mg, 7.5mg, 10mg, 15mg* **Zyprexa Zydis** *Tab (orally disint) 5mg, 10mg, 15mg, 20mg*	**Psychotic DO** →344: ini 5-10mg PO qd, incr prn by 5mg/d qwk to usual effective dose of 10-15mg/d, max 20mg/d; DARF: see Prod Info
Quetiapine	EHL 6h, PRC C, Lact ?
Seroquel *Tab 25mg, 100mgSV, 150mg, 200mg*	**Psychotic DO** →344: ini 25mg PO bid, incr by 25-50mg bid to 300-400mg/d (div bid-tid), range 150-750mg/d, max 800mg/d
Risperidone	EHL 20-30h, PRC C, Lact ?
Risperdal *Tab 0.25mg, 0.5mg, 1mg, 2mg, 3mg, 4mg,* *Sol (oral) 1mg/ml*	**Psychotic DO** →344: ini 1mg PO bid, incr prn by 1mg bid on d 2 + d 3, then at intervals >1wk, maint 4-6mg/d, max 16mg/d; DARF: ini 0.5mg bid, incr prn by 0.5-1.5mg bid, then by 0.5mg bid qwk; see Prod Info
Ziprasidone	EHL 6-7h, PRC C, Lact -
Geodon *Tab 20mg, 40mg, 60mg, 80mg*	**Schizophrenia** →344: ini 20mg PO bid, incr prn q >2d to maint 20-80mg bid; DARF: not req

12 A.3.2 Antipsychotics: D_2 Antagonists - Low Potency

MA (D_2-Antagonists): antagonism at central dopamine receptors
EF (D_2-Antagonists): antipsychotic and sedating (the higher the antipsychotic effect, the lower the sedating effect, and vice versa), sympatholytic, anticholinergic, antihistaminergic, antiserotoninergic
AE (D_2-Antagonists): early and late dyskinesias, parkinsonism, acathisia, restlessness, excitement, depression, lethargy, hyperprolactinemia, amenorrhea, mydriasis, accommodation disturbances, micturition disturbances, constipation, glaucoma, rise in spasmophilia, hypotension, tachycardia, conduction disturbances, allergic reactions, complete blood count changes, cholestasis
CI (D_2-Antagonists): M. Parkinson, severe hepatic dysfunction, micturition DO, glaucoma, acute intoxications with sedating drugs
AE (chlorprom): hypotension, akathisia, tardive dyskinesia, arrhythmias, constipation
AE (mesorid.): tardive dyskinesia, drowsiness, seizures, dry mouth, myelosuppression
AE (thioridazine): myelosuppression, arrhythmias, QT interval↑, N/V, NMS, extrapyramidal effects
CI (chlorpromazine): hypersensitivity to chlorpromazine, myelosuppression, coma
CI (thioridazine): severe CNS depression, circulatory collapse, hypersensitivity to thioridazine products, HTN/hypotension/heart disease, QT interval↑, patients on drugs that prolong the QT interval, patients on drugs that inhibit cytochrome p450-2D6
CI (mesoridazine): hypersensitivity to mesoridazine products, coma

Chlorpromazine
EHL 6h, PRC C, Lact ?

Sonazine *Conc (oral) 30mg/ml, 100mg/ml, Syr 10mg/5ml*
Sparine *Tab 25mg, 50mg, Inj 50mg/ml*
Thorazine *Tab 10mg, 25mg, 50mg, 100mg, 200mg, Cap ext.rel. 30mg, 75mg, 150mg, 200mg, 300mg, Conc (oral) 30mg/ml, 100mg/ml, Syr 10mg/5ml, Supp 25mg, 100mg, Inj 25mg/ml*
Generics *Tab 10mg, 25mg, 50mg, 100mg, 200mg, Conc (oral) 30mg/ml, 100mg/ml, Inj 25mg/ml*

Psychotic DO →344: outpatients: dose range 50-400mg/d; inpatients: ini 25mg tid, incr gradually until effective dose is reached, max 800mg/d; **IM**: 25mg IM, can repeat with 25-50mg in 1h (severe cases: may be gradually incr over several d up to a max of 400mg q4-6h; a dose of 500mg/d is generally sufficient); **CH 6mo-12y: severe behavioral/psychotic DO**: 0.5mg/kg PO q4-6h prn or 1mg/kg PR q6-8h prn or 0.5mg/kg IM q6-8h prn

Mesoridazine
EHL no data, PRC C, Lact ? (adverse data)

Serentil *Tab 10mg, 25mg, 50mg, 100mg Conc (oral) 25mg/ml*

Alcoholism →341: ini 25mg PO bid, usual dose 50-200mg/d; **chronic brain syndrome**: ini 25mg PO tid, usual dose 75-300mg/d; **schizophrenia** →344: ini 50mg PO tid, usual dose 100-400mg/d

Thioridazine
EHL 21-24h , PRC C, Lact ?

Mellaril *Tab 10mg, 15mg, 25mg, 50mg, 100mg, 150mg, 200mg, Conc (oral) 30mg/ml, 100mg/ml*
Thioridazine HCL Intensol *Conc (oral) 30mg/ml, 100mg/ml*
Generics *Tab 10mg, 15mg, 25mg, 50mg, 100mg, 150mg, 200mg, Conc (oral) 30mg/ml, 100mg/ml*

Psychotic DO →344: ini 50-100mg PO tid, gradual incr prn, maint 200-800mg/d div bid-qid, max 800mg/d; doses > 300mg/d are only rec for patients with severe psychoses; **CII 2-12y** (if unresponsive to other agents): 0.5mg/kg/d PO div bid-tid, titrate to optimum clinical response or to max 3mg/kg/d

12 A.3.3 Antipsychotics: D$_2$ Antagonists – Mid Potency

MA, EF, AE, CI (D$_2$ Antagonists): see: low potency neuroleptic drugs →327
AE (loxapine): hypotension, extrapyramidal effects, blurred vision, weight gain, sedation
AE (molindone): CVS effects, NMS, anticholinergic effects, extrapyramidal effect
CI (loxapine): coma, hypersensitivity to loxapine products
CI (molindone): coma, hypersensitivity to molindone products

Loxapine	EHL 4h (oral), 12h (IM), PRC C, Lact ?
Loxitane *Cap 5mg, 10mg, 25mg, 50mg* **Loxitane C** *Conc (oral) 25mg/ml* **Loxitane IM** *Inj 50mg/ml* **Generics** *Cap 5mg, 10mg, 25mg, 50mg*	**Psychosis** →344: ini 10mg PO bid or up to 50mg/d in severe cases, maint 60-100mg/d div bid-qid, max 250mg/d; IM: 12.5-50mg IM q4-12h, according to response

Molindone	EHL no data, PRC C, Lact ?
Moban *Tab 5mg, 10mg, 25mg, 50mg, 100mg,* *Conc (oral) 20mg/ml*	**Psychotic DO** →344: ini 50-75mg/d PO, incr prn to 100mg/d after 3-4d, max 225mg/d; maint 5-15mg tid-qid (mild), 10-25mg tid-qid (moderate), up to 225mg/d (severe symptoms)

12 A.3.4 Antipsychotics: D$_2$ Antagonists – High Potency

MA, EF, AE, CI (D$_2$ Antagonists): see: low potency neuroleptic drugs →327
AE (fluphenazine hydrochloride): agranulocytosis, akathisia, weight gain, hepatotoxicity, extrapyramidal effects, neuroleptic malignant syndrome
AE (haloperidol): sedation, dystonic/extrapyramidal reactions, hypotension, arrhythmias
AE (perphenazine): extrapyramidal, anticholinergic + CVS effects, seizures, sedation
AE (pimozide): extrapyramidal + CVS effects, nausea, seizures
AE (thiothixene): restlessness, blurred vision, extrapyramidal effects, N/V, myelosuppression
AE (trifluoperazine): seizures, NMS, extrapyramidal effects, blood dyscrasias
CI (fluphenazine): coma, hypersensitivity to fluphenazine products
CI (haloperidol): hypersensitivity to haloperidol products, Parkinson's disease
CI (perphenazine): blood dyscrasias, subcortical brain damage, coma, hypersensitivity to perphenazine products, severe liver disease
CI (pimozide): QT interval ↑, concomitant macrolides, hypersensitivity to pimozide, coma
CI (thiothixene): hypersensitivity to thiothixene products
CI (trifluoperazine): coma, bone marrow depression, hypersensitivity to trifluoperazine

Fluphenazine Hydrochloride	EHL 33h, PRC C, Lact ?
Permitil *Tab 2.5mg, 5mg, 10mg,* *Conc (oral) 5mg/ml* **Prolixin** *Tab 1mg, 2.5mg, 5mg, 10mg,* *Conc (oral) 5mg/ml, Elixir 2.5mg/5ml,* *Inj 2.5mg/ml* **Generics** *Tab 1mg, 2.5mg, 5mg, 10mg,* *Conc (oral) 5mg/ml, Elixir 2.5mg/5ml,* *Inj 2.5mg/ml*	**Psychosis** →344: 0.5-10mg/d PO div q6-8h; usual effective doses 1-20mg/d, max 40mg/d PO; IM: 1.25-10mg/d IM div q6-8h, max 10mg/d IM

Haloperidol

EHL 21h, IM: approx. 3wk; PRC C, Lact ?

Haldol *Tab 0.5mg, 1mg, 2mg, 5mg, 10mg, Conc (oral) 2mg/ml, Inj 5mg/ml*
Haldol Decanoate *Inj 50mg/ml, 100mg/ml*
Generics *Tab 0.5mg, 1mg, 2mg, 5mg, 10mg*

IM (non depot): acutely agitated patients →338: ini 2-5mg IM, may repeat q1-8h; **psychotic DO** →344: ini 1-6mg/d PO (moderate) and 6-15mg/d (severe symptoms) div bid-tid; usual range 1-15mg/d, max100mg/d; **Haldol decanoate** (oral to depot conversion): ini: 10-20 x the previous daily oral dose, but 100mg max ini dose, at monthly intervals; **CH 3-12 y psychotic DO:** 0.05-0.15mg/kg/d PO div bid-tid, **non-psychotic DO:** 0.05-0.075mg/kg/d PO div bid-tid; DARF: not req

Perphenazine

EHL 8.4-12.3h, PRC C, Lact -

Trilafon *Tab 2mg, 4mg, 8mg, 16mg, Conc (oral) 16mg/5ml, Inj 5mg/ml*
Generics *Tab 2mg, 4mg, 8mg, 16mg*

Psychotic symptoms →344: ini 4-8mg PO tid (moderately disturbed outpatients) or 8-16mg PO bid-qid (inpatients); IM: ini 5-10mg IM, then 5mg IM q6h prn, max 15mg/d IM (out-), max 30mg/d IM (inpatients)

Pimozide

EHL 53-55h, PRC C, Lact ?

Orap *Tab 1mg, 2mg*

Tourette's syndrome: ini 1-2mg/d PO in div doses, incr q2d prn; max 0.2mg/kg/d up to 10mg/d; **Tourette's syndrome + CH >12y: ini** 0.05mg/kg PO hs, incr prn q3d to max 0.2mg/kg up to 10mg/d; DARF: probably not req; see Prod Info

Thiothixene

EHL 34h, PRC C, Lact ?

Navane *Cap 1mg, 2mg, 5mg, 10mg, 20mg, Conc (oral) 5mg/ml, Inj 10mg/vial*
Generics *Cap 1mg, 2mg, 5mg, 10mg, Conc (oral) 5mg/ml*

Schizophrenia →344: ini 6mg PO div tid (milder conditions) and 5mg bid (severe conditions); usual effective dose range 20-30mg/d, max 60mg/d; IM: ini 4mg bid-qid, max 30mg/d

Trifluoperazine

EHL 24h, PRC C, Lact ?

Stelazine *Tab (oral) 1mg, 2mg, 5mg, 10mg, Conc (oral) 10mg/ml, Inj 2mg/ml*

Non-psychotic anxiety →345: 1-2mg PO bid for up to 12wk, max 6mg/d; **psychotic DO** →344: ini 2-5mg PO bid, usual dose is 15-20mg/d, sometimes up to 40mg/d; IM: 1-2mg q4-6h prn; **CH 6-12y** (hospitalized or under close supervision): 1mg PO qd-bid, prn gradually incr, max 15mg/d; IM: 1mg IM qd-bid

12 A.4 Anxiolytics, Hypnotics
12 A.4.1 Benzodiazepines

MA: opening of Cl^- channels $\Rightarrow$ inhibition of GABA neurons↑, especially in limbic system
EF: sedative, sleep inducing, anxiolytic, anti-aggressive, anti-convulsive, muscle relaxing
AE: tiredness, sleepiness, drowsiness, confusion, paradox reactions, anterograde amnesia, respiratory depression, psychic and physical addiction
CI: myasthenia gravis, severe hepatic damage, respiratory insufficiency, ataxia

Alprazolam
EHL 11.23h, PRC D, Lact ?

Xanax *Tab 0.25mg, 0.5mg, 1mg, 2mg*
Generics *Tab 0.25mg, 0.5mg, 1mg, 2mg, Conc (oral) 1mg/ml, Sol (oral) 0.5mg/5ml*

Anxiety →345 ini 0.25-0.5mg PO tid, incr prn q3-4d to max 4mg/d, usual effective dose 0.5-4mg/d in div doses; **panic DO** →345: ini 0.5mg PO tid, incr prn by max 1mg/d q3-4d, slower titration may be needed at doses > 4mg/d, usual effective dose 1-10mg/d (mean 5-6mg/d), max 10mg/d

Chlordiazepoxide
EHL 10-48h, PRC D, Lact ?

Chlordiazachel *Cap 5mg, 10mg, 25mg*
Librium *Cap 5mg, 10mg, 25mg,*
Inj 100mg/amp
Generics *Cap 5mg, 10mg, 25mg*

Anxiety →345: usual oral dose range is 5-10mg PO tid-qid (mild to moderate anxiety + tension) or 20-25mg tid-qid (severe anxiety + tension); **IV/IM: acute or severe anxiety:** 25-50mg IM/IV tid-qid; **CH > 6y + anxiety:** ini with lowest dose, incr prn, maint 5mg PO bid-qid, max 10mg bid-tid; **acute alcohol withdrawal** →339: 50-100mg IM/IV, repeat q2-4h prn up to 300mg/d; DARF: mild to moderate RF: not req; CrCl (ml/min) <10: 50%; see Prod Info

Clonazepam
EHL 30-40h, PRC C, Lact -
serum-level (ng/ml): 25-30

Klonopin *Tab 0.125mg, 0.25mg, 0.5mg, 1mg, 2mg, Tab (orally disint), 0.125mg , 0.25mg, 0.5mg, 1mg, 2mg*
Generics *Tab 0.5mg, 1mg, 2mg*

Panic DO →345: ini 0.25mg PO bid, gradually incr prn after 3d, max 4mg/d; (gradually decr by 0.125mg twice daily, q3d);
epilepsy →312, **neuralgias** →286

Clorazepate
EHL 2.29h, PRC D, Lact ?

Gen-xene *Tab 3.75mg, 7.5mg, 15mg*
Tranxene *Tab 3.75mg, 7.5mg, 15mg*
Tranxene sd *Tab 11.25mg, 22.5mg*
Generics *Cap 3.75mg, 7.5mg, 15mg*

Anxiety →345: ini 7.5-15mg/d PO, maint. 15-60mg/d according to patients response; DARF: not req

Diazepam
EHL 0.83-2.25d, PRC D, Lact ?

Diazepam Intensol *Conc (oral) 5mg/ml*
Valium *Tab 2mg, 5mg, 10mg*
Generics *Tab 2mg, 5mg, 10mg, Sol (oral) 5mg/5ml, Inj 5mg/ml*

Anxiety →345: 2-10mg PO bid-qid; IM/IV: 2-5mg IM/IV, repeat in 3-4h prn (moderate anxiety); 5-10mg IM/IV, repeat q3-4h prn (severe DO); DARF: see Prod Info; **epilepsy** →312; **muscle spasm** →304

Estazolam
EHL 10-24h, PRC X, Lact ?

Prosom *Tab 1mg, 2mg*
Generics *Tab 1mg, 2mg*

Insomnia: 1-2mg PO hs prn, reduce dose to 0.5mg in elderly, small, debilitated patients, incr prn with caution; DARF: not req

Flurazepam	EHL 2.3h, PRC X, Lact ?
Dalmane *Cap 15mg, 30mg* **Generics** *Cap 15mg, 30mg*	**Short term Tx of insomnia:** 15-30mg PO hs; DARF: see Prod Info
Lorazepam	EHL 10-20h (mean 12h) , PRC D, Lact ?
Ativan *Tab 0.5mg, 1mg, 2mg* **Lorazepam Intensol** *Conc (oral) 2mg/ml* **Generics** *Tab 0.5mg, 1mg, 2mg,* *Sol (oral) 0.5mg/5ml*	**Anxiety** →345: ini 0.5-1mg PO bid-tid, maint 2-6mg/d in div doses, max 10mg/d (div) **insomnia:** 2-4mg PO hs prn; DARF: see Prod Info
Oxazepam	EHL 2.8-8.6h, PRC D, Lact ?
Serax *Tab 15mg, Cap 10mg, 15mg, 30mg* **Generics** *Cap 10mg, 15mg, 30mg*	**Anxiety** →345: 10-15mg PO tid-qid (mild-to-moderate anxiety), 15-30mg tid-qid (severe anxiety and agitation with depression); **alcoholics with acute inebriation, tremulousness, or anxiety on alcohol withdrawal** →339: 15-30mg tid-qid; DARF: not req, see Prod Info
Temazepam	EHL 3.5-18.4h, PRC X, Lact ?
Restoril *Cap 7.5mg, 15mg, 30mg* **Generics** *Cap 15mg, 30mg*	**Insomnia:** 7.5-30mg PO hs
Triazolam	EHL 2.3h, PRC X, Lact ?
Halcion *Tab 0.125mg, 0.25mg* **Generics** *Tab 0.125mg, 0.25mg*	**Insomnia:** 0.125-0.25mg PO hs prn, max 0.5mg/d

12 A.4.2 Sedating Antihistamines

MA (diphenhydramine): antihistamine with sedative and hypnotic effect (see other antihistamines →124, →408, →409)
AE (diphenhydramine): dizziness, headache, convulsions, cardiac arrhythmia, oral dryness, micturition disturbances, paralytic ileus
CI (diphenhydramine): glaucoma, prostate hypertrophy with residual urine, acute asthma attacks, pheochromocytoma, epilepsy

Diphenhydramine	EHL 4-8h (prolonged with age), PRC B, Lact -
Allermax *Tab 25mg, 50mg, Sol (oral) 12.5mg/5ml* **Benadryl** *Cap 25mg, 50mg, Elixir (oral) 12.5mg/5ml* **Diphen** *Elixir (oral) 12.5mg/5ml* **Sominex** *Tab 25mg, 50mg* **Generics** *Cap 25mg, 50mg, Elixir (oral) 12.5mg/5ml*	**Insomnia:** 50mg PO hs; **anaphylaxis** →16, **allergic rhinitis, rhinorrhea** →408, DARF: GFR (ml/min) >50: q6h, 10-50: q6-12h, < 10: q12-18h; see Prod Info

12 A.4.3 Barbiturates

MA (barbiturat.): reinforcement of the inhibitory effect caused by GABA in the CNS
EF (barbiturates): sedative, sleep inducing, anxiolytic, anti-aggressive, anti-convulsive, muscle relaxing
AE (barbiturates): tiredness, dizziness, anterograde amnesia, dizziness, ataxia, dysopias, porphyria, N/V, hepatic dysfunction, bradycardia, respiratory depression, skin reactions, complete blood count changes, enzyme induction, addiction
AE (butabarbital): somnolence, agitation, confusion, dizziness, hypoventilation
AE (pentobarbital): respiratory depression, tachycardia, myasthenia gravis, drowsiness
AE (secobarbital): vertigo, excitation, respiratory depression, CNS depression
CI (barbiturates): porphyria, severe hepatic and renal dysfunction, status asthmaticus, respiratory insufficiency, barbiturate sensitivity

Butabarbital	EHL 34–100h, PRC D, Lact ?
Butisol Sodium *Tab 15mg, 30mg, 50mg, 100mg, Elixir (oral) 30mg/5ml* **Generics** *Tab 15mg, 30mg*	**Sedation:** 15-30mg PO tid-qid **insomnia:** 50-100mg PO hs prn

Mephobarbital	EHL 11–67h, PRC D, Lact -
Mebaral *Tab 32mg, 50mg, 100mg*	**Sedation:** 32-100mg PO tid-qid; **CH** sedation: 16-32mg PO tid-qid; DARF: administer with caution, see Prod Info

Pentobarbital	EHL 15–48h, PRC D, Lact ?
Nembutal *Supp 30mg, 60mg, 120mg, 200mg* **Nembutal Sodium** *Cap 30mg, 50mg, 100mg, Inj 50mg/ml* **Generics** *Cap 100mg, Inj 50mg/ml*	**Hypnotic:** 100mg PO hs; 120mg or 200mg PR (for patients < 110 lb.); 150-200mg IM; **CH hypnotic:** 10-20 lb. (2mo-1y): 30mg PR; 20-40 lb. (1-4y): 30mg or 60mg PR; 40-80 lb. (5-12y): 60mg PR; 80-110 lb. (12-14y): 60mg or 120mg PR; IM (**CH**, hypnotic): 2-6mg/kg/dose IM, not to exceed 100mg; DARF: see Prod Info

Secobarbital	EHL 19–34h, PRC D, Lact +
Seconal Sodium *Cap 50mg, 100mg* **Sodium Secobarbital** *Cap 100mg, Inj 50mg/ml* **Generics** *Cap 100mg, Inj 100mg/vial*	**Hypnotic:** 100mg PO hs prn; 100-200mg IM hs prn ; DARF: not req

12 A.4.4 Other Anxiolytics, Hypnotics

MA (buspirone): unknown, high affinity for 5-HT_{1A}-receptors
MA (chloral hydrate): hypnotic without influence on REM sleep
MA (zaleplon, zolpidem): benzodiazepin-like effect
AE (buspirone): sedation, dizziness
AE (chloral hydrate): arrhythmias, hallucinations, disorientation, N/V, diarrhea
AE (zaleplon, zolpidem): allergic reactions, tiredness, headache, dizziness, somnolence, nausea, development of addiction
CI (buspirone): hypersensitivity to buspirone products
CI (chloral hydrate): hypersensitivity to chloral hydrate products
CI (zaleplon, zolpidem): Myasthenia gravis, severe liver impairment, hypersensitivity to product ingredients

Buspirone	EHL 2.4-2.7h, PRC B, Lact ?
Buspar *Tab 5mg, 10mg, 15mg, 30mg, Cap 5mg, 7.5mg, 10mg, 15mg* **Generics** *Tab 5mg, 7.5mg, 10mg, 15mg*	**Anxiety** →345: ini 7.5mg PO bid, incr by 5mg/d q2-3d prn, usual effective dose 20-30mg/d (in div doses), max 60mg/d DARF: see Prod Info
Chloral Hydrate	EHL no data, PRC C, Lact ?
Aquachloral Supprettes *Supp 325mg, 650mg* **Somnote** *Cap 500mg*	**Alcohol withdrawal** →339: 0.5g-1g PO q6h prn; **insomnia** (short-term Tx): 0.5g-1g PO/PR hs; **sedation:** 250mg PO/PR tid pc; **CH insomnia** (short-term Tx): 50mg/kg/d PO/PR, max 1g/single dose; **CH sedation:** 8mg/kg/d PO/PR tid, max 0.5g tid; DARF: GFR (ml/min): >50: 100%, < 50: not recommend.; see Prod Info
Zaleplon	EHL 1h, PRC C, Lact -
Sonata *Cap 5mg, 10mg*	**Short-term Tx of insomnia:** 5-10mg PO hs prn; DARF: see Prod Info
Zolpidem	EHL 2-2.6h, PRC B, Lact ?
Ambien *Tab 5mg, 10mg*	**Insomnia:** 5-10mg PO hs prn (limit to 7-10d), max 10mg PO; DARF: see Prod Info

12 A.4.5 Anxiolytics, Hypnotics – Combinations

AE (amitriptyline + chlordiazepoxide): drowsiness, anticholinergic + CVS effects, seizures, myelosuppression; **AE** (perphenazine): extrapyramidal, anticholinergic + CVS effects, sedation, seizures; **CI** (amitriptyline + chlordiazepoxide): hypersensitivity to benzodiazepines or TCAs, concomitant use with MAO inhibitors, recovery following an MI
CI (amitriptyline + perphenazine): CVS disease, recovery period after MI, MAO Inhibitor usage, large doses of other CNS depressants, blood dyscrasias, bone marrow depression or hepatic damage, hypersensitivity to perphenazine, other piperazine phenothiazines, amitriptyline, or other TCA, subcortical brain damage, coma

Chlordiazepoxide + Amitriptyline	
Limbitrol, Generics *Tab 5mg + 12.5mg, 10mg + 25mg*	**Anxiety** →345/**depression** →341: 1 Tab PO tid-qid, max 6 Tab/d; DARF see Prod Info
Perphenazine + Amitriptyline	
Etrafon *Tab 2mg + 10mg, 2mg + 25mg* **Etrafon-forte** *Tab 4mg + 25mg* **Triavil** *Tab 2mg + 10mg, 2mg + 25mg, 4mg + 10mg, 4mg + 25mg, 4mg + 50mg* **Generics** *Tab 2mg + 10mg, 4mg + 10mg, 2mg + 25mg, 4mg + 25mg, 4mg + 50mg*	**Depression** →341/**anxiety** →345: ini 2-4mg perphen. + 25mg amitript. tid-qid, use lowest effective level for maint; max daily dose 16mg perphenazine + 200mg amitriptyline

12 A.5 Drugs used in Substance Dependence
12 A.5.1 Smoking Cessation

MA/EF (bupropion): catecholamine reuptake in CNS↓ ⇒ local concentrations of noradrenaline + dopamine ↑ ⇒ nicotine withdrawal symptoms↓, urge to smoke ↓
MA/EF (nicotine products): ganglionic (nicotinic) cholinergic-receptor agonists; used for nicotine replacement therapy as temporary adjunct in cessation of cigarette smoking
AE (nicotine products): tachycardia, diarrhea, nausea/indigestion, dizziness, insomnia, headache, nasal irritation with spray, skin irritation with patch, mouth irritation (gum)
AE (bupropion): fever, oral dryness, N/V, stomachache, constipation, insomnia, difficulty concentrating, headache, tachycardia, BP↑, depression, restlessness, fear, seizures/tremors, agitation, insomnia, hypersensitivity reactions
CI (nicotine products): angina, arrhythmias, active temporomandibular joint disease (gum), immediately post-MI, continued use of tobacco products, gastric ulcer, uncontrolled HTN, hypersensitivity to nicotine products
CI (bupropion): epilepsy, bulimia, anorexia, bipolar psychosis, severe liver cirrhosis, combination with MAO inhibitors, children and adolescents < 18, hypersensitivity to bupropion products, concomitant use of other bupropion products

Bupropion	EHL 14h (chronic dosing 21h), PRC B, Lact ?
Zyban *Tab ext.rel. 150mg*	**Smoking cessation:** ini 150mg PO qd x 3d, incr to 150mg PO bid x 7–12wk, max 150mg PO bid; DARF: see Prod Info
Nicotine Gum	EHL 30–120min, PRC C, Lact ?
Nicorette *Gum (chew, buccal) 2mg, 4mg*	**Smoking cessation:** 1 piece (2mg) q1–2h for 6wk, then 1 piece (2mg) q2–4h for 3wk, then 1 piece (2mg) q4–8h for 3wk, max 30 pieces/d of 2mg or 24 pieces/d of 4mg; 4mg pieces for high cigarette use (> 24 cigarettes/d)
Nicotine Inhalation System	PRC (nicotine) D, Lact (nicotine): ?
Nicotrol *Inhalant 4mg/cartridge*	**Smoking cessation:** 6–16 cartridges/d x 12wk, then reduction; max. 16 cartridges/d
Nicotine Nasal Spray	PRC (nicotine): D, Lact (nicotine): ?
Nicotrol *Spray (nasal) 0.5mg/Spray*	**Smoking cessation:** 1–2 doses/h (each dose = 2 sprays, 1 in each nostril), max 5doses/h or 40 doses/24h
Nicotine Patches	PRC (nicotine): D, Lact (nicotine): ?
Habitrol *Film (ext.rel, TD) 7mg/24h, 14mg/24h, 21mg/24h* **Nicoderm** *Film (ext.rel, TD) 7mg/24h, 14mg/24h, 21mg/24hr* **Nicotrol** *Film (ext.rel, TD) 15mg/16h* **Generics** *Film (ext.rel, TD) 7mg/24h, 14mg/24h, 21mg/24h*	**Smoking cessation:** see Prod Info

12 A.5.2 Alcohol Dependence

MA/EF: enzymatic oxidation of acetaldehyde to acetate ↓, during normal alcohol catabolism ⇒ acetaldehyde ↑ ⇒ unpleasant symptoms, hypersensitivity to alcohol
AE: psychotic reactions, neuropathy, blurred vision, seizures, hepatitis
CI: hypersensitivity to disulfiram, recent use of paraldehyde, metronidazole, ethanol, exposure to ethylene dibromide (pesticides), myocardial disease, psychoses

Disulfiram	EHL 12hPRC C, Lact ?
Antabuse *Tab 250mg, 500mg*	**Alcoholism** →341: **ini** up to max 500mg/d PO for 1–2wk, maint 125–250mg/d, max 500mg/d

see **Diazepam**→330, **Chloral Hydrate**→332, **Chlordiazepoxide**→330, **Oxazepam**→330

12 A.5.3 Opioid Dependence

AE (methadone): respiratory depression, dizziness, N/V, sweating, constipation
AE (naltrexone): opioid withdrawal-like syndrome, nausea, headache, dizziness, anxiety
CI (methadone): hypersensitivity to metha4done
CI (naltrexone): concomitant opioid analgesics, opioid dependency or withdrawal, hypersensitivity to naltrexone, acute hepatitis or liver failure

Methadone	EHL 23h (IV), 22h (chronic PO), PRC C, Lact ?
Dolophine HCT *Tab 5mg, 10mg,* *Syr (oral) 10mg/30ml* **Methadose** *Tab 5mg, 10mg, Tab (dispersible) 40mg,* *Conc (oral) 10mg/ml* **Generics** *Tab 5mg, 10mg, Tab (dispersible) 40mg,* *Conc (oral) 10mg/ml, Sol (oral) 5mg/5ml, 10mg/5ml*	**Narcotic addiction:** 40–180mg/d PO (div), taper dose as appropriate to avoid withdrawal symptoms; DARF: see Prod Info, (GFR (ml/min): > 50: q6h; 10–50: q8h, severe RF: q8–12h)

Naltrexone	EHL 4h, PRC C, Lact ?
Revia *Tab 50mg* **Generics** *Tab 50mg*	**Alcohol dependence** →341: 50mg PO qd **narcotic dependence:** ini 25mg PO qd, incr to 50mg PO qd if no signs of withdrawal

12 A.6 CNS Stimulants

MA/EF (amphetamine): CNS/respiratory stimulation; sympathomimetic activity ↑ ⇒ pressor response, mydriasis, bronchodilation, contraction of urinary bladder sphincter;
MA/EF (atomoxetine): selective inhibition of norepinephrine reuptake
MA/EF (caffeine): competitive inhibition of phosphodiesterase ⇒ intracellular cyclic AMP↑ ⇒ CNS stimulation at all levels (thought flow↑, wakefulness);
MA/EF (methylphenidate): amphetamine derivate → release of catecholamines ⇒ centrally stimulating;
MA/EF (modafinil): potentiation of cerebral α_1-adrenergic activity ⇒ improvement of vigilance↑, number of sudden sleep episodes ↓;
MA/EF (Pemoline): CNS and respiratory stimulation and weak sympathomimetic activity
AE (amphetamine): restlessness, palpitations/tachycardia, dizziness, HTN; **AE** (atomoxetine): headache, insomnia, dry mouth, nausea, decreased appetite, constipation, upper abdominal pain, vomiting, cough;
AE (caffeine): restlessness, vomiting, tachycardia; **AE** (dextroamphetamine): insomnia, tachycardia, dry mouth, dependence, anorexia; **AE** (methylphenidate): restlessness, behavior DO, slurred speech, dermatitis, skin rashes, convulsions, insomnia, states of excitability, psychoses, development of addiction;
AE (modafinil): headache, nausea, nervousness, loss of appetite, sleep DO; **AE** (pemoline): anorexia, insomnia, dizziness, LFT abnormalities, Tourette's syndr.;
AE (sodium oxybate): headche, nausea, dizziness, pain, somnolence, pharyngitis, infection, flu-syndrome
CI (amphetamine): MAOI therapy, drug abuse, HTN, glaucoma, CAD, hyperthyroidism
CI (atomoxetine): hypersens. to atom., MAOI therapy, narrow angle glaucoma
CI (dextroamphetamine): hypersens. to dextroamphetamine, concomitant MAOI, CVS disease, hyperthyroidism; **CI** (methylphenidate): glaucoma, marked anxiety, tension, agitation, depression, psychoses, addictions, hypersens. to methylphenidate, hyperthyroidism, prostate hypertrophy, pheochromocytoma;
CI (modafinil): combination with prazosin, addictions; **CI** (pemoline): hypersens. to pemoline, liver disease, ADD with concomitant Tourette's syndrome/tics
CI (sodium oxybate): treatment with sedative hypnotic agents, succinic semialdehyde dehydrogenase deficiency

Amphetamine + Dextroamphetamine

Adderall *Tab 2.5 + 2.5mg, 3.75 + 3.75mg, 6.25 + 6.25mg, 10 + 10mg, 15 + 15mg;* *Tab ext.rel. 5 + 5mg, 10 + 10mg, 15 + 15mg*	**Narcolepsy:** 5–60mg/d in div doses, **CH 6–12y:** ini 5mg PO qd, incr by 5mg qwk prn; **>12y:** ini 10mg PO qd, incr by 10mg qwk prn; **attention deficit DO, hyperactivity: CH 3–5y:** ini 2.5mg PO qd, incr by 2.5mg qwk prn; **age >6y:** ini 5mg PO qd-bid, incr by 5mg qwk prn; max 40mg/d; ext.rel.: ini 10mg PO qd, incr prn by 10mg qwk, max 30mg/d; DARF: see Prod Info

Atomoxetine

	EHL 22h, PRC C, Lact ?
Strattera *Cap 10mg, 18mg, 25mg, 40mg, 60mg*	**Attention deficit hyperactivity DO:** >70kg: ini 40mg/d PO, incr after 3d to 80mg/d div qd-bid; max 100mg/d after 2–4wk; <70kg: ini 0.5mg/kg/d PO, incr. after 3d to 1.2mg/kg/d div qd-bid; max 1.4mg/d; DARF: not req

Caffeine

	EHL 4–5h, PRC C, Lact +
Caffedrine *Cap ext. rel. 200mg* **NoDoz** *Tab 100mg, 200mg, Tab (chew) 100mg* **Vivarin** *Tab 200mg*	**Fatigue:** 100–200mg PO q3-4h prn

Dextroamphetamine — EHL 7-34h, PRC C, Lact -

Dexedrine *Tab 5mg, Cap ext.rel. 5mg, 15mg, 10mg*
Dextrostat *Tab 5mg, 10mg*
Generics *Tab 5mg, 10mg*

Narcolepsy: usual 5-60mg/d (div. qd-tid) **6-12y + narcolepsy:** ini 5mg/d PO, incr qwk by 5mg prn; **>12y:** ini 10mg PO qd, incr qwk by 10mg/d prn; **attention deficit hyperactivity DO**: 3-5y: ini 2.5mg PO qd, incr by 2.5mg qwk prn; $\geq$ **6y:** ini 5mg PO qd-bid, incr by 5mg qwk prn, max 40mg/d div qd-tid at 4-6h intervals

Dexmethylphenidate — EHL 2.2h, PRC C, Lact ?

Focalin *Tab 2.5mg, 5mg, 10mg*

Attention deficit hyperactivity DO: 6-17y: ini 2.5mg PO bid, incr by 2.5-5mg qwk prn to max 10mg bid

Methylphenidate — EHL PO 2-7h; IV 1-2h, PRC C, Lact ?

Metadate ER *Tab ext.rel. 10mg, 20mg*
Metadate CD *Cap ext.rel. 20mg*
Methylin ER *Tab ext.rel. 10mg, 20mg*
Ritalin *Tab 5mg, 10mg, 20mg; Tab ext.rel. 20mg, 30mg, 40mg*
Generics *Tab 5mg, 10mg, 20mg*

Narcolepsy: narcolepsy 10-60mg/d in 2-3 div doses (mean 20-30mg/d); **attention deficit DO: CH > 6y:** ini 2.5-5mg PO bid before breakfast and lunch, incr gradually by 5-10mg qwk prn to max 60mg/d

Modafinil — EHL 7.5-15h, PRC C, Lact ?

Provigil *Tab 100mg, 200mg*

Narcolepsy: 200mg PO qam; DARF: ini 100-200mg/d, gradual incr based on safety and tolerability, see Prod Info

Pemoline — EHL 7-13h, PRC B, Lact ?

Cylert, Generics *Tab 10.75mg, 37.5mg, 75mg, Tab (chew) 37.5mg*

Attention deficit DO: CH > 6y: ini 37.5mg/d PO qam, incr by 18.75mg qwk prn, maint 56.25-75mg/d, max 112.5mg/d

Sodium oxybate — EHL 22min, PRC B, Lact ?

Xyrem *Sol (oral) 500mg/ml*

Cataplexy with narcolepsy: to be taken at bedtime and 2.5-4h later, ini 4.5g/d, may incr. to max. 9g/d in increments of 1.5g/d; **DARF** not req

12 B. Psychiatry – Therapies

John H. Krystal, MD, Professor
D. Cyril D'Souza, MD, Associate Professor
Department of Psychiatry, School of Medicine
Yale University School of Medicine, New Haven, CT

12 B.1 Psychiatric Emergencies
12 B.1.1 Acute Agitation or Excitement

Acute Agitation or Excitement (e.g. in manic, schizophrenic disorder, schizoaffective psychosis). **Combine psychopharmacological approach** with **reducing environmental stimulation** e.g., seclusion room and in rare instances mechanical restraints until psychopharmacological treatment takes effect

prim. Tx	**Benzodiazepine** →330 (facilitation of inhibitory GABA-A receptor transmission)	**Lorazepam** (Ativan, Gens)	1–2mg IM or slowly IV
		Diazepam (Diastat, Valium, Gens)	5mg slowly IV
		Midazolam (Versed, Gens)	1–2mg slowly IV, rep after 30–45min sos
	Caution: beware of respiratory depression!		
poss. augm. with	**High potency antipsychotic** →328 (dopamine antagonism)	**Haloperidol** (Haldol, Gens)	5mg PO or IM, rep after 30–45 min sos; synerg EF, less AE poss, if co-admin with benzodiazepine
or	**Atypical antipsychotic** →326 (D2–5HT2 antagonist)	**Olanzapine** (Zyprexa)	5mg IM
		Ziprasidone (Geodon)	5–10mg IM (less extrapyram. side effects)

12 B.1.2 Acute Suicidality

Secure patient in a **safe environment** e.g., in-patient unit, emergency room and assess for imminent risk and choose appropriate level of **monitoring**, including one-to-one observation. Treat underlying disorder e.g., psychosis or depression.

	Benzodiazepine →330 (inhibitory transmitter GABA ↑)	**Lorazepam** (Ativan, Gens)	1–2mg PO tid-qid (non-specific relief of distress)
		Diazepam (Diastat, Valium, Gens)	5–10mg PO tid-qid
		Clonazepam (Klonopin)	0.5–1mg PO bid (long-acting!)

12 B.1.3 Catatonia

Secure patient in a **safe environment**.

prim. Tx	**Benzodiazepine** →330 (inhibitory transmitter GABA ↑)	**Lorazepam** (Ativan, Gens)	2.5mg PO or 1–2mg slowly IV, rep sos
augm. with	**Atypical antipsychotic** →326 (D_2-/5-HT_2-antagonist)	**Olanzapine** (Zyprexa)	10–20mg PO
		Risperidone (Risperdal)	1–4mg PO

12 B.1.4 Acute Alcohol Withdrawal (Delirium)

In general

Secure patient in a **safe environment** e.g., in-patient unit, emergency room and monitor for physiologic signs and symptoms of alcohol withdrawal.

Tx of choice	**Benzodiazepine** →330 (facilitation of GABA receptor function)	**Lorazepam** (Ativan, Gens)	*1-2mg q1-4h titrated according to autonomic signs of withdrawal*
		Oxazepam (Serax)	*15-30mg tid to qid*
		Chlordiazepoxide (Chlordiazachel, Librium)	*50-100mg IM/IV, rep q2-4h prn up to 300mg/d*
	Adjust dose to the point at which withdrawal symptoms are subsiding and eventually taper slowly by 25-50% qd after symptoms have stabilized. Chlordiazepoxide (Librium) or other benzodiazepines may also be used.		
2nd line	**Anticonvulsant** →286 (facilitation of GABA receptor function)	**Valproic acid** (Depakote)	*500mg tid x 4d, then taper by 250-500mg/d*
suppl. Tx	**Vitamin B$_1$** →145 (PRO of Wernicke's encephalopathy)	**Thiamine** (Gens)	*5-10mg PO qd; 100mg PO/IM qd in suspected begin of Wernicke's encephalopathy*
		Folate	*1mg qd*
suppl. Tx	**Magnesium** →140 (PRO of hypomagnesemia and seizures)	**Magnesium sulfate**	*1g/d IV or IM in sympt. hypomagnesemia or inablity to tolerate PO Tx*

If psychotic symptoms

	Atypical antipsychotic →326 (D$_2$-/5-HT$_2$-antagonist)	**Olanzapine** (Zyprexa)	*10-20mg PO qd*
		Risperidone (Risperdal)	*0.5-2mg PO bid (less AE)*
or	**Typical antipsychotic** →328	**Haloperidol** (Haldol, Gens)	*5-15mg PO qd*

If autonomic symptoms (BP > 180/120mmHg, tachycardia > 120/min) are not sufficiently treatable with benzodiazepines

poss. plus	**Antihypertensive** →30 (central alpha$_2$-receptor agonist)	**Clonidine** (Catapres, Catapres-TTS, Gens)	*Ini 0.1mg bid, incr slowly sos by 0.1-0.2mg/d, up to 0.3-0.6mg q6h; Caution: monitor vital signs cosely!*

If seizures

plus	**Anticonvulsant** →286	**Diphenylhydantoin** (Dilantin, Gens)	*Ini 10-15mg/kg IV, max rate 50mg/min, then 100mg IV/PO q6-8h*

12 B.2 Dementia

12 B.2.1 In General

Investigate cause of dementia i.e., vascular, Alzheimers. For vascular dementia also treat hypertension, reduction of platelet aggregation, etc.

12 B.2.2 First Line

In Alzheimers dementia and possibly vascular dementia

1st	**Reversible competitive-noncompetitive ACI** →293	**Donepezil** (Aricept)	*5mg PO qd over 1mo, then 10mg qd; discont if no change after 2mo*
	Pseudoreversible ACI + butylcholine esterase inhibitor →293	**Rivastigmine** (Exelon)	*Ini 2mg PO qd, then titrate slowly over 12wk to 6-12mg*
	Reversible, competitive ACI + nicotinic agonist →293	**Galantamine** (Reminyl)	*Ini 4mg PO bid, incr by 8mg q4wk up to 16-32mg*

EF/MA of ACI (= acetyl cholinesterase inhibitor): inhibition of centrally-active acetylcholinesterase ⇒ concentration of acetylcholine ↑ ⇒ synaptic transmission ↑ ⇒ cognitive function ↑. With all ACIs: the slower the titration the less GI side effects

12 B.2.3 Second Line (Weak Evidence)

In mild to moderate dementia

	Noncompetitive NMDA receptor antagonist	**Memantine** (Akatinol)	*Wk1: 5mg qd, wk2: 10mg qd, then 15-20mg qd*

In mild to moderate vascular dementias

	Ca^{++} channel blocker (brain vessel dilation + modulation of neuronal Ca^{++} homeostasis) →28	**Nimodipine** (Nimotop)	*30mg tid*

12 B.2.4 Psychosis associated with Dementias

	Atypical antipsychotic, low dose →326 (D$_2$-/5-HT$_2$-antagonist)	**Olanzapine** (Zyprexa, Zyprexa Zydis)	*1.25–2.5mg qd; Zydis, if Pat unable to swallow*
		Quetiapine (Seroquel)	*25mg bid up to max 200mg bid; Caution: monitor BP and pulse!*
		Risperidone (Risperdal)	*0.5-1.0mg qd*
or	**Typical antipsychotic, low dose, high potency** →328 (dopamine antagonism)	**Haloperidol** (Haldol, Gens)	*0.5-2mg PO qd*

Caution: since the elderly are more vulnerable to develop tardive dyskinesia, chronic Tx with typical antipsychotics should be avoided

poss.	**Benzodiazepine** →330	**Lorazepam** (Ativan, Gens)	*Low doses; Caution: paradoxical effects poss*

12 B.3 Alcoholism

12 B.3.1 Acute Alcohol Withdrawal

See Acute Alcohol Withdrawal (Delirium) →339

12 B.3.2 Chronic Alcoholism

Deterrent →335 (deterrant acetaldehyde formed during normal catabolism of alcohol ⇒ unpleasant symptoms)	**Disulfiram** (Antabuse)	*250–500mg qd PO after discussion of interactions with alcohol and alcohol containing preparations*
Glutamate modulating (craving↓ ⇒ period of abstinence↑)	**Acamprosate** (Campral)	*BW <60kg: 1.3g/d; >60kg: 2g/d div bid; available as 333mg enteric-coated Tab*
Opioid antagonism →335 (craving↓)	**Naltrexone** (Revia)	*50mg PO qd*

12 B.4 Depressive Disorders

12 B.4.1 Acute Treatment

With all antidepressants assessment of success at the earliest after 2-3 wk of Tx with target/Tx dose! After depressive symptoms cease, cont drug Tx for at least 6 mo.

	SSRI →323 (selective serotonin reuptake inhibition)	**Citalopram** (Celexa)	*Incr slowly to 20-60mg PO qd*
		Fluoxetine (Prozac)	
		Paroxetine (Paxil, Paxil CR)	
		Sertraline (Zoloft)	*Incr slowly to 50-150mg PO qd*
		Fluvoxamine (Luvox, Gens)	
		Escitalopram (Lexapro)	*Incr slowly to 10-20mg PO qd*
or	**NASA** →325 (norepinephrine and serotonin antagonism)	**Mirtazapine** (Remeron, Remeron Soltab)	*Incr slowly to 15-45mg PO qd*
or	**Non-Tricyclic SNRI** →322 (serotonin-norepinephrine reuptake inhibition)	**Venlafaxine** (Effexor, Effexor-XR)	*Incr slowly to 75-225mg PO qd*

or	**Tricyclic SNRI** →320, →321 (serotonin-norepinephrine reuptake inhibition plus additional (side)effects due to cholinergic and histaminergic actions)	**Amitriptyline** (Clavil, Elavil, Endep, Gens)	*Incr slowly to 150-200mg/d in div doses prn*
		Clomipramine (Anafranil, Gens)	*Incr slowly to 150-200mg/d in div doses prn*
		Desipramine (Norpramin, Gens)	*Incr slowly to 50-200mg in div doses prn*
		Doxepin (Sinequan, Gens)	*Incr slowly to 150-200mg in div doses prn*
		Nortriptyline (Aventyl, Pamelor, Gens)	*Incr slowly to 150-200mg in div doses prn*
		Protrlptylline (Vivacty)	*Incr slowly to 15-40mg in div doses prn*
		Trimipramine (Surmontil)	*Incr slowly to 150-200mg in div doses prn*
		Amoxapine (Asendin)	*Incr slowly to 150-200mg in div doses prn*
		Maprotiline (Ludiomil)	*Incr slowly to 100-150mg in div doses prn*
or	**DRI** →322 (dopamine reuptake inhibition)	**Bupropion** (Wellbutrin)	*Incr slowly to 150-450mg PO qd (div tid); seizures at higher doses*
or	**SARI** →324 (serotonin 5-HT$_2$-antagonism and reuptake inhibition)	**Trazodone** (Desyrel, Gens)	*Incr slowly to 200-600mg qd in div doses*
		Nefazodone (Serzone)	*Incr slowly to 200-500mg qd in div doses*
or	**Irreversible MAO inhibitor** →322 (norepinephrine and serotonine breakdown ↓)	**Tranylcypromine** (Parnate)	*Incr slowly to 20-50mg qd in div doses prn*
		Phenelizine (Nardil)	*45-60 mg qd; low tyramine diet req!*

12 B.4.2 If no response or partial response

	Change to an antidepressant from a different substance class (s.a.)
or	Augment with: **SSRI, tricyclic SNRI** or **previously described antidepressant. Caution**: do not combine with MAOIs!
or	**Lithium augmentation** →325 (complex mechanism of action) **Lithium** (Eskalith, Eskalith CR, Lithane, Lithobid, Gens) *Ini 300mg bid, titrate to serum level of 0.4-0.8meq/l*
or	**Stimulant** →336 (DA release) **Dextroamphetamine** *5-30mg/d in div doses*
or	**Electroconvulsive Tx** (induction of a grand mal seizure in anesthesia) *e.g. three times a week*

12 B.4.3 Psychotic Depression

plus	**Atypical antipsychotic** →326 (D_2-/5-HT$_2$-antagonist)	**Olanzapine** (Zyprexa)	*Incr slowly to 5-20mg/d PO*
		Risperidone (Risperdal)	*Incr slowly to 2-6mg/d PO*
		Quetiapine (Seroquel)	*Incr slowly to 200-400mg PO bid*
		Ziprasidone (Geodon)	*Incr slowly to 40-80mg PO bid*

12 B.5 Manic Disorders

12 B.5.1 Acute Mania

First line

either	**Lithium** →325 (complex mechanism of action)	**Lithium** (Eskalith, Eskalith CR, Lithane, Lithobid, Gens)	*Ini 300mg bid, then titrate to serum level of 0.8–1.2meq/l; Caution overdose!*
or	**Anticonvulsant** →286 (facilitation of GABA receptor function)	**Valproic acid** (Depakene, Depakote, Myproic Acid, Gens)	*Titrate to serum level of 75-100mg/l; "IV-loading" also poss: 20mg/kg/d*

Second line

	Atypical antipsychotic →326 (D_2-/5-HT$_2$-antagonist)	**Olanzapine** (Zyprexa)	*Incr slowly to 5-20mg/d PO*
		Risperidone (Risperdal)	*Incr slowly to 2-6mg/d PO*
		Quetiapine (Seroquel)	*Incr slowly to 200-400mg/d PO (div bid-tid)*
		Ziprasidone (Geodon)	*Incr slowly to 40-80mg/d PO bid*

May be used as standalone Tx (without mood stabilizer) regardless of whether the patient has psychotic symptoms

Supplementary Tx for agitation, excitement, insomnia

	Benzodiazepine →330 (increase in inhibitory transmitter GABA)	**Lorazepam** (Ativan, Gens)	*1-2mg IM or slowly IV*
		Diazepam (Diastat, Valium, Gens)	*5-10mg slowly IV, rep prn*

12 B.5.2 Prophylaxis, Maintenance

Continue mood stabilizer, but lower dose

either	**Lithium** →325 (established antimanic effects, complex MA)	**Lithium** (Eskalith, Eskalith CR, Lithane, Lithobid, Gens)	*Titrate dose for serum level of 4-8meq/l*
or	**Anticonvulsant** →286 (facilitation of GABA function)	**Valproic acid** (Depakene, Depakote, Myproic acid, Gens)	*Titrate dose for serum level of 50-100mg/l*

12 B.6 Psychotic Disorders (Schizophrenia, Delusional Disorder)
12 B.6.1 Acute or Subacute Psychosis

First line

Atypical antipsychotic →326 (Balanced D_2- : 5-HT_2-receptor antagonism)	**Risperidone** (Risperdal)	*Incr slowly to 4-8mg PO qd; in higher dose more frequently extrapyram. symptoms*
	Olanzapine (Zyprexa, Zyprexa Zydis)	*Incr slowly to 5-20mg PO qd*
	Quetiapine (Seroquel)	*Incr slowly to 200-400mg PO bid*
	Ziprasidone (Geodon)	*Incr slowly to 40-80mg PO bid*
	Zotepine (Zoleptil)	*Ini 75-150mg (div tid), incr to 300mg/d sos*
	Amisulpride (Solian)	*400-800mg PO qd*

Second line (in order of decreasing potency)

Typical antipsychotic →328 (central dopamine receptor antagonism)	**Haloperidol** (Haldol, Gens)	*5-20mg qd PO*
	Fluphenazine (Prolixin)	*5-20mg*
	Pimozide (Orap)	*1-8mg PO qd*
	Perphenazine (Trilafon, Gens)	*16-64mg PO qd*

In drug-induced dose-related extrapyramidal disorder (dystonia, parkinsonism)

Anticholinergic Parkinsonian drug →293 (inhibition of central cholinergic neurons)	**Biperiden** (Akineton)	*2mg PO or 5mg slowly IV*
	Benztropine mesylate (Cogentin)	*1-2mg PO or IM/IV*

In dose-related akathisia

Betablocker →23 (central sympathic activity ↓)	**Propranolol** (Inderal, Inderal LA, Gens)	*10-30mg PO tid*

12 B.6.2 Treatment-resistant Psychosis or Intolerable Side-effects (e.g. treatment failure with at least 2 other antipsychotics)

SDA →326 (serotonin dopamine receptor antagonist)	**Clozapine** (Clozaril, Gens)	*Ini 12.5-25mg qd, then titrate up to 300-600mg qd; Caution: monitor granulocyte (neutrophil) count (agranulocytosis!)*
or	**Electroconvulsive Tx** (Induction of a grand mal seizure in anesthesia)	*e.g. 3 x per wk*
or	Combination of antipsychotics	

12 B.6.3 Acute Catatonia

Benzodiazepine →330 (inhibitory transmitter GABA ↑)	**Lorazepam** (Ativan, Gens)	*1–2.5mg PO or IM, rep sos*

plus Treat as for acute psychosis with **atypical** or **typical antipsychotics:**
- **If negative symptoms predominant, lower doses and atypical antipsychotics preferred**
- **Comorbid substance abuse disorders: atypical antipsychotics preferred**
- **Relapse prophylaxis, maintenance of remission: consider reducing dose to minimum effective dose**

12 B.6.4 In Noncompliant Patients

Depot Neuroleptic →328 (delayed release after IM-injection through bond to oily medium)	**Haloperidol Decanoate** (Haldol Decanoate)	*50–200mg IM q3–4wk*
	Fluphenazine Decanoate (Prolixin Decanoate)	*12.5–50mg IM q2wk*
	Flupentixol (Fluanxol)	*20–40mg IM q2wk*

12 B.7 Anxiety Disorders

12 B.7.1 Acute Fear or Acute Panic Attack

Benzodiazepine →330 (inhibitory transmitter GABA ↑)	**Lorazepam** (Ativan, Gens)	*1–2mg PO*
	Diazepam (Diastat, Valium, Gens)	*5–10mg PO*

12 B.7.2 Generalized Anxiety Disorder (GAD)

either	**SSRI antidepressant** →323 (selective serotonin reuptake inhibition)	**Citalopram** (Celexa)	*Incr slowly to 20–60mg PO qd*
		Fluoxetine (Prozac)	*Incr slowly to 20–60mg PO qd*
		Paroxetine (Paxil, Paxil CR)	*Incr slowly to 20–60mg PO qd*
		Sertraline (Zoloft)	*Incr slowly to 50–150mg PO qd*
		Fluvoxamine (Luvox, Gens)	*Incr slowly to 50–150mg PO qd*
		Escitalopram (Lexapro)	*Incr slowly to 10–20mg PO qd*
	Effects often seen only after several weeks of treatment.		
or	**Non-Tricyclic SNRI** →322 (serotonin-norepineph-rine reuptake inhibition)	**Venlafaxine** (Effexor, Effexor XR)	*Incr slowly to 225–375mg PO qd*
	Effects often seen only after several weeks of treatment.		
and/ or	**Benzodiazepine** →330 (inhibitory transmitter GABA ↑)	**Clonazepam** (Klonopin)	*1–4 mg PO qd*
		Lorazepam (Ativan, Gens)	*up to 1–2mg tid PO*
		Diazepam (Diastat, Valium, Gens)	*5–10mg PO tid*
		Alprazolam (Xanax)	*0.5–1 mg PO tid–qid*
	Tolerance and dependence may emerge over time.		

and/ or	**Anxiolytic** →332 (partial serotonin 5-HT1a receptor agonism)	**Buspirone** (Buspar, Gens)	*Ini 5mg tid, incr up to 20mg tid*

12 B.7.3 Panic Disorder and Agoraphobia

	SSRI antidepressant →323 (selective serotonin reuptake inhibitor)	**Paroxetine** (Paxil, Paxil CR)	*40-80mg qd; effects often only after several wks' Ts*
or	**Tricyclic SNRI antidepressant** →320 (especially serotonin reuptake inhibition)	**Imipramine** (Tofranil, Gens)	*100-300mg qd*
		Clomipramine (Anafranil, Gens)	*150-225mg qd*
	Effects often only after several weeks' treatment. Tricyclics may lead to cardiac toxicity.		
and/ or	**Benzodiazepine** →330 (inhibitory transmitter GABA ↑)	**Clonazepam** (Klonopin)	*1-4 mg PO qd*
		Lorazepam (Ativan, Gens)	*up to 1-2mg tid PO*
		Diazepam (Diastat, Valium, Gens)	*5-10mg PO tid*
		Alprazolam (Xanax)	*0.5-1 mg PO qid*
	Tolerance and dependence may emerge over time.		

12 B.7.4 Social Phobia

	SSRI antidepressant →323 (selective serotonin reuptake inhibitor)	**Paroxetine** (Paxil, Paxil CR)	*40-60mg qd; effects often only after several weeks' treatment*
or	**Reversible MAO inhibitor** (inhibition of MAO ⇒ norepinephrine and serotonine breakdown ↓)	**Moclobemide** (Manerix)	*Ini 300mg qd, incr to 300mg bid; effects often only after several weeks' Tx*

12 B.8 Obsessive-Compulsive Disorders

either	**SSRI** →323 (selective serotonin reuptake inhibition)	**Fluvoxamine** (Luvox, Gens)	*Incr slowly to 100-300mg PO qd*
		Fluoxetine (Prozac)	*Incr slowly to 20-80mg PO qd*
		Sertraline (Zoloft)	*Incr slowly to 75-225mg PO qd*
		Paroxetine (Paxil, Paxil CR)	*Incr slowly to 40-80mg PO qd*
or	**Tricyclic Antidepressant** →320 (reuptake inhibition of serotonin and norepinephrine)	**Clomipramine** (Anafranil, Gens)	*Incr slowly to 150-300mg qd*

Improvement takes 5-10 weeks of treatment.

13 A. Dermatology – Drugs

13 A.1 Acne Preparations
13 A.1.1 Anti-Infectives

S, R, AE, CI see Antibiotics →186

Clindamycin	PRC B, Lact -
Cleocin, Clindets *Swab 1%* **CleocinT** *Sol, Gel, Lot (top) 1%* **Clinda-derm** *Sol (top) 1%* **Generics** *Sol (top)1%, Gel (top)1%*	**Acne** →361: apply bid; **rosacea** →373: apply lotion bid
Doxycycline	PRC D, Lact -
Doryx *Cap 100mg* **Vibramycin** *Susp 25mg/5ml, 50mg/5ml, Cap 50mg, 100mg* **Generics** *Tab 100mg, 50mg, Cap 20mg, 50mg, 100mg*	**Acne vulgaris** →361: 100mg PO bid; **CH** >8y: 2.2mg/kg PO qd or div bid, max 100mg PO bid; DARF: not req
Erythromycin	PRC B, Lact +
Akne-mycin *Oint 2%* **Benzamycin** *Gel (top) 3%, 5%* **Emgel** *Gel 2%* **Generics** *Sol (top)2%, Gel (top)2%, Swab 2%*	**Acne** →361: apply bid
Sodium Sulfacetamide	PRC C, Lact ?
Klaron *Lot (top) 10%*	**Acne** →361: apply bid
Sodium Sulfacetamide and Sulfur	PRC C, Lact ?
Plexion *Lot (top) 10% + 5%, Cleanser 10% + 5%* **Sulfacet-R** *Lot (top) 10% + 5%*	**Acne** →361, **rosacea** →373, **seborrheic dermatitis** →366: apply qd-tid, cleanser: qd-bid; DARF: contraind. in RF

13 A.1.2 Dicarboxylic Acid

AE (azelaic acid): pruritus, tingling feeling, burning/stinging
CI (azelaic acid): hypersensitivity to azelaic acid products

Azelaic Acid	PRC B, Lact ?
Azelex *Crm 20%* **Finevin** *Crm 20%*	**Acne** →361: apply bid, therapeutic results in 4wk

13 A.1.3 Keratolytics

AE (benzoyl peroxide): burning/stinging, contact dermatitis, redness
CI (benzoyl peroxide): hypersensitivity to benzoyl peroxide products

Benzoyl Peroxide	PRC C, Lact ?
Benzac *Sol (top) 2.5%, 5%, 10 %, Liquid (top) 5%, 10%, Gel (top) 2.5%, 5%, 10 %* **Buf–Oxal** *Cleanser 5%, 10%* **Desquam** *Sol (top) 10%, Liquid (top) 4%, 10%, Gel (top) 2.5%, 5%, 10%, Cleanser 5%, 10%, Soap 10%*	**Acne** →361: cleansers: wash qd/bid, cream/gel/sol: ini apply qd, prn gradually incr to bid/tid

13 A.1.4 Retinoids

MA/EF (acitretin): normalizes growth and differentiation of skin and mucosa cells
MA/EF (isotretinoin, tazarotene, tretinoin): mitotic rate of epidermal cells↑, keratolysis, sebaceous production↓
AE (acitretin, isotretinoin): dryness of skin and mucous membranes, lip infx, hair loss, transaminases↑, blood count changes, hyperlipidemia; **AE** (isotretinoin): visual disturbances, epistaxis, conjunctivits; **AE** (tazarotene): burning, itching, photosensitivity; **AE** (tretinoin): leukocytosis (PO), arrhythmias (PO), headache (PO), dry skin
CI (acitretin, isotretionin): renal/hepatic insufficiency, DM, **CI** (acitretin)women of childbearing age; **CI** (tazarotene): hypersensitivity to tazarotene products, vitamin A/retinoids; **CI** (tretinoin): hypersensitivity to tretinoin or parabens

Acitretin	PRC X, Lact ?
Soriatane *Cap 10mg, 25mg*	**Severe psoriasis** →372: 25–50mg PO qd; **lichen planus** →369: 30mg/d PO x 4wk, then titrate to 10–50mg/d x 12wk total; **Sjogren–Larsson syndr.:** 0.47mg/kg/d PO

Isotretinoin	PRC X, Lact –
Accutane *Cap 10mg, 20mg, 40mg*	**Severe, recalcitrant cystic acne** →361: 0.5-2 mg/kg/d PO div bid x 15-20wk, rep prn 2nd course of Tx after >2mo; **prevention of second primary tumors in patients treated for squamous–cell CA of head and neck:** 50-100mg/m^2/d PO; **neuroblastoma** (maint Tx): 100-250mg/m^2/d PO div bid

Tazarotene	PRC X, Lact ?
Tazorac Bile X *Crm 0.05%, 0.1%* *Gel (top) 0.05%, 0.1%*	**Acne** →361, **psoriasis** →372: apply qhs, max x 3mo

13 A.1.5 Retinoid–Like Drugs

AE (adapalene): skin irritation
CI (adapalene): hypersensitivity to adapalene

Adapalene	PRC C, Lact ?
Differin Bile *Sol (top) 0.1%, Gel (top) 0.1%, Crm 0.1%*	**Acne** →361: apply qhs, therapeutic results in 8-12wk

13 A.2 Anti-Infectives
13 A.2.1 Antibacterials (topical)

AE (bacitracin): contact dermatitis
AE (mafenide): burning sensation, rash/pruritus
AE (mupirocin): headache (nasal), rhinitis/pharyngitis (nasal), taste DO (nasal), stinging/burning, pruritus
AE (silver sulfadiazine): local skin irritation, skin rash, itching
CI (bacitracin): hypersensitivity to bacitracin products
CI (mafenide): hypersensitivity to mafenide products, hypersensitivity to sulfites (metabisulfite in cream)
CI (mupirocin): hypersensitivity to mupirocin products, avoid contact with the eyes, avoid products with polyethylene glycol on open wounds
CI (silver sulfadiazine): hypersensitivity to silver or sulfonamide products, preterm or newborn infants < 2mo

Bacitracin	PRC C, Lact ?
Baciquent, Generics *Oint 500 U/g*	**Minor cuts, wounds, burns or skin abrasions:** apply qd-tid
Gentamicin	PRC C, Lact ?
Garamycin, Generics *Crm 0.1%, Oint 0.1%*	**Skin infx:** apply tid-qid, **CH** >1y: apply tid-qid
Mafenide	PRC C, Lact ?
Sulfamylon *Sol (top) 5%, Crm 85mg/g*	**Adj Tx of burns:** apply qd-bid
Metronidazole	PRC B/X in 1st trimester Lact -
Noritate *Crm 1%* **MetroCream** *Crm 0.75%* **MetroGel** *Gel (top) 0.75%* **MetroLotion** *Lot (top) 0.75%*	**Rosacea** →373: apply bid, therapeutical effects in 3-9wk
Mupirocin	PRC B, Lact -
Bactroban *Crm (augmented) 2%,* *Oint (nasal) 2%*	**Impetigo** →369: apply tid x 3-5d; **wound infx:** tid x 10d; **nasal MRSA eradication:** 1g div between nostrils bid x 5 d
Neomycin + Polymyxin + Bacitracin Zinc	PRC C, Lact ?
Neosporin *Oint 3.5mg/g + 5,000 U/g + 400mg/g*	**Minor cuts, wounds, burns or skin abrasions:** apply qd-tid
Silver Sulfadiazine	PRC B, Lact -
Silvadene, SSD, Thermazene *Crm 1%*	**Burns:** apply qd-bid; DARF: measurement of sulfadiazine levels in severe RF

13 A.2.2 Antifungals (topical) – Polyene Group

see systemic Antifungals →217

Amphotericin B
PRC B, Lact ?

Fungizone *Lot (top) 3%, Susp 100mg/ml, Crm 3%, Inj 50mg/vial (bladder irrigation)*
Generics *Inj 50mg/vial (bladder irrigation)*

Oral candidiasis: 1ml swish and swallow qid between meals for ≥2wk; **candidal cystitis:** bladder irrigation with 50µg/ml sol periodically or continuous-ly x 5-10d;
cutaneous and mucocutaneous Candida infx: apply bid-qid;
candidiasis of diaper area: apply bid-qid

Nystatin
PRC C, Lact ?

Mycostatin *Pastille (Troches, oral) 200,000 U, Susp 100,000 U/ml, Crm 100,000 U/g, Powder (top) 100,000 U/g*
Generics *Susp 100,000 U/ml, Oint 100,000 U/g*

Cutaneous or mucocutaneous Candida infx: apply bid-tid; **fungal infx of the feet, dust feet and footwear:** powder applied bid-tid; **thrush:** 4-6ml PO swish and swallow qid or suck on 1-2 troches 4-5 x/d, infants: 2ml/dose PO with 1ml in each cheek qid

13 A.2.3 Antifungals (topical) – Azole Group

see systemic Antifungals →217

Clotrimazole
PRC B, Lact ?

Lotrimin *Sol(top) 1%, Lot(top) 1%, Crm 1%*
Mycelex *Sol (top) 1%, Crm 1%*
Generics *Sol (top)1%*

Tinea pedis, cruris, corporis, versicolor/cutaneous candidiasis →364, →374: apply bid

Econazole
PRC C, Lact ?

Spectazole *Crm 1%*

Tinea pedis, cruris, corporis →364, **versi-color** →374: apply qd x 2wk, tinea pedis x 4wk; **cutaneous candidiasis:** apply bid x 2wk

Ketoconazole
PRC C, Lact ?

Nizoral *Crm 2%, Shampoo 1%, 2%*
Generics *Crm 2%*

Tinea versicolor →374: apply shampoo 2% to affected area, leave on x 5min, rinse, treat x 2wk; **cutaneous candidiasis, tinea coporis, cruris** →364, **versicolor** →374: apply crm qd, treat x 2wk, tinea pedis x 6wk; **seborrheic dermatitis** →366: apply crm (2%) bid x 4wk; **dandruff:** apply shampoo (1%) biw

Miconazole
PRC, Lact ?

Desenex *Spray (liquid) 2%, Spray (powder) 2%, Shake Powder 2%, Jock Itch Spray Powder 2%*
Monistat-derm *Crm 2%*
Generics *Sol (top) 2%, Crm 2%, Spray 2%*

Tinea pedis, cruris, corporis →364, **versicolor** →374/ **cutaneous candidiasis:** apply bid x 2wk, tinea pedis x 1mo

Oxiconazole
PRC B, Lact ?

Oxistat *Lot (top) 1%, Crm 1%*

Tinea pedis, cruris, corporis →364: apply qd-bid; **tinea versicolor** →374: apply cream qd

13 A.2.4 Antifungals (topical) - Allylamine Group

AF (naftifine): local burning or stinging, contact dermatitis
AE (terbinafine): local irritation, N/V, LFT's↑
CI (naftifine, terbinafine): hypersensitivity to product ingredients

Naftifine	PRC B, Lact ?
Naftin *Gel 1%, Crm 1%*	**Tinea pedis, cruris, corporis** →364: apply qd (cream) or bid (gel)
Terbinafine	PRC B, Lact -
Lamisil *Tab 250mg, Sol (top) 1%, Gel (top) 1%, Crm 1%*	**Tinea pedis** →364: apply bid x 1-4wk; **tinea cruris, corporis** →364: apply qd-bid x 1-4wk; **tinea versicolor** →374: apply sol bid x 1-4wk; **onychomycosis** (fingernails): 250mg PO qd x 6wk; **onychomycosis** (toenails): 250mg PO qd x 12wk; **CH** <20kg: 67.5mg PO qd, 20-40kg: 125mg PO qd, >40kg: 250mg PO qd, x 6wk for fingernails, x 12wk for toenails; **onychomycosis "pulse dosing"**: 500mg PO qd for 1st wk of mo x 2mo for fingernails, 4mo for toenails; DARF: CrCl (ml/min):<50: contraind.

13 A.2.5 Other Topical Antifungals

AE (butenafine): burning/stinging
AE (ciclopirox): periungual erythema, burning of surrounding skin
AE (haloprogin): dermal allergic reactions
AE (tolnaftate): irritation, contact dermatitis
CI (butenafine, ciclopirox, haloprogin, tolnaftate): hypersensitivity to product ingredients

Butenafine	PRC B, Lact ?
Mentax *Crm 1%*	**Tinea pedis** →364: apply qd x 4wk or bid x 7d; **tinea coporis/cruris** →364: apply qd x 2wk
Ciclopirox	PRC B, Lact ?
Loprox *Gel (top) 0.77%, Lot (top) 0.77%, Crm 0.77%* **Penlac** *Sol (nail) 8%*	**Tinea pedis, cruris, corporis** →364, **versicolor/candidiasis:** cream, lotion: apply bid; **onchomycosis of fingernails/toenails:** apply nail sol qd to affected nails, over previous coat, remove with alcohol q7d
Haloprogin	PRC B, Lact ?
Halotex *Sol (top) 1%, Crm 1%*	**Tinea pedis, cruris, corporis, manuum** →364, **versicolor.** apply bid x 2-3wk, intertriginous areas x 4wk
Tolnaftate	PRC N, Lact ?
Aftate *Gel (top) 1%, Powder (top) 1%, Aerosol (liquid/powder, top) 1%* **Dr Scholl's Athlete's Foot** *Sol (top) 1% Crm, Spray (top) 1%, Powder (top) 1%, Aerosol (liquid/powder, top)* **Tinactin** *Sol (top) 1%, Crm 1%, Spray (liquid/powder, top) 1%, Powder 1%*	**Tinea pedis, cruris, corporis** →364, **versicolor** →374: apply bid, **CH** >2y: apply bid; **prevention of tinea pedis:** apply powder/aerosol prn

13 A.2.6 Antivirals

AE (acyclovir): N/V, headache, renal impairment, rash, phlebitis; **AE** (imiquimod): erosion, flaking, edema, erythema; **AE** (penciclovir): erythema; **AE** (podofilox): local irritation, inflammation, itching; **CI** (podophyllin): see Prod Info; **CI** (acyclovir, imiquimod, penciclovir, podofilox): hypersensitivity to product ingredients; **CI** (podophyllin): DM, patients using steroids or with poor blood circulation, not on bleeding warts, moles, birthmarks or unusual warts with hair growing from them

Acyclovir	PRC C (top)/B (oral) Lact +
Zovirax *Tab 400mg, 800mg, Cap 200mg Susp 40mg/ml, Oint 5%* **Generics** *Tab 400mg, 800mg, Cap 200mg, Susp 40mg/ml*	**Herpes genitalis** (ini episodes): apply q3h (6x/d) x 7d or 200mg PO q4h (5x/d) x 10d for 1st episode, x 5d for recurrent episodes, **CH** 80mg/kg/d PO div tid (max 1.2g/d) x 7-10d; **mucocutaneous herpes simplex in immunocompromised patients** (non-life threatening): apply q3h (6x/d) x 7d; **herpes PRO:** 400mg PO bid; **herpes zoster:** 800mg PO q4h (5x/d) x 7-10d; **varicella:** 800mg PO qid x 5d, IV: 5-10mg/kg IV q8h, each dose x 1h, **CH** >2y: 20mg/kg PO qid x 5d, >40kg: adult dose; **primary gingivostomatitis:** 15mg/kg PO 5x/d x 7d; DARF: CrCl (ml/min) 10-25, 800mg: q8h, <10, 800mg: q12h, <10, 400mg: 50% q12h, <10, 200mg: q12h
Imiquimod	PRC B, Lact ?
Aldara *Crm 5%*	**External genital and perianal warts** →363: apply tiw hs, wash off in 6-10h; **giant molluscum contagiosum:** apply tiw x 6-10h
Penciclovir	PRC B, Lact -
Denavir *Crm 1%*	**Herpes labialis** (cold sores): apply cream q2h while awake x 4d, ini at prodrome signs
Podofilox	PRC C, Lact ?
Condylox *Sol (top) 0.5%* *Gel (top) 0.5%*	**External genital warts** (gel/sol)/**perianal warts** (gel only) →363: apply bid x 3 consecutive d/wk, rep x max 4wk
Podophyllin	PRC N, Lact -
Podocon-25 *Sol (top) 25%*	**Genital wart removal** →363: ini apply to wart and leave on x 30-40min to determine patient's sensitivity, then use minimum contact time necessary (1-4h), then remove dried podophyllin with alcohol or soap + water

13 A.2.7 Antiparasitics (topical)

AE (crotamiton): dermatitis, skin irritation
AE (lindane): dermatitis, anxiety, dizziness, insomnia, myelosuppression
AE (malathion): mild eye irritation or conjunctivits may occur with direct eye contact, scalp and/or eye irritation, mild skin rash and/or skin irritation on the scalp, temporary increase in dandruff
AE (permethrin): pruritus, burning, stinging, rash
CI (crotamiton): hypersensitivity to crotamiton
CI (lindane): hypersensitivity to lindane products, premature neonates, seizure DO
CI (malathion): neonates + infants, known sensitivity to malathion or any of the vehicle ingredients
CI (permethrin): hypersensitivity to permethrin/chrysanthemums

Crotamiton	PRC C, Lact ?
Eurax *Lot (top) 10%, Crm 10%*	**Scabies** →370: massage cream/lotion into entire body from chin down, rep in 24h, then bathe in 48h; **pruritus:** massage into affected areas prn
Lindane	PRC B, Lact ?
Kwell *Lot (top) 1%, Crm 1%* *Shampoo 1%* **Lindane** *Lot (top) 1%, Shampoo 1%*	**Head/crab lice** →371: apply lotion 30-60ml to affected area, wash off in 12h or apply shampoo 30-60ml, wash off in 4min, then comb to remove nits, prn rep in 7d; **scabies** →371: apply lotion to total body from neck down, wash off in 8-12h
Malathion	PRC B, Lact ?
Ovide *Lot (top) 0.5%*	**Head lice** →371: apply to dry hair, let dry naturally, wash off in 8-12h, then comb to remove nits, rep in 7-9d, **CII** > 6y: adult application
Permethrin	PRC B, Lact ?
Acticin, Elimite *Crm 5%* **Nix** *Crm (rinse) 1%* **Generics** *Lot (top) 1%*	**Scabies** →371: massage 30g (cream) into entire body, wash off in 8-14h, **CH** >2mo: <30g of cream needed; **head lice:** apply liquid to clean, towel-dried hair, saturate hair, scalp, wash off in 10min, **CH** >2mo: adult applic.
Pyrethrins, Piperonyl Butoxide	PRC C, Lact ?
A-200 *Shampoo 0.33% + 4%* **RID Maximum Strength** *Shampoo 0.33% + 4%,* *Foam 0.33% + 4%*	**Head/crab/body lice** →371: apply shampoo/foam on dry hair, wash after 10min, rep in 5-7d

13 A.2.8 Anti-Infective Combinations

Neomycin + Polymyxin + Hydrocortisone	PRC C, Lact ?
Cortisporin *Crm 3.5mg/g +* *10,000 U/g + 5mg/g*	**Corticosteroid-responsive dermatoses with secondary infx:** apply bid-qid
Betamethasone + Clotrimazole	PRC C, Lact ?
Lotrisone *Lot (top) 0.05% + 1%,* *Crm 0.05% + 1%*	**Tinea pedis, cruris, corporis** →364: apply bid x 2wk, tinea pedis x 4wk

Nystatin + Trimacinolone — PRC C, Lact ?

Mycolog-II, Myco-triacet II, Mykacet, Mytrex f, Generics *Crm 100,000 U/g + 0.1%, Oint 100,000 U/g + 0.1%* — **Cutaneous candidiasis:** apply bid

13 A.3 Antipsoriatics

MA/EF (alefacept): immunosupressive dimeric fusion protein binding to lymphocyte antigen $\Rightarrow$ reduction in CD4, CD8 and T-lymphocyte counts; **MA/EF** (calcipotriene): vitamin D_3 derivate; **AE** (alefacept): lymphopenia, malignancies, serious infections, hypersensitivity reactions, pharyngitis, cough, nausea, dizziness, chills; **AE** (anthralin): skin inflammation, irritiation, rash; **AE** (calcipotriene): skin irritation; **AE** (coal tar): rash; **CI** (alefacept): hypersensitivity to a.; **CI** (anthralin): hypersens. to anthralin, erythroderma, psoriasis pustulosa, type Zumbusch (full-body psoriasis), inflammatory + acute psoriasis, renal DO, flexures; **CI** (calcipotriene): vitamin D toxicity, hypercalcemia, hypersensitivity to calcipotriene; **CI** (coal tar): hypersensitivity to coal tar

Alefacept — EHL 270h PRC B, Lact ?

Amevive *Inj 7.5mg/vial, 15mg/vial* — **Moderate-severe psoriasis** →372: 7.5mg IV or 15mg IM qwk; course of 12 weekly injections is recommended, may repeat after minimum 12wk

Anthralin — PRC C, Lact ?

Anthra-Derm *Oint 0.1%, 0.25%, 0.5%, 1%*
Drithocreme *Crm 0.1%, 0.25%, 0.5%*
Lasan *Oint 0.4%, Paste (top) 0.4%* — **Quiescent/chronic psoriasis** →372: apply qd

Coal Tar — PRC N, Lact ?

Tegrin *Crm 5%, Shampoo 7%* — **Dandruff, seborrheic dermatitis** →366: shampoo $\geq$ biw; **psoriasis** →372: apply cream qd-qid or shampoo affected areas, **CH** >2y: as adults

Calcipotriene — PRC C, Lact ?

Dovonex *Sol (top) 0.005%, Crm 0.005%, Oint 0.005%* — **Moderate plaque psoriasis** →372s: apply bid

see Retinoids →348

13 A.4 Corticosteroids (topical)
13 A.4.1 Topical Corticosteroids - Very High Potency

Augmented Betamethasone Dipropionate — PRC C, Lact ?

Diprolene *Gel (top) 0.05%, Lot (top) 0.05%, Oint 0.05%, Crm 0.05%* — **Dermatoses:** apply qd-bid, max x 2wk, max 50g/wk resp. 50ml/wk

Clobetasol Propionate — PRC C, Lact ?

Cormax *Crm 0.05%*
Temovate *Sol (top) 0.05%, Gel (top) 0.05%, Crm 0.05%, Oint (top) 0.05%*
Generics *Sol (top) 0.05%, Gel (top) 0.05%, Crm 0.05%, Oint 0.05%* — **Dermatoses:** apply bid, max x 2wk, max 50g/wk

Diflorasone Diacetate
Psorcon *Oint 0.05%*

PRC C, Lact ?
Dermatoses: apply qd-qid

Halobetasol Propionate
Ultravate *Crm 0.05%, Oint 0.05%*

PRC C, Lact ?
Dermatoses: apply qd-bid, max x 2wk, max 50g cream or oint/wk

13 A.4.2 Topical Corticosteroids – High Potency

Amcinonide
Cyclocort *Lot (top) 0.1%, Crm 0.1%, Oint 0.1%*

PRC C, Lact ?
Dermatoses: apply bid-tid

Betamethasone Dipropionate
Diprosone *Lot (top) 0.05%, Crm 0.05%, Oint 0.05%*

PRC C, Lact ?
Dermatoses: apply qd-bid

Desoximetasone
Topicort *Crm 0.25%, Oint 0.25%, Gel (top) 0.05%*

PRC C, Lact ?
Dermatoses: apply bid

Fluocinonide
Lidex *Sol (top) 0.05%, Gel (top) 0.05%, Crm 0.05%, Oint 0.05%*

PRC C, Lact ?
Dermatoses: apply bid-qid

Halcinonide
Halog *Sol (top) 0.1%, Crm 0.1%, Oint 0.1%*

PRC C, Lact ?
Dermatoses: apply bid-tid

Triamcinolone Acetonide
Aristocort *Crm 0.5%, Oint 0.5%*
Kenalog *Crm 0.5%*

PRC C, Lact ?
Dermatoses: apply tid-qid

13 A.4.3 Topical Corticosteroids – Medium Potency

Betamethasone Valerate
Betatrex, Beta-Val *Lot (top) 0.1%, Crm 0.1%*
Luxiq *Foam 0.12%*

PRC C, Lact ?
Dermatoses: apply qd-bid, for skalp: foam

Desoximetasone
Topicort *Crm 0.05%*

PRC C, Lact ?
Dermatoses: apply bid

Flurandrenolide
Cordran *Lot (top) 0.05%, Crm 0.025%, 0.05%, Oint 0.025%, 0.05%, Tape (top) 0.004mg/cm^2*
Cordran SP *Crm 0.025%, 0.05%*
Generics *Lot (top) 0.05%*

PRC C, Lact ?
Dermatoses: apply bid-tid

Fluocinolone Acetonide
Synalar *Sol (top) 0.01%, Crm 0.01%, 0.025%, 0.2%, Oint 0.025%*

PRC C, Lact ?
Dermatoses: apply bid-qid

Flurandrenolide	PRC C, Lact ?
Cordran *Lot (top) 0.05%, Crm 0.025%, 0.05%, Oint 0.025%, 0.05%, Tape (top) 0.004mg/cm²*	**Dermatoses:** apply bid-tid
Fluticasone Propionate	PRC C, Lact ?
Cutivate *Crm 0.05%, Oint 0.005%*	**Eczema** →366: apply qd-bid, **CH** >3mo: adult application; **other dermatoses:** apply bid, **CH** >3mo: adult application
Hydrocortisone Butyrate	PRC C, Lact ?
Locoid *Sol (top) 0.1%, Crm 0.1%, Oint 0.1%*	**Dermatoses:** apply bid-tid; **seborrheic dermatitis** →366: apply sol bid-tid
Hydrocortisone Valerate	PRC C, Lact ?
Westcort, Generics *Crm 0.2%, Oint 0.2%*	**Dermatoses:** apply bid-tid
Mometasone Furoate	PRC C, Lact ?
Elocon *Lot (top) 0.1%, Crm 0.1%, Oint 0.1%*	**Dermatoses:** apply qd, **CH** ≥ 2y: adult application
Prednicarbate	PRC C, Lact ?
Dermatop *Crm 0.1%*	**Dermatoses:** apply bid, **CH** ≥ 1y: adult application
Triamcinolone Acetonide	PRC C, Lact ?
Aristocort *Crm 0.025%, 0.1%, Oint 0.025%, 0.1%* **Kenalog** *Lot (top) 0.025%, 0.1%, Crm 0.025%, 0.1%*	**Dermatoses:** apply tid-qid

13 A.4.4 Topical Corticosteroids – Low Potency

Alclometasone Dipropionate	PRC C, Lact ?
Aclovate *Crm 0.05%, Oint 0.05%*	**Dermatoses:** apply bid-tid, **CH** ≥ 1y: adult application
Clocortolone Pivalate	PRC C, Lact ?
Cloderm *Crm 0.1%*	**Dermatoses:** apply tid
Desonide	PRC C, Lact ?
Tridesilon *Crm 0.05%, Oint 0.05%* **Desowen** *Lot (top) 0.05%, Crm 0.05%, Oint 0.05%*	**Dermatoses:** apply bid-tid
Hydrocortisone	PRC C (top) Lact ?
Generics *Sol (top) 1%, Lot (top) 0.5%, 1%, 2%, 2.5%, Crm 0.5%, 1%, 2.5%, Oint 1%, 2.5%*	**Dermatoses:** apply bid-qid
Hydrocortisone Acetate	PRC C, Lact ?
Dricort *Lot (top) 0.5%* **Micort–HC, Generics** *Crm 2.5%* **OraBase hca** *Paste (top) 0.5%*	**Dermatoses:** apply bid-qid

13 A.5 Antipruritics
13 A.5.1 Histamine Receptor Blockers and Combinations

AE (doxepin): burning/stinging (cream), drowsiness, CVS/anticholin. effects, seizures
CI (doxepin): hypersensitivity to doxepin products, glaucoma, urinary retention, concomitant MAO inhibitors

Calamine + Pramoxine	PRC N, Lact ?
Caladryl *Lot 8% + 1%*	**Itching due to poison ivy/oak/sumac, insect bites, minor irritation:** apply prn, max tid-qid
Doxepin	PRC B (top) Lact -
Zonalon *Crm 5%*	**Pruritus associated with atopic dermatitis, lichen simplex chronicus, eczematous dermatitis:** qid x max 8d

13 A.5.2 Other Antipruritics

Oatmeal	PRC N, Lact +
Aveeno *Bath Packets 100% colloidal oatmeal*	**Pruritus from poison ivy/oak, varicella:** add packet to bath qd prn

13 A.6 Hemorrhoid Care

AE (dibucaine): contact dermatitis, photosensitivity reactions
AE (witch hazel): mild itching or burning
CI (dibucaine): hypersensitivity to dibucaine
CI (witch hazel): hypersensitivity to Witch Hazel, internal consumption is not rec

Pramoxine + Zinc Oxide + Mineral Oil	PRC N, Lact ?
Anusol Hemorrhoidal Ointment *Oint 1% + 12.5% + 46.7%* **ProctoFoam** *Foam (pramoxine) 1%*	**Hemorrhoids:** apply oint prn, max 5 x/d
Dibucaine	PRC N, Lact ?
Nupercainal, Generics *Oint 1%*	**Hemorrhoids, other anorectal DO:** apply prn tid-qid, **CH** see adults
Hydrocortisone	PRC C, Lact ?
Anusol-HC *Crm 2.5%, Supp 25mg* **Anusol-HC-1 Anti Itch** *Crm 1%*	**External anal itching:** apply cream tid-qid prn or supp PR bid
Starch	PRC N, Lact +
Anusol Suppositories *Supp 51%*	**Hemorrhoids:** 1 Supp PR prn, max 6 x/d or after each bowel movement
Witch Hazel	PRC N, Lact +
Preparation H Medical Wipes *Pads 50% witch hazel* **Tucks Pre-moistered Pads** *Pads 50% witch hazel*	**Hemorrhoids:** pads for anus/perineum prn, max 6x/d

13 A.7 Hair Restorers

MA/EF (finasteride): inhibition of 5-α-reductase $\Rightarrow$ testosterone cannot be transformed to dihydro-testosterone $\Rightarrow$ hair loss $\downarrow$, prostatic hyperplasia $\downarrow$
AE (finasteride): libido and erection disturbances, gynecomastia, lip swelling, skin rash; pregnant women may not touch tablet brittle!; **AE** (minoxidil): hypertrichosis, pleural/pericardial effusion, reflex tachycardia, fluid retention; **CI** (finasteride): women or children, hypersensitivity to finasteride products; **CI** (minoxidil): hypersensitivity to minoxidil

Finasteride	EHL 6h, PRC X, Lact -
Propecia *Tab 1mg*	**Androgenetic alopecia in men** →362: 1mg PO qd; **androgenetic alopecia in postmeno-pausal women** →362: 1mg PO

Minoxidil	EHL 2.3-28.9h, PRC C, Lact +
Rogaine for Women/for Men *Sol (top) 2%* **Rogaine Extra Strength for Men** *Sol (top) 5%* **Generics** *Sol (top) 2%, 5%*	**Androgenetic alopecia in men or women** →362: apply 1ml bid (to dry scalp)

13 A.8 Anesthetics

Lidocaine HCl	EHL 1.5-2h, PRC B, Lact +
Lta II kit *Sol (top) 4%* **Laryng-o-jet kit** *Sol (top) 4%* **Pediatric Lta kit** *Sol (top) 2%* **Xylocaine** *Jelly (top) 2%, Sol (top) 4%* **Generics** *Jelly (top) 2%, Sol (top) 4%*	**Topical anesthesia for minor dermal procedures** (eg, IV cannulation, venipuncture): apply 2.5g over 20-25cm^2 area or 1 disc $\geq$ 1h prior to procedure; **topical anesthesia for major dermal procedures** (ie, skin grafting harvesting): apply 2g per 10cm^2 area $\geq$ 2h prior to procedure; **topical anesthesia in CH:** 1-3mo or <5kg: apply max 1g over max 10cm^2, 4-12mo and >5kg: apply max 2g over max 20cm^2, 1-6y and >10kg: apply max 10g over max 100cm^2, 7-12y and >20kg: apply max 20g over max 200cm^2; **prior to circumcision in infants >37wk gestation:** apply ma 1g over max 10cm^2;

Lidocaine + Prilocaine

EMLA *Crm 2.5% + 2.5%, Disc (top) 2.5% + 2.5%*

Topical anesthesia for minor dermal procedures: apply 2.5g/20-25cm^2 area or 1 disc $\geq$ 1h prior to procedure; **topical anesthesia for major dermal procedures:** apply 2g/10cm^2 area $\geq$ 2h prior to procedure; **topical anesthesia in CH** 1-3mo or <5kg: apply max 1g over max 10cm^2, 4-12mo and >5kg: apply max 2g over max 20cm^2, 1-6y and >10kg: apply max 10g over max 100cm^2, 7-12y and >20kg: apply max 20g over max 200cm^2; **prior to circumcision in infants > 37 wk gestation:** apply max 1g over max 10cm^2

see Local Anesthetics, →285

13 A.9 Other Dermatologic Agents

AE (alitretinoin): rash, pain (application site), exfoliative dermatitis, pruritus, edema; **AE** (azelaic acid): burning, pruritus, dry skin, erythema, contact dermatitis, acne, seborrhea
AE (becaplermin): rash; **AE** (capsaicin): cough with inhalation, local irritation
AE (hydroquinone): urine discoloration, ochronosis, fingernail staining, local irritation
AE (masoprocol): local skin irritation; **AE** (selenium sulfide): skin irritation, hair loss or disoloration, oily or dry scalp; **CI** (alitretinoin): hypersensitivity to retinoids/alitretinoin; **CI** (azelaic acid): hypersensitivity to a. and propylene glycol; **CI** (becaplermin): hypersensitivity to bacaplermin or parabens, neoplasm at application site; **CI** (capsaicin, hydroquinone, masoprocol, selenium sulfide): hypersensitivity to product

Alitretinoin	PRC D, Lact –
Panretin *Gel (top) 0.1%*	**Cutaneous lesions of AIDS–related Kaposi's sarcoma:** apply bid-qid
Aminolevulinic Acid	PRC C, Lact ?
Levulan *Sol (top) 20%*	**Photodynamic Tx of actinic keratoses:** apply sol 20% directly to the target lesions, rep after ini application has dried, in 14-18h ini photoactivation of aminolevulinic acid by a 1,000sec exposure to blue light (light dose: 10 Joules/cm^2), rep prn q8wk
Azelaic acid	PRC B, Lact ?
Finacea *Gel (top) 15%*	**Rosacea →373:** apply bid to affected areas
Becaplermin	PRC C, Lact ?
Regranex Gel *Gel 0.01%*	**Diabetic neuropathic ulcers:** apply qd (length x width x 0.6=amount of gel in inches), cover with saline-moistened gauze x 12h, then rinse and cover with saline gauze without medication

Capsaicin	PRC N, Lact ?
Zostrix *Crm 0.025%, 0.075%, Oint 0.025%, 0.075%, Stick 0.075%* **Generics** *Crm 0.025%, 0.075%*	**Pain due to rheumatoid arthritis** →276, **osteoarthritis** →275, **neuralgias (zoster)** →304: apply prn, max tid-qid, **CH** >2y: adult application
Fluorouracil	PRC X, Lact -
Efudex *Sol (top) 2%, 5%, Crm 5%* **Fluoroplex** *Sol (top) 1%, Crm 1%* **Generics** *Crm 0.5%*	**Actinic/solar keratoses:** apply bid to lesions x 2-6wk; **superficial basal cell CA:** cover lesions with 5% bid x 3-6wk, max 12wk
Hydroquinone	PRC C, Lact ?
Eldoquin Forte, Eldopaque Forte, Lustra AF *Crm 4%* **Melanex** *Sol (top) 3%* **Solaquin Forte** *Gel (top) 4%, Crm 4%*	**Temporary bleaching of hyperpigmented skin conditions** →370: (i.e. chloasma, discoloration from oral contraceptives, pregnancy): apply bid to affected area
Lactic Acid	PRC C, Lact ?
Lac-Hydrin *Lot (top) 12%, Crm 12%*	**Ichthyosis vulgaris** →369, **xerosis** (dry, scaly skin): apply bid to affected area
Masoprocol	PRC B, Lact ?
Actinex *Crm 10%*	**Actinic keratoses:** apply bid x 2-4wk
Pimecrolimus	PRC C, Lact ?
Elidel *Crm 1%*	**Atopic dermatitis** →366: apply to lesions bid
Selenium Sulfide	PRC C, Lact ?
Head and Shoulders Intensive Treatment *Shampoo 1%* **Selsun Rx** *Lot (top) 2.5%* **Thames, Zenith Goldline, Generics** *Shampoo 2.5%*	**Dandruff, seborrheic dermatitis** →366: massage 5-10ml of shampoo into wet scalp, allow to remain 2-3min, rinse, apply biw x 2wk, maint 1x/wk; **tinea versicolor** →374: apply 2.5% shampoo/lotion to affected area, allow to remain on skin 10min, rinse, rep qd x 7d
Mequinol + Tretinoin	PRC C, Lact ?
Solage *Sol (top) 2% + 0.01%*	**Solar lentigines:** apply bid separated >8h

13 B. Dermatology – Therapies

Norman Levine, MD
Professor, Chief, Dermatology Section, Department of Medicine,
Arizona Health Sciences Center, University of Arizona, Tucson, AZ

13 B.1 Abscess

	Penicillin – penicillinase resistant →188	**Oxacillin** (Bactocill)	*Adults, Ped > 40kg: 500mg PO q6h for 10d;* **Ped** *< 40kg: 25mg/kg PO qid for 10d*
or		**Dicloxacillin** (Dycill, Pathocil, Gens)	*Adults,* **Ped** *> 40kg: 250mg PO qid for 10d;* **Ped** *< 40kg: 6.25mg/kg PO q6h for 10d*
or	**Oral cephalosporin** →192	**Cephalexin** (Keflet, Keflex, Keftab, Gens)	*500mg PO tid for 10d;* **Ped***: 12.5-25mg/kg PO tid for 10d*

13 B.2 Acne Vulgaris
13 B.2.1 Comedonal Acne

	Retinoid →348 (sebaceous gland size ↓, sebum production ↓)	**Tretinoin** (Avita, Renova, Retin-A, Gens)	*Apply gel/crm/sol qpm until clear*
or		**Adapalene** (Differin)	*Apply gel/crm qpm until clear*
or		**Tazarotene** (Avage, Tazorac)	*Apply crm/gel qpm until clear*

13 B.2.2 Papulopustular Acne

Topical agents

	Retinoid →348 (sebaceous gland size ↓, sebum production ↓)	**Tretinoin** (Avita, Renova, Retin-A, Gens)	*Apply gel/crm/sol qhs until clear*
or		**Adapalene** (Differin)	*Apply gel/crm qhs until clear*
or		**Tazarotene** (Avage, Tazorac)	*Apply crm/gel qhs until clear*
Plus	**Antibiotic** →348 (oxidization of bacterial proteins, keratolytic, comedolytic)	**Benzoyl peroxide** (Benzac, Buf-Oxal, Desquam)	*Apply sol/gel bid until clear*
or	**Dicarboxylic acid** →347 (antimicrobial, normalization of keratinization)	**Azelaic acid** (Azelex, Finevin)	*Apply crm bid until clear*
Plus	**Macrolide** →347	**Erythromycin 2%** (Akne-mycin, E-glades, Emgel, Erygel, Gens)	*Apply crm/gel bid until clear*
or	**Lincosamide** →347	**Clindamycin 1%** (Cleocin T, Clinda-Derm, Clindets, Gens)	*Apply sol/gel bid until clear*
Or	**Antibiotic + Macrolide** →347	**Benzoyl peroxide + Erythromycin** (Benzamycin)	*Apply gel bid until clear*
or	**Antibiotic + Lincosamide** →347	**Benzoyl peroxide + Clindamycin** (Benzaclin, Duac)	*Apply gel bid until clear*

Systemic agents

1.	**Tetracycline** →198	**Tetracycline** (Achromycin, Bristacycline, Panmycin, Robitet, Sumycin, Gens)	*500mg PO bid until improvement, maint Tx 250-500mg PO qd indef.*
or		**Minocycline** (Dynacin, Minocin, Vectrin, Gens)	*50-100mg PO bid until improvement, maint Tx 50-100mg PO qd indef.*
or		**Doxycycline** (Doryx, Monodox, Periostat, Vibramycin, Gens)	*100mg PO bid until improvement, maint Tx 50-100mg PO qd indef.*
2.	**Oral contraceptive** →442	**Desogestrel + Ethinyl Estradiol** (Desogen, Ortho-Cept, Gens)	*1 Tab PO qd for 21d indef. (monophasic)*
or		**Ethinyl Estradiol + Norgestimate** (Ortho Tri-Cyclen)	*1 Tab PO qd for 21d indef. (triphasic)*

13 B.2.3 Nodulocystic Acne

Retinoid →348 (sebaceous gland size ↓, sebum production ↓)	**Isotretinoin** (Accutane, Amnesteem, Gens)	*1mg/kg PO qd for 5mo*

Caution: in women of childbearing potential mandatory oral contraception during Tx and until 4wk after Tx!

13 B.3 Alopecia
13 B.3.1 Androgenetic in Men

	Topical hair growth stimulator →358 (vasodilation ⇒ hair growth ↑)	**Minoxidil 5%** (Rogaine)	*Apply sol bid indef.*
and/or	**Systemic 5-α-reductase inhibitor** →358 (conversion of testosterone to dihydrotestosterone ↓)	**Finasteride** (Propecia)	*1mg PO qd indefintely*

13 B.3.2 Androgenetic in Women

Topical hair growth stimulator →358 (vasodilation ⇒ hair growth ↑)	**Minoxidil 2%** (Rogaine)	*Apply sol bid indef.*

13 B.3.3 Alopecia Areata

	Intralesional corticosteroid →355 (locally immunosuppressive)	**Triamcinolone** (Kenalog)	*3-4mg/ml intralesional Inj q6wk until hair regrowth*
or	**Systemic corticosteroid** →148 (antiinflammatory, immunosuppressive)	**Prednisone** (Deltasone, Meticorten, Prednisone Intensol, Gens)	*20-60mg PO qd until full regrowth; Caution: AE of chronic Tx!*

13 B.4 Bullous Pemphigoid

Topical therapy

	Topical corticosteroid, very high potency →354 (antiinflammatory)	**Clobetasol 0.05%** (Cormax, Temovate, Gens)	*Apply crm/oint bid for max 2wk, then 1wk rest, rep cycle until clear*
or		**Diflorasone 0.05%** (Psorcon)	*Apply crm/oint bid for max 2wk, then 1wk rest, rep cycle until clear*
or		**Halobetasol 0.05%** (Ultravate)	*Apply crm/oint bid for max 2wk, then 1wk rest, rep cycle until clear*

Systemic therapy

	Systemic corticosteroid →148 (antiinflammatory, immunosuppressive)	**Prednisone** (Deltasone, Meticorten, Prednisone Intensol, Gens)	*0.5-1.5mg/kg PO qd until clear; Caution: AE of chronic corticosteroid Tx!*
OR	**Tetracycline** →198 (antiinflammatory)	**Tetracycline** (Achromycin, Bristacycline, Panmycin, Robitet, Sumycin, Gens)	*500mg PO bid-tid until clear*
or		**Minocycline** (Dynacin, Minocin, Vectrin, Gens)	*50-100mg PO bid until clear*
or		**Doxycycline** (Doryx, Monodox, Periostat, Vibramycin, Gens)	*100mg PO bid until clear*
Poss plus	**Vitamin B3** →145	**Niacinamide** (Nicotinamide)	*500mg PO bid-tid until clear*
OR	**Anti-inflammatory** →209	**Dapsone** (Gens)	*25-200mg PO qd until clear*

13 B.5 Condyloma Acuminata

	Antiviral →352 (antimitotic)	**Podofilox 0.5%** (=Podophyllotoxin) (Condylox, Gens)	*Apply sol/gel bid for 3d, hold for 4d, then rep for 4 cycles*
or	**Antiviral, immune response modifier** →352 (secretion of cytokines/ interferon alpha↑)	**Imiquimod 5%** (Aldara)	*Apply crm tiw for max 6wk*

13 B.6 Dermatophytosis (superficial fungal infection)
13 B.6.1 Tinea Capitis

Topical therapy

	Antifungal, azole →350 (change in membrane fluidity, fungistatic)	**Clotrimazole 1%** (Lotrimin, Mycelex, Gens)	*Apply crm/sol bid for 6-8wk*
or		**Miconazole 2%** (Monistat-Derm, Gens)	*Apply crm/sol bid for 6-8wk*
or		**Ketoconazole 2%** (Ketozole, Nizoral, Gens)	*Apply crm bid for 6-8wk*
or		**Oxiconazole 1%** (Oxistat)	*Apply crm/lot bid for 6-8wk*
or	**Antifungal, allylamine** →351 (keratophilic, chitin synthesis↓, fungicidal)	**Terbinafine 1%** (Lamisil)	*Apply crm/sol bid for 1-4wk*
or		**Naftifine 1%** (Naftin)	*Apply crm/gel bid for 6-8wk*

Plus systemic therapy

	Antifungal →219 (keratophilic, inhibition of cell wall synthesis)	**Griseofulvin** (Fulvicin, Grifulvin-V, Grisactin, Gris-Peg, Ultragris, Gens)	*500mg PO bid for 6-8wk,* **Ped** *20mg/kg qd for 6-8wk*
or	**Antifungal, allylamine** →351 (keratophilic, chitin synthesis↓, fungicidal)	**Terbinafine** (Lamisil)	*250mg PO qd for 3-4wk,* **Ped** *125mg PO qd for 3-4wk*
or	**Antifungal, azole** →350 (change in membrane fluidity, fungistatic)	**Itraconazole** (Sporanox)	*200mg PO qd for 3-4wk,* **Ped** *200mg PO qd for 3-4wk*

13 B.6.2 Tinea Cruris, Tinea Pedis, Tinea Corporis

Topical therapy

	Antifungal, azole (change in membrane fluidity, fungistatic) →350	**Clotrimazole 1%** (Lotrimin, Mycelex, Gens)	*Apply crm/sol bid for 3-4wk*
or		**Miconazole 2%** (Monistat-Derm, Gens)	*Apply crm/sol bid for 3-4wk*
or		**Ketoconazole 2%** (Ketozole, Nizoral, Gens)	*Apply crm bid for 3-4wk*
or		**Oxiconazole 1%** (Oxistat)	*Apply crm/lot bid for 3-4wk*
or	**Antifungal, allylamine** (keratophilic, chitin synthesis↓, fungicidal) →351	**Terbinafine 1%** (Lamisil)	*Apply crm/sol bid for 1wk*
or		**Naftifine 1%** (Naftin)	*Apply crm/gel bid for 3-4wk*

Or systemic therapy in severe or recurrent disease

	Antifungal →219 (keratophilic, inhibition of cell wall synthesis)	**Griseofulvin** (Fulvicin, Grifulvin-V, Grisactin, Gris-Peg, Ultragris, Gens)	*500mg PO bid for 4-6wk,* **Ped** *20mg/kg PO qd for 6-8wk*
or	**Antifungal, allylamine** →351 (keratophilic, chitin synthesis↓, fungicidal)	**Terbinafine** (Lamisil)	*250mg PO qd for 3-4wk,* **Ped** *125mg PO qd for 3-4wk*

or	**Antifungal, azole** (change in membrane fluidity, fungistatic) →350	**Itraconazole** (Sporanox)	*200mg PO qd for 3-4wk,* **Ped** *200mg PO qd for 3-4wk*

13 B.6.3 Onychomycosis (Tinea Unguium)

Topical therapy

	Antifungal, pyridone →351 (Inhibit synthesis of DNA, RNA, protein)	**Ciclopirox 12%** (Loprox, Penlac)	*Apply qd for 48wk*

Plus systemic therapy

	Antifungal →219 (keratophilic, inhibition of cell wall synthesis)	**Griseofulvin** (Fulvicin, Grifulvin-V, Grisactin, Gris-Peg, Ultragris, Gens)	*1000mg PO qd for 6-12mo,* **Ped** *20mg/kg PO qd for 6-12mo*
or	**Antifungal, allylamine** →351 (keratophilic, chitin synthesis↓, fungicidal)	**Terbinafine** (Lamisil)	*250mg PO qd for 3mo,* **Ped** *125mg PO qd for 3mo*
or	**Antifungal, azole** →350 (change in membrane fluidity, fungistatic)	**Itraconazole** (Sporanox)	*400mg PO qd for 7d, hold for 21d, then rep for 2 cycles,* **Ped** *200mg PO qd for 7d, hold for 21d, then rep for 2 cycles*

13 B.6.4 Candidiasis, Including Candida Vulvovaginitis

Topical therapy

	Antifungal, azole →350 (change in membrane fluidity, fungistatic)	**Clotrimazole 1%** (Lotrimin, Mycelex, Gens)	*Apply crm/sol bid for 3-4wk*
or		**Miconazole 2%** (Monistat-Derm, Gens)	*Apply crm/sol bid for 3-4wk*
or		**Ketoconazole 2%** (Ketozole, Nizoral, Gens)	*Apply crm bid for 3-4wk*
or		**Oxiconazole 1%** (Oxistat)	*Apply crm/sol bid for 3-4wk*
or	**Antifungal, allylamine** →351 (keratophilic, chitin synthesis↓, fungicidal)	**Terbinafine 1%** (Lamisil)	*Apply crm/sol bid for 1wk*
or		**Naftifine 1%** (Naftin)	*Apply crm/gel bid for 3-4wk*

Systemic therapy in severe or extensive disease

	Antifungal, azole →350 (change in membrane fluidity, fungistatic)	**Fluconazole** (Diflucan)	*150mg PO once*
or		**Itraconazole** (Sporanox)	*200mg PO qd for 1-2wk*

13 B.7 Eczema
13 B.7.1 Contact, Stasis, Atopic, Xerotic, Nummular, Dyshidrotic Eczema

Topical Agents

	Topical corticosteroid, medium potency →355 **(antiinflammatory)**	**Hydrocortisone 1%** (Alphaderm, Anusol-HC, Cetacort, Cortaid, Texacort, Locoid, Nutracort)	*In mild disease or facial involvement: apply crm/oint bid until clear*
or	**Topical corticosteroid, high potency** →355 **(antiinflammatory)**	**Triamcinolone 0.1%** (Aristocort, Kenalog)	*In moderate disease: apply crm/oint bid until clear*
or		**Fluocinonide 0.05%** (Lidex)	*In severe disease: apply crm/oint bid until clear*
OR	**Topical immunomodulator** →260 (humoral immunity/ T-lymphocyte activity↓)	**Tacrolimus 0.03% or 0.1%** (Protopic)	*Apply oint bid until clear*
or		**Pimecrolimus** (Elidel)	*Apply crm bid until clear*

Systemic Agents in severe, recalcitrant, extensive disease

	Antipruritic, oral antihistamine →357, →331 (relief of pruritus)	**Diphenhydramine** (AllerMax, Benadryl, Diphen, Sominex, Gens)	*25-50mg PO qhs prn*
or		**Hydroxyzine** (Atarax, Vistaril, Gens)	*10-25mg PO tid prn*
or		**Doxepin** (Sinequan, Gens)	*10-25mg PO qhs prn*
	Systemic corticosteroid →148 (antiinflammatory, immunosuppressive)	**Prednisone** (Deltasone, Meticorten, Prednisone Intensol, Gens)	*1mg/kg PO qd for max 3wk; Caution: AE of chronic corticosteroid Tx!*
or		**Triamcinolone** (Kenalog, Gens)	*40-80mg IM, not > q6-8wk*
or	**Immunosuppressant** →260	**Cyclosporine** (Neoral, Sandimmune, Gens)	*3-5mg/kg PO qd for max 6mo; Caution: potent drug to be used only in severe cases!*

13 B.7.2 Seborrheic Eczema

	Shampoo	**Zinc pyrithione** (Head and Shoulders, Zincon, ZNP)	*Use shampoo qd indef.*
or	**Shampoo, antifungal** →350	**Ketoconazole** (Nizoral)	*Use shampoo biw indef.*
or	**Shampoo, keratolytic** →354	**Coal Tar** (Polytar, T Gel, Zetar, Gens)	*Use shampoo qd indef.*
poss	**Topical corticosteroid, medium potency** →355 **(antiinflammatory)**	**Hydrocortisone 1%** (Alphaderm, Anusol-HC, Cetacort, Cortaid, Texacort, Locoid, Nutracort)	*In mild disease or facial involvement: apply crm/oint qd-bid prn*

or	**Topical corticosteroid, high potency** →355 (antiinflammatory)	**Triamcinolone 0.1%** (Aristocort, Kenalog)	*In moderate disease: apply crm/oint/lotion qd-bid prn*
or	**Topical corticosteroid, medium potency** →355 (antiinflammatory)	**Betamethasone** (Betatrex, Betaval, Luxiq)	*In scalp involvement: apply lot (0.1%) qd-bid prn; apply aerosol (0.12%, Luxiq) qd-bid prn*

13 B.8 Erysipelas

Oral antibiotic therapy

	Oral penicillin - penicillinase resistant →188	**Dicloxacillin** (Dycill, Pathocil, Gens)	*Adults, Ped > 40kg: 500mg PO qid for 10d, Ped < 40kg: 6.25mg/kg PO q6h for 10d*
or	**Oral cephalosporin** →192	**Cephalexin** (Keflet, Keflex, Keftab, Gens)	*500mg PO qid for 10d, Ped 12.5-25mg/kg PO qid for 10d*
or	**Oral macrolide** →199	**Azithromycin** (Zithromax)	*500mg PO on d1; 250mg qd on d2-5, Ped 10mg/kg PO on d1; 5mg/kg PO on d2-5*
or		**Clarithromycin** (Biaxin)	*250mg PO q12h for 5-7d*

Intravenous antibiotic therapy, when systemically ill

	IV penicillin, penicillinase resistant →188	**Nafcillin** (Nallpen, Unipen, Gens)	*0.5-1.5g IV q4h for 3-7d, Ped 10-20mg/kg IV q4h for 3-7d*
or	**IV cephalosporin** →197	**Cefotaxime** (Claforan, Gens)	*1g IV q12h for 3-7d, Ped 12.5-45mg/kg IV q6h for 3-7d*

13 B.9 Erythrasma

	Topical antifungal, azole →350 **(change in membrane fluidity, fungistatic)**	**Miconazole 2%** (Monistat-Derm, Gens)	*Apply crm/sol bid for 14d*
or	**Topical macrolide** →347	**Erythromycin 2%** (Akne-mycin, E-glades, Emgel, Erygel, Gens)	*Apply crm/gel bid for 7-10d*
or	**Systemic macrolide** →199	**Erythromycin base** (E-base, E-Mycin, Eryc, Ery-Tab, Ilotycin, PCE, Gens)	*250mg PO qid for 7-10d*
or		**Clarithromycin** (Biaxin)	*1g PO once*

13 B.10 Folliculitis
13 B.10.1 Bacterial Folliculitis

Topical therapy

	Topical antiseptic	**Povidone-iodine** (Betadine)	*Cleanse (sol) qd-bid until clear*
or		**Chlorhexidine** (Hibiclens)	*Cleanse (sol) qd-bid until clear*

Systemic antibiotic therapy in extensive disease

	Penicillin – penicillinase resistant →188	**Dicloxacillin** (Dycill, Pathocil, Gens)	**Adults, Ped** > 40kg: 500mg PO qid for 10d; **Ped** < 40kg: 6.25mg/kg PO q6h for 10d
or	**Oral cephalosporin** →192	**Cephalexin** (Keflet, Keflex, Keftab, Gens)	500mg PO qid for 10d; **Ped** 12.5-25mg/kg PO qid for 10d

13 B.10.2 Inflammatory Folliculitis

Topical therapy

	Topical antiseptic	**Povidone–iodine** (Betadine)	Cleanse (sol) qd-bid until clear
or		**Chlorhexidine** (Hibiclens)	Cleanse (sol) qd-bid until clear

Systemic therapy in extensive or chronic disease

	Systemic tetracycline →198	**Tetracycline** (Achromycin, Bristacycline, Panmycin, Robitet, Sumycin, Gens)	500mg PO bid until improvement, maint Tx 250-500mg PO qd indef.
or		**Minocycline** (Dynacin, Minocin, Vectrin, Gens)	50-100mg PO bid until improvement, maint Tx 50-100mg PO qd indef.
or		**Doxycycline** (Doryx, Monodox, Periostat, Vibramycin, Gens)	100mg PO bid until improvement, maint Tx 50-100mg PO qd indef.

13 B.11 Herpes Simplex Virus Infection (Including Herpes Vulvovaginitis)

Topical therapy

	Virostatic →352 (purine antagonist, inhibits DNA polymerase)	**Acyclovir 0.5%** (Zovirax)	Apply oint q4h for 5-7d (only useful in primary infection)
or		**Penciclovir 1%** (Denavir)	Apply crm q2h for 4d, while awake

Plus systemic therapy

	Virostatic →211 (purine antagonist, inhibits DNA polymerase)	**Acyclovir** (Zovirax, Gens)	200mg PO 5x/d for 7d
or		**Valacyclovir** (Valtrex)	500mg PO q12h for 7d
or		**Famciclovir** (Famvir)	500mg PO tid for 7d

Systemic prophylaxis

	Virostatic →211 (purine antagonist, inhibits DNA polymerase)	**Acyclovir** (Zovirax, Gens)	200mg PO bid-tid indef.
or		**Valacyclovir** (Valtrex)	500mg PO qd-bid indef.
or		**Famciclovir** (Famvir)	250mg PO bid indef.

13 B.12 Ichthyosis

Topical therapy

Emollients	**Lotion, cream**	*Apply at least bid indef.*
Desquamating agent →348 (epidermal keratinization ↓)	**Ammonium lactate** (AmLactin, Lac–Hydrin)	*Apply crm/lot bid indef.*

Systemic therapy in severe disease, lamellar ichthyosis or epidermolytic hyperkeratosis

Retinoid →348 (normalizes skin/ mucosa cell differentiation)	**Acitretin** (Soriatane)	*25–75mg PO qd indef.*

Caution: in women of childbearing potential mandatory oral contraception!

13 B.13 Impetigo

Topical therapy

Topical antibiotic →349	**Mupirocin** (Bactroban)	*Apply oint tid for 7–10d*
Antibacterial soap	(Lever 2000, Dial, Hibiclens)	*Use at least bid for 7–10d*

Systemic antibiotic therapy, if multiple lesions

Penicillin = penicillinase resistant →188	**Oxacillin** (Bactocill)	**Adults, Ped > 40kg:** 500mg PO q6h for 10d, **Ped < 40kg: 25mg/kg PO qid for 10d**
or	**Dicloxacillin** (Dycill, Pathocil, Gens)	**Adults, Ped > 40kg: 250mg PO qid for 10d, Ped < 40kg: 6.25mg/kg PO q6h for 10d**
or **Ural cephalosporin** →192	**Cephalexin** (Keflet, Keflex, Keftab, Gens)	*500mg PO tid for 10d, **Ped** 12.5–25mg/kg PO tid for 10d*

13 B.14 Lichen Planus

Topical therapy

Topical corticosteroid, high potency →355 (antiinflammatory)	**Triamcinolone 0.1%** (Kenalog, Aristocort)	*In moderate disease: apply crm/oint bid until clear*
or	**Fluocinonide 0.05%** (Lidex)	*In severe disease: apply crm/oint bid until clear*
or **Topical corticosteroid, very high potency** →354 (antiinflammatory)	**Clobetasol 0.05%** (Cormax, Temovate, Gens)	*In severe disease: apply crm/oint bid for max 2wk, then 1wk rest, then rep cycle*
or	**Diflorasone 0.05%** (Psorcon)	*In severe disease: apply crm/oint bid for max 2wk, then 1wk rest, then rep cycle*
or	**Halobetasol 0.05%** (Ultravate)	*In severe disease: apply crm/oint bid for max 2wk, then 1wk rest, then rep cycle*

Systemic therapy in severe, widespread disease

	Systemic corticosteroid →148 (antiinflammatory, immunosuppressive)	**Prednisone** (Deltasone, Meticorten, Prednisone Intensol, Gens)	*20-60mg PO qd for max 3wk per course, Caution: AE of chronic Tx!*
or		**Triamcinolone** (Kenalog, Gens)	*40-60mg IM, not > q8wk*
	Retinoid →348 (normalizes skin/ mucosa cell differentiation)	**Acitretin** (Soriatane)	*25-75mg PO qd until clear*
	Caution: in women of childbearing potential mandatory oral contraception!		

13 B.15 Lyme Disease (Lyme Borreliosis)

	Tetracycline →198	**Doxycycline** (Doryx, Monodox, Periostat, Vibramycin, Gens)	*100mg PO bid for 3wk*
or	**Amoxicillin** →189	**Amoxicillin** (Amoxil, Polymox, Trimox)	*250-500mg PO tid for 3wk,* **Ped** *20-50mg/kg PO tid for 3wk*
or	**Oral cephalosporin, 2nd gen.** →194	**Cefuroxime-Axetil** (Ceftin, Veftin)	*500mg PO bid for 3wk,* **Ped** *250mg PO bid for 3wk*
or	**Macrolide** →199	**Erythromycin base** (E-base, E-Mycin, Eryc, Ery-Tab, Ilotycin, PCE, Gens)	*250mg PO qid for 3wk,* **Ped** *30-50mg/kg qd PO (div tid) for 3wk*

13 B.16 Melasma

	Depigmenting agent →359 (melanocyte metabolic processes ↓ ⇒ reversible depigmentation)	**Hydroquinone 4%** (Eldopaque Forte, Eldoquin Forte, Lustra AF, Solaquin Forte)	*Apply crm/gel to affected areas bid until clear*
and/or	**Dicarboxylic acid** →347 (antimicrobial)	**Azelaic acid** (Azelex, Finevin)	*Apply crm bid until clear*
and/or	**Retinoid** →348 (regulate cell growth/ proliferation, formation of microcomedos ↓)	**Tretinoin** (Avita, Renova, Retin-A, Gens)	*Apply gel/crm/sol qpm until clear*
		Adapalene (Differin)	*Apply gel/crm qpm until clear*
		Tazarotene (Avage, Tazorac)	*Apply crm/gel qpm until clear*

13 B.17 Parasitic Infestation
13 B.17.1 Scabies

	Topical anti-parasitic →353	**Permethrin** (Elimite)	*Apply overnight; rep in 7d*
or		**Lindane** (Kwell, Scabene, Kwildane, Thionex)	*Apply overnight; rep in 7d*
OR	**Systemic anti-parasitic** →220	**Ivermectin** (Stromectol)	*200µg/kg PO once, rep in 7d*

13 B.17.2 Pediculosis

	Topical Anti-parasitic →353	**Lindane** (Kwell, Scabene, Kwildane, Thionex)	*Apply to wet hair, rinse in 30min; rep in 7d sos*
or		**Malathion** (Ovide)	*Apply to dry hair; wash out in 8-12h*
or		**Permethrin 1%** (Nix)	*Apply crm to dry hair; rinse in 10-15min*
or		**Pyrethrin 4% shampoo/foam** (A-200, Rid)	*Apply to dry hair; rinse in 10-15min*

13 B.18 Pemphigus Vulgaris

Topical therapy

	Topical corticosteroid, high potency →355 (antiinflammatory)	**Triamcinolone 0.1%** (Aristocort, Kenalog)	*In moderate disease: apply crm/oint bid until clear*
or		**Fluocinonide 0.05%** (Lidex)	*In severe disease: apply crm/oint bid until clear*
or	Topical corticosteroid, very high potency →354 (antiinflammatory)	**Clobetasol 0.05%** (Cormax, Temovate, Gens)	*In severe disease: apply crm/oint bid for max 2wk per course, hold for 1wk, then rep until clear*
or		**Diflorasone 0.05%** (Psorcon)	
or		**Halobetasol 0.05%** (Ultravate)	

Systemic therapy

	Systemic corticosteroid →148 (antiinflammatory, immunosuppressive)	**Prednisone** (Deltasone, Meticorten, Prednisone Intensol, Gens)	*1-2mg/kg PO qd until clear; Caution: AE of chronic Tx!*
Plus	Immunosuppressant →260 (synthesis of DNA, RNA, proteins↓, proliferation of immune cells↓)	**Azathioprine** (Imuran, Gens)	*100-150mg PO qd until clear*
or	(cytokine synthesis↓) →263	**Methotrexate** (Folex, Rheumatrex, Gens)	*10-25mg PO per wk until clear*
or	(alkylating agent)	**Cyclophosphamide** (Cytoxan, Neosar)	*75-200mg PO qd until clear*
or	→262	**Aurothioglucose** (Solganal)	*25-50mg IM qwk until clear*
or	(proliferation of immune cells↓) →260	**Mycophenolate Mofetil** (CellCept)	*2-3g PO qd until clear*
or	(cytokine synthesis ↓) →260	**Cyclosporine** (Neoral, Sandimmune, Gens)	*3-5mg/kg PO qd until clear*

13 B.19 Pityriasis Rosea

Macrolide →199	**Erythromycin base** (E-base, E-Mycin, Eryc, Ery-Tab, Ilotycin, PCE, Gens)	*250mg PO qid for 2wk,* **Ped** *30-50mg/kg PO qd (div tid) for 2wk*

13 B.20 Psoriasis

Topical therapy

	Topical corticosteroid, high potency →355 (antiinflammatory)	**Triamcinolone 0.1%** (Aristocort, Kenalog)	*In mild disease: apply crm/oint bid until clear*
or		**Fluocinonide 0.05%** (Lidex)	*In moderate disease: apply crm/oint bid until clear*
or	**Topical corticosteroid, very high potency** →354 (antiinflammatory)	**Clobetasol 0.05%** (Cormax, Temovate, Gens)	*In severe disease: apply crm/oint bid for max 2wk per course, hold for 1wk, then rep until clear*
or		**Diflorasone 0.05%** (Psorcon)	
or		**Halobetasol 0.05%** (Ultravate)	
and/or	**Antiproliferative** →354 (cell proliferation ↓, keratolytic)	**Anthralin** (Anthra-Derm, Drithocreme, Lasan)	*Apply for 10-30min qd until clear*
and/or	(vitamin D3 analog, regulate skin cell production) →354	**Calcipotriene 0.005%** (Dovonex)	*Apply crm/sol/oint qd-bid until clear*
and/or	**Retinoid** →348 (regulate cell growth/ proliferation)	**Tazarotene** (Avage, Tazorac)	*Apply crm/gel qd-bid until clear*
and/or	**Tar** →354 (antimitotic)	**Coal Tar** (Estar)	*Apply gel qd until clear*
or		**LCD (Liquor carbonis detergens) 5%**	*Apply qd until clear*

Systemic Therapy

	Retinoid →348 (normalizes skin/ mucos a cell differentiation)	**Acitretin** (Soriatane)	*25-75mg PO qd until clear*
	Caution: in women of childbearing potential mandatory oral contraception!		
or	**Immunosuppressant** →263 (cytokine synthesis ↓)	**Methotrexate** (Folex, Rheumatrex, Gens)	*5-25mg PO qwk indef.*
or		**Thioguanine**	*120-160mg PO biw-tiw indef.*
or	(cytokine synthesis ↓) →260	**Cyclosporine** (Neoral, Sandimmune, Gens)	*3-5mg/kg PO qd for max 6mo*
or	(proliferation of immune cells ↓) →260	**Mycophenolate Mofetil** (CellCept)	*2-3g PO qd indef.*

13 B.21 Rosacea

Topical therapy

	Antiinfective →349	**Metronidazole** (Noritate, MetroCream, MetroGel, MetroLotion)	*Apply crm/lot/gel qd indef.*
or		**Sulfur + Sodium Sulfacetamide** (Plexion, Sulfacet-R)	*Apply lot bid indef.*
or	**Retinoid** →348 (regulate cell growth/ proliferation)	**Tretinoin** (Avita, Renova, Retin-A, Gens)	*Apply gel/crm/sol qpm indef.*
or		**Adapalene** (Differin)	*Apply gel/crm qpm indef.*

Systemic Therapy

	Tetracycline →198	**Tetracycline** (Achromycin, Bristacycline, Panmycin, Robitet, Sumycin, Gens)	*500mg PO bid until improvement, then maint Tx 250-500mg PO qd indef*
or		**Minocycline** (Dynacin, Minocin, Vectrin, Gens)	*50-100mg PO bid until improvement, then maint Tx 50-100mg PO qd indef*
or		**Doxycycline** (Doryx, Monodox, Periostat, Vibramycin, Gens)	*100mg PO bid until improvement, then maint Tx 50-100mg PO qd indef*

13 B.22 Sexually Transmitted Diseases

13 B.22.1 Syphilis (Treponema pallidum)

	Depot Benzylpenicillin →187	**Benzathine Penicillin** (Bicillin L-A, Permapen)	*<1y of infection: 2.4 M U IM; >1y of infection: 2.4 M U IM qwk for 3 wk*
or	**Tetracycline** →198	**Tetracycline** (Achromycin, Bristacycline, Panmycin, Robitet, Sumycin, Gens)	*Prim./sec. or early latent disease: 500mg PO tid for 14d; late latent or tertiary disease: 500mg PO qid for 28d*

13 B.22.2 Chancroid (Haemophilus ducreyi)

	Macrolide →199	**Azithromycin** (Zithromax)	*1g PO once*
or	**Cephalosporin 3rd Gen.** →195	**Ceftriaxone** (Rocephin)	*250mq IM once*
or	**Fluoroquinolone** →203	**Ciprofloxacin** (Cipro)	*500mg PO bid for 3d*

13 B.22.3 Granuloma Inguinale (Calymmatobacterium granulomatis)

	Folate antagonist + p-Aminobenzoic acid antagonist →206	**Sulfamethoxazole + Trimethoprim** (Bactrim, Cotrim, Septra, Sulfamethoprim, Sulfatrim, Gens)	*800+160mg PO bid for 14d*
or	**Tetracycline** →198	**Doxycycline** (Doryx, Monodox, Periostat, Vibramycin, Gens)	*100mg PO bid for 14d*
or	**Fluoroquinolone** →203	**Ciprofloxacin** (Cipro)	*500mg PO bid for 3d*

13 B.22.4 Lymphogranuloma Venereum (Chlamydia trachomatis)

	Tetracycline →198	**Doxycycline** (Doryx, Monodox, Periostat, Vibramycin, Gens)	*100mg PO bid for 21d*
or	**Macrolide** →199	**Erythromycin base** (E-base, E-Mycin, Eryc, Ery-Tab, Ilotycin, PCE, Gens)	*500mg PO qid for 21d*

13 B.22.5 Chlamydia Urethritis (Chlamydia trachomatis)

	Tetracycline →198	**Tetracycline** (Achromycin, Bristacycline, Panmycin, Robitet, Sumycin, Gens)	*500mg PO bid until improvement, then 250-500mg qd indef.*
or		**Minocycline** (Dynacin, Minocin, Vectrin, Gens)	*50-100mg PO bid until improvement, then 50-100mg qd indef.*
or		**Doxycycline** (Doryx, Monodox, Periostat, Vibramycin, Gens)	*100mg PO bid until improvement, then 50-100mg qd indef.*

13 B.23 Tinea Versicolor (Malassezia furfur)

Topical therapy

or	**Antifungal, azole** →350 (change in membrane fluidity, fungistatic)	**Clotrimazole 1%** (Lotrimin, Mycelex, Gens)	*Apply crm/sol bid for 3-4wk*
or		**Miconazole 2%** (Monistat-Derm, Gens)	*Apply crm/sol bid for 3-4wk*
or		**Ketoconazole 2%** (Ketozole, Nizoral, Gens)	*Apply crm bid for 3-4wk*
or		**Oxiconazole 1%** (Oxistat)	*Apply crm/lot bid for 3-4wk*
or	**Antifungal, allylamine** →351 (keratophilic, chitin synthesis↓, fungicidal)	**Terbinafine 1%** (Lamisil)	*Apply crm bid for 1wk*
or		**Naftifine 1%** (Naftin)	*Apply crm/gel bid for 3-4wk*
or	**Selenium sulfide** →359	**Selenium sulfide** (Selsun Blue, Exsel, Head abd Shoulders)	*Apply shampoo qod for 2wk; apply lot qd for 2wk*
or	**Zinc pyrithione**	**Zinc pyrithione shampoo** (Zincon, ZNP)	*Apply shampoo qod for 2wk*

Systemic therapy in extensive disease

	Antifungal, azole →217 (fungistatic)	Ketoconazole (Nizoral, Gens)	400mg PO once; rep in 7d
or		Itraconazole (Sporanox)	200mg PO qd for 7-10d

13 B.24 Urticaria
13 B.24.1 Acute Urticaria

	Antihistamine →357, →408 (suppress histamine activity)	Diphenhydramine (AllerMax, Benadryl, Diphen, Sominex, Gens)	25-50mg PO qid 7-21d
or		Hydroxyzine (Atarax, Vistaril, Gens)	10-25mg PO tid 7-21d
or		Doxepin (Sinequan, Gens)	10-25mg PO qhs 7-21d
or		Cetirizine (Zyrtec)	10mg PO qd for 7-21d
or	(nosedating)	Loratadine (Claritin)	10mg PO qd 7-21d

13 B.24.2 Chronic Urticaria

	Antihistamine →357, →408 (suppress histamine activity)	Diphenhydramine (AllerMax, Benadryl, Diphen, Sominex, Gens)	25-50mg PO qhs indef.
or		Hydroxyzine (Atarax, Vistaril, Gens)	10-25mg PO tid indef.
or		Doxepin (Sinequan, Gens)	10-25mg PO qhs indef.
or		Cetirizine (Zyrtec)	10mg PO qd indef.
or	(nosedating)	Loratadine (Claritin)	10mg PO qd indef.
poss plus	Ca++ channel blocker →28 (stabilize mast cells and inhibit degranulation)	Nifedipine (Adalat, Procardia, Gens)	20-30mg PO bid indef.
poss plus	Systemic corticosteroid →148 (antiinflammatory, immunosuppressive)	Prednisone (Deltasone, Meticorten, Prednisone Intensol, Gens)	0.5-1.0mg/kg PO qd indef.; Caution: AE of chronic Tx!

13 B.25 Varicella Zoster Virus Infection
13 B.25.1 Varicella

	Virostatic →211 (purine antagonist, inhibits DNA polymerase)	Valacyclovir (Valtrex)	1000mg PO tid for 7d
or		Famciclovir (Famvir)	500mg PO tid for 7d

13 B.25.2 Herpes Zoster (Shingles)

	Virostatic →211 (purine antagonist, inhibits DNA polymerase)	Valacyclovir (Valtrex)	1000mg PO tid for 7d
or		Famciclovir (Famvir)	500mg PO tid for 7d

13 B.26 Warts (Verruca; human papilloma virus, HPV)

	Keratolytic (dissolving intercellular cement, desquamating horny layer of skin)	**Salicylic acid +/−** **Lactic acid** (Duofilm, Occlusal-HP, Wart-Off, Medi-Plast)	*Apply qd until clear*
or	**Retinoid** →348 (regulate cell growth/ proliferation, formation of microcomedos ↓)	**Tretinoin** (Avita, Renova, Retin-A, Gens)	*Apply gel/crm/sol qpm (flat warts only) until clear*
or		**Adapalene** (Differin)	*Apply gel/crm qpm (flat warts only) until clear*
or		**Tazarotene** (Avage, Tazorac)	*Apply crm/gel qpm (flat warts only) until clear*
or	**Vesicating agent** (epidermal necrosis and blistering)	**Cantharidin** (Cantharone)	*Apply 0.7% sol once; rep in 4-6wk prn*
or	**Cytotoxic agent** (inhibit cell growth and proliferation)	**Bleomycin** (Blenoxane, Gens)	*0.5-1U/ml sol intralesional Inj, not to exceed 1.5 U/Tx; rep prn*

14 A. Ophthalmology – Drugs

14 A.1 Anti-Infectives
14 A.1.1 Antibacterials – Single Ingredient Drugs

S, R, AE, CI see Antibiotics →186

Bacitracin	PRC C, Lact ?
Generics *Oint 500 U/g*	**Ocular infx:** apply ½ inch ribbon of oint q3-4h or bid-qid
Ciprofloxacin	PRC C, Lact ?
Ciloxan *Sol/Gtt (oph) 0.3%* *Oint (oph) 0.3%*	**Corneal ulcers/keratitis** →392: 2 Gtt q15min x 6h, then 2 Gtt q30min x 1d, then 2 Gtt q1h x 1d and 2 Gtt q4h x 3-14d; **CH** adult dose, if ≥ 1 y use sol, ≥ 2 y use oint; **conjunctivitis** →391: 1-2 Gtt q2h while awake x 2d, then 1-2 Gtt q4h while awakefferve x 5d, or ½ inch ribbon of oint tid x 2d, then ½ inch ribbon bid x 5d; **CH** adult dose, if ≥ 1 y use sol, if ≥ 2 y use oint
Erythromycin Gluceptate	PRC B, Lact +
Ilotycin *Oint 0.5%*	**Ocular infx:** ½ inch ribbon of oint to affected eye(s) q3-4h; **chlamydial infx:** ½ inch ribbon of oint bid x 2mo or bid x 5d/mo x 6mo; **ophthalmia neonatorum PRO:** ½ inch ribbon of oint to eyes within 1h of birth
Gentamicin	PRC C, Lact ?
Garamycin *Sol (oph) 0.3%,* *Oint (oph) 0.3%* **GentAcidin, Genoptic** *Sol/Gtt (oph) 0.3%*	**Ocular infx:** 1-2 Gtt q4h or ½ inch ribbon of oint bid- tid, for severe infx max 2 Gtt qh
Levofloxacin	PRC C, Lact ?
Quixin *Sol (oph) 0.5%*	**Ocular infx:** 1-2 Gtt q2-4h x7d
Norfloxacin	PRC C, Lact -
Chibroxin *Sol/Gtt (oph) 0.3%*	**Ocular infx:** 1-2 Gtt qid x 7d, prn for severe infx 1-2 Gtt q2h x 1-2d, then qid; **CH** >1 y: 1-2 Gtt qid x 7d
Ofloxacin	PRC C, Lact -
Ocuflox *Sol/Gtt (oph) 0.3%*	**Corneal ulcers/keratitis** →392: 1-2 Gtt q30min while awake and 1-2 Gtt 4h and 6h after retiring x 2d, then 1-2 Gtt q1h while awake x 5d, then 1-2 Gtt qid x 3d; **conjunctivitis** →391: 1-2 Gtt q2-4h x 2d, then 1-2 Gtt qid x 5d; **CH** ≥ 1 y: adult dose

Sulfacetamide — PRC C, Lact -

Bleph-10 *Oint(oph) 10%, Sol/Gtt(oph) 10%*
Bleph-30 *Sol/Gtt (oph) 30%*
Cetamide *Oint (oph) 10%*
Isopto Cetamide, Sulf-15, Sulfacel-15 *Sol/Gtt (oph) 15%*
Ocusulf-10 *Sol/Gtt 10%*
Generics *Oint (oph) 10%, Sol/Gtt (oph) 10%, 30%*

Ocular infx: ini 1-2 Gtt q2-3h, then taper x 7-10d, or ini ½ inch ribbon of oint q3-4h, then taper x 7-10d; **CH** ≥ 2 mo: adult dose; **trachoma:** 2 Gtt q2h with systemic sulfonamide; **CH** ≥ 2 mo: adult dose

Tobramycin — PRC B, Lact -

Aktob *Sol/Gtt (oph) 0.3%*
Tobrex *Oint (oph) 0.3%, Sol/Gtt (oph)0.3%*
Generics *Sol/Gtt (oph) 0.3%*

Ocular infx: 1-2 Gtt q2h x 1-2d, then 1-2 Gtt q4-6h or ½ inch ribbon of oint bid-qid

14 A.1.2 Antibacterials – Combinations

Bacitracin + Polymyxin B — PRC C, Lact ?

Polysporin, Generics *Oint (oph) 500 U/g + 10,000 U/g*

Ocular infx: ½ inch ribbon of oint qd or q3-4h x 7-10d

Polymyxin B + Bacitracin + Neomycin — PRC C, Lact ?

Neosporin, Generics *Oint (oph) 10,000 U/g + 400 U/g + 3.5mg/g*

Ocular infx: ½ inch ribbon of oint q3-4 h x 7-10d

Polymyxin + Gramicidin + Neomycin — PRC C, Lact ?

Neosporin, Generics *Sol/Gtt (oph) 10,000 U/ml + 0.025mg/ml + 1.75mg/ml*

Ocular infx: 1-2 Gtt q1-6h x 7-10d, for severe infx max 1-2 Gtt q1h

Polymyxin B + Trimethoprim — PRC C, Lact ?

Polytrim, Generics *Sol/Gtt (oph) 10,000 U/ml + 1mg/ml*

Ocular infx: 1 Gtt q3-6h x 7-10d, max 6 Gtt/d; **CH** ≥ 2 mo: adult dose

14 A.1.3 Antivirals

Fomivirsen — EHL 78h, PRC C, Lact -

Vitravene Exonuclease C *Inj 6.6mg/ml*

CMV retinitis in AIDS patients →244 (failure/intolerance to other Tx): 330µg by intravitreal Inj q2wk x 2 doses, then q4wk

Trifluridine — EHL 12min, PRC C, Lact ?

Viroptic *Sol/Gtt (oph) 1%*

HSV keratitis/keratoconjunctivitis →393: 1 Gtt q2h, max 9 Gtt/d, after re-epithelialization, decr to 1 Gtt q4h (min 5 Gtt/d) while awake x 7-14d, max contin use: 21d; **CH** ≥ 6 y: adult dose

Vidarabine — EHL 2.4-3.3h, PRC C, Lact ?

Vira-A *Oint (oph) 3%*

HSV keratitis/keratoconjunctivitis →393: ½ inch of oint q3h while awake (5x/d), after re-epithelialization, decr to ½ inch bid x 5-7d, max contin. use: 21d; **CH** ≥ 2 y: adult dose

14 A.1.4 Antifungals

Natamycin — PRC C, Lact ?

Natacyn *Sol (oph) 5%* — **Fungal blepharitis, conjunctivitis, keratitis** →393: 1Gtt q1-2h for 3-4d, then 6-8 times daily

14 A.2 Ophthalmic Anti-Inflammatory Agents
14 A.2.1 Corticosteroids – Single Ingredient Drugs

AE (corticosteroids): glaucoma, cataracts, corneal ulcers, secondary infections
CI (corticosteroids): bacterial, viral and fungal diseases of the eyes, injuries, corneal ulcers

Fluorometholone — PRC C, Lact ?

Fluor-Op *Susp/Gtt (oph) 0.1%*
Fml *Oint (oph) 0.1%, Susp/Gtt (oph) 0.1%*
Fml Forte *Susp/Gtt (oph) 0.25%* — **Anti-inflammatory:** prn ini 1 Gtt q4h or ½ inch of oint q4h x 1-2d, then 1 Gtt bid-qid or ½ inch of oint qd-tid; **CH** ≧ 2 y: adult dos.

Loteprednol — EHL 2.8h, PRC C, Lact ?

Altrex *Susp/Gtt (oph) 0.2%*
Lotemax *Susp/Gtt (oph) 0.5%* — **Anti-inflammatory:** 1-2 Gtt qid, prn incr to 1 Gtt q1h during 1st wk of Tx prn

Prednisolone — EHL 2.6-3h, PRC C, Lact -

Econopred *Susp/Gtt (oph) 0.125%*
Pred Forte, Econopred plus *Susp/Gtt (oph) 1%*
Pred Mild *Susp/Gtt (oph) 0.12%* — **Anti-inflammatory:** ini 1-2 Gtt q1h during the day and q2h during the night, then 1-2 Gtt q3-12h

Rimexolone — EHL 1-2h, PRC C, Lact ?

Vexol *Susp/Gtt (oph) 1%* — **Postop inflammation:** 1-2 Gtt qid x 2wk, ini 24h after surgery; **uveitis** →397: 1-2 Gtt q1h while awake x 1wk, then 1 Gtt q2h while awake x 1wk, then taper

14 A.2.2 Corticosteroids – Combinations

Dexamethasone, Tobramycin — PRC C, Lact ?

Tobradex *Oint (oph) 0.1% + 0.3%*
Susp/Gtt (oph) 0.1% + 0.3%
Generics *Susp/Gtt (oph) 0.1% + 0.3%* — **Anti-inflammatory:** 1-2 Gtt q2h x 1-2d, then 1-2 Gtt q4-6h or ½ inch ribbon of oint bid-qid, gradually taper when discontinuing

Neomycin, Polymyxin, Hydrocortisone, (Bacitracin Zinc) PRC C, Lact ?

Cortisporin *Oint (oph) 1% + 3.5mg/g + 10,000 U/g + 400 U/g, Susp/Gtt (oph) 1% + 3.5mg/ml + 10,000 U/ml* — **Anti-inflammatory:** 1-2 Gtt or ½ inch ribbon of oint q3-4h, prn more frequently, gradually taper when discontinuing

Polymyxin, Dexamethasone, Neomycin — PRC C, Lact ?

DexAcidin, Dexasporin *Susp/Gtt (oph) 10,000 U/ml + 0.1% + 3.5mg/ml*
Maxitrol *Oint (oph) 10,000 U/g + 0.1% + 3.5mg/g, Susp/Gtt (oph) 10,000 U/ml + 0.1% + 3.5mg/ml*
Generics *Oint (oph) 10,000 U/g + 0.1% + 3.5mg/g* — **Anti-inflammatory:** ini 1-2 Gtt q1h during the day and q2h during the night, then 1 Gtt q4-8h or ini ½ -1 inch ribbon (oint) tid-qid, then qd-bid, gradually taper when discontinuing

Prednisolone Acetate + Sulfacetamide Sodium	PRC C, Lact -
Blephamide *Susp (oph) 0.2% + 10%, Oint (oph) 0.2% + 10%* **Cetapred** *Oint (oph) 0.25% + 10%* **Isopto Cetapred** *Susp (oph) 0.25% + 10%* **Metimyd** *Oint (oph) 0.5% + 10%,* *Susp/Gtt (oph) 0.5% + 10%* **Vasocidin** *Oint (oph) 0.5% + 10%*	**Anti-inflammatory**: 2 Gtt q4h while awake and hs or ½ inch ribbon of oint tid-qid (during the day) and 1–2x during the night, gradually taper when discontinuing

14 A.2.3 Nonsteroidal Anti-Inflammatory Agents

Diclofenac	EHL 2h, PRC B, Lact ?
Voltaren *Sol/Gtt (oph) 0.1%*	**Postop inflammation following cataract removal:** 1 Gtt qid x 2wk, ini 24h postop; **photophobia associated with incisional refractive surgery:** 1 Gtt to operative eye(s) 1h prior to surgery and 1 Gtt 15min postop, then 1 Gtt qid prn x max 3 d

Ketorolac	EHL 5.3h, PRC C, Lact ?
Acular, Acular preservative free *Sol/Gtt (oph) 0.5%*	**Allergic conjunctivitis** →390: 1 Gtt (0.25 mg) qid; **inflammation after cataract removal:** 1 Gtt (0.25 mg) to affected eye(s) qid, ini 24h postop x 2wk; **CH** ≥ 12 y: adult dose

14 A.3 Glaucoma Agents
14 A.3.1 Glaucoma Agents – Adrenergic Agonists

AE (dipivefrin): burning, mydriasis, blurred vision, follicular conjunctivitis
CI (dipivefrin): narrow angle glaucoma, hypersensitivity to dipivefrin

Dipivefrin	PRC B, Lact ?
Akpro,Propine,Generics *Sol/Gtt (oph)0.1%*	**Glaucoma** →403: 1 Gtt q12h

14 A.3.2 Glaucoma Agents – Alpha$_2$ Agonists

AE (apraclonidine): upper lid elevation, conjunctival blanching, mydriasis, irregular heart beat; **AE** (brimonidine): lid retraction, headache, drowsiness, conjunctival blanching
CI (apraclonidine): hypersensitivity to apraclonidine or clonidine
CI (brimonidine): hypersensitivity to brimonidine, concomitant MAOI therapy

Apraclonidine	EHL 8h, PRC C, Lact ?
Iopidine *Sol/Gtt (oph) 0.5%, 1%*	**Glaucoma** →403: 1–2 Gtt (0.5%) tid; **perioperative IOP** ↑: 1 Gtt (1%) 1h prior to surgery, then 1 Gtt immediately after surgery

Brimonidine	EHL 3h, PRC B, Lact -
Alphagan *Sol/Gtt (oph) 0.15%, 0.2%*	**Glaucoma** →403: 1 Gtt tid

14 A.3.3 Glaucoma Agents - Beta Blockers

AE (beta blockers): eye: conjunctival irritation, dry eyes, decline of papillary blood supply; systemic: bronchospasm, bradycardia, hypotension, cardiac failure ↑
CI (beta blockers): cardiac insufficiency (NYHA III and IV), bradycardia, asthma

Betaxolol — EHL 12-22h, PRC C, Lact ?

Betoptic *Sol/Gtt (oph) 0.5%, Susp/Gtt (oph) 0.25%*
Generics *Sol/Gtt (oph) 0.5%*
Glaucoma →403: 1-2 Gtt bid

Carteolol — EHL 4.7-8.5h, PRC C, Lact ?

Ocupress, Generics *Sol/Gtt (oph) 1%*
Glaucoma →403: 1 Gtt bid

Levobunolol — EHL 6.1h, PRC C, Lact -

Akbeta, Betagan, Generics *Sol/Gtt (oph) 0.25%, 0.5%*
Glaucoma →403: 1-2 Gtt (0.5%) qd-bid or 1-2 Gtt (0.25%) bid

Timolol — EHL 4h, PRC C, Lact -

Betimol *Sol/Gtt (oph) 0.25%, 0.5%*
Timoptic *Sol/Gtt (oph) 0.25%, 0.5%*
Timoptic-XE *Sol (gel forming)/Gtt (oph) 0.25%, 0.5%*
Generics *Sol/Gtt (oph) 0.25%, 0.5%*
Sol (gel forming)/Gtt (oph) 0.25%, 0.5%
Glaucoma →403: 1 Gtt (0.25 or 0.5%) bid or 1 Gtt of gel (0.25 or 0.5% Timoptic XE) qd

14 A.3.4 Glaucoma Agents - Carbonic Anhydrase Inhibitors

AE (acetazolamide): taste ÐÐ, paresthesia, metabolic acidosis, tinnitus; **AE** (brinzolamide): blurred vision, bitter taste; **AE** (dorzolamide): bitter taste, superficial punctate keratitis, blurred vision, ocular burning, photophobia, conjunctivitis; **CI** (acetazolamide): hyponatremia/hypokalemia, severe hepatic disease, hyperchloremic acidosis, hypersens. to acetazolamide; **CI** (brinzolamide, dorzolamide): hypersens. to product ingredients

Acetazolamide — EHL 4-8h, PRC C, Lact -

Diamox *Tab 125mg, 250mg, Cap ext.rel. 500mg, Inj 500mg/vial*
Generics *Tab 125mg, 250mg, Inj 500mg/vial*
Glaucoma →405: 250mg PO qd-qid (immediate release) or 500mg PO qd-bid (ext.rel);
acute glaucoma: ini 250mg IV q4h, then PO, or ini 500mg PO, then 125-250mg PO q4h; DARF: GFR (ml/min) >50: q6h, 10-50: q12h, <10: contraind.

Brinzolamide — EHL 111d, PRC C, Lact

Azopt *Susp/Gtt (oph) 1%*
Glaucoma →403: 1 Gtt tid; DARF: CrCl (ml/min) <30: contraind., caution in moderate RF

Dorzolamide — EHL 4mo, PRC C, Lact -

Trusopt *Sol/Gtt (oph) 2%*
Glaucoma →403: 1 Gtt tid; DARF: CrCl (ml/min) <30: contraind., caution in moderate RF

Dorzolamide + Timolol — PRC C, Lact -

Cosopt *Sol/Gtt (oph) 2% + 0.5%*
Glaucoma →403: 1 Gtt bid; DARF: CrCl (ml/min)<30: contraind., caution in moderate RF

14 A.3.5 Glaucoma Agents - Cholinergic Agonists

AE (cholinergics): conjunctival reddening, accommodation disturbances, transient myopia, spasms of ciliary muscle, (headache, aching eyes), iridocysts, retinal detachment, cataracts
AE (pilocarpine): blurred vision, difficulty in night vision, burning or itching of eyes
CI (cholinergics): malignant glaucoma, secondary glaucoma, iritis, corneal damage
CI (pilocarpine): hypersensitivity to pilocarpine products, acute iritis or glaucoma after cataract extraction, uncontrolled asthma

Pilocarpine	EHL 0.76-1.35h, PRC C, Lact ?
Isopto Carpine *Sol (oph) 1%, 2%, 4%, 6%, 8%* **Ocusert Pilo-40** *Drug Delivery System (oph) 11mg (40µg/h x 1wk)* **Ocusert Pilo-20** *Drug Delivery System (oph) 5mg (20µg/h x 1wk)* **Pilopine HS** *Gel (oph) 4%*	**Glaucoma** →403: 1-2 Gtt up to tid-qid or ½ inch ribbon (4% gel) hs; for drug delivery system see Prod Info

14 A.3.6 Glaucoma Agents - Cholinesterase-Inhibitors

AE (echothiophate iodide): headache/browache, burning/stinging, night vision↓
CI (echothiophate iodide): active uveal inflammation, angle-closure glaucoma (most cases), hypersensitivity to echothiophate products

Echothiophate Iodide	PRC C, Lact -
Phospholine Iodide *Sol (oph) 0.03%, 0.06%, 0.125%, 0.25%*	**Glaucoma** →403: 1 Gtt (0.03%) bid (qam + hs); **convergent strabismus, diagnosis and ini Tx:** 1 Gtt (0.125%) in both eyes hs x 2-3wk; **convergent strabismus, Tx:** 1 Gtt (0.125%) in both eyes qod or 1 Gtt (0.06%) qd, max 1 Gtt (0.125%) qd, taper gradually to lowest possible conc

14 A.3.7 Glaucoma Agents - Prostaglandin F_2 (Alpha) Analogues

AE (prostaglandin analogues): conjunctival hyperemia, growth of eyelashes, ocular pruritus, iris pigmentation, ocular irritation; **CI** (prostaglandin analogues): known hypersensitivity

Bimatoprost	EHL 45min, PRC C, Lact ?
Lumigan *Sol/Gtt (oph) 0.03%*	**Glaucoma** →403: 1 Gtt hs
Latanoprost	EHL 17min, PRC C, Lact ?
Xalatan *Sol/Gtt (oph) 0.005%*	**Glaucoma** →403: 1 Gtt hs
Travoprost	EHL no data, PRC C, Lact ?
Travatan *Sol/Gtt (oph) 0.004%*	**Glaucoma** →403: 1 Gtt hs

14 A.4 Mydriatics, Cycloplegics
14 A.4.1 Anticholinergics

AE (cyclopentolate): IOP↑, burning, photophobia, blurred vision, conjunctivitis; **AE** (homatropine): stinging/burning, keratitis, IOP↑, eye pain; **AE** (tropicamide): ocular irritation, blurred vision; **CI** (cyclopentolate): glaucoma, hypersensitivity to cyclopentolate products; **CI** (homatropine): hypersensitivity to homatropine products, primary glaucoma
CI (tropicamide): narrow angle glaucoma, sensitivity to tropicamide

Atropine	PRC C, Lact ?
Atropine care *Sol/Gtt 1%* **Atropisol** *Sol/Gtt (oph) 0.5%, 1%, 2%* **Isopto Atropine** *Sol/Gtt (oph) 0.5%, 1%, 3%* **Generics** *Sol/Gtt (oph) 1%* *Oint (oph) 1%*	**Anterior uveitis** →397/**postop mydriasis:** 1 Gtt (1–2% sol) up to tid or ¼ inch ribbon (1% oint) up to tid; mydriasis lasts 7–14d; **preoperative mydriasis/ refraction:** 1 Gtt (1% sol) with 1 Gtt phenylephrine (2.5% or 10%) prior to surgery; **ciliary block glaucoma:** ini 1 Gtt (1–2% sol) with 1Gtt phenylephrine 10% tid-qid, red to maint 1Gtt 1–2% sol qd-qod; **posterior synechiae:** 1 Gtt 2% alternately with phenylephrine 10% q5-10min x 5 applications each
Cyclopentolate	PRC C, Lact ?
AK-Pentolate *Sol/Gtt (oph) 1%, 2%* **Cyclogyl** *Sol/Gtt (oph) 0.5%, 1%, 2%* **Pentolair, Generics** *Sol/Gtt (oph) 1%*	**Refraction:** 1–2 Gtt (1–2%), rep prn in 5–10min, apply 45min prior to procedure; mydriasis lasts 6–24h; →397
Homatropine	PRC C, Lact ?
Isopto Homatropine *Sol/Gtt (oph) 2%, 5%*	**Refraction:** 1–2 Gtt (sol 2%) or 1 Gtt (sol 5%) in eye(s) prior to procedure, rep prn q5-10min; **uveitis** →397: 1–2 Gtt (2–5%), rep up to max q3-4h; mydriasis lasts 1–3d
Tropicamide	PRC N, Lact ?
Mydriacyl, Tropicacyl, Generics *Sol/Gtt (oph) 0.5%, 1%*	**Fundus exam:** 1–2 Gtt (0.5%) in eye(s) 15–20min prior to exam, rep prn q30min; mydriasis lasts 6h; →397

14 A.4.2 Sympathomimetics

AE (phenylephrine): tachycardia, HTN, MI, SAH
CI (phenylephrine): hypersensitivity to phenylephrine products, narrow angle glaucoma, HTN, CAD, BPH

Phenylephrine	PRC C, Lact ?
Neo-Synephrine *Sol/Gtt (oph) 2.5%, 10%*	**Ophthalmologic exams:** 1–2 Gtt (2.5 or 10%) prior to procedure; **ocular surgery:** 1–2 Gtt (2.5 or 10%) prior to surgery; **glaucoma** →406: 1 Gtt (10%) qid with atropine; **uveitis** →397: 1–2 Gtt (2.5 or 10%) tid with atropine; **minor eye irritation:** 1–2 Gtt (0.12%) qid prn; **refraction:** 1 Gtt (2.5%) after atropine; mydriasis lasts 5h

14 A.5 Ocular Decongestants, Anti-Allergics
14 A.5.1 H$_1$-Receptor Antagonists

AE (levocabastine): ocular irritation, headache, drowsiness; **AE** (olopatadine): headache, ocular burning, dryness, cold syndrome, rhinopharyngitis, dysgeusia
CI (levocabastine): hypersensitivity to levocabastine products, soft contact lenses
CI (olopatadine): hypersensitivity to olopatadine

Levocabastine	EHL 33-40h, PRC C, Lact ?
Livostin *Susp/Gtt (oph) 0.05%*	**Seasonal allergic conjunctivitis** →390: 1 Gtt in each eye bid-qid x up to 2wk; **CH** ≥ 12 y: adult dose
Olopatadine	EHL 3h, PRC C, Lact ?
Patanol *Sol/Gtt (oph) 0.1%*	**Allergic conjunctivitis** →390: 1-2 Gtt bid in each eye within 6-8h; **CH** >3 y: adult dose

14 A.5.2 H$_1$-Antagonist, Mast Cell Stabilizer

CI (ketotifen fumarate): hypersensitivity to ketotifen products or benzoate compounds

Ketotifen Fumarate	EHL 21h, PRC C, Lact ?
Zaditor *Sol/Gtt (oph) 0.025%*	**Allergic conjunctivitis** →390: 1 Gtt q8-12h in each eye; **CH** > 3 y: adult dose

14 A.5.3 Mast Cell Stabilizers

AE (iodoxamide tromethamine): burning, stinging, blurred vision, dry eye, ocular itching/pruritus
AE (pemirolast): burning, dry eyes, foreign body sensation
CI (iodoxamide tromethamine, pemirolast): hypersensitivity to product ingredients

Cromolyn Sodium	EHL 80-90min, PRC B, Lact ?
Crolom, Cromoptic, Opticrom, Generics *Sol/Gtt (oph) 4%*	**Allergic ocular DO:** 1-2 Gtt in each eye 4-6 x/d; **CH** ≥ 4 y: adult dose
Lodoxamide Tromethamine	EHL 8.5h, PRC B, Lact ?
Alomide *Sol/Gtt (oph) 0.1%*	**Allergic ocular DO:** 1-2 Gtt qid x up to 3mo; **CH** ≥ 2 y: adult dose
Nedocromil	EHL 1.5-3.3h, PRC B, Lact ?
Alocril *Sol/Gtt (oph) 2%*	**Allergic conjunctivitis** →390: 1-2 Gtt bid; **CH** ≥ 3 y: adult dose
Pemirolast	EHL 4-5h, PRC C, Lact ?
Alamast *Sol/Gtt (oph) 0.1%*	**Allergic conjunctivitis** →390: 2 Gtt in affected eyes qid; **CH** ≥ 3 y: adult dose

14 A.5.4 Sympathomimetics

AE (naphazoline): local mucosal irritation, HTN, CNS effects, tremor, eye irritation and redness
CI (naphazoline): hypersensitivity to naphazoline products, narrow angle glaucoma, hyperthyroidism, CAD, BPH, HTN

Naphazoline	PRC C, Lact ?
Albalon, Naphcon fort, Nafazair, Opcon, Vasocon, Generics *Sol/Gtt (oph) 0.1%*	**Ocular vasoconstrictor/decongestant:** 1 Gtt q3-4h prn up to qid

14 A.5.5 Sympathomimetics + H_1-Receptor Antagonists

Naphazoline + Pheniramine	PRC C, Lact ?
Naphcon-A, Visine-A *Sol/Gtt (oph) 0.025% + 0.3%* **Opcon-A** *Sol/Gtt (oph) 0.02675% + 0.315%*	**Ocular decongestant:** 1-2 Gtt bid-qid prn; **CH** $\geq$ 6 y: adult dose

14 A.6 Local Anesthetics

AE: allergic reactions, corneal damage after long-term use

Proparacaine	PRC C, Lact ?
Alcaine, Ophthaine, Ophthetic, Paracaine, Generics *Sol/Gtt (oph) 0.5%*	**Local anesthetic:** 1-2 Gtt prior to procedure, rep q5-10min x 1-3 doses (suture or foreign body removal) or x 5-7 doses (cataract or glaucoma surgery)
Tetracaine	PRC C, Lact ?
Opticaine, Pontocaine *Sol/Gtt (oph) 0.5%*	**Local anesthetic:** 1-2 Gtt prior to procedure

14 A.7 Other Ophthalmologic Drugs

Artifical Tears	PRC N, Lact ?
Hypotears *Sol/Gtt (oph) Polyvinyl alcohol 1% + Polyethylene glycol 1%* **Tears Naturale** *Sol/Gtt (oph) Hydroxypropyl methylcellulose 0.3% + Dextran 70 0.1%*	**Ophthalmic lubricant:** 1-2 Gtt tid-qid prn
Cyclosporine	PRC C, Lact ?
Restasis *Sol/Gtt (oph) 0.05%*	**Keratoconjunctivitis sicca:** 1 Gtt bid

14 B. Ophthalmology – Therapies

Daniel S. Casper, MD, Assistant Clinical Professor
Department of Ophthalmology, College of Physicians & Surgeons
Columbia University, New York, NY
Pamela Cheung, MD, Assistant Professor
Department of Ophthalmology, University of Tennessee Health Science
Center, Memphis, TN

14 B.1 Hordeolum, Chalazion

	- **Warm compresses** - **Massage** - **Lid hygiene**		
plus or	**Topical Antibiotic** →377 (broad-spectrum)	**Bacitracin oint** (Gens)	*apply ½ inch ribbon tid-qid for 7-10d*
		Erythromycin oint 0.5% (Ilotycin)	
con- sider	**Intralesional Corticosteroid** →355	**Triamcinolone 40mg/ml** (Kenalog, Aristocort)	*0.2-1.0ml Inj directly into lesion*

Intralesional corticosteroid may be associated with localized permanent skin depigmentation. If these measures do not eliminate the lesion, then **incision with drainage and curettage** may be considered.

14 B.2 Blepharitis
14 B.2.1 Anterior Blepharitis

	Lid hygiene with eyelid scrubs + warm compresses		
Plus	**Artificial Tears, Lubricant** →385 (lubricate ocular surface, maintain ocular tonicity)	**Methyl, ethyl, and propyl cellulose preparations; Glycerin** (Celluvisc, GenTeal, Hypo Tears, Ref resh Tears, Tears Naturale II, Gens)	*1 Gtt qid-qh (short or longterm)*
or		**Preservative-free Tears** (Bion Tears, GenTeal, Hypo Tears PF, OcuCoat PF, Refresh Plus, Tears Naturale Free, Thera Tears)	*1 Gtt qid-qh (long-term)*
or		**Petrolatum/lanolin/mineral oil oint comb.** (Lacri-lube, Duolube, Duratears Naturale, Refresh PM, Gens)	*½ inch qhs-qid*
Plus	**Topical Antibiotic** →377 (gram-positive coverage)	**Bacitracin oint** (Gens)	*apply ½ inch ribbon qhs- tid*
or	**Topical Macrolide** →377	**Erythromycin oint 0.5%** (Ilotycin)	
Or	**Topical Antibiotic + Corticosteroid** →379	**Tobramycin + Dexamethasone 0.1%** (Tobradex aq or oint)	*1 Gtt qd-qid or ½ inch oint qhs*

14 B.2.2 Posterior Blepharitis, Meibomianitis

	Topical Antibiotic →377 (gram-positive coverage)	**Bacitracin oint** (Gens)	*apply ½ inch ribbon qhs- tid*
or	**Topical Macrolide** →377	**Erythromycin oint 0.5%** (Ilotycin)	
Plus	**Oral Tetracycline** →198	**Doxycycline** (Doryx, Periostat, Vibramycin, Gens)	*100mg PO bid for 2wk, then decr slowly*
or		**Minocycline** (Dynacin, Minocin, Vectrin, Gens)	
or		**Tetracycline** (Achromycin, Sumycin, Gens)	*250mg PO qid for 2wk, then decr slowly*
or	**Oral Macrolide** →199	**Erythromycin** (e-Base, E-mycin, Eryc, Gens)	

Note: Doxycycline, minocycline and tetracycline are contraindicated in children, pregnant women and nursing women.

144.   Cohen EJ: Cornea and external disease in the new millennium. Arch Ophthalmol 2000; 118(7): 979-981
145.   Fraunfelder FT, Roy FH, Steinemann TL: Current Ocular Therapy. 5th ed, 2000: 72, 374, 378, 450.
146.   Lederman C, Miller M: Hordeola and chalazia Pediatr Rev 1999; 20(8): 283-284.

14 B.3   Abscess, Furuncle of the Eyelids
14 B.3.1 In General

- Warm compresses
- Debridement (prn)
- Incision and drainage (prn)

plus	**Topical Antibiotic** →377	**Bacitracin + Polymyxin B oint** (Polysporin, Gens)	*½ inch tid-qid*
or		**Tobramycin oint 0.3%** (Tobrex)	
plus	**Systemic Cephalosporin** →194	**Cefaclor** (Ceclor, Gens)	*250-500mg PO q8h,* **Ped** *20-40mg/kg PO qd (div tid), for 7-10d*
or	**Systemic broad-spectrum penicillin + beta-lactamase Inhibit.** →191	**Amoxicillin + Clavulanate** (Augmentin)	*250-500mg PO q8h,* **Ped** *20-40mg/kg qd (div tid) for 7-10d*

14 B.3.2 In Severe Cases in Adults

Systemic Cephalosporin →194	**Cefuroxime** (Kefurox, Zinacef, Gens)	*750-1500mg IM/IV q8h*

14 B.3.3 In Severe Cases in Children

Systemic broad-spectrum penicillin →189	**Ampicillin** (Omnipen, Principen, Totacillin, Gens)	**Ped** *50-100mg/kg PO qd (div q6h), or 100-200mg/kg IM/IV qd (div q6h)*

147. Barza m, Baum J: Ocular infections. Med Clin North Am 1983;67(1):131–152.
Schwartz G: Etiology, Diagnosis, and Treatment of Orbital Infections. Curr Infect Dis Rep 2002;4(3):201–205.
148. Weiss A, Friendly D, Eglin K, et al: Bacterial periorbital and orbital cellulitis in childhood. Ophthalmology 1983; 90(3): 195-203.

14 B.4 Viral Infections of the Eyelids
14 B.4.1 Herpes Simplex

Warm compresses to lesions tid

Plus	**Topical Antiviral** →378	**Trifluridine 1%** (Viroptic)	*1 Gtt 5x/d for 7-14d*
or		**Vidarabine oint 3%** (Vira-A)	*½ inch 5x/d*
+/–	**Oral Antiviral** →211	**Acyclovir** (Zovirax, Gens)	*400mg PO 5x/d for 7-14d; systemic in primary herpetic infection*

14 B.4.2 Herpes Zoster

Warm compresses to lesions tid

Plus	**Topical Antibiotic** →377	**Bacitracin oint** (Gens)	*½ inch bid-tid;*
or		**Erythromycin oint 0.5%** (Ilotycin)	*Note: trifluridine not effective in HZV*
Plus	**Oral Antiviral** →211	**Acyclovir** (Zovirax, Gens)	*800mg PO 5x/d for 7d*
or		**Famciclovir** (Famvir)	*500mg PO tid for 7d*
or		**Valacyclovir** (Valtrex)	*1g PO tid for 7d*

149. Chern KC, Margolis TP: Varicella zoster virus ocular disease. Int Ophthalmol Clin 1998; 38(4): 149-160.
150. Pavan-Langston D: Viral diseases of the cornea and external eye. In: Albert DM, Jakobiec FA, eds.
151. Principles and Practices of Ophthalmology. Vol. 1. 1994: 117-161.

14 B.5 Dacryoadenitis
14 B.5.1 Acute Bacterial Dacryoadenitis

In general

	Systemic broad-spectrum penicillin + beta-lactamase Inhibit. →191	**Amoxicillin + Clavulanate** (Augmentin)	*250-500mg PO q8h,* **Ped** *20-40mg/kg PO qd (div tid) for ca. 7-14d*
or	Systemic Cephalosporin →192	**Cephalexin** (Keflex, Keftab, Gens)	*250-500mg PO q6h,* **Ped** *20-50mg/kg PO qd (div qid) for ca. 7-14d*

In severe cases IV Tx

	Systemic Cephalosporin →191	**Cefazolin** (Ancef, Kefzol, Gens)	*1g IV tid-qid for 7-14d,* **Ped** *50-100mg/kg qd (div tid-qid) for 7-14d*

In Gonococci

Systemic Cephalosporin →195	**Ceftriaxone** (Rocephin)	*125mg IM once*

In Staphylococci

Systemic Penicillin →188	**Oxacillin** (Bactocill)	*1g IM/IV q6h,* **Ped** *50-100mg/kg qd (div qid) for 7-14d*

In Streptococci

Systemic broad-spectrum penicillin →189	**Ampicillin** (Omnipen, Principen, Totacillin, Gens)	*500mg q6h,* **Ped** *50-100mg/kg PO qd (div q6h), or 100-200mg/kg IM/IV qd (div q6h)*

14 B.5.2 Acute Viral Dacryoadenitis

- Mumps, Mononucleosis, EBV, HZV, CMV
- Supportive measures: cool compresses, analgesics prn

14 B.5.3 Chronic Dacryoadenitis in Tuberculosis

Tuberculostatic →208	**Isoniazid** (Gens)	*300mg PO qd for 2mo; PRO of isoniazid neuropathy:* **Pyridoxine** *(Gens) 25-50mg PO qd suppl*
or	**Rifampin** (Rifadin, Rimactane, Gens)	*600mg PO qd for 2mo*
or	**Pyrazinamide** (Gens)	*2g PO qd for 2mo*
or	**Ethambutol** (Myambutol, Gens)	*15mg/kg PO qd, max 2500mg qd*

152. Boruchoff SA, Boruchoff SE: Infections of the lacrimal system. Infect Dis Clin North Am 1992; 6(4): 925-932.
153. Fitzsimmons TD, Wilson SE, Kennedy RH: Infectious dacryoadenitis. In: Ocular Infection and Immunity. St. Louis: CV Mosby; 1996:1341-1345.
154. Massaro BM, Tabbara KF: Infections of lacrimal apparatus. In: Infections of the Eye. Boston: Little Brown & Co; 1996:551-558.

14 B.6 Dacryocystitis

14 B.6.1 In General

- Warm compresses
- Massage
- Poss incision/drainage if abscess

14 B.6.2 Acute Dacryocystitis in Adults (modify depending on etiology)

Systemic Cephalosporin →192	**Cephalexin** (Keflex, Keftab, Gens)	*500mg PO q6h for 10-14d*
or	Systemic penicillin + beta-lactamase Inhibit. →191 / **Amoxicillin + Clavulanate** (Augmentin)	*500mg PO q8h for 10-14d*
severe	Systemic Cephalosporin →191 / **Cefazolin** (Ancef, Kefzol, Gens)	*1g IV q8h*
or	Systemic penicillin + beta-lactamase Inhibit. →191 / **Ampicillin + Sulbactam** (Unasyn)	*1.5g IV q6h*

14 B.6.3 Acute Dacryocystitis in Children

	Systemic penicillin + beta-lactamase Inhibit. →191	**Amoxicillin + Clavulanate** (Augmentin)	*20-40mg/kg qd (div tid) for 10-14d*
severe	**Systemic Cephalosporin** →193	**Cefuroxime** (Kefurox, Zinacef, Gens)	*50-100mg/kg IV qd (div tid) for 10-14d*

155. Dryden RM, Wulc AE: Lacrimal inflammations and infections. In: Oculoplastic, Orbital and Reconstructive Surgery. Vol. 2. 1417-1423.
156. Hurwitz JJ, Rodgers KJ: Management of acquired dacryocystitis. Can J Ophthalmol 1983; 18(5): 213-216.

14 B.7 Conjunctivitis

14 B.7.1 Keratoconjunctivitis Sicca

	Artificial Tears, Lubricant →385 (lubricate ocular surface, maintain ocular tonicity)	**Methyl, ethyl, and propyl cellulose preparations; Glycerin** (Celluvisc, GenTeal, Hypo Tears, Refresh Tears, Tears Naturale II, Gens)	*1 Gtt qid-qh (long-term)*
or		**Preservative-free Tears** (Bion Tears, GenTeal, Hypo Tears PF, OcuCoat PF, Refresh Plus, Tears Naturale Free, Thera Tears)	*1 Gtt qid-qh (long-term)*
or		**Petrolatum/lanolin/mineral oil oint comb.** (Lacri-lube, Duolube, Duratears Naturale, Refresh PM, Gens)	*½ inch qhs-qid*

Consider placement of punctal plugs in punctae of nasolacrimal ducts to decrease tear egress and prolong tear presence in conjunctival sac

14 B.7.2 Allergic Conjunctivitis

	Vasoconstrictor + Antihistamine →385	**Naphazoline + Pheniramine** (Naphcon-A, Opcon-A, Visine-A)	*1 Gtt qid prn*
or	**Topical mast cell stabilizer** →384	**Cromolyn sodium** (Crolom, Opticrom, Gens)	*1 Gtt qid* *may take wk for effect*
or		**Nedocromil** (Alocril)	*1 Gtt bid prn*
or		**Pemirolast** (Alamast)	*1 Gtt qid prn*
or		**Lodoxamide** (Alomide)	*1 Gtt bid-qid prn*
+/ or	**Topical Antihistamine** →384 (H1 receptor antagonist)	**Levocabastine** (Livostin)	*1 Gtt bid-qid prn*
		Azelastine (Optivar)	*1 Gtt bid prn*

or	**Antihistamine/ Mast cell stabilizer** →384	**Olopatadine** (Patanol)	*1 Gtt bid prn*
		Ketotifen (Zaditor)	*1 Gtt bid prn*
or	**Topical Corticosteroid** →379 (low-medium potency)	**Loteprednol** (Alrex, Lotemax)	*1 Gtt bid-qid*
+/–	**Oral Antihistamine** →408	**Diphenhydramine** (Benadryl, Gens)	*25-50mg q4-6h*

14 B.7.3 Bacterial Conjunctivitis

In general

	Topical Antibiotic →377, →378	**Polymyxin B + Trimethoprim** (Polytrim, Gens)	*1 Gtt qid for 5-7d*
or	(broad-spectrum)	**Bacitracin oint** (Gens)	*½ inch qid for 5-7d*
or		**Erythromycin oint 0.5%** (Ilotycin)	
or	**Topical Fluoroquinolone** →377	**Ciprofloxacin** (Ciloxan)	*1 Gtt (0.3%) qid for 5-7d*
		Ofloxacin (Ocuflox)	

In Gonococci

- Irrigate with saline QID
- Treat concurrent Chlamydia

	Topical Antibiotic →377 (broad-spectrum)	**Bacitracin oint** (Gens)	*½ inch q2-4h*
	Systemic Cephalosporin →195	**Ceftriaxone** (Rocephin)	*1g IM once, Neonatal: 125mg IM once*

Chlamydia conjunctivitis

	Topical Antibiotic →377	**Erythromycin oint 0.5%** (Ilotycin)	*½ inch qid*
or		**Sulfacetamide oint** (Bleph-10, Gens)	
Plus	**Systemic Antibiotic** →198	**Tetracycline** (Achromycin, Sumycin, Gens)	*250-500mg qid for 3-6wk*
or		**Doxycycline** (Doryx, Periostat, Vibramycin, Gens)	*100mg bid for 3-6wk*

Note: Doxycycline and tetracycline are contraindicated in children, pregnant women and nursing women

or	**Systemic Macrolide** →199	**Erythromycin** (e-Base, E-mycin, Eryc, Gens)	*250-500mg qid, Neonate: 50mg/kg qd (div qid) for 3-6wk*

14 B.7.4 Viral Conjunctivitis

- Cool compresses
- Spread precautions

	Artificial Tear preparations and lubricants →385	**Methyl, ethyl, and propyl cellulose preparations; Glycerin** (Celluvisc, GenTeal, Hypo Tears, Refresh Tears, Tears Naturale II, Gens)	*1 Gtt qid-qh*
+/-	**Vasoconstrictor + Antihistamine** →385	**Naphazoline + Pheniramine** (Naphcon-A, Opcon-A, Visine-A)	*1 Gtt qid prn*
+/-	**Topical NSAID** →380 (anti-inflammatory)	**Diclofenac** (Voltaren)	*1 Gtt qid prn*

157. Allansmith MR, Ross RN: Ocular allergy and mast cell stabilizers. Surv Ophthalmol 1986; 30(4): 229-244.
158. Friedlaender MH: A review of the causes and treatment of bacterial and allergic conjunctivitis. Clin Ther 1995;17(5):800-810.
159. Hingorani M, Lightman S: Therapeutic options in ocular allergic disease. Drugs 1995;50(2):208-221.
160. Nelson JD: Diagnosis of keratoconjunctivitis sicca. Int Ophthalmol Clin 1994; 34(1): 37-56.
161. Pavan-Langston D: Viral diseases of the cornea and external eye. In: Albert DM, Jakobiec FA, eds.
162. Principles and Practices of Ophthalmology. Vol. 1. 1994:117-161.

14 B.8 Keratitis
14 B.8.1 Bacterial Ulcers

Note: Any ulcer at or near the visual axis, and > 1mm in diameter, or any lesion > 2-3mm in diameter requires culturing.

Topical therapy

or	**Topical broad–spectrum antibiotic** →377	**Ciprofloxacin** (Ciloxan)	*1 Gtt (0.3%) qid–qh (may use loading dose as directed)*
or		**Ofloxacin** (Ocuflox)	
or		**Tobramycin** (Tobrex)	
+/-		**Ciprofloxacin oint** (Ciloxan)	*½ inch (0.3%) qhs*
or		**Tobramycin oint** (Tobrex)	
or if severe	**Fortified Topical Antibiotics** (-gram-positive coverage)	**Fortified Cefazolin** (50mg/ml)	*1 Gtt q1-2h*
or		**Fortified Vancomycin** (25-50mg/ml)	*1 Gtt q1-2h*
or	**Fortified Topical Antibiotics** (-gram-neg. coverage)	**Fortified Tobramycin** (15mg/ml)	*1 Gtt q1-2h alternating*
plus	**Cycloplegic** →383 (ciliary spasm ↓)	**Cyclopentolate 1–2%** (AK-Pentolate, Cyclogyl, Gens)	*1 Gtt bid-tid*
or		**Homatropine 2%, 5%** (Isopto Homatropine)	
or		**Atropine 1.0%** (Atropine care, Atropisol, Isopto Atropine, Gens)	

+/-	Topical Corticosteroid →379 (anti-inflammatory)	Prednisolone 1% (Predforte, Econopred Plus)	*1 Gtt qd-qid; recommend referral to ophthalmologist*

Systemic therapy in Gonococci, Haemophilus, +/- Pseudomonas

	Systemic Cephalosporin →191, →195	Cefazolin (Ancef, Kefzol, Gens)	*1-2g IV bid*
or		Ceftriaxone (Rocephin)	*1g IV qd*
H. Flu	Systemic broad-spectrum penicillin + beta-lactamase Inhibit. →191	Amoxicillin + Clavulanate (Augmentin)	*500mg PO q8h for 10-14d,* **Ped** *20-40mg/kg qd (div tid) for 10-14d*

14 B.8.2 Fungal Keratitis

	Topical Antifungal →379 (molds: ex/Fusarium)	Natamycin 5% (Natacyn)	*1 Gtt q1-2h; Note: only topical antifungal commercially available*
or	Topical Antifungal (-yeasts: ex/Candida)	Amphotericin B 0.15% (Fungizone)	*1 Gtt q1-2h*
or	Topical Antifungal	Clotrimazole 0.1-1% (Mycelex)	*1 Gtt q1-2h*
or		Miconazole 0.1-1% (Monistat)	
+/-	Oral Antifungal →217	Ketoconazole (Nizoral, Gens)	*200-400mg PO qd*
or		Fluconazole (Diflucan)	*100-400mg PO qd*
or		Itraconazole (Sporanox)	*200mg PO qd-bid*
plus	Cycloplegic →383 (ciliary spasm ↓; see bacterial ulcer, →392)	Cyclopentolate 1-2% (AK-Pentolate, Cyclogyl, Gens)	*1 Gtt bid-tid*
or		Homatropine 2%, 5% (Isopto Homatropine)	

14 B.8.3 Herpes Simplex Keratitis

Epithelial HSV keratitis

	Topical Antiviral →378	Trifluridine 1% (Viroptic)	*1 Gtt 9x/d*
or		Vidarabine oint 3% (Vira-A)	*½ inch 5x/d*
+/-	Cycloplegic →383 (ciliary spasm ↓; see bacterial ulcer, →392)	Cyclopentolate 1-2% (AK-Pentolate, Cyclogyl, Gens)	*1 Gtt bid-tid*
or		Homatropine 2%, 5% (Isopto Homatropine)	

Stromal HSV keratitis

	Antiviral prophylaxis →378	Trifluridine 1% (Viroptic)	*1 Gtt tid-qid*
plus	Topical Corticosteroid →379 (anti-inflammatory)	Prednisolone 1% (Predforte, Econopred Plus)	*1 Gtt qid*
+/-	Cycloplegic →383 (ciliary spasm ↓; see bacterial ulcer, →392)	Cyclopentolate 0.5-2% (AK-Pentolate, Cyclogyl, Gens)	*1 Gtt bid-tid*
or		Homatropine 2%, 5% (Isopto Homatropine)	

HSV keratouveitis, in addition to above:

+/-	**Systemic Antiviral** →211	**Acyclovir** (Zovirax, Gens)	*400mg PO 5x/d*

Neurotrophic/Metaherpetic keratopathy

	Artificial Tears, Lubricant →385 (lubricate ocular surface, maintain ocular tonicity; see Keratoconjunctivitis →390)	**Preservative-free Tears** (Bion Tears, GenTeal, Hypo Tears PF, OcuCoat PF, Refresh Plus, Tears Naturale Free, Thera Tears)	*1 Gtt q1-2h*
+/- or	**Topical Antibiotic** →377 (broad-spectrum)	**Bacitracin oint** (Gens)	*½ inch tid-qid*
		Erythromycin oint 0.5% (Ilotycin)	

14 B.8.4 Herpes Zoster Keratitis

or	**Topical Antibiotic** →377 (broad-spectrum)	**Bacitracin oint** (Gens)	*½ inch tid-qid*
		Erythromycin oint 0.5% (Ilotycin)	
plus	**Artificial Tears, Lubricant** →385 (lubricate ocular surface, maintain ocular tonicity; see Keratoconjunctivitis sicca →390)	**Preservative-free Tears** (Bion Tears, GenTeal, Hypo Tears PF, OcuCoat PF, Refresh Plus, Tears Naturale Free, Thera Tears)	*1 Gtt q1-2h*
plus	**Systemic Virostatic** →211 (purine antagonist, DNA polymerase inhibit.)	**Acyclovir** (Zovirax, Gens)	*800mg PO 5x/d for 7d*

In HZV disciform keratitis

+/-	**Topical Corticosteroid** →379 (anti-inflammatory)	**Prednisolone 1%** (Predforte, Econopred Plus)	*1 Gtt q1-4h*

N.B A biomicroscopic exam must precede any **use of topical corticosteroids**, which should be used only with extreme caution in the presence of a corneal epithelial defect, or evidence of ocular viral, fungal, or bacterial infection. Some clinicians feel that topical steroids are absolutely contraindicated for many corneal infections, particularly active HSV, viral epithelial keratitis, and fungal keratitis. Long-term effects of topical steroids can include cataract formation, and glaucoma.

163. Baum J, Barza M: The evolution of antibiotic therapy for bacterial conjunctivitis and keratitis: 1970-2000. Cornea 2000;19(5): 659-672.
164. Chern KC, Margolis TP: Varicella zoster virus ocular disease. Int Ophthalmol Clin 1998 Fall; 38(4):149-160.
165. Herpetic Eye Disease Study Group: Oral acyclovir for herpes simplex virus eye disease: effect on prevention of epithelial keratitis and stromal keratitis. Arch Ophthalmol 2000;118(8): 1030-1036.
166. Mabon M: Fungal keratitis. Int Ophthalmol Clin 1998; 38(4): 115-23.
167. Stern GA, Buttross M: Use of corticosteroids in combination with antimicrobial drugs in the treatment of infectious corneal disease. Ophthalmology 1991 Jun; 98(6): 847-853.
168. Wilhelmus KR et al: Herpetic Eye Disease Study. A controlled trial of topical corticosteroids for herpes simplex stromal keratitis. Ophthalmology 1994;101(12):1883-95; discussion 1895-1896.

14 B.9 Chemical Burns of the Conjunctiva and Cornea
14 B.9.1 Immediate Treatment

Topical Anesthetic →385	**Proparacaine** (Alcaine, Ophthaine, Ophthetic, Gens)	*1 Gtt; apply topical anesthetic prior to irrigation*
Caution: do not prescribe topical anesthetic for patient use, due to potential for corneal infections or toxicity		
Irrigation (dilutes substance, flushes it away)	**Saline 0.9%, Ringer's lactate**	*Irrigate conjunctival sac and fornices for >½h until neutral pH=7.0; may use IV tubing*

14 B.9.2 Further Treatment

Depending on severity of burns

	Artificial Tears, Lubricant →385 (lubricate ocular surface)	**Preservative-free Tears** (Bion Tears, GenTeal, Hypo Tears PF, OcuCoat PF, Refresh Plus, Tears Naturale Free, Thera Tears)	*1 Gtt qh*
plus	**Topical Antibiotic** →377 (broad-spectrum)	**Bacitracin oint** (Gens)	*½ inch qid*
or		**Erythromycin oint 0.5%** (Ilotycin)	
plus	**Topical Corticosteroid** →377 (anti-inflammatory)	**Prednisolone 1%** (Pred Forte, Econopred Plus)	*1 Gtt qid-q2h for 7d*
or	**Topical Antibiotic + Corticosteroid** →379	**Tobramycin + Dexamethasone 0.1%** (Tobradex)	*1 Gtt qid-q2h*
plus	**Cycloplegic** →383 (ciliary spasm↓; see bacterial ulcer, →392)	**Cyclopentolate 1-2%** (AK-Pentolate, Cyclogyl, Gens)	*1 Gtt bid-tid*
or		**Homatropine 2%, 5%** (Isopto Homatropine)	
+/- severe	**Oral Anti-collagenase** →198 (inhibits breakdown of collagen fibers)	**Doxycycline** (Doryx, Periostat, Vibramycin, Gens)	*100mg PO bid*
+/- severe	**Oral Vitamin C** →145	**Ascorbic acid** (Gens)	*1g PO bid*
Plus	**Oral Analgesic** →266, →269	**Indomethacin** (Indocin, Indocin SR, Gens)	*25-50mg PO tid prn*
or		**Acetaminophen 300mg + Codeine 30mg** (Tylenol, Gens)	*1-2 tabs PO q4h prn*

Avoid phenylephrine, lyse symblepharon, and treat glaucoma

169. Pfister RR, Pfister DA: Alkali injuries of the eye. In: Fundamentals of Cornea and External Disease. Cornea. Vol 1. 1997: 1443-1451.

170. Wagoner MD: Chemical injuries of the eye: current concepts in pathophysiology and therapy. Surv Ophthalmol 1997; 41(4): 275-313.

14 B.10 Episcleritis

mild	**Artificial Tears, Lubricant** →385 (lubricate ocular surface)	**Methyl, ethyl, and propyl cellulose preparations; Glycerin** (Celluvisc, GenTeal, Hypo Tears, Refresh Tears, Tears Naturale II, Gens)	*Gtt qid-6x/d (chilling of tear preparations may provide relief)*
or	**Topical Corticosteroid** →379 (anti-inflammatory)	**Fluorometholone 0.1%** (Flarex, Fluor-Op, FML)	*1 Gtt bid-qid*
or	**Topical NSAID** →380 (anti-inflammatory)	**Diclofenac 0.1%** (Voltaren)	*1 Gtt qid*
or		**Ketorolac 0.5%** (Acular, Acular preservative free)	
+/-	**Oral NSAID** →265, →266 (anti-inflammatory)	**Ibuprofen** (Advil, Children's advil, Motrin, Gens)	*200-600mg PO tid-qid*
or		**Indomethacin** (Indocin, Indocin SR, Gens)	*25mg PO tid*

14 B.11 Scleritis

	Oral NSAID →265, →266 (inhibits cyclooxygenase ⇒ prostaglandins ↓ ⇒ anti-inflammatory, analgesic)	**Ibuprofen** (Advil, Children's advil, Motrin, Gens)	*400-600mg PO qid*
or		**Naproxen** (Anaprox, Naprelan, Naprosyn, Gens)	*250-500mg PO bid*
or		**Indomethacin** (Indocin, Indocin SR, Gens)	*25mg PO tid, 75mg SR PO qd-bid*
or		**Diclofenac** (Voltaren, Voltaren-XR, Gens)	*75mg PO bid-tid*
plus	**Plus** antacid or H_2-blocker, →131		
+/-	**Oral Corticosteroid** →148 (anti-inflammatory)	**Prednisone** (Deltasone, Meticorten, Gens)	*1-1.5mg/kg PO qd for 1wk, then taper slowly*
+/-	**Systemic Immunosuppressant** →263 (Antimetabolite, cytokine synthesis ↓)	**Methotrexate** (Rheumatrex)	*7.5-15mg PO qwk, or 15mg IM qwk;* **Plus** *folate suppl.*
or		**Azathioprine** (Imuran, Gens)	*1-2mg/kg PO/IV qd for 6-8wk*
or	(Cytotoxic agent)	**Cyclophosphamide** (Cytoxan, Neosar)	*1-3mg/kg PO qd*
or	(T-Cell Suppressor) →260	**Cyclosporine** (Neoral, Sandimmune, Gens)	*2.5mg/kg PO qd (div bid)*

Note: systemic immunosuppressant in consultation with internist

Note: Sub-conjunctival/tenon's corticosteroid injection is contraindicated. If scleritis progresses or worsens despite Tx, an underlying cause, such as Lupus, or Wegener's Granulomatosis must be suspected, and would require aggressive systemic Tx.

171. Jabs DA et al: Episcleritis and scleritis: clinical features and treatment results. Am J Ophthalmol 2000;130(4):469-476.
172. Sainz de la Maza M, Jabbur NS, Foster CS: An analysis of therapeutic decision for scleritis. Ophthalmology 1993;100(9):1372-1376.
173. Watson PG: Episcleritis. Current Ocular Therapy. 5th ed. 809.

14 B.12 Anterior Uveitis

14 B.12.1 Mild to Moderate Anterior Uveitis

con-sider	**Topical Corticosteroid, medium potency** →379 (anti-inflammatory)	**Fluorometholone** (Flarex, Fluor-Op, FML)	*1 Gtt bid-qid*
or		**Loteprednol** (0.2%, Alrex; 0.5%. Lotemax)	
or		**Prednisolone 0.12%** (Econopred, Pred Mild)	
or	**Topical Corticosteroid, high potency** →379 (anti-inflammatory)	**Dexamethasone 0.1%** (Decadron, Maxidex, Gens)	*1 Gtt qid-6x/d*
or		**Prednisolone 1%** (Pred Forte, Inflamase Forte, Econopred Plus)	
Plus con-sider	**Cycloplegic** →385 (pain of ciliary muscle spasm↓, posterior synechiae formation↓)	**Tropicamide 0.5–1.0%** (Mydriacyl, Tropicacyl, Gens)	*1 Gtt qd-tid*
or		**Cyclopentolate 0.5–2%** (AK-Pentolate, Cyclogyl, Gens)	
or		**Homatropine 2%, 5%** (Isopto Homatropine)	

14 B.12.2 Moderate to Severe Anterior Uveitis

	Topical Corticosteroid, high potency →379 (anti-inflammatory)	**Prednisolone 1%** (Pred Forte, Inflamase Forte, Econopred Plus)	*1 Gtt 6-10x/d*
Plus	**Cycloplegic** →385 (ciliary spasm↓; see bacterial ulcer, →392)	**Tropicamide 0.5–1.0%** (Mydriacyl, Tropicacyl, Gens)	*1 Gtt qd-qid*
or		**Cyclopentolate 0.5–2%** (AK-Pentolate, Cyclogyl, Gens)	
or		**Homatropine 2%, 5%** (Isopto Homatropine)	
or		**Atropine 1.0%** (Atropine care, Atropisol, Isopto Atropine, Gens)	*1 Gtt qd-bid*

14 B.12.3 Severe Anterior Uveitis

	Topical Corticosteroid →379 (anti-inflammatory)	**Prednisolone 1%** (Pred Forte, Inflamase Forte, Econopred Plus)	*qh when awake; consider adding corticosteroid oint hs*
Con-sider	**Local Corticosteroid, subconjunctival or sub-Tenon Injection** →148 (anti-inflammatory)	**Triamcinolone** (Kenalog, Aristocort)	*20-40mg Inj (0.5-1ml) q2-4wk*
or		**Methylprednisolone 80mg/ml** (Depo-Medrol, Solu-Medrol)	*40mg Inj (0.5ml) q2-4wk*

Plus	**Cycloplegic** →385 (ciliary spasm ↓; see bacterial ulcer, →392)	**Tropicamide 0.5–1.0%** (Mydriacyl, Tropicacyl, Gens)	*1 Gtt bid-qid*
or		**Cyclopentolate 0.5–2%** (AK-Pentolate, Cyclogyl, Gens)	
or		**Homatropine 2%, 5%** (Isopto Homatropine)	
or		**Atropine + Phenylephrine 2.5%** (Neo-Synephrine)	
con-sider	**Systemic Corticosteroid** →148 (anti-inflammatory)	**Prednisone** (Deltasone, Meticorten, Gens)	*1-1.5mg/kg PO qam, taper over 2-4wk*
and/ or	**Oral NSAID** →266 (inhibits cyclooxygenase ⇒ prostaglandins ↓ ⇒ anti-inflammatory, analgesic)	**Diclofenac** (Voltaren, Voltaren-XR, Gens)	*75mg bid-tid*
		Indomethacin (Indocin, Indocin SR, Gens)	*25-50mg PO tid prn*

14 B.12.4 Very Severe Anterior Uveitis

Systemic immunosuppressive Tx (in addition to above)

Consider in consultation with internist (!)

	Systemic Immunosuppressant →260 (cytokine synthesis ↓, T-Cell Suppressors)	**Cyclosporine** (Neoral, Sandimmune, Gens)	*Ini 5mg/kg PO qd (div bid), taper according to disease activity*
or	(alkylating agent, cytotoxic agent)	**Cyclophosphamide** (Cytoxan, Neosar)	*1-3mg/kg PO qd*
or	(antimetabolite, cytokine synthesis ↓) →260, →263	**Azathioprine** (Imuran, Gens)	*1-2 mg/kg PO qd, max 2.5 mg/kg qd; keep dose as low as possible*
or		**Methotrexate** (Rheumatrex, Gens)	*7.5mg PO qwk, incr grad to 17.5-20 mg/wk prn;* **Plus** *folate suppl.*
or		**Mycophenolate** (CellCept)	*Ini 500mg PO bid, max 1.5g bid*

In addition, if herpetic kerato-uveitis

| con-sider | **Topical Antiviral** →378 | **Trifluridine 1%** (Viroptic) | *1Gtt tid-5x/d* |
| | **Systemic Antiviral** →211 | **Acyclovir** (Zovirax, Gens) | *400mg PO 5x/d* |

If secondary glaucoma (see glaucoma for more details, →403)

| sos | **Topical Carbonic Anhydrase Inhibitor** →381 (aqueous humor prod. ↓ ⇒ IOP↓) | **Dorzolamide** (Trusopt) | *Gtt bid-tid* |
| plus | **Topical Betablocker** →381 (aqueous humor production↓ or inflow↓) | **Timolol 0.25-0.5%** (Betimol, Timoptic, Timoptic-XE, Gens) | *1 Gtt bid (avoid metipranolol and prostaglandin analogues with intraocular inflam.)* |

Note: In all cases of recurrent or bilateral uveitis, a determination of etiology must be attempted. If a treatable cause is determined, such as an infection (e.g. syphilis, tuberculosis), this must be treated initially, sometimes prior to institution of uveitis medications.

174. American Academy of Ophthalmology: Intraocular inflammation and uveitis. In: Basic and Clinical Science Course, Section 9. San Francisco: American Academy of Ophthalmology; 1999-2000.
175. Bloch-Michel E, Nussenblatt RB: International Uveitis Study Group recommendations for the evaluation of intraocular inflammatory disease. Am J Ophthalmol 1987; 103(2): 234-235.
176. Herndon LW: Glaucoma associated with anterior uveitis. Current Ocular Therapy 2000;5:470-471.
177. Nussenblatt RB, Whitcup SM, Palestine AG: Uveitis: Fundamentals and Clinical Practice. 2nd ed. St. Louis: CV Mosby, 1996.

14 B.13 Intermediate and Posterior Uveitis

14 B.13.1 Mild Intermediate/Posterior Uveitis

- No significant visual impairment (20/40 or worse)
- No macular edema
- No significant vasculitis
- No peripheral retinal neovascularization
⇒ No therapy required

14 B.13.2 Moderate Intermediate/Posterior Uveitis, if Associated Iritis

con-sider	**Topical Corticosteroid** →379	**Prednisolone 1%** (Pred Forte, Inflamase Forte, Econopred Plus)	*1 Gtt tid-qh*

14 B.13.3 Severe Intermediate/Posterior Uveitis, or if Cystoid Macular Edema

	Depot Corticosteroid or sub-Tenon Injection →148 (anti-inflammatory)	**Triamcinolone** (Kenalog, Aristocort)	*20-40mg Inj (0.5-1ml) q2-4wk*
		Methylprednisolone 80mg/ml (Depo-Medrol, Solu-Medrol)	*40mg Inj (0.5ml) q2-4wk*

If insufficient response, consider

	Systemic Corticosteroid →148 (anti-inflammatory)	**Prednisone** (Deltasone, Meticorten, Gens)	*1mg/kg PO qd*
sos	**Systemic Immunosuppressive** →260	**Cyclosporine, Methotrexate, or Azathioprine** (→398; in consultation with internist)	
sos	**Surgical therapy** (cryotherapy, vitrectomy) **Specific therapy** (e.g., antibiotics, chemotherapy) to treat underlying diseases)		
sos	**Topical Betablocker and Carbonic Anhydrase inhibitor, as above** (may be required in future if secondary glaucoma develops; see glaucoma section for further medications and guidelines, →403)		
sos	**Topical Carbonic Anhydrase Inhibitor** →381 (aqueous humor prod. ↓ ⇒ IOP↓)	**Dorzolamide** (Trusopt)	*1 Gtt bid-tid*
plus	**Topical Betablocker** →381 (aqueous humor production ↓ or intlow↓)	**Timolol 0.25-0.5%** (Betimol, Timoptic, Timoptic-XE, Gens)	*1 Gtt bid (avoid metipranolol and prostaglandin analogues with intraocular inflam.)*

178. American Academy of Ophthalmology: Intraocular inflammation and uveitis. In: Basic and Clinical Science Course, Section 9. San Francisco: American Academy of Ophthalmology; 1999-2000.
179. Bloch-Michel E, Nussenblatt RB: International Uveitis Study Group recommendations for the evaluation of intraocular inflammatory disease. Am J Ophthalmol 1987; 103(2): 234-235.
180. Henderly DE, Genstler AJ, Smith RE, Rao NA: Changing patterns of uveitis. Am J Ophthalmol 1987; 103(2): 131-136.
181. Jabs DA et al: Guidelines for the use of immunosuppressive in patients with ocular inflammatory disorders: recommendations of an expert panel. Am J Ophthalmol 2000;130(4): 492-513.
182. Kaplan HJ: Intermediate Uveitis- A four step approach to treatment. In: Saari KM, ed. Uveitis Update. Amsterdam: Excerpta Medica; 1984: 169-172.
183. Moorthy RS et al: Glaucoma associated with uveitis. Surv Ophthalmol 1997;41(5):361-394.
184. Opremcek EM: Uveitis: A Clinical Manual for Ocular Inflammation. New York: Springer-Verlag; 1995.
185. Smith RE, Nozik RA: Uveitis: A Clinical Approach to Diagnosis and Management. 2nd ed. Baltimore: Williams & Wilkins; 1988.

14 B.14 Optic Neuritis
14 B.14.1 With Acute Visual Loss

N.B.: Corticosteroid treatment is controversial, and although there is evidence that high doses of IV methylprednisolone given for an isolated acute attack of optic neuritis reduces the rate at which multiple sclerosis develops over a 2-year period, there is no evidence that long-term outcome is enhanced. IV steroid is instituted to decrease the likelihood of developing clinical multiple sclerosis if brain lesions are already noted on MRI. Oral steroid use alone, however, has been shown to be associated with increased rate of recurrence

Con-sider	**Systemic Corticosteroid** →148 (anti-inflammatory)	**Methylprednisolone** (Solu-Medrol, Gens)	*Pulse Tx: 250mg IV q6h for 3d (if brain lesions are also noted on MRI), followed by Prednisone*
then		**Prednisone** (Deltasone, Meticorten, Gens)	*1mg/kg qd PO for taper for 12d*

186. Beck R et al: A randomized controlled trial of corticosteroids in the treatment of acute optic neuritis. N Engl J Med 1992;326:581-588.
187. Beck R et al: The effect of corticosteroids for acute optic neuritis on the subsequent development of multiple sclerosis.The Optic Neuritis Study Group. N Engl J Med 1993;329(4):1764-1769.
188. Optic Neuritis Study Group: The clinical profile of optic neuritis. Experience of the Optic Neuritis Treatment Trial. Arch Ophthalmol 1991; 109(12): 1673-1678.
189. Trobe JD, et al: The impact of the optic neuritis treatment trial on the practices of ophthalmologists and neurologists. Ophthalmology 1999;106(11):2047-2053.

14 B.15 Ischemic Optic Neuropathy
14 B.15.1 Non-arteritic

	Antiplatelet Drug →74 (phosphodiesterase/platelet aggregation-adhesion inhibition)	**Aspirin – ASA** (Ascriptin, Asprimox, Bayer Aspirin, Bufferin, Easprin, Ecotrin, Empirin, Genprin, Halfprin, St. Joseph Pain Reliever, ZORprin, Gens)	*80-325mg PO qd;* **Note**: *use contorversial*
plus	**Oral Corticosteroid** →148 (anti-inflammatory) (controversial; usually not recommended)	**Prednisone** (Deltasone, Meticorten, Gens)	*100mg PO qd*

14 B.15.2 Arteritic (Giant Cell Arteritis, Temporal Arteritis)

Consider initial pulse	**Systemic Corticosteroid** →148 (anti-inflammatory)	**Methylprednisolone** (Solu-Medrol, Gens)	*0.5-1g IV bid for 3-5d (followed by Prednisone)*
then		**Prednisone** (Deltasone, Meticorten, Gens)	*80-100mg PO qd; taper slowly (over months) based on symptoms and lab results*

190. Ghanchi FD, Dutton GN: Current concepts in giant cell (temporal) arteritis. Surv Ophthalmol 1997; 42(2): 99-123.
191. Hoffman GS et al: A multicenter, randomized, double-blind, placebo-controlled trial of adjuvant methotrexate treatment for giant cell arteritis. Arthritis Rheum 2002;46(5):1309-1318.
192. Neff AG, Greifenstein EM: Giant cell arteritis update. Semin Ophthalmol 1999 ;14(2): 109-112.
193. Weyand CM, Bartley GB: Giant cell arteritis: new concepts in pathogenesis and implications for management. Am J Ophthalmol 1997; 123(3):392-395.

14 B.16 Central Retinal Artery Occlusion
14 B.16.1 Acute Measures

Reduction of intraocular pressure (see section on glaucoma, →403)

plus/or	**Topical Carbonic Anhydrase inhibitor** →381 (aqueous humor prod.↓)	**Dorzolamide 2%** (Trusopt)	*1 Gtt bid-tid*
		Acetazolamide (Diamox, Gens)	*500mg PO/IV qd, max 1g/d*
plus	**Topical Betablocker** →381 (aqueous humor production ↓ or inflow↓, IOP↓)	**Timolol 0.25-0.5%** (Betimol, Timoptic, Timoptic-XE, Gens)	*1 Gtt qd or bid*
or		**Levobunolol** (Akbeta, Betagan, Gens)	

- Immediate digital ocular massage
- Consider anterior chamber paracentesis

14 B.16.2 Additional Measures

Inhalation of carbogen (5% CO2, 95% O2) or hyperbaric oxygen

plus	**Antiplatelet Drug** →74 (phosphodiesterase/platelet aggregation-adhesion inhibition)	**Aspirin - ASA** (Ascriptin, Asprimox, Bayer Aspirin, Bufferin, Easprin, Ecotrin, Empirin, Genprin, Halfprin, St. Joseph Pain Reliever, Zorprin, Gens)	*80-325mg PO qd*

In suspected giant cell arteritis (→401) additionally

	Systemic Corticosteroid →148 (anti-inflammatory)	**Methylprednisolone** (Solu-Medrol, Gens)	*1000mg IV (once, followed by Prednisone)*
then		**Prednisone** (Deltasone, Meticorten, Gens)	*60-100mg PO qd*

plus	- Obtain CBC with platelets + - Sedimentation Rate (ESR) + - C-Reactive protein + - Consider temporal artery biopsy.

194. Atebara NH, Brown GC, Cater J: Efficacy of anterior chamber paracentesis and Carbogen in treating acute nonarteritic central retinal artery occlusion. Ophthalmology 1995; 102(12): 2029-2034.
195. Augsburger JJ, Magargal LE: Visual prognosis following treatment of acute central retinal artery obstruction. Br J Ophthalmol 1980 ; 64(12): 913-917.
196. Brown G: Retinal arterial occlusive disease. In: Guyer DR, ed. Retina-Vitreous-Macula. Vol. 1. WB Saunders; 1999: 271-285.
197. Mangat HS: Retinal artery occlusion. Surv Ophthalmol 1995;40(2): 145-156.

14 B.17 Central Retinal Vein Occlusion

Most practitioners do not treat CRVO with any medications except aspirin.
Close follow-up is required to monitor for secondary glaucoma.

Possible treatments (controversial)

con- sider	**Antiplatelet Drug** →74 (phosphodiesterase/platelet aggregation-adhesion inhibition)	**Aspirin - ASA** (Ascriptin, Asprimox, Bayer Aspirin, Bufferin, Easprin, Ecotrin, Empirin, Genprin, Halfprin, St. Joseph Pain Reliever, Zorprin, Gens)	*80-325mg PO qd*
or	**IV Anticoagulant** →70 (unfractionated Heparin ⇒ coagulation factor inhibition↑, embolism prophylaxis)	**Heparin** (Gens)	*With primary care MD*
then	**Oral Anticoagulant** →72 (vit. K antagonism ⇒ clotting factors II, VII, IX, X↓ ⇒ longterm anticoag.)	**Warfarin** (Coumadin, Gens)	*With primary care MD*
con- sider or	**Oral NSAID** →265, →266 (inhibits cyclooxygenase ⇒ prostaglandins ↓ ⇒ anti-inflammatory,analgesic)	**Ibuprofen** (Advil, Children's advil, Motrin, Gens)	*400-600mg PO qid*
or		**Naproxen** (Anaprox, Naprelan, Naprosyn, Gens)	*250-500mg PO bid*
or		**Indomethacin** (Indocin, Indocin SR, Gens)	*25mg PO tid,* *75mg SR PO qd-bid*
or		**Diclofenac** (Voltaren, Voltaren-XR, Gens)	*75mg PO bid-tid*
or	**Plus** antacid or H$_2$-blocker, →131		
or	**Systemic Corticosteroid** →148 (anti-inflammatory)	**Prednisone** (Deltasone, Meticorten, Gens)	*Recommended dose not established (e.g. 5-60 mg PO qd (div qd-qid), max 80 mg/d, taper over 2wk as symptoms resolve)*

or	**Intravitreal Corticosteroid** →148 (PRO of macular edema after CRVO, recently reported, controversial)	**Triamcinolone** (Kenalog, Aristocort)	*4mg intravitreal Inj*
sos	**Topical Betablocker** →381 (aqueous humor production↓, IOP↓)	**Timolol 0.25– 0.5%** (Betimol, Timoptic, Timoptic-XE, Gens)	*1 Gtt bid*
plus/or	**Topical Carbonic Anhydrase Inhibitor** →381 (aqueous humor prod.↓)	**Dorzolamide 2%** (Trusopt)	*1 Gtt bid-tid*
	Note: may be required in future if secondary neovascularization glaucoma develops; see glaucoma section for further medications and guidelines, →403		

198. Central Vein Occlusion Study: Baseline and early natural history report. Arch Ophthalmol 1993; 111(8): 1087-1095.
199. Central Vein Occlusion Study Group: Natural history and clinical management of central retinal vein occlusion. Arch Ophthalmol 1997; 115(4): 486-491.
200. Hayreh SS: Classification of central retinal vein occlusion. Ophthalmology 1983; 90(5): 458-474.
201. Ip MS: Intravitreal triamcinolone acetonide as treatment for macular edema from central retinal vein occlusion. Arch Ophthalmol.2002;120:1217-1219.

14 B.18 Glaucoma
14 B.18.1 Primary Open-Angle Glaucoma

Stage 1: Monotherapy

	Topical Betablocker, non-selective →381 (aqueous humor prod.↓)	**Timolol 0.25% or 0.5%** (Betimol, Timoptic, Timoptic-XE, Gens)	*1 Gtt qd or bid*
or		**Levobunolol** (Betagan, Gens)	
or		**Carteolol 1%** (Ocupress, Gens)	
or		**Metipranolol 0.3%** (Optipranolol)	*1 Gtt bid*
or	**Topical Betablocker, β-1 selective** →381 (aqueous humor prod.↓)	**Betaxolol 0.25%** (Betoptic S, Gens)	*1 Gtt bid*

If intolerance, insufficient pressure reduction, contraindication or unstable visual field situation, → Stage 2

Stage 2: Alternative Monotherapy

	Topical Carbonic Anhydrase Inhibitor →381 (aqueous humor prod.↓ ⇒ IOP↓)	**Dorzolamide 2%** (Trusopt)	*1 Gtt bid-tid*
or		**Brinzolamide 1%** (Azopt)	*1 Gtt (1%) bid-tid*
or	**Topical Prostaglandin Analogue** →382 (uveoscleral outflow/drainage of aqueous↑)	**Latanoprost 0.005%** (Xalatan)	*1 Gtt qhs*
or		**Unoprostone 0.15%** (Rescula)	*1 Gtt bid*
or		**Travoprost 0.004%** (Travatan)	*1 Gtt qhs*
or		**Bimatoprost 0.03%** (Lumigan)	*1 Gtt qhs*

or	**Topical alpha–2 selective adrenergic agonist** →380 (aqueous production ↓)	**Apraclonidine 1%** (Iopidine)	*1 Gtt bid-tid*
or		**Brimonidine 0.15%** (Alphagan P)	*1 Gtt bid-tid*
or	**Topical Miotic, Cholinergic** →382 (ciliary muscle contraction ⇒ outflow of aqueous↑)	**Pilocarpine 0.5, 1, 2, 3, 4, 6%** (Isopto Carpine, Ocusert Pilo-40, Ocusert Pilo-20, Gens)	*1 Gtt tid-qid*
or		**Carbachol 0.75, 1.5, 2.25, 3%** (Carbastat, Miostat)	*1 Gtt up to tid*
or	**Topical adrenergic agonist** →380 (outflow of aqueous↑, aqueous production↓)	**Dipivefrin 0.1%** (Akpro, Propine, Gens)	*1 Gtt bid*
or		**Epinephrine 0.5, 1, 2%** (Epinal, Epifrin, Glaucon)	*1Gtt qd-bid*
or	**Topical Cholinesterase Inhibitor** →382 (aqueous humor drainage↑)	**Echothiophate Iodide** (Phospholine Iodide)	*Gtt qd-bid; absolutely contraindicated prior to general anesthesia with succinylcholine*
or		**Physostigmine** (Eserine)	*1 Gtt or ½ inch oint qhs-tid*
or		**Demecarium** (Humorsol)	*Up to 1 Gtt bid*

Note: Anticholinesterase inhibitors are no longer commonly used!

If insufficient pressure reduction, progression of visual field defects, optic nerve deterioration, ⇒ Stage 3

Stage 3: Fixed Combination Therapy (2 Drugs)

	Topical Betablocker + Carb. Anhydr. Inhibitor (aqueous humor prod.↓)	**Timolol + Dorzolamide** (Cosopt 0.5/2%)	*1 Gtt bid*

If insufficient pressure reduction, progression of visual field defects, optic nerve deterioration, ⇒ Stage 4

Stage 4: Combination Therapy (3 drugs)

	Topical Betablocker + Carb. Anhydr. Inhib. + Alpha–2 Agonist	Timolol/Metipranolol + Dorzolamide/Brinzolamide + Brimonidine
or	**Topical Prostaglandin + Betablocker + Sympathomimetic**	Latanoprost + Timolol + Brimonidine
or	**Topical Prostaglandin + Carb. Anhydr. Inhib. + Alpha–2 Agonist**	Latanoprost + Dorzolamide + Brimonidine
or	**Topical Betablocker + Cholinergic + Carb. Anhydr. Inhib.**	Timolol/Metipranolol + Pilocarpine + Dorzolamide/Brinzolamide

If persistent high pressure, progressive visual field and/or optic nerve deterioration, on maximal topical therapy, or if intolerant of topical therapy:

	Systemic Carbonic Anhydrase inhibitor →35 (aqueous humor prod. ↓)	Acetazolamide 125, 250, 500mg (Diamox, Diamox Sequels, Gens)	250-1000mg, PO qd, split dosage bid or qid
or		Methazolamide 25, 50, 100mg (Neptazane)	25-100mg PO, bid to tid

Note: **topical** carbonic anhydrase inhibitors should be stopped.

If persistent high pressure, progressive visual field and/or optic nerve deterioration, on maximal medical therapy, → Stage 5

Stage 5: Non-Medical Treatments

sos	**Laser procedures** - e.g., trabeculoplasty **Surgical procedures** - e.g., trabeculectomy - shunt/valve placement)

202. American Academy of Ophthalmology Preferred Practice Pattern: Primary Open-Angle Glaucoma. 2000.
203. Foundation of the American Academy of Ophthalmology: Medical management of glaucoma. In: Basic and Clinical Science Course, Section 10. San Francisco: American Academy of Ophthalmology;2000-2001; 130-146.
204. David, R: Changing therapeutic paradigms in glaucoma management. Exp Opin Invest Drugs. 1998;7(7):1063-1066.
205. Hugues FC, Jeunne CL, Munera Y: Systemic effects of topical antiglaucomatous drugs. Glaucoma. 1992;14:100-104.
206. Hutzelmann J et al, and International Clinical Equivalence Study Group:Comparison of the safety and efficacy of the fixed combination of dorzolamide/timolol and the concomitant administration of dorzolamide and timolol: A clinical equivalence study. Br J Ophthalmol. 1998;02.1249-1253.
207. The Advanced Glaucoma Intervention Study (AGIS): The relationship between control of intaocular pressure and visual field deterioration. The AGIS Investigators. Am J Ophthalmol. 2000; 130:429-440.

14 B.18.2 Angle-Closure Glaucoma

In General

	Miotic, Cholinergic →382 (ciliary muscle contraction ⇒ miosis, outflow of aqueous ↑)	Pilocarpine 0.5-1% (Isopto Carpine, Pilo, Gens)	1 Gtt q15min for 1h (during attack); also 1 Gtt 0.5 or 1% once in contralateral eye
	Systemic Carbonic Anhydrase inhibitor →35 (aqueous humor prod. ↓)	Acetazolamide (Diamox, Gens)	500 mg PO, then 125-250mg q4h; in nausea IV (during attack)
con-sider	Topical Betablocker, non-selective →381 (aqueous humor prod. ↓)	Timolol 0.25% or 0.5% (Betimol, Timoptic, Timoptic-XE, Gens)	1 Gtt qd or bid (caution with obstructive pulmonary disease)
or		Levobunolol (Betagan, Gens)	
or		Carteolol 1% (Ocupress, Gens)	
or		Metipranolol 0.3% (Optipranolol)	1 Gtt bid

con-sider	**Topical Alpha$_2$ Agonist** →380 (alpha-2 sympathomimetic)	**Apraclonidine 1%** (Iopidine)	*1 Gtt once*
or		**Brimonidine 0.15%** (Alphagan)	
con-sider	**Systemic Analgesic** →270	**Meperidine** (Demerol, Gens)	*50-150mg PO/SC/IM q3-h prn*
con-sider	**Systemic Antiemetic** →124	**Trimethobenzamide** (Tigan)	*200mg PR/IM tid prn*
poss.	**Systemic Hyperosmotic** →296 (osmotic gradient blood-ocular fluids↑ ⇒ H$_2$O loss from vitreous ⇒ IOP↓)	**Mannitol 20%** (Osmitrol, Gens)	*1-2g/kg IV Inf (during attack); extreme caution with diabetics*
or		**Glycerin 50% solution** (Osmoglyn)	*1-1.5g/kg PO*
or		**Isosorbide 45% solution** (Ismotic)	*1.5g/kg PO*
consider	**Topical Corticosteroid** →379	**Prednisolone acetate** (Pred Forte)	*1% q15min for 1h, then qh*

N.B.: If medical Tx of angle-closure glaucoma does not sufficiently lower intraocular pressure, an emergency laser iridotomy or surgical iridotomy may be necessary.

Malignant Glaucoma (Aqueous Misdirection Syndrome)

	Topical Anticholinergic →383 (mydriasis and cycloplegia)	**Atropine + Phenylephrine 2.5%** (Neo-Synephrine)	*1 Gtt tid-qid (during attack), then qd 1 Gtt qid*
plus	**Systemic Carbonic Anhydrase inhibitor** →35 (aqueous humor prod.↓)	**Acetazolamide** (Diamox, Gens)	*250-500 mg PO, then 250mg qid; in nausea IV (during attack)*
plus	**Systemic Hyperosmotic agent** →296 (osmotic gradient blood-ocular fluids↑ ⇒ H$_2$O loss from vitreous ⇒ IOP↓)	**Mannitol 20%** (Osmitrol, Gens)	*0.5-2g/kg IV Inf*
or		**Glycerin 50% solution** (Osmoglyn)	*1-1.5g/kg PO*
or		**Isosorbide 45% solution** (Ismotic)	*1.5g/kg PO*
Plus	**Topical Betablocker, non-selective** →381 (aqueous humor prod.↓)	**Timolol 0.25% or 0.5%** (Betimol, Timoptic, Timoptic-XE, Gens)	*1 Gtt qd or bid (caution with obstructive pulmonary disease)*
or		**Levobunolol** (Betagan, Gens)	
or		**Carteolol 1%** (Ocupress, Gens)	
or		**Metipranolol 0.3%** (Optipranolol)	*1 Gtt bid*
or	**Topical Alpha$_2$ Agonist** →380 (alpha-2 selective sympathomimetic)	**Apraclonidine** (Iopidine)	*1 Gtt once*
		Brimonidine (Alphagan)	

208. American Academy of Ophthalmology:Laser peripheral iridotomy for pupillary-block glaucoma. Ophthalmology.1994;101(10):1749-1758.
209. Fourman S: Malignant glaucoma. Surv Ophthalmol. 1987;32(2):73-93.
210. Foundation of the American Academy of Ophthalmology: Angle-Closure Glaucoma In: Basic and Clinical Science Course, Section 10. San Francisco: American Academy of Ophthalmology;2000-2001; 100-121.
211. Foundation of the American Academy of Ophthalmology: Medical management of glaucoma. In: Basic and Clinical Science Course, Section 10. San Francisco: American Academy of Ophthalmology;2000-2001; 130-146.
212. Ching-Costa A, Chen TC: Malignant glaucoma. Int Ophthalmol Clin. 2000; 40(1):117-125.

14 B.19 Thyroid–Related Exophthalmos

Treatment of thyroid dysfunction (Graves' thyroid ophthalmopathy)

See Endocrinology, →175

Lid retraction, exposure keratopathy, keratoconjunctivitis sicca

Artificial Tears, Lubricant →385 (lubricate ocular surface, maintain ocular tonicity)	**Methyl, ethyl, and propyl cellulose preparations; Glycerin** (Celluvisc, GenTeal, Hypo Tears, Refresh Tears, Tears Naturale II, Gens)	*1 Gtt qid-qh (short or long-term); Caution: avoid any drops containing vasoconstrictive components!*
or	**Preservative-free Tears** (Bion Tears, GenTeal, Hypo Tears PF, OcuCoat PF, Refresh Plus, Tears Naturale Free, Thera Tears)	*1 Gtt qid-qh (long-term)*
or	**Petrolatum/lanolin/mineral oil oint comb.** (Lacri-lube, Duolube, Duratears Naturale, Refresh PM, Gens)	*½ inch qhs-qid*

Note: Used to treat dry eye irritation. Many types of artificial tears are available over the counter. In mild cases, preserved tears can be used. In severe cases, only nonpreserved tears should be used. **N.B.**: Most orbitologists agree that smoking cessation is critical for the treatment of thyroid orbitopathy.

Exophthalmos; acute diplopia; optic neuropathy w/visual loss

	Systemic Corticosteroid →148 (anti-inflammatory)	**Prednisone** (Deltasone, Meticorten, Gens)	*80-100mg PO qd; Note: in consultation with internist, use is controversial!*
plus	**Systemic Immunosuppressive** →260 (reduction of dosage of corticosteroid possible)	**Azathioprine** (Imuran, Gens) **Cyclosporine** (Neoral, Sandimmune, Gens) *Dosage in consultation with internist or rheumatologist. Note: use is controversial!*
poss. plus	**Megavolt Radiotherapy:** *2000 cGy in fractionated doses over 10d*
sos	Acute thyroid ophthalmopathy with severe exposure or visual loss from optic neuropathy may require emergent orbital decompression surgery.

213. Brennan MW, Leone C, Janaki L: Radiation therapy for Graves' disease. Am J Ophthalmol 1983;96:195-199.
214. Day RM, Carroll RD: Corticosteroids in the treatment of optic nerve involvement associated with thyroid dysfunction. Arch Ophthalmol 1968;79:279-282.
215. Feldon SE, Weiner JM: Clinical significance of extraocular muscle volume in Graves' ophthalmopathy. Arch Ophthalmol 1982;100:1266-1269.
216. Kazim M, Trokel, SL, Moore, S: Treatment of acute Graves orbitopathy. Ophthalmology 1991;98:1443-1448.
217. Sergott RC et al: Graves' ophthalmopathy. Immunologic parameters related to corticosteroid therapy. Invest Ophthalmol Vis Sci 1981; 20:173-182.

15 A. ENT – Drugs

15 A.1 Antihistamines
15 A.1.1 Sedating Antihistamines

MA: competitive blockage of H_1-receptors (see antihistamines →124, →331, →409)
AE (antihistamines): sedation, excitatory appearances (small children), dry mouth, glaucoma, micturition DO; **AE** (azatadine): drowsiness, epigastric distress, urinary retention or frequency; **AE** (brompheniramine): dry mouth, nasal congestion, drowsiness, blurred vision,; **AE** (cetirizine): drowsiness, fatigue (mild sedation), dry mouth, headache
AE (clemastine): sedation, shortness of breath; **AE** (chlorpheniramine): drowsiness, N/V
AE (cyproheptadine): drowsiness, N/V, anticholinergic effects, diarrhea
AE (dexchlorphenir.): drowsiness, dryness of mouth/nose, epigastric distress
AE (diphenhydramine): dyskinesias, anaphylaxis, sedation; **AE** (hydroxyzine): xerostomia, drowsiness, headache; **CI** (antihistamines): urinary retention, glaucoma; **CI** (azatadine): hypersens. to azatadine/related antihistamines, use of MAOI, narrow-angle glaucoma or urinary retention; **CI** (brompheniramine): MAOI Tx, focal CNS lesions, hypersens. to brompheniramine; **CI** (cetirizine): hypersens. to cetirizine or hydroxyzine
CI (clemastine): hypersens. to clemastine, MAOI therapy, lower resp tract symptoms; **CI** (chlorpheniramine, dexchlorpheniramine): hypersens. to product ingredeints; **CI** (cyproheptadine): hypersens. to cyproheptadine, newborn or premature infants, nursing mothers
CI (diphenhydramine): hypersens. to diphenhydramine, MAOI Tx, chicken pox, measles, blisters (topical use), topical use on eyes; **CI** (hydroxyzine): hypersens. to hydroxyzine

Azatadine	EHL 9h, PRC B, Lact ?
Optimine *Tab 1mg*	**Allergic rhinitis** →417, **urticaria** →375: 1-2mg PO bid; **CH** >12y: 1-2mg PO bid; DARF not req

Brompheniramine	EHL 25h, PRC C, Lact -
Veltane *Tab 4mg* **Generics** *Tab 4mg, Elixir 5mg/5ml, Inj 10mg/ml*	**Allergic reactions**: 4mg PO q4-6h or ext.rel 8mg PO q8-12h or 12mg q12h, max 24mg/d or 5-10mg IV/SC/IM q6-12h, max 40mg/d; **CH** 2-6y: 1mg PO q4-6h, 6-12y: 2mg PO q4-6h, >12y: 4mg PO q4-6h, <12y: 0.5mg/kg/d IV/SC/IM

Cetirizine	EHL 7.4-9h, PRC B, Lact ?
Zyrtec *Tab 5mg, 10mg, Syr 5mg/5ml*	**Allergic rhinitis** →417, **urticaria** →375: 5-10mg PO qd, max 20mg/d; **CH** 2-6y: 2.5mg PO qd, max 5mg/d, >6y: 5-10mg PO qd, max 10mg/d; DARF: GFR (ml/min): <30: max 5mg/d

Clemastine	EHL 21h, PRC B, Lact -
Tavist *Tab 1.34mg, 2.68mg, Syr 0.5mg/5ml* **Generics** *Tab 1.34mg, 2.68mg, Syr 5mg/5ml*	**Allergic rhinitis** →417, **urticaria** →375: 1.34-2.68mg PO bid-tid, max 8.04mg/d; **CH** 6-12y: 0.5mg PO bid, max 6mg/d

Chlorpheniramine	EHL 20h, PRC B, Lact -
Chlor-Trimeton *Tab ext.rel. 8mg, 12mg* **Efidac 24** *Tab ext.rel. 16mg* **Generics** *Tab 4mg, Tab ext.rel. 12mg, Inj 10mg/ml*	**Allergic rhinitis** →417: 4mg PO q4-6h; ext.rel 8mg PO q8-12h or 12mg PO q12h, max 24mg/d; **CH** 6-11y: 2mg PO q4-6h, max 12mg/d, >12y: adult dose; DARF: not req

Cyproheptadine | EHL 16h, PRC B, Lact -
Periactin, Generics *Tab 4mg,* *Syr 2mg/5ml* | **Allergic rhinitis** →417, **urticaria** →375: 4mg PO tid, max 0.5mg/kg/d; **CH** 2-6y: 2mg PO bid-tid, max 12mg/d, 7-14y: 4mg PO bid-tid, max16mg/d

Dexchlorpheniramine | EHL 20h, PRC B, Lact ?
Mylaramine *Syr 2mg/5ml* **Polaramine** *Tab 2mg, Syr 2mg/5ml* **Generics** *Tab 2mg* | **Allergic rhinitis** →417, **urticaria** →375: 2mg PO q4-6h; ext.rel 4-6mg PO q8-10h; **CH** 6-11y: 1mg PO q4-6h, 2-5y: 0.5mg PO q4-6h, or 6-12y: 4mg ext.rel PO hs; DARF: not req,

Diphenhydramine | EHL 4-8h, PRC B, Lact -
Benadryl *Inj 50mg/ml* **Generics** *Cap 25mg, 50mg, Elixir 12.5mg/5ml, Inj 10mg/ml, 50mg/ml* | **Allergic rhinitis** →417, **rhinorrhea**: 25-50mg PO/IV/IM q4-6h, max 0.4g/d; **motion sickness**: 25-50mg PO 30min before exposure, then prn q4-6h; **CH** 1.25mg PO qid, max 0.3g/d; **anaphylaxis** →16, **insomnia** →331, DARF: GFR (ml/min) >50: q6h, 10-50: q6-12h, < 10: q12-18h; see Prod Info

Hydroxyzine | EHL 3-20h, PRC C, Lact -
Atarax *Tab 10mg, 25mg, 50mg, 100mg* *Syr 10mg/5ml* **Vistaril** *Cap 25mg, 50mg, 100mg, Susp 25mg/5ml, Inj 25mg/ml, 50mg/ml* **Generics** *Tab 10mg, 25mg, 50mg, 100mg, Syr 10mg/5ml, Inj 25mg/ml, 50mg/ml* | **Allergic reactions, pruritus**: 25-100mg PO/IM tid-qid; **CH** <6y: 50mg/d PO div tid-qid, >6y: 50-100mg/d PO div tid-qid; →366, →375

15 A.1.2 Nonsedating Antihistamines

MA, AE, CI (antihistamines): see antihistamines→124, →331, →409
AE (fexofenadine): nausea, dyspepsia, fatigue; **AE** (loratadine): sedation, dizziness, dry mouth, headache, nausea; **CI** (fexofenadine): hypersensitivity to fexofenadine;
CI (loratadine): hypersensitivity to loratadine

Desloratadine | EHL 27h, PRC C, Lact ?
Clarinex *Tab 5mg* | **Allergic rhinitis** →417, **urticaria** →375: 5mg PO qd; DARF: 5mg PO qod

Fexofenadine | EHL 14-18h, PRC C, Lact -
Allegra *Tab 30mg, 60mg, 180mg,* *Cap 60mg* | **Allergic rhinitis** →417, **urticaria** →375: 60mg PO bid or 180mg qd; **CH** 6-11y: 30mg PO bid, >12y: adult dose, DARF: 60mg PO qd

Loratadine | EHL 12-15h, PRC B, Lact ?
Claritin *Tab 10mg, Tab (orally disint) 10mg,* *Syr 1mg/ml* | **Allergic rhinitis** →417, **urticaria** →375: 10mg PO qd; **CH** 6-11y: adult dose; DARF: GFR (ml/min) <30: 10mg PO qod

15 A.2 Nasal Preparations
15 A.2.1 Anticholinergics

AE: dry mouth, bitter taste, epistaxis, nasal dryness, nasal congestion
CI: hypersensitivity to ipratropium products

Ipratropium Bromide — EHL 1.6h (IV), PRC B, Lact ?

Atrovent *Spray (metered, nasal) 0.03% (0.021mg/spray), 0.06% (0.042mg/spray)*

Rhinorrhea associated with allergic rhinitis: 2 sprays (0.03%) in each nostril bid-tid; **CH** ≥ 6y: adult dose; **rhinorrhea associated with common cold/vasomotor rhinitis:** 2 sprays (0.06%) in each nostril tid-qid; **CH** ≥ 12y: adult dose

15 A.2.2 Antihistamines, Mast Cell Stabilizers

MA/EF: see antihistamines →124, →331, →409
AE (azelastine): drowsiness, altered taste, dry mouth/nose, nosebleeds
CI (azelastine): hypersensitivity to azelastine products

Azelastine — EHL 22-25h, PRC C, Lact -

Astelin *Spray (metered, nasal) 0.125mg/spray*

Allergic rhinitis →417: 2 sprays in each nostril bid; **CH** ≥ 12y: adult dose

Cromolyn — EHL 22-25h, PRC C, Lact -

NasalCrom *Spray (metered, nasal) 5.2mg/spray*
Generics *Spray (metered, nasal) 5.2mg/spray*

Allergic rhinitis →417: 1 spray in each nostril q4-h; **CH** ≥ 6y: adult dose

15 A.2.3 Corticosteroids

AE (beclomethasone): adrenal suppression, candidiasis, nasopharyngeal irritation
AE (budesonide): nasal stinging, throat irritation, nasal dryness, epistaxis, headache
AE (flunisolide): nasal irritation, dysphonia, headache
AE (fluticasone): hoarseness, nasal burning/epistaxis, nasal congestion, pruritus/burning, eosinophilia
AE (mometasone): burning, atrophy, pruritus, headache
AE (triamcinolone): GI distress, fluid and electrolyte disturbances, HPA axis suppression, mild euphoria/depression
CI (beclomethasone, budesonide, flunisolide, fluticasone): hypersensitivity to product ingredients/corticosteroids, status asthmaticus or other acute episodes of asthma
CI (mometasone): hypersensitivity to mometasone or other corticosteroids
CI (triamcinolone): systemic fungal infections

Beclomethasone — EHL 3h, PRC C, Lact ?

Beconase AQ *Spray (metered, nasal) 0.042mg/spray*
Vancenase AQ *Spray (metered, nasal) 0.042mg/spray, 0.084mg/spray*

Allergic rhinitis →417/**nasal polyp PRO:** 1-2 spray(s) (0.042-0.084mg) in each nostril bid; **CH** >12y: adult dose, 6-12y: 1 spray (0.042mg) in each nostril bid, max 0.084mg bid

Budesonide — EHL 2-3h PRC C, Lact ?

Rhinocort *Aerosol (metered, nasal) 0.032mg, Spray (metered, nasal) 0.032mg/spray, 0.064mg/spray*

Allergic rhinitis →417: 2 sprays in each nostril bid or 4 sprays qd; **CH** ≥ 6y: adult dose, max 4 sprays/d (0.032mg/spray) or 2 sprays/d (0.064mg/spray)

Flunisolide — EHL 1-2h, PRC C, Lact ?

Nasalide, Nasarel *Spray (metered, nasal) 0.025mg/spray*
Allergic rhinitis →417: 2 sprays in each nostril bid, prn incr to 2 sprays in each nostril tid, max 8 sprays/nostril/d; **CH** 6-14y: 1 spray in each nostril tid or 2 sprays in each nostril bid, max 4 sprays/nostril/d

Fluticasone — EHL 7.8h, PRC C, Lact ?

Flonase *Spray (metered, nasal) 0.05mg/spray*
Allergic rhinitis →417: 2 sprays in each nostril qd or 1 spray in each nostril bid, decr to 1 spray in each nostril qd when appropriate; **CH** >4y: 1-2 sprays in each nostril qd, max 2 sprays/nostril/d

Mometasone — EHL 5.8h, PRC C, Lact ?

Nasonex *Spray (metered, nasal) 0.05mg/spray*
Allergic rhinitis →417: 2 sprays in each nostril qd; **CH** ≥ 12y: adult dose, 3-11y: 1 spray in each nostril qd

Triamcinolone — EHL 2-3hPRC C, Lact ?

Nasacort *Aerosol (met.nas.) 0.055mg/spray*
Nasacort AQ *Spray (met.nas.) 0.055mg/spray*
Tri-Nasal *Spray (met.nas.) 0.05mg/spray*
Allergic rhinitis →417: ini 2 sprays in each nostril bid, prn decr to 2 sprays/nostril qd, max 8 sprays/d; **CH** ≥ 12y: adult dose, 6-12y: 1-2 sprays in each nostril qd

15 A.2.4 Nasal (Topical) Decongestants

AE (sympathomimetic decongestants): reactive hyperemia, mucus membrane burning, dryness, tachycardia, BP ↑. Long use: epithelial damage, chronic stuffy nose
AE (oxymetazoline): rebound congestion, mucosal irritation, CNS effects, tremors
AE (phenylephrine): tachycardia, HTN, MI, SAII
AE (phenylpropanolamine): headache, tremor, visual disturbances, HTN, arrhythmias
AE (pseudoephedrine): restlessness, HTN, arrhythmias
CI (sympathomimetic decongestants): rhinitis sicca, severe coronary diseases
CI (oxymetazoline, phenylephrine): hypersensitivity to product ingredients, narrow angle glaucoma, hyperthyroidism, CAD, BPH, HTN
CI (phenylpropanolamine, pseudoephedrine): hypersensitivity to product ingredients or sympathomimetics, MAOI therapy, severe HTN/CAD

Oxymetazoline — EHL 5-8h, PRC C, Lact ?

Afrin *Gtt (nasal) 0.05%, 0.025%, Spray (nasal) 0.05%*
Neo-Synephrine *Spray (nasal) 0.05%*
Vicks Sinex *Spray (nasal) 0.05%*
Nasal congestion: 2-3 sprays/Gtt (0.05%) in each nostril bid x 3d; **CH** ≥ 6y: adult dose, 2-5y: 2-3 Gtt (0.025%) in each nostril bid x 3d

Phenylephrine — EHL 2-3h, PRC C, Lact +

Neo-Synephrine *Gtt (nasal) 0.5%, 1%, Spray (nasal) 0.25%, 0.5%, 1%*
St Joseph *Gtt (nasal) 0.125%*
Generics *Gtt (nasal) 0.25%, 0.5%, 1%, Spray (nasal) 0.25%, 0.5%, 1%*
Nasal congestion: 2-3 sprays/Gtt (0.25 or 0.5%) in each nostril q4h prn x 3d, sol 1% for severe congestion; **CH** >12y: adult dose, 6-12y: 2-3 sprays/Gtt (0.25%) in each nostril q4h prn x 3d, 1-5y: 2-3 Gtt (0.125% or 0.16%) in each nostril q4h prn x 3d, 6-11 mo: 1-2 Gtt (0.125% or 0.16%) in each nostril q4h prn x 3d

Phenylpropanolamine + Brompheniramine	EHL 5.6hPRC C, Lact ?
Bromatapp *Tab ext.rel 75mg + 12mg* **Contac** *Tab ext.rel 75mg + 12mg,* *Cap ext.rel 75mg + 8mg* **Demazin** *Tab 25mg + 4mg,* *Cap ext.rel 75mg + 12mg* **Dimetapp** *Tab ext.rel 75mg + 12mg,* *Elixir 12.5mg/5ml + 2mg/5ml*	**Allergic rhinitis** →417/**nasal congestion:** 1 Tab/Cap or 10ml PO q4h, max 6 doses/d or 1 Tab ext.rel PO q12h, max 2 Tab/d; **CH** >12y: adult dose, 6–11y: ½ Tab (12.5mg) or 5ml PO q4h, 2–5y: 2.5ml PO q4h, max 6 doses/d
Pseudoephedrine	EHL 9–16hPRC C, Lact ?
Pediacare, Triaminic *Gtt (oral, pediatric)* *7.5mg/0.8ml* **Sudafed** *Tab 30mg, 60mg,* *Tab (chew) 15mg, Tab ext.rel 120mg, 240mg, Liquid* *(oral) 30mg/5ml* **Generics** *Tab 30mg, 60mg,* *Tab ext.rel 120mg, Syr 30mg/5ml*	**Nasal congestion:** 60mg PO q4–6h or 120mg PO q12h (ext.rel) or 240mg PO qd (ext.rel), max 240mg/d; **CH** >12y: adult dose, 6–11y: 30mg PO q4–6h, max 120mg/d, 2–5y: 15mg PO q4–6h, max 60mg/d, 2–3y: 1.6ml; pediatric Gtt PO q4–6h: 12–23 mo: 1.2ml, 4–11 mo: 0.8ml, 0–3 mo: 0.4ml, max 4 doses/d

15 A.2.5 Other Nasal Preparations

Saline Nasal Spray	EHLPRC A, Lact +
Natru-Vent *Spray (nasal) 0.9%* **Afrin Extra Moisturizing Saline Mist** *Spray (nasal)* **Neo–Synephrine Nasal Saline** *Spray (nasal) 0.65%*	**Nasal dryness:** 1–3 sprays/Gtt in each nostril prn

15 A.3 Ear Preparations
15 A.3.1 Antibacterial/Antifungal Combinations

AE (acetic acid): local stinging or burning
CI (acetic acid): hypersensitivity to acetic acid products, perforated tympanic membranes, vaccinia and varicella (steroid-containing ear drops)

Acetic Acid + Aluminium Acetate	PRC C, Lact ?
Domeboro *Sol/Gtt (otic) 2% + 0.79%* **Generics** *Sol/Gtt (otic) 2% + 0.79%*	**Otitis externa** →420: 4–6 Gtt in affected ear(s) q2–3h, keep moist (cotton plug) x 24h
Acetic Acid/Propylene Glycol	PRC C, Lact ?
VoSol otic *Sol/Gtt (otic) 2% acetic acid*	**Otitis externa** →420: 5 Gtt in affected ear(s) tid-qid, keep moist (cotton plug) with 3–5 Gtt q4–6h x 24 h; **CH** >3y: 3–4 Gtt in affected ear(s) tid-qid, keep moist (cotton plug) with 3–4 Gtt q4–6h x 24h

15 A.3.2 Agents for Otitis Externa Prophylaxis

Isopropyl Alcohol + Anhydrous Glycerins	PRC N, Lact ?
Swim-Ear *Sol/Gtt (otic) 95% + 5%*	**Otitis externa** (PRO) →420: 4–5 Gtt in ears after swimming, bathing; **CH** adult dose

15 A.3.3 Antibacterial/Corticosteroid Combinations

Ciprofloxacin + Hydrocortisone — PRC C, Lact -

Cipro HC Otic *Susp/Gtt (otic) 0.2% + 1%* — **Otitis externa** →420: 3 Gtt into affected ear(s) bid x 7d; **CH** ≥ 1y: adult dose

Hydrocortisone + Neomycin + Thozonium Bromide + Colistin PRC N, Lact ?

Cortisporin TC, Coly-mycin S *Susp (otic) 1% + 3.3 + 0.5 + 3mg/ml* — **Otitis externa** →420: 5 Gtt in affected ear(s) tid-qid; **CH** 4 Gtt in affected ear(s) tid-qid

Hydrocortisone + Polymyxin + Neomycin — PRC C, Lact ?

Neo-Otosol-HC, Cortisporin, Oticair, Pediotic, Generics *Sol/Gtt (otic) 1% + 3.5mg/ml + 10,000 U/ml* — **Otitis externa** →420: 4 Gtt in affected ear(s) tid-qid; **CH** 3 Gtt in affected ear(s) tid-qid

Polymyxin B + Hydrocortisone — PRC C, Lact ?

Otobiotic *Sol/Gtt (otic) 10,000 U/ml + 5mg/ml* — **Otitis externa** →420: 4 Gtt in affected ear(s) tid-qid; **CH** 3 Gtt in affected ear(s) tid-qid

15 A.3.4 Antibiotics

AE (ofloxacin): all application forms: N/V, insomnia, headache, dizziness, diarrhea
CI (ofloxacin): hypersensitivity to ofloxacin or other fluoroquinolones

Ofloxacin — EHL 5-7.5h, PRC C, Lact ?

Floxin *Sol/Gtt (otic) 0.3%* — **Otitis externa** →420: 10 Gtt in affected ear(s) bid x 10d; **CH** >12y: adult dose, 1-12y: 5 Gtt in affected ear(s) bid x 10d; **chronic suppurative otitis media:** 10 Gtt in affected ear(s) bid x 14d; **CH** >12y: adult dose; **acute otitis media with tympanostomy tubes; CH** 1-12y: 5 Gtt in affected ear(s) bid x 10d

15 A.3.5 Decongestant/Analgesic Combinations

Benzocaine + Antipyrine — PRC C, Lact ?

Auralgan *Sol (otic) 14mg/ml + 54mg/ml* — **Otitis media** (adjunct) →421: 2-4 Gtt tid-qid or q1-2h prn; **cerumen removal:** 2-4 Gtt tid x 2-3d to detach cerumen, then prn for discomfort, insert moistened cotton plug (with sol)

15 A.3.6 Surfactants, Ceruminolytics

AE (cerumenex eardrops): localized dermatitis reactions, allergic contact dermatitis, skin ulcerations, burning and pain at the application site and skin rash
CI (carbamide peroxide): hypersensitivity to carbamide peroxide products, ear drainage or discharge, perforated tympanic membrane
CI (cerumenex eardrops): perforated tympanic membrane, otitis media, history of hypersensitivity to cerumenex eardrops or to any of its components

Carbamide Peroxide	PRC N, Lact ?
Debrox *Sol/Gtt (otic) 6.5%* **Gly-Oxide** *Sol/Gtt (otic) 10%*	**Cerumen removal:** 5-10 Gtt into ear bid, max x 4d
Triethanolamine	PRC C, Lact ?
Cerumenex *Sol/Gtt (otic) 10%*	**Cerumen removal:** fill ear canal with sol, insert cotton plug x 15-30min, then flush, max x 4d

15 A.4 Mouth and Lip Preparations
15 A.4.1 Antifungals

AE (clotrimazole): N/V, LFT's ↑ (transient), contact dermatitis
AE (nystatin): diarrhea, vaginal irritation/pain, N/V, rash
CI (clotrimazole, nystatin): hypersensitivity to product ingredietns

Clotrimazole	EHL 3.5-5h, PRC C, Lact ?
Mycelex *Troche/Lozenge 10mg*	**Oral candidiasis:** 1 troche dissolved slowly in mouth 5x/d x 14d; **CH ≥ 3y:** adult dose; **prevention of oropharyngeal candidiasis in immunocompromised patients:** 1 troche dissolved slowly in mouth tid until end of chemotherapy/ high-dose corticosteroids
Nystatin	PRC C, Lact +
Mycostatin *Pastille/Lozenge 200,000 U* *Susp 100,000 U/ml* **Nilstat, Generics** *Susp 100,000 U/ml*	**Thrush:** 5ml PO swish and swallow qid with ½ of dose in each cheek or 1-2 lozenges 4-5x/d, max 14d; **CH** 2ml PO swish and swallow qid with 1ml in each cheek or use a cotton sqab, premature and low birth weight infants: 0.5ml PO in each cheek qid or use a cotton squab

15 A.4.2 Antivirals

AE (penciclovir): erythema
CI (penciclovir): hypersensitivity to penciclovir or famciclovir

Penciclovir	PRC B, Lact ?
Denavir *Crm 1%*	**Herpes labialis** →368 **(cold sores):** apply q2h while awake x 4d, ini during prodrome

15 A.4.3 Other Mouth and Lip Preparations

AE (amlexanox): stinging and/or burning sensations or transient pain at the application site, contact mucositis/dermatitis
AE (chlorhexidine gluconate): skin irritation, tooth staining, altered taste
CI (chlorhexidine gluconate): hypersensitivity to chlorhexidine products
CI (amlexanox): hypersensitivity to amlexanox

Amlexanox	EHL 3.5h, PRC B, Lact ?
Aphthasol *Paste (dental) 5%*	**Aphthous ulcers:** apply ¼ inch paste to ulcer in mouth qid after oral hygiene
Chlorhexidine Gluconate	PRC B, Lact ?
Periogard, Peridex, Generics *Sol (dental) 0.12%*	**Gingivitis:** apply 15ml x 30sec bid as oral rinse (qam and qpm after brushing teeth), expectorate after rinsing
Lidocaine Viscous	PRC B, Lact +
Xylocaine *Sol (top) 5%*	**Mouth or lip pain:** 15ml topically or swish and spit q3h, max 8 doses/24h or 4.5mg/kg or max 300mg, use lowest effective dose, prn apply to small sore places with cotton-tipped applicator; **CH** >3y: 3.75-5ml topically or swish and spit up to q3h
Triamcinolone Acetonide	PRC C, Lact ?
Kenalog in Orabase, Oracort, Oralone *Paste 0.1%*	Apply bid-tid with finger, apply about 0.5cm of paste to the oral lesion

15 B. ENT – Therapies

Gayle Ellen Woodson, MD, FACS, FRCS (C)
Professor, Department of Otolaryngology
University of Florida, Gainesville, FL

15 B.1 Rhinosinusiitis

15 B.1.1 Acute Viral Rhinosinusiitis

	Topical alpha–Sympathomimetic →411 (mucosal detumescence, nasal decongestant)	**Oxymetazoline** (Afrin)	*2-3 sprays/nostril bid; Caution: do not use > 5d, may cause rebound!*
and/or	**Systemic sympathomimetic** →411 (nasal decongestant)	**Pseudoephedrine** (Pediacare, Sudafed, Triaminic, Gens)	*30-60mg PO q4-6h prn*
plus/ or	**Anticholinergic** →97 (antisecretory)	**Ipratropium bromide** (Atrovent)	*1-2 sprays tid*

15 B.1.2 Acute Bacterial Rhinosinusiitis

	Aminopenicillin →189	**Amoxicillin** (Amoxil, Larotid, Trimox, Wymox, Gens)	*250-500mg PO q8h for 10-14d*
or	**Aminopenicillin + Betalactamase inhibitor** →191	**Amocxicillin + Clavulanate** (Augmentin)	*500-875mg PO bid for 10-14d*
or	**Macrolide** →199	**Azithromycin** (Zithromax)	*500mg PO for 1d, then 250mg PO qd for 4d*
		Clarithromycin (Biaxin)	*250-500mg PO bid for 10-14d*
or	**Oral Cephalosporin** →194	**Cefuroxime–Axetil** (Ceftin, Veftin)	*250-500mg PO bid for 10-14d*
		Cefprozil (Cefzil)	*150-500mg PO bid for 10-14d*
		Loracarbef (Lorabid)	*200-400mg PO bid for 10-14d*
or	**Folate antagonist + p-Aminobenzoic acid antagonist** →206	**Sulfamethoxazole + Trimethoprim** (Cotrimoxazole) (Bactrim, Cotrim, Septra, Sulfamethoprim, Sulfatrim, Gens)	*800+160mg PO bid for 10-14d*

15 B.1.3 Chronic Sinusitis

	Aminopenicillin + Betalactamase inhibitor →191	**Amoxicillin + Clavulanate** (Augmentin)	*500-875mg PO bid for 3-6wk*
or	**Fluoroquinolone** →203	**Ciprofloxacin** (Cipro)	*750mg PO bid for 3-6wk*
or	**Lincosamide** →201	**Clindamycin** (Cleocin, Gens)	*300mg PO qid for 3-6wk*
or	**Nitroimidazole** →206	**Metronidazole** (Flagyl)	*500mg PO q6-8h for 3-6wk*

Plus	Topical Glucocorticoid →410	Beclomethasone (Beconase AQ, Vancenase AQ)	*1 spray each nostril bid-qid*
		Flunisolide (Nasalide, Nasarel)	*2 sprays in each nostril bid-tid*
		Fluticasone (Flonase)	*2 sprays each nostril qd or 1 spray each nostr. bid*
		Mometason (Nasonex)	*2 sprays each nostril qd*
		Triamcinolone (Nasacort/AQ, Tri-nasal)	*2 sprays each nostril bid, prn decr to 2 sprays/nostril qd*

218. Benninger MS, Anon, J, Mabry RL: The medical management of rhinosinusitis. Otolaryngology-Head & Neck Surgery 1997;117:41-49.

15 B.1.4 Allergic Rhinitis

	Topical Antihistamine →410 (histamine release in allergic response ↓)	Azelastine (Astelin)	*2 sprays each nostril bid*
and/or	Mast Cell Stabilizer →410 (degranulation of mast cells after Ag exposure ↓)	Cromolyn (NasalCrom, Gens)	*1 spray each nostril tid-qid*
plus	Topical Glucocorticoid →410 (anti-inflammatory)	Beclomethasone (Beconase AQ, Vancenase AQ)	*1 spray each nostril bid-qid*
		Flunisolide (Nasalide, Nasarel)	*2 sprays in each nostril bid-tid*
		Fluticasone (Flonase)	*2 sprays each nostril qd or 1 spray each nostr. bid*
		Mometasone (Nasonex)	*2 sprays each nostril qd*
		Triamcinolone (Nasacort/AQ, Tri-nasal)	*2 sprays each nostril bid, prn decr to 2 sprays/nostril qd*
plus/or	Systemic Antihistamine →408 (histamine release in allergic response ↓)	Cetirizine (Zyrtec)	*5-10mg PO qd*
		Fexofenadine (Allegra)	*60-80mg PO bid*

15 B.2 Furuncles of the Nose

Initially

	Tetracycline →198	Doxycycline (Doryx, Monodox, Periostat, Vibramycin, Gens)	*d1: 200mg PO, d2-8(10): 100mg PO qd for 8-10d*

In betalactam allergy

	Macrolide →199	Clarithromycin (Biaxin)	*250mg PO bid for 10-14d*

219. Recommendations of the Paul-Ehrlich Society, Chemother J, 1999, 8, 2-49

15 B.3 Tonsillitis
15 B.3.1 Acute Tonsillitis

Initially

	Benzylpenicillin →187	**Penicillin V** (Pen-vee K, Veetids, Gens)	*250-500mg PO q6-8h for 10d*
or	**Oral Cephalosporin** →194	**Cefuroxime-Axetil** (Ceftin, Veftin)	*250-500mg PO bid for 10d*
or	**Macrolide** →199	**Azithromycin** (Zithromax)	*500mg PO for 1d, then 250mg PO qd for 4d*
		Clarithromycin (Biaxin)	*500mg PO qd for 10d;* **Ped** *12mg/kg PO qd*
or	**IM Penicillin** →187	**Benzathine Penicillin** (Bicillin L-A, Permapen)	*<27.3kg: 600,000 U IM, >27.3kg:1,200,000 U IM, as single dose*
poss.	**Analgesic – aniline derivative** →269 (inhibits cyclooxygenase ⇒ prostaglandins ↓, analgesic, antipyretic)	**Acetaminophen** (Acephen, Infants' feverall, Neopap, Tylenol, Gens)	*In pain or fever: 500-1000mg PO/PR tid-qid; infants max 125mg/d, toddler 250mg/d,* **Ped** *500mg/d*

In resistance to therapy

	Aminopenicillin + Betalactamase inhibitor →191	**Amoxicillin + Clavulanate** (Augmentin)	*500-875mg PO bid for 10d*
or	**Lincosamide** →201	**Clindamycin** (Cleocin, Gens)	*300mg PO qid for 10d*

15 B.4 Pharyngitis
15 B.4.1 Viral Pharyngitis, Symptomatic

	Salicylate →264 (analgesic, anti-inflammatory, antipyretic)	**Aspirin – ASA** (Ascriptin, Asprimox, Bayer Aspirin, Bufferin, Easprin, Ecotrin, Empirin, Genprin, Halfprin, St. Joseph Pain Reliever, Zorprin, Gens)	*0.5-1g PO bid-tid*

15 B.4.2 Bacterial Pharyngitis, Superinfection

1sr Choice

	Benzylpenicillin →187	**Penicillin V** (Pen-vee K, Veetids, Gens)	*250-500mg PO q6-8h for 10d*

In penicillin allergy

or	**Macrolide** →199	**Axithromycin** (Zithromax)	*500mg PO on d1, then 250mg PO qd for 4d*
		Clarithromycin (Biaxin)	*250mg PO bid for 10-14d*

15 B.5 Laryngitis
15 B.5.1 Symptomatic

poss.	**Expectorant** →99 (sputum viscosity↓)	**Guaifenesin** (Humibid, Robitussin, Gens)	*200-400mg PO q4h, max 2400mg/d*
or		**Guaifenesin - sustained release** (Humibid, Gens)	*SR: 600-1200mg PO q12h, plenty of water, max 2400mg/d*
poss.	**Antitussive** →99 (acts on cough center in medulla oblongata)	**Dextromethorphan** (Benylin, Delsym, Hold, Pertussin, Robitussin DM, Sucrets, Vicks, Gens)	*10-20mg PO q4h prn, or 30-60mg SR q12h*
poss.	**Glucocorticoid** →148 (anti-inflammatory, immunosuppressive)	**Methylprednisolone** (Medrol, Depo-Medrol, Solu-Medrol, Gens)	*2-60mg PO qd*
		Prednisone (Deltasone, Meticorten, Prednisone Intensol, Gens)	*5-60mg PO qd*

15 B.5.2 Bacterial Superinfection, Epiglottitis

Initially

	Cephalosporin 2nd gen. →194	**Cefuroxime-Axetil** (Ceftin, Veftin)	*0.75-1.5g IV tid for 7d*
or	**Cephalosporin 3rd gen.** →195	**Ceftriaxone** (Rocephin)	*1-2g IV qd for 7d,* **Ped** *75mg/kg IV qd for 7d*

For tuberculous laryngitis

poss.	**Tuberculostatic** →208	**Rifampin** (Rifadin, Rimactane, Gens)	*10mg/kg PO qd (div bid) for 4d*

For diphtheria

	Antitoxin (from horse serum, passive immunization)	**Diphtheria antitoxin**	*30,000-50,000 IU IV inf over 1h, max 120,000 IU*
Plus	**Benzylpenicillin** →187	**Penicillin G** (Penicillin, Penicillin G Potassium, Pfizerpen, Gens)	*0.5-10 M IU IV qid-6x/d for 14d*
or	**Macrolide** →199	**Clarithromycin** (Biaxin)	*250mg PO bid for 10d*

15 B.6 Perichondritis

	Fluoroquinolone →203	**Ciprofloxacin** (Cipro)	*500mg PO bid for 14d*

15 B.7 External Otitis

15 B.7.1 Acute Otitis Externa

	Fluoroquinolone →203	**Ciprofloxacin** (Cipro)	*3 Gtt qd for 14d*
		Ofloxacin (Floxin)	*1 Gtt tid for 14d*
Plus	**Glucocorticoid** →410 (anti-inflammatory, immunosuppressive)	**Triamcinolone acetonide** (Aristocort, Kenalog, Oracort, Oralone)	*Apply qd-bid with finger*
or	**Antibiotic + Glucocorticoid** →413	**Polymyxin B + Hydrocortisone** (Otobiotic)	*5 Gtt tid-qid*
or	**Anti–bacterial** →412	**Acetic acid Sol 2%** (Acetasol, Domeboro, VoSol)	*4-6 Gtt q2-3h in canal or on ear wick*
Plus poss	**NSAID - proprionic acid derivate** →265 (inhibits cyclooxygenase ⇒ prostaglandins ↓ ⇒ anti-inflamm., analgesic)	**Ibuprofen** (Advil, Children's advil, Ibu, Ibu-Tab, Motrin, Gens)	*400mg PO tid*

15 B.7.2 Otitis Externa Circumscripta (Acoustic Duct Furuncle)

	Oral Cephalosporin →192	**Cephalexin** (Keflet, Keflex, Keftab, Gens)	*1g PO tid for 7d*
	NSAID - proprionic acid derivate →265 (inhibits cyclooxygenase ⇒ prostaglandins ↓ ⇒ anti-inflammatory, analgesic)	**Ibuprofen** (Advil, Children's advil, Ibu, Ibu-Tab, Motrin, Gens)	*400mg PO tid*

15 B.7.3 Chronic Otitis Externa

	Anti–bacterial + Glucocorticoid →412	**Acetic acid 2% + Hydrocortisone 1%** (VoSol HC)	*5 Gtt tid-qid*

15 B.7.4 Fungal Otitis Externa

	Antifungal →414	**Clotrimazole Sol 1%** (Lotrimin, Mycelex, Gens)	*3 Gtt tid*
or		**Nystatin cream** (Mycostatin, Gens)	*Fill canal, leave 5-7d*
or	**Anti–bacterial + Glucocorticoid** →412	**Acetic acid 2% + Hydrocortisone 1%** (VoSol HC)	*5 Gtt tid-qid*

15 B.7.5 Otitis Externa Maligna

	Fluoroquinolone →203	**Ciprofloxacin** (Cipro)	*1000-1500mg PO qd*
poss plus	**Fluoroquinolone + Glucocorticoid** →413	**Ciprofloxacin + Hydrocortisone** (Cipro HC Otic)	*Instill Gtt tid-5x/d*

poss plus	**NSAID - proprionic acid derivate** →265 (inhibits cyclooxygenase ⇒ prostaglandins ↓ ⇒ anti inflammatory, analgesic)	**Ibuprofen** (Advil, Children's advil, Ibu, Ibu-Tab, Motrin, Gens)	*400mg PO tid*

220. Louie TJ: Ciprofloxacin: and oral quinolone for the treatment of infections with gram-negative pathogens. Committee on Antimicrobial Agents. Canadian Infectious Disease Society. CMAJ 1994; 150:669-76.

15 B.8 Herpes Zoster Oticus

poss. plus	**Virostatic** →211 (purine antagonist, DNA polymerase inhibitor)	**Acyclovir** (Zovirax, Gens)	*Moderately severe: 800mg PO 5x/d; severe: 10mg/kg IV qd (div tid-5x/d)*

15 B.9 Otitis Media

Symptomatic

	Analgesic - aniline derivative →269 (inhibits cyclooxygenase ⇒ prostaglandins ↓, analgesic, antipyretic)	**Acetaminophen** (Acephen, Infants' feverall, Neopap, Tylenol, Gens)	*500-1000mg PO/PR tid-qid prn; Infants: 125mg/d; toddler. 250mg/d; **Ped** 500mg/d PR; max dose 4g in adults and 90 mg/kg in CH*

Initially

	Aminopenicillin →189	**Amoxicillin** (Amoxil, Larotid, Trimox, Wymox, Gens)	*250-500mg PO tid for 7-10d; **Ped** 80-90mg/kg PO qd (div q8h) for 7-10d*
or	**Oral Cephalosporin** →194, →196	**Cefixime** (Suprax)	*400mg PO qd for 7-10d; **Ped** 8mg/kg PO qd for 7-10d*
		Cefuroxime-Axetil (Ceftin, Veftin)	*250-500mg PO bid for 7-10d*
or	**Aminopenicillin + Betalactamase inhibitor** →191	**Amoxicillin + Clavulanate** (Augmentin)	*500+250mg tid for 10d; **Ped** 50-100mg/kg PO qd for 10d*
or	**Cephalosporin 3rd gen.** →195	**Ceftriaxone** (Rocephin)	***Ped** 60mg/kg IV/IM qd (single dose)*
or	**Folate antagonist + p-Aminobenzoic acid antagonist** →206	**Sulfamethoxazole + Trimethoprim** (Cotrimoxazole) (Bactrim, Cotrim, Septra, Sulfamethoprim, Sulfatrim, Gens)	*800+160mg PO bid for 10d*

In resistance to therapy, complications

	Fluoroquinolone →203	**Ciprofloxacin** (Cipro)	*500mg PO bid for 14d*
plus	**Lincosamide** →201	**Clindamycin** (Cleocin, Gens)	*150-450mg PO tid-qid; 200-600mg IV tid-qid, for 14d*

15 B.10 Mastoiditis

Acute empiric treatment, pending culture

	Aminopenicillin + Betalactamase inhibitor →191	**Ampicillin + Sulbactam** (Unasyn)	*1-3g IV q6h;* **Ped** *100-200mg/kg qd (div q6h)*
or	**Cephalosporin 3rd gen.** →195	**Cefotaxime** (Claforan, Gens)	*6g IV qd,* **Ped** *50mg/kg IV q12h*

Treatment should be adjusted based on culture & sensitivity

15 B.11 Ménière Disease
15 B.11.1 During Acute Attack

	Antiemetic, antihistamine →124 (inhibition of histamine receptors ⇒ antiemetic)	**Dimenhydrinate** (Dramamine, Marmine, Gens)	*50-100mg PO/IM/IV q4-6h*
or	**Benzodiazepine** →330 (sedation)	**Diazepam** (Diastat, Diazepam Intensol, Valium, Gens)	*2-10mg PO/IM q4h*
poss.	**Loop diuretic** →33 (volume relief)	**Furosemide** (Lasix, Gens)	*40mg IV*

15 B.11.2 Prevention

	Diuretic →33 (excretion of Na^+, H_2O, K^+, H^+ ↑, volume relief)	**Hydrochlorothiazide** (Esidrix, Hydrodiuril, Microzide, Oretic, Gens)	*50mg PO qd*
poss.	**Vestibulosuppressant** →124 (excitability of middle ear labyrinth ↓)	**Meclizine** (Antivert, Gens)	*25-50mg PO bid-tid*
or	**Anticholinergic** →124 (suppressing conduction in vestibular cerebellar pathways)	**Scopolamine** (Transderm Scop)	*Transdermal patch: apply 2.5cm² patch to hairless area behind the ear q3d*
plus	– Reduce salt intake, Stop smoking, Avoid significant noise exposure, Reduce stress		

15 B.12 Sudden Deafness

	Glucocorticoid →148 (anti-inflammatory immunosuppressive)	**Prednisolone** (Onapred, Pediapred, Prelone, Gens)	*IV inf in 500ml Ringer's solution over >4-6h on d1-8, then PO on d9-14, d1: 250mg, d2: 200mg, d3-4: 150mg, d5-6: 100mg, d7: 75mg, d8: 50mg, d9: 40mg, d10: 20mg, d11: 16mg, d12: 12mg, d13: 8mg, d14: 4mg (14d)*

15 B.13 Inflammation of the Salivary Glands (Sialadenitis)

poss.	**Oral Cephalosporin** →194	**Cefuroxime-Axetil** (Ceftin, Veftin)	*250-500mg PO bid for 7-14d*

16 A. Urology – Drugs

16 A.1 Bladder Agents
16 A.1.1 Antispasmodics (Parasympatholytics)

MA/EF (parasympatholytics): blockage of muscarine receptors, mainly direct action on smooth muscles (papaverine-like) ⇒ tonicity of smooth muscles↓ in GI + urinary tract
AE: sweat secretion↓, dry mouth, tachycardia, accommodation DO, glaucoma
AE (hyoscyamine): dry mouth, urinary hesitancy, blurred vision, tachycardia, headache
AE (oxybutynin): tachycardia, anticholinergic EF, insomnia, somnolence, sexual dysfunction
AE (tolterodine): dry mouth, headache, dyspepsia, constipation, xerophthalmia
CI: glaucoma, urinary retention, tachyarrhythmia, GI stenosis, toxic megacolon, myasthenia gravis
CI (hyoscyamine): hypersensitivity to hyoscyamine products, glaucoma, intestinal obstruction, severe liver/renal disease
CI (oxybutynin): glaucoma, GI obstruction, obstructive uropathy, myasthenia gravis, colitis
CI (tolterodine): urinary/gastric retention, glaucoma, hypersensitivity to tolterodine

Hyoscyamine	EHL 3.5h, PRC C, Lact -
Cystospaz *Tab 0.15mg* **Cystospaz-M** *Cap 0.375mg* **Levbid** *Tab ext.rel. 0.375mg* **Levsin** *Tab 0.125mg, Inj 0.5mg/vial* **Levsinex Timecaps** *Tab ext.rel. 0.375mg* **NuLev** *Tab (orally disintegr.) 0.125mg*	**Bladder spasm** →436: 0.125-0.3mg PO qid; ext.rel.: 0.375-0.75mg bid; max 1.5 g/d; **CH** 2-12y: 0.0625-0.125mg PO qid; ext.rel.: 0.375mg PO bid, >12y: 0.125-0.25mg PO qid; ext.rel.: see adults; **GI** →127
Oxybutynin	EHL 1.1-2.3h, PRC B, Lact ?
Ditropan *Syr 5mg/5ml, Tab 5mg* **Ditropan XL** *Tab ext.rel. 5mg, 15mg, 10mg* **Oxytrol** *Film (ext.rel, TD) 3.9mg/24h* **Generics** *Syr 5mg/5ml, Tab 5mg*	**Bladder spasm** →436: 5mg PO bid-tid, max 5mg PO qid; ext.rel.: 5-15mg PO qd, max 30mg PO qd; TD: 1 patch q3-4d; **CH** >5y: 5mg PO bid, max 5mg PO tid
Propantheline	EHL (biphasic) 57.9min, 2.93h, PRC C, Lact ?
Pro-Banthine *Tab 7.5mg, 15mg* **Generics** *Tab 7.5mg, 15mg*	**Urinary incontinence** →436, **neurogenic bladder**: 15mg q4-6h, max 90mg PO qid; **GI, peptic ulcer** →127
Tolterodine	EHL 1.9-3.7h, PRC C, Lact -
Detrol *Tab 1mg, 2mg, Cap ext.rel. 2mg, 4mg*	**Overactive bladder** →436: 2mg PO bid; 1mg PO if reduced hepatic function

16 A.1.2 Bladder Spasm

AE (flavoxate): nervousness, headache, blurred vision, drowsiness, N/V
AE (prosed/DS): rapid pulse, flushing, blurred vision, dizziness, shortness of breath or troubled breathing, difficult micturition, acute urinary retention, dry mouth, N/V
AE (urised): generalized skin rash, dry mouth, flushing, difficulty in initiating micturition, rapid pulse, dizziness, blurring of vision, acute urinary retention
CI (flavoxate): intestinal obstruction, obstructive uropathy
CI (prosed/DS, urised): glaucoma, urinary bladder neck obstruction, pyloric or duodenal obstruction or cardiospasm, hypersensitivity to any of the ingredients

Flavoxate	EHL no data, PRC B, Lact ?
Urispas *Tab 100mg*	**Incontinence, bladder spasm** →436: 100-200mg PO tid-qid; **CH** >12y: see adults
Methenamine + Phenyl salicylate + Methylene blue + Benzoic acid + Atropine sulfate + Hyoscyamine	
Prosed/DS *Tab ext.rel. 81.6mg + 36.2mg + 10.8mg + 9.0mg + 0.06mg + 0.06mg* **Urised** *Tab ext.rel. 40.8mg + 18.1mg + 5.4mg + 4.5mg + 0.03mg + 0.03mg*	**Bladder spasm** →436: Prosed: 1 Tab PO qid; Urised: 2 Tab PO qid

16 A.1.3 Other Bladder Agents

AE (pentosan polysulfate): peripheral edema, headache, dizziness, nausea
AE (phenazopyridine): GI DO, headache, rash, hemolytic anemia, nephrotoxicity, hepatitis
CI (pentosan polysulfate): hypersensitivity to pentosan polysulfate sodium
CI (phenazopyridine): hypersensitivity to phenazopyridine, hepatitis, renal insufficiency

Pentosan Polysulfate	EHL 4.8h, PRC B, Lact ?
Elmiron *Cap 100mg*	**Interstitial cystitis**: 100mg PO tid
Phenazopyridine	EHL no data, PRC B, Lact ?
Azo-Standard *Tab 95mg* **Phenazodine** *Tab 100, 200mg* **Pyridiate** *Tab 100, 200mg* **Pyridium** *Tab 100mg, 200mg* **Urobiotic-250** *Cap 250mg* **Urodine** *Tab 100mg, 200mg*	**Dysuria**: 200mg PO tid for 2d; **CH** 6-12y: 12mg/kg/d PO div tid for 2d

16 A.2 Erectile Dysfunction

MA/E (alprostadil): identical to prostaglandin E1 ⇒ vasodilation
MA/EF (sildenafil): specific phosphodiesterase inhibitor ⇒ relaxation of corpus cavernosal smooth muscle cells ⇒ blood flow into cavernosal spaces ↑
MA/EF (yohimbine): alpha$_2$-adrenergic blocker ⇒ erectogenic
AE (alprostadil): penile pain, neonatal apnea, bradycardia, fever
AE (sildenafil): headache, flushing, dyspepsia, abnormal vision, nasal congestion
AE (yohimbine): anxiety, nervousness, tremor, irritability, agitation, manic reactions, bronchospasm, cough, antidiuresis, dizziness, headache, HTN, tachycardia, N/V, flushes
CI (alprostadil): priapism, hypersensitivity to alprostadil, neonatal respir. distress syndrome
CI (sildenafil): hypersensitivity to sildenafil, concurrent use of nitrates
CI (yohimbine): chronic inflammation of sexual organs, prostatitis, antidepressants, tyramine-containing food, gastric/duodenal ulcers, hypersensitivity to yohimbine, children, psychiatric patients, renal or liver disease

Alprostadil	EHL 5-10min, PRC X, Lact -
Caverject *Inj 5µg/vial, 10µg/vial, 20µg/vial, 40µg/vial, Inj 10µg/ml 20µg/ml* **Edex** *Inj 10µg/vial, 20µg/vial, 40µg/vial* **Muse** *Supp (urethral) 125µg, 250µg, 500µg, 1000µg*	**Erectile dysfunction**: 2.5µg intracavernosal injection, incr prn stepwise by 2.5, 5, 10µg to max 40µg; 125-250µg intraurethral, incr decrease dose prn; max 1000µg; max 2 uses in 24h

Sildenafil	EHL 4h, PRC B , Lact -
Viagra *Tab 25mg, 50mg, 100mg*	**Erectile dysfunction**: 50mg PO 0.5-4h before intercourse, incr prn to max 100mg PO; max 1dose/d; >65y: reduce dose
Yohimbine	EHL 0.6h, PRC N, Lact -
Aphrodyne *Tab 5.4mg*	**Erectile dysfunction**: 5.4mg PO tid up to 10wk

16 A.3 Benign Prostatic Hyperplasia
16 A.3.1 Alpha-Reductase Inhibitors

MA/EF (dutasteride, finasteride): inhibition of the 5-α-reductase $\Rightarrow$ inhibition of transformation of testosterone into dihydrotestosterone $\Rightarrow$ prostatic hyperplasia $\downarrow$
AE (dutasteride, finasteride): sexual dysfunction, breast tenderness/enlargement
CI (dutasteride, finasteride): severe hepatic insufficiency, hypersensitivity to finasteride products, women, children

Dutasteride	EHL 5wk, PRC X, Lact -
Avodart *Cap 0.5mg*	**Benign prostatic hypertrophy** →435: 0.5mg PO qd; DARF: not req
Finasteride	EHL 6h, PRC X, Lact -
Proscar *Tab 5mg*	**Benign prostatic hypertrophy** →435: 5mg PO qd; DARF: not req

16 A.3.2 Peripheral Antiadrenergic Agents

MA/EF (tamsulosin, terazosin): selective blockage of α_1-receptors in the smooth musculature of the prostate and the bladder neck → urine flow ↑
AF (doxazosin): hypotension, dizziness, vertigo, headache
AE (tamsulosin, terazosin): dizziness, postural hypotension, headache, palpitations, retrograde ejaculation
CI (doxazosin): hypersensitivity to doxazosin products or other quinazolines
CI (tamsulosin, terazosin): postural dysregulation, severe hepatic insufficiency

Doxazosin	EHL 8.8-22hPRC C, Lact ?
Cardura *Tab 1mg, 2mg, 4mg, 8mg* **Generics** *Tab 1mg, 2mg, 4mg, 8mg*	**Benign prostatic hypertrophy** →435: ini 1mg PO qd, incr prn to max 8mg PO qd
Tamsulosin	EHL 9-13h, PRC B, Lact -
Flomax *Cap 0.4mg*	**Benign prostatic hypertrophy** →435: 0.4mg PO qd, incr prn after 2-4wk to 0.8mg PO qd; DARF: not req
Terazosin	EHL 9-12h, PRC C, Lact ?
Hytrin *Tab 1mg, 2mg, 5mg, 10mg* *Cap 1mg, 2mg, 5mg, 10mg* **Generics** *Tab 1mg, 2mg, 5mg, 10mg* *Cap 1mg, 2mg, 5mg, 10mg*	**Benign prostatic hypertrophy** →435: ini 1mg PO qd, incr prn to 2-10mg PO qd, max 20mg/d; DARF: not req

16 A.4 Prostate Cancer

MA/EF (bicalutamide, flutamide, nilutamide): competitive blocker of nuclear androgen receptors ⇒ action of androgens ↓; pure antiandrogen without gestagen-like effects
MA/EF (leuprolide, goserelin): GnRH agonist ⇒ gonadotropin secretion ↓, ovarian/testicular steroidogenesis ↓
AE (bicalutamide): hot flashes, diarrhea, pain; **AE** (flutamide): diarrhea, cystitis, rectal bleeding, hot flashes, liver injury; **AE** (goserelin): bone pain, hot flashes, gynecomastia, impotence, breakthrough bleeding; **AE** (leuprolide): amenorrhea, hot flashes, vaginal spotting, bone pain, N/V, edema; **AE** (nilutamide): hot flashes, gynecomastia, N/V, LFT ↑, blurred vision; **CI** (bicalutamide): hypersensitivity to bicalutamide products; **CI** (flutamide): hypersensitivity to flutamide products, severe hepatic impairment; **CI** (goserelin): hypersensitivity to goserelin products; **CI** (leuprolide): hypersensitivity to leuprolide products/GnRH agonists; **CI** (nilutamide): hypersensitivity to nilutamide, severe hepatic impairment, severe respiratory insufficiency

Bicalutamide	EHL 5.8d, PRC X, Lact ?
Casodex *Tab 50mg*	**Prostate CA** →468: 50mg PO qd
Flutamide	EHL 9.6h, PRC D, Lact ?
Eulexin *Cap 125mg*	**Prostate CA** →468: 250mg PO tid
Goserelin	EHL 2.3-4.2h, PRC X, Lact -
Zoladex *Implants 3.6mg, 10.8mg*	**Prostate CA** →468: 3.6mg implant SC q4wk or 10.8mg implant SC q12wk
Leuprolide	EHL 3h, PRC X, Lact -
Eligard *Inj 7.5mg/vial* **Lupron** *Inj 1mg/0.2ml* **Lupron Depot** *Inj 7.5mg/vial, 22.5mg/vial, 30mg/vial* **Viadur** *Implant 65mg (deliv. 120µg/d)* **Generics** *Inj 1mg/0.2ml*	**Prostate CA** →468: 1mg SC qd or 7.5mg IM qmo or 22.5mg IM q3mo or 30mg IM q4mo; **implant**: 65mg SC q12mo
Nilutamide	EHL 38-59.1h, PRC C, Lact ?
Nilandron *Tab 50mg, 150mg*	**Prostate CA** →468: 300mg PO qd for 30d, then 150mg PO qd
Triptorelin	EHL 3h, PRC X, Lact -
Trelstar Depot *Inj 3.75mg/vial* **Trelstar LA** *Inj. 11.25mg/vial*	**Prostate CA** →468: 3.75mg IM q4wk; 11.25mg IM q3mo

16 A.5 Nephrolithiasis

MA/EF (allopurinol): inhibition of xanthine oxidase $\Rightarrow$ uric acid formation $\downarrow$ $\Rightarrow$ uricostatic
AE (acetoh. acid): N/V, headache; **AE** (allopurinol): pruritus, rash, allergic reactions, N/V, myelosuppression, leukopenia, hepatotoxicity, xanthic calculus; **AE** (K^+ citrate): metabolic alkalosis, hyperkalemia, N/V, diarrhea; **CI** (acetoh. acid): serum creatinine > 2.5mg/dL, urine infected by non-urease-producing organism, patients amenable to surgery/antimicrobials; **CI** (allopurinol): allergy to allopurinol; **CI** (potassium citrate): severe renal impairment

Acetohydroxamic Acid	EHL 5-10h, PRC X, Lact ?
Lithostat *Tab 250mg*	**Chronic UTI**: 250mg PO tid-qid (12mg/kg/d), max 1.5g/d; **CH** 10mg/kg/d PO; DARF: CrCl (mg/dl) >1.8: 500mg bid, >2.5: not recomm.
Allopurinol	EHL 1-2h, PRC C, Lact ?
Aloprim *Inj 500mg/vial* **Lopurin** *Tab 100mg, 300mg* **Zyloprim** *Tab 100mg, 300mg* **Generics** *Tab 100mg, 300mg*	**Recurrent calcium oxalate stones** →433: 200-300mg PO qd; DARF: GFR (ml/min): 10-20: 200mg/d; <10: 100mg/d
Potassium Citrate	EHL no data, PRC C, Lact ?
Urocit K *Tab 540mg (=5mEq), 1080mg(=10mEq)* **Generics** *Tab ext.rel. 5mEq, 10mEq*	**Nephrolithiasis** →433: 10-20mEq PO tid-qid, max 100mEq/d

16 A.6 Other Urologic Drugs

AE (bethan.): diarrhea, miosis, excessive lacrimation, flushing of skin; **AE** (desm.): nausea, flushing, headache; **CI** (bethan.): hyperthyroidism, peptic ulcer, asthma, bradycardia, hypo-tension, vasomotor instability, CAD, epilepsy, Parkinsonism, GI inflamm./spasms, peritonitis, vagotonia; **CI** (desm.): hypersens. to desmopressin, **CH** < 3mo, Type IIB von Willebrand's

Bethanechol	EHL no data, PRC C, Lact ?
Urecholine *Tab 5mg, 10mg, 25mg, 50mg;* *Inj 5mg/ml*	**Urinary retention**: 10-50mg PO tid-qid; 2.5-5mg SC tid-qid
Desmopressin	EHL IV 75.5min, PO 90-150min, PRC B, Lact ?
DDAVP *Spray (nasal) 0.01mg/Spray* **Generics** *Spray (nasal) 0.01mg/Spray*	**Nocturnal enuresis**: >6y: ini 20µg, intranasally hs, maint 10-40µg; **diabetes insipidus** →183: →159; **hemophilia A** →79: →78

16 B. Urology – Therapies

Y. Howard Lien, MD
Professor, Section of Nephrology, College of Medicine,
University of Arizona, Tucson, AZ

16 B.1 Cystitis

16 B.1.1 Acute Urinary Tract Infection (UTI, Cystitis–Urethritis)

	Fluoroquinolone →203	**Ciprofloxacin** (Cipro)	*250mg PO bid x 3d*
		Ofloxacin (Floxin)	*200mg PO bid x 3d* *7d for preg and DM*
or	**p-Aminobenzoic acid antagonist** →206	**Sulfamethoxazole + Trimethoprim** (Bactrim, Cotrim, Septra, Sulfatrim, Sulfamethoprim, Gens)	*800+160mg PO bid x 3d. 7d for preg and DM. Avoid in last 2wk of preg. E coli resist. 18% in US*
or	**Macrolide** →199	**Azithromycin** (Zithromax)	*1g PO qd (once) for pos-sible STD (C.trachomatis)*

16 B.1.2 Recurrent Urinary Tract Infection

ini	**Initial treatment as acute UTI**		
then	**Folate + p-Aminobenzoic acid antagonist** →206	**Sulfamethoxazole + Trimethoprim** (Bactrim, Cotrim, Septra, Sulfatrim, Sulfamethoprim, Gens)	*400+80mg qd as long-term Tx*

16 B.2 Pyelonephritis

16 B.2.1 Outpatient, Mild Clinical Course, without Predisposing Factors

	Fluoroquinolone →203	**Ciprofloxacin** (Cipro)	*500mg PO bid x 7d*
		Ofloxacin (Floxin)	*400mg PO bid x 7d*
or	**Aminopenicillin + β-Lactamase inhibitor** →191	**Amoxicillin + Clavulanic acid** (Augmentin)	*500+125mg PO tid x 14d*
or	**Folate + p-Aminobenzoic acid antagonist** →206	**Sulfamethoxazole + Trimethoprim** (Bactrim, Cotrim, Septra, Sulfatrim, Sulfamethoprim, Gens)	*800+160mg PO bid x 14d*
or	**Cephalosporin 2nd Gen.** →193	**Cefuroxime** (Ceftin)	*500mg PO bid x 14d*

16 B.2.2 Nosocomial, Severe Clinical Course, with Predisposing Factors

Initial treatment (adjust antibiotics according to culture results; switch to PO 1–2d after defervescence)

	Fluoroquinolone →203	**Ciprofloxacin** (Cipro)	*400mg IV bid*
		Ofloxacin (Floxin)	
or	Cephalosporin 3rd Gen. →195	**Ceftriaxone** (Rocephin)	*2g IV qd. Do not use if suspect enterococcus*
or	Penicillin 4th Gen. →190	**Piperacillin** (Pipracil)	*3g IV q6h*

After defervescence, continue with PO antibiotics based on culture and sensitivity results to complete 2wk course

	Fluoroquinolone →203	**Ciprofloxacin** (Cipro)	*500mg PO bid*
		Ofloxacin (Floxin)	*400mg PO bid*
or	Aminopenicillin + β-Lactamase inhibitor →191	**Amoxicillin + Clavulanic acid** (Augmentin)	*500mg + 125mg PO tid*
or	Folate + p-Aminobenzoic acid antagonist →206	**Sulfamethoxazole + Trimethoprim** (Bactrim, Cotrim, Septra, Sulfatrim, Sulfamethoprim, Gens)	*800+160mg PO bid*

16 B.3 Urosepsis

Initial treatment (adjust antibiotics according to culture results)

	Cephalosporin 3rd Gen. →195	**Ceftriaxone** (Rocephin)	*2g IV q8h*
plus	Aminoglycoside →200	**Gentamicin** (Garamycin, U-gencin, Gens)	*5mg/kg IV qd;*
	Caution: nephrotoxic, follow blood levels!		
Or			
	Fluoroquinolone →203	**Ciprofloxacin** (Cipro)	*400mg IV q12h*
Or			
	Penicillin 4th Gen. + β-lactamase inhibitor →191	**Piperacillin + Tazobactam** (Zosyn)	*4g+0.5g IV q8h*
Or			
	Carbapenem →197	**Imipenem** (Primaxin)	*0.5g IV q6h*

16 B.4 Glomerulonephritis (GN)

16 B.4.1 Acute Post-streptococcal GN (in active Strep. infection)

	Penicillin →187	**Penicillin V** (Beepen VK, Betapen VK, Ledercill in VK, Pen-vee K, Uticillin VK, V-cillin VK, Veetids)	*500mg PO bid x 10d*
or	Macrolide →199	**Erythromycin** (e-Base, E-mycin, Eryc, Ery-tab, Ilosone, Ilotycin, PCE, Gens)	*500mg PO qid x10d, in penicillin allergy*

16 B.4.2 Minimal Change GN

Initial treatment

	Glucocorticoid →148 (anti-inflammatory, immunosuppressive)	**Prednisone** (Deltasone, Meticorten, Prednisone Intensol, Gens)	*1mg/kg PO qd until 1wk after remission, then 1mg/kg PO qod x 1mo, then taper over mo*

Glucocorticoid-resistant or glucocorticoid-dependent

	Immunosuppressant →260 (calcineurin inhibitor, cytokine synthesis ↓)	**Cyclosporine** (Neoral, Sandimmune, Gens)	*5mg/kg PO qd x 6mo, taper 25% q3mo. Caution: nephrotoxic, follow blood level*
or	**Alkylating agent** (immunosuppressive)	**Cyclophosphamide** (Cytoxan, Neosar)	*2mg/kg PO qd x 8wk*

16 B.4.3 Membranous GN

	Glucocorticoid →148 (anti-inflammatory, immunosuppressive)	**Prednisone** (Deltasone, Meticorten, Prednisone Intensol, Gens)	*2mg/kg PO qod x 6mo, then taper over several mo*
plus sos	**Alkylating agent** (immunosuppressive)	**Cyclophosphamide** (Cytoxan, Neosar)	*1.5mg/kg PO qd x 6m*
or (Ponti-celli prot.)	**Glucocorticoid** →148 (anti-inflammatory, immunosuppressive)	**Methylprednisolone** (Medrol, Depo-Medrol, Solu-Medrol, Gens)	*1g IV qd x 3d, then Prednisone 0.5mg/kg qd until 30d (1st, 3rd, 5th m)*
		Prednisone (Deltasone, Meticorten, Prednisone Intensol, Gens)	
plus	**Cytotoxic** (immunosuppressive)	**Chlorambucil** (Leukeran)	*0.2mg/kg qd for 30d (in 2nd, 4th and 6th m)*
or	**Immunosuppressant** →260 (calcineurin inhibitor, cytokine synthesis ↓)	**Cyclosporine** (Neoral, Sandimmune, Gens)	*5mg/kg PO qd x 6mo, taper 25% q3m; Caution: nephrotoxic, ⇒blood level*

16 B.4.4 Focal Segmental Sclerosing GN

Initial treatment

	Glucocorticoid →148 (anti-inflammatory, immunosuppressive)	**Prednisone** (Deltasone, Meticorten, Prednisone Intensol, Gens)	*2mg/kg PO qd x 6-9mo, then taper over several months*

Glucocorticoid-resistant

	Immunosuppressant →260 (calcineurin inhibitor, cytokine synthesis ↓)	**Cyclosporine** (Neoral, Sandimmune, Gens)	*5mg/kg PO qd x 6mo, taper 25% q3m; Caution: nephrotoxic, ⇒blood level*
or	**Alkylating agent** (immunosuppressive)	**Cyclophosphamide** (Cytoxan, Neosar)	*2mg/kg qd for 8wk; Caution: leukopenia*

16 B.4.5 Rapid Progressive GN

Goodpasture's syndrome

	Glucocorticoid →148 (anti-inflammatory, immunosuppressive)	**Methylprednisolone** (Medrol, Depo-Medrol, Solu-Medrol, Gens)	*1g IV qd for 3d, then Prednisone 1mg/kg PO qd until remission, then taper slowly*
		Prednisone (Deltasone, Meticorten, Prednisone Intensol, Gens)	
plus	**Alkylating agent** (immunosuppressive)	**Cyclophosphamide** (Cytoxan, Neosar)	*2mg/kg PO qd x 6-12mo, Caution: leukopenia*
plus	**Plasmaphoresis** (removes anti-GBM Abs)	**Plasmaphoresis**	*qd till anti-GBM not detected (usu. 1-2wk)*

Immune complex-GN, Lupus nephritis

	Glucocorticoid →148 (anti-inflammatory, immunosuppressive)	**Methylprednisolone** (Medrol, Depo-Medrol, Solu-Medrol, Gens)	*1g IV qd for 3d, then Prednisone 1mg/kg PO qd until remission, then taper slowly*
		Prednisone (Deltasone, Meticorten, Gens)	
plus	**Alkylating agent** (immunosuppressive)	**Cyclophosphamide** (Cytoxan, Neosar)	*Bolus Tx with 0.5-0.75g/m² IV q1mo x 6, then q3mo x 6 (2yr course); Caution: leukopenia*
or	**Purine synthesis inhibitor** →260 (immunosuppressive)	**Azathioprine** (Imuran, Gens)	*50-100mg PO qd*
		Mycophenolate Mofetil (CellCept)	*500-750mg PO bid;*
	Caution: bone marrow suppression, diarrhea (Cellcept)		

Lupus nephritis WHO classification: Class I: no Tx, Class II + V: only glucocorticoids, Class III + IV: see plan

Pauci-immune GN (Wegener's granulomatosis, microscopic polyangiitis)

	Glucocorticoid →148 (anti-inflammatory, immunosuppressive)	**Methylprednisolone** (Medrol, Depo-Medrol, Solu-Medrol, Gens)	*1g IV qd for 3d, then Prednisone 1mg/kg PO qd until remission, then slow taper*
		Prednisone (Deltasone, Meticorten, Prednisone Intensol, Gens)	
plus	**Alkylating agent** (immunosuppressive)	**Cyclophosphamide** (Cytoxan, Neosar)	*2mg/kg PO qd x 6-12mo, Caution: leukopenia*

16 B.5 Diabetic Nephropathy

	ACE inhibitor →25 (renoprotective, antihypertensive)	**Benazepril** (Lotensin)	*2.5-20mg PO qd. Caution: coughing. Follow renal function*
		Lisinopril (Prinivil, Zestril)	
		Quinapril (Accupril)	
		Ramipril (Altace)	

Angiotensin II receptor blocker →27 (renoprotective, antihypertensive)	Candesartan (Atacand)	*16-32mg PO qd*
	Irbesartan (Avapro)	*75-200mg PO qd*
	Losartan (Cozaar)	*25-100mg PO qd*
	Valsartan (Diovan)	*80-320mg PO qd*

Blood pressure and blood sugar control important! Follow renal function!

16 B.6 Renal Failure
16 B.6.1 Acute Renal Failure

poss.	Loop diuretic →33	Furosemide (Lasix)	*50-500mg IV bolus or 40-100mg/h IV infusion*
poss.	Cation exchanger →144 (remove K$^+$ from GI)	Polystyrene sulfonate (Kayexalate, Kionex, SPS, Gens)	*20g in 100ml 20% sorbitol every 4-6h*
or	Redistribution (intracellular shift of K$^+$)	Glucose 50% + Regular insulin	*50ml + 10U IV over 20min*
or	Redistribution →18 (intracellular shift of K$^+$)	Sodium bicarbonate (8.4%, 1meq/ml)	*50ml IV over 5min*
or	Membrane antagonism →139 (inhibition of depolarization)	Calcium gluconate 10% (4.5meq/ml)	*10ml IV over 2-3min Caution: digitalis toxicity↑*
poss.	Buffer →18 (pH neutralization)	Sodium bicarbonate (8.4%, 1meq/ml)	*Ini Tx (meq)= (12-bicarb) x 0.7 x kg IV over 4-8h*

16 B.6.2 Chronic Renal Failure

	Erythrocyte colony stimulating factor →76 (RBC production ↑, maturation, activation)	Erythropoietin (Epogen, Procrit)	*50-100U/kg SC qwk; iron suppl if iron def., follow hematocrit*
or		Darbepoetin (Aranesp)	*0.45µg/kg/wk SC*
poss.	Vitamin D →146 (parathyroid hormone ↓)	Calcitriol (Rocaltrol)	*0.25-1µg PO tiw. Caution: hypercalcemia*
poss.	Phosphate binder →139 (reduce phosphorus)	Calcium carbonate (Mylanta, Titralac, Tums)	*500-1000mg PO tid with meals*

Other possible therapies: antihypertensives (esp. ACE inhibitors, caution: hyperkalemia), protein restriction, antilipidemics

16 B.7 Nephrotic Syndrome

	Loop diuretic →33	Furosemide (Lasix)	*40-80mg PO bid. IV if not responding to PO*
plus sos	Thiazide diuretic →33	Metolazone (Zaroxolyn)	*2.5-5mg PO given same time as PO furosemide. Caution: hypokalemia*
	HMG–CoA reductase inhibitor →42 **(Lipid reduction)**	Simvastatin (Zocor)	*10-40mg PO qd Caution: rhabdomyelysis*
		Atorvastatin (Lipitor)	

ACE inhibitor →25 (renoprotective, antihypertensive)	**Benazepril** (Lotensin) **Lisinopril** (Prinivil, Zestril) **Quinapril** (Accupril) **Ramipril** (Altace)	*2.5-20mg PO qd. Caution: coughing. Follow renal function*
Angiotensin II receptor blocker →27 (renoprotective, antihypertensive)	**Candesartan** (Atacand)	*16-32mg PO qd*
	Irbesartan (Avapro)	*75-200mg PO qd*
	Losartan (Cozaar)	*25-100mg PO qd*
	Valsartan (Diovan)	*80-320mg PO qd*

Blood pressure and blood sugar control important! Follow renal function!

16 B.8 Nephrolithiasis

16 B.8.1 Urate Stone

	Urine alkalinization →427 (Litholysis)	**K⁺ citrate** (Urocit K)	*10-20meq PO tid. keep urine pH > 6.5*
plus	**Xanthine oxidase inhibitor →138** (uric acid synthesis ↓)	**Allopurinol** (Zyloprim, Gens)	*100-300mg PO qd*

Water intake >2l/d for all stones!

16 B.8.2 Cystine Stone

	Urine alkalization →427 (Litholysis)	**K⁺ citrate** (Urocit K)	*20-30meq PO tid keep urine pH > 7.0*
poss plus	**Disulfide formation with Cysteine →25, →471** (cystine formation ↓)	**Captopril** (Capoten, Gens)	*25-75mg PO bid Caution: ↑ PO intake to avoid hypotension*
or		**Alpha-Mercapto-propionylglycine** (Tiopronin)	*0.5-4g qd*
final resort		**D-Penicillamine** (Cuprimine, Depen)	*150mg qid*

Water intake >2l/d for all stones!

16 B.8.3 Calcium Oxalate Stone

	Thiazide diuretic →33 (Ca secretion ↓)	**Chlorthalidone** (Hygroton, Thalitone, Gens)	*25-50mg PO qd*
poss.	**K⁺ sparing diuretic →34** (Ca secretion ↓)	**Amiloride** (Midamor, Gens)	*5-10mg PO qd*
poss.	**Xanthine oxidase inhibitor →138** (uric acid synthesis ↓)	**Allopurinol** (Zyloprim, Gens)	*100-300mg PO qd*
poss.	**Citrate replacement →427** (litholysis)	**K⁺ citrate** (Urocit K)	*10-20meq PO tid. keep urine citrate >320mg/d*

Water intake >2l/d for all stones!

16 B.8.4 Calcium Phosphate Stone (associated with renal tubular acidosis)

poss.	**Citrate replacement** →427 (litholysis)	**K⁺ citrate** (Urocit K)	*10-20meq PO tid. keep urine citrate >320mg/d*
	Water intake >2l/d for all stones!		

16 B.9 Renal Colic
16 B.9.1 Basic Therapy

	Non-steroid anti-inflammatory drug →265, →266	**Ketorolac** (Acular PF, Toradol, Gens	*60mg IV or IM, 100mg PR, then cont with PO NSAID. Stop 3d before lithotripsy. Caution: renal failure if dehydrated*
		Indomethacin (Indocin SR, Indocin, Gens)	
or	**Narcotic analgesic** →270	**Morphine sulfate**	*4-10mg IV slowly or 5-20mg IM, q4h prn*
or	**Narcotic analgesic** →272	**Hydrocodone/Acetaminophen** (Vicodin, Norco)	*5-10mg +325-650mg PO q4-6h prn*

16 B.9.2 Renal Colic with UTI

	Fluoroquinolone →203	**Ciprofloxacin** (Cipro)	*250mg bid x 3d*
		Ofloxacin (Floxin)	*200mg bid x 3d 7d for preg and DM*
or	**Folate + p-Aminobenzoic acid antagonist** →206	**Sulfamethoxazole + Trimethoprim** (Bactrim, Cotrim, Septra, Sulfatrim, Sulfamethoprim, Gens)	*800+160mg PO bid x 3d. 7d for preg and DM, avoid in last 2wk of preg. E coli resist. 18% in US.*

16 B.10 Urethritis
16 B.10.1 Initial Treatment

	Fluoroquinolone →203	**Ciprofloxacin** (Cipro)	*250mg bid x 3d*
		Ofloxacin (Floxin)	*200mg bid x 3d*
or	**Folate + p-Aminobenzoic acid antagonist** →206	**Sulfamethoxazole + Trimethoprim** (Bactrim, Cotrim, Septra, Sulfatrim, Sulfamethoprim, Gens)	*800+160mg PO bid x 3d*

16 B.10.2 Mycoplasma

	Macrolide →199	**Clarithromycin** (Biaxin)	*250mg PO bid x 7d*
or		**Azithromycin** (Zithromax)	*500mg PO qd x 3d*
or	**Tetracycline** →198	**Doxycycline** (Doryx, Vibramycin)	*100mg PO qd x 7d*

16 B.10.3 Chlamydia trachomatis

	Macrolide →199	**Azithromycin** (Zithromax)	*1g PO qd (once)*
or	**Tetracycline** →198	**Doxycycline** (Doryx, Vibramycin)	*100mg PO qd x 7d*

16 B.10.4 Candida

Imidazole derivative →217 (antimycotic)	**Fluconazole** (Diflucan)	*100-200mg PO qd x 10-14d*

16 B.10.5 Trichomonas vaginalis

Nitroimidazole →206 (antiparasitic)	**Metronidazole** (Flagyl, Metro, Metryl, Protostat, Gens)	*2g PO x 1d or 500mg PO bid x 7d*

16 B.11 Prostatitis
16 B.11.1 Acute Bacterial Prostatitis

	Fluoroquinolone →203	**Ofloxacin** (Floxin)	*400mg PO x 1d then 300mg bid x 10d*
or	**Cephalosporin 3rd Gen.** →195	**Ceftriaxone** (Rocephin)	*250mg IM x 1d*
plus	**Tetracycline** →198	**Doxycycline** (Doryx, Vibramycin)	*100mg PO qd x 10d*

16 B.11.2 Chronic Bacterial Prostatitis

	Fluoroquinolone →203	**Ciprofloxacin** (Cipro)	*500mg bid x 4wk*
		Ofloxacin (Floxin)	*300mg bid x 6wk*
or	**Folate + p-Aminobenzoic acid antagonist** →206	**Sulfamethoxazole + Trimethoprim** (Bactrim, Cotrim, Septra, Sulfatrim, Sulfamethoprim, Gens)	*800+160mg PO bid x 1-3mo*

16 B.11.3 Nonbacterial Prostatitis

	Tetracycline →198	**Doxycycline** (Doryx, Vibramycin)	*100mg PO qd x 10d*
poss. cont. with	**Nitroimidazole** →206 (anti-protozoa drug)	**Metronidazole** (Flagyl, Metro, Metryl, Protostat, Gens)	*500mg PO bid x 10d*
or	**Macrolide** →199	**Erythromycin** (e-Base, E-mycin, Eryc, Ery-tab, Ilosone, Ilotycin, PCE, Gens)	*500mg PO qid x 10d*

16 B.12 Prostate Hyperplasia

	Alpha-1-blocker →30 (makes urination easier)	**Doxazosin** (Cardura, Gens)	*Start 1mg PO hs, then incr to 2-5mg PO bid. Caution: orthostatic hypotension with ini Tx*
		Prazosin (Minipress, Minipress XL, Gens)	
		Terazosin (Hytrin, Gens)	
or	**5-alpha-Reductase inhibitor** (hyperplasia↓) →425	**Finasteride** (Proscar)	*5mg PO qd (long-term Tx)*

16 B.13 Epididymitis

	Fluoroquinolone →203	**Ofloxacin** (Floxin)	*300mg bid x 10d*
or	**Cephalosporin 3ʳᵈ Gen.** →195	**Ceftriaxone** (Rocephin)	*250mg IM x 1d*
plus	**Tetracycline** →198	**Doxycycline** (Doryx, Vibramycin)	*100mg PO qd x 10d*

16 B.14 Urinary Incontinence
16 B.14.1 Stress Incontinence

poss.	**Estrogen** →437	**Conjugated estrogen** (Premarin)	*0.3 -0.6mg PO qd or vaginal crm 2g topically qd*
poss.	**Alpha–Sympathomim.** →22 (bladder neck toning)	**Midodrine** (ProAmatine)	*2.5-5mg PO bid Caution: hypertension*

16 B.14.2 Urge Incontinence

poss.	**Antispasmodic** →423 (parasympatholytic, spasmolytic)	**Oxybutynin** (Ditropan, Ditropan XL, Gens)	*5mg PO bid-tid*
or poss.		**Tolterodine** (Detrol, Detrol LA)	*1-2mg PO bid*
or poss.	**Spasmolytic** →423 (detrusor hyperactivity ↓)	**Flavoxate** (Urispas)	*200mg PO tid-qid*
poss.	**Tricycl. Antidepressant** →320 (modulation of urinary urgency feeling)	**Imipramine** (Tofranil, Gens)	*25-100mg PO qhs*

17 A. Gynecology, Obstetrics – Drugs

17 A.1 Sex Hormones, Hormone Drugs
17 A.1.1 Estrogens

MA/EF: sec. female sexual characteristics ↑, proliferation of endometrium, liquefying of cervical mucus, protein anabolism, mineralocorticoid EF, Ca^{2+} resorption ↑, Ca^{2+} uptake in bone ↑; **AE:** thrombosis, skin reactions, edema, glucose tolerance ↓; **CI:** hepatic DO, hormone dependent breast/uterus CA, previous thromboembolism, pancreatitis, severe HTN

Esterified Estrogens — EHL no data, PRC X, Lact -

Estratab *Tab 0.3mg, 0.625mg*
Menest *Tab 0.3mg, 0.625mg, 1.25mg, 2.5mg*

Menopausal vasomotor symptoms: 1.25mg PO qd, cyclically 3wk on/1wk off or contin. + progestin qd; **atrophic vaginitis:** 0.3-1.25mg PO qd, cyclically, if no response, >1.25mg/d; **female hypogonadism:** 2.5-7.5mg PO qd div x 20d followed by a 10d rest period; rep until bleeding; **female castration, primary ovarian failure:** 1.25mg PO qd, cyclically; **breast CA palliation in certain patients:** 10mg PO tid ≥ 3mo; **PRO of postmenopausal osteoporosis** →172: 0.3-1.25mg PO qd, estrogen qd + progestin for last 10-12d of cycle

---

Estradiol — EHL 1h, PRC X, Lact -

Estrace *Tab 0.5mg, 1mg, 2mg, Crm (vag) 0.01%*
Estring *Insert (ext.rel, vag) 0.0075mg/24h*

Menopausal vasomotor symptoms and atrophic vaginitis, female hypogonadism, female castration and primary ovarian failure: 1-2mg PO qd, cyclically 3wk on/1wk off or continuous + progestin qd; **breast CA palliation in certain patients:** 10mg PO tid ≥ 3mo; **PRO of postmenopausal osteoporosis** →172: 0.5mg PO qd, cyclically 3 wk on/1 wk off or contin. with progestin qd, estrogen qd + progestin for last 10-12d of cycle; **atrophic vaginitis:** local application

---

Estradiol Cypionate — EHL no data, PRC X, Lact -

Depo-Estradiol *Inj 5mg/ml*
Generics *Inj 5mg/ml*

Menopausal vasomotor symptoms: 1–5mg IM/wk, cyclically 3wk on and 1wk off; **female hypogonadism:** 1.5–2mg IM/mo, cyclically

Estradiol Transdermal System

Alora Transdermal System *Film (ext.rel, TD) 0.05, 0.075, 0.1mg/d*
Climara *Film (ext.rel, TD) 0.05, 0.075, 0.1mg/d*
Esclim *Film (ext.rel, TD) 0.025, 0.0375, 0.05, 0.075, 0.1mg/d*
Estraderm *Film (ext.rel, TD) 0.05, 0.1mg/d*
Estring *Film (ext.rel, TD) 0.0075mg/d*
Fempatch *Film (ext.rel, TD) 0.025mg/d*
Vivelle *Film (ext.rel, TD) 0.025, 0.0375, 0.05, 0.075, 0.1mg/d*
Vivelle-Dot *Film (ext.rel, TD) 0.0375, 0.05, 0.075, 0.1mg/d*
Generics *Film (ext.rel, TD) 0.05, 0.1mg/d*

EHL no data, PRC X, Lact -

Menopausal vasomotor symptoms and atrophic vaginitis, female hypogonadism, female castration and primary ovarian failure: ini 0.025-0.05mg/d patch 1-2/wk, depending on the product, typical regimen: 3wk on and 1wk off or continuously + progestin qd,
postmenopausal osteoporosis (PRO) →172: 0.025 mg/d–0.1mg/d patch

Estradiol Valerate

Delestrogen *Inj 10mg/ml, 20mg/ml, 40mg/ml*
Generics *Inj 20mg/ml, 40mg/ml*

EHL no data, PRC X, Lact -

Menopausal vasomotor symptoms and atrophic vaginitis, female hypogonadism, female castration and primary ovarian failure: 10–20mg IM q4wk

Estrogens, Conjugated

Premarin *Tab 0.3mg, 0.625mg, 0.9mg, 1.25mg, 2.5mg, Crm (vag) 0.625mg/gm, Inj 25mg/vial*

EHL 4-18.5h, PRC X, Lact -

Menopausal vasomotor symptoms, atrophic vaginitis, and urethritis: 0.3-1.25mg PO qd, cyclically 3wk on/1wk off or contin. + progestin qd, locally (cream); **female hypogonadism:** 2.5-7.5mg PO qd div x 20d, then x 10d rest period; **female castration, primary ovarian failure:** 1.25mg PO qd cyclically; **PRO of postmeno-pausal osteoporosis** →172: 0.625mg PO qd cycl.; **breast CA palliation:** 10mg PO tid ≥ 3mo;

abnormal uterine bleeding: 25mg IV/IM q6-12h, **normalizing bleeding time in AV malformations and underlying renal impairment:** 30–70mg IV/PO qd until normal, estrogen qd + progestin for last 10-12d of cycle

Estrogens, Synthetic, Conjugated

Cenestin *Tab 0.625mg, 0.9mg, 1.25mg*

EHL 4-18.5h, PRC X, Lact -

Menopausal vasomotor symptoms: 0.625-1.25mg PO qd, cyclically 3wk on/1wk off or contin. + progestin qd; estrogen qd + progestin for last 10-12d of cycle

Estrone

Estrone *Inj 5mg/ml*

EHL no data, PRC X, Lact -

Menopausal vasomotor symptoms, female hypogonadism, female castration, primary ovarian failure: 0.1-1mg IM qwk, max 2mg/wk; **senile vaginitis and vulvitis:** 0.1-0.5mg IM 2-3Inj/wk; **abnormal uterine bleeding:** 2–5mg IM qd x several d; **breast CA palliation:** 5mg IM ≥ tiw

Estropipate — EHL no data, PRC X, Lact -

Ogen *Crm (vag) 1.5mg/g*
Ogen 0.625 *Tab 0.75mg*
Ogen 1.25 *Tab 1.5mg*
Ogen 2.5 *Tab 3mg*
Ogen 5 *Tab 6mg*
Ortho-Est *Tab 0.75mg, 1.5mg*
Generics *Tab 0.75mg, 1.5mg, 3mg, 6mg*

Menopausal vasomotor symptoms, vulvar and vaginal atrophy: 0.625-5mg PO qd cyclically 3wk on/1wk off or contin. + progestin qd; **female hypogonadism, female castration, primary ovarian failure:** 1.25-7.5mg PO qd cyclically 3wk on and 8-10d off; **PRO of osteoporosis** →172: 0.625mg PO qd x 25d/31d cycle; estrogen qd + progestin for the last 10-12d of the cycle

Ethinyl Estradiol — EHL no data, PRC X, Lact -

Estinyl *Tab 0.02mg, 0.05mg, 0.5mg*

Postcoital contraception: 0.1mg ethinyl estradiol + 1mg levonorgestrel, rep in 12h within 72h after sexual intercourse
menopausal vasomotor symptoms: 0.02–0.05mg PO qd, cyclically 3wk on and 1 wk off or continuous + progestin qd;
female hypogonadism: 0.05mg PO qd–tid cyclically x 2wk, followed by progesterone x 2wk;
breast CA palliation in certain patients →455: 1mg PO tid; typical regimen: estrogen qd + progestin for the last 10-12d of the cycle

17 A.1.2 Selective Estrogen Receptor Modulators

MA/EF: bind on estrogen receptors ⇒ selective expression of estrogen regulating genes ⇒ bone density ↑, total + LDL cholesterol ↓; **AE:** hot flashes, leg cramps, higher risk of thromboembolic illnesses; **CI:** women of childbearing age, history of thromboembolism, hypersensitivity to raloxifene, severe hepatic/renal insufficiency, endometrial or breast CA

Raloxifene — EHL 27.7h, PRC X, Lact ?

Evista *Tab 60mg*

Osteoporosis PRO/Tx →172: 60mg PO qd; **breast CA PRO** →455: 60–120mg PO qd

17 A.1.3 Antiestrogens

MA/EF (tamoxifen): blockage of peripheral estrogen receptors; **AE** (tamoxifen): alopecia, bone pain, hot flashes, vaginal bleeding, cycle DO, hyperplasia of endometrium, N/V, hypercalcemia; **CI** (tamoxifen): severe leuko- and thrombopenia, severe hypercalcemia

Aminoglutethimide — EHL 9-15h,

Cytadren *Tab 250mg*

Metastatic breast CA →455: 250mg PO bid, give with hydrcortisone 15mg PO bid

Anastrozole — EHL 50h, PRC D, Lact ?

Arimidex *Tab 1mg*

Breast CA; adjuvant Tx →455: 1mg PO qd

Exemestane — EHL 24h, PRC D, Lact ?

Aromasin *Tab 25mg*

Breast CA; adjuvant Tx →455: 25mg PO qd

Fulvestrant — EHL 40d, PRC D, Lact ?

Faslodex *Syr 250mg/5ml; Syr 125mg/2.5ml*

Metastatic breast CA →455: 250mg IM qmo

Letrozole	EHL 2d, PRC D, Lact ?
Femara *Tab 2.5mg*	**Advanced or metastatic breast CA** →455: 2.5mg PO qd
Tamoxifen	EHL 5-7d, PRC D, Lact ?
Nolvadex *Tab 10mg, 20mg*	**Breast CA, adjuvant Tx/PRO in high-risk women** →455: 20mg PO qd x 5 y
Toremifene	EHL 5d, PRC D, Lact ?
Fareston *Tab 60mg*	**Breast CA; adjuvant Tx** →455: 60mg PO qd

17 A.1.4 Progestins

MA/EF: secretive transformation of endometrium, pregnancy maintenance, inhibition of ovulation, thickening of cervical mucus, body temperature ↑
AE: acne, hepatic dysfunction, edema, weight gain, nausea, headache, dysmenorrhea
CI: hepatic diseases, cholestasis, retained abort, vesicular mole

Hydroxyprogesterone Caproate	EHL no data, PRC D, Lact ?
Duralutin *Inj 250mg/ml* **Gesterol LA 250** *Inj 250mg/ml* **Pro-Depo** *Inj 125mg/ml, 250mg/ml* **Generics** *Inj 125mg/ml, 250mg/ml*	**Amenorrhea, dysfunctional uterine bleeding, metrorrhagia:** 375mg IM; **production of secretory endometrium and desquamation:** 125-250mg IM on d 10 of cycle, rep q7d prn; **endometrial hyperplasia:** 500mg IM/wk
Levonorgestrel	EHL 11-45h, PRC X, Lact ?
Norplant II *Implant of 2 covered rods (75mg/rod)* **Norplant system** *Implant 6 Cap (36mg/Cap)* **Mirena** *Intrauterine device (IUD) 52mg* **Plan B** *Tab 0.75mg* **Generics** *Implant 75mg/implant*	**Contraception:** implant complete system subdermal 8-10cm above the elbow crease within 7d after onset of menses (Implant) or fundal insertion of IUD; **postcoital contraception:** 1 Tab PO, rep in 12h, Tx within 24-72h after sexual intercourse
Medroxyprogesterone Acetate	EHL 38-46 h, PRC D, Lact +
Depo-provera *Inj 150mg/ml, 400mg/ml* **Amen** *Tab 10mg* **Provera** *Tab 2.5mg, 5mg, 10mg* **Generics** *Tab 2.5mg, 5mg, 10mg*	**Contraception:** 150mg IM q13wk, inj only during first 5d after onset of menses or within 5d postpartum if not breastfeeding or, if breastfeeding, at 6wk postpartum; **secondary amenorrhea:** 5-10mg PO qd x 5-10d; **abnormal uterine bleeding:** 5-10mg PO qd x 5-10d beginning on the 16th or 21st day of the cycle (after estrogen priming); **hormone replacement Tx to prevent endometrial hyperplasia:** 10mg PO qd for the last 12d mo, or 2.5-5mg PO qd continuously; **endometrial hyperplasia:** 10-30mg PO qd (long-term) or 40-100mg PO qd (short-term) or 500mg IM twice/wk

Megestrol	EHL 13-105h, PRC D (Tab), X (Susp) Lact ?
Megace *Tab 20mg, 40mg, Susp 40mg/ml* **Generics** *Tab 20mg, 40mg*	**AIDS anorexia:** 800mg Susp PO qd; **palliative Tx of advanced breast CA** →455: 40mg PO qid; **endometrial CA:** Tab 40-320mg/d in div doses; **endometrial hyperplasia:** 40-160mg PO qd x 3-4mo; **CA-associated anorexia/cachexia:** 80-160mg PO qid
Norethindrone	EHL 4-13h, PRC X, Lact -
Aygestin *Tab 5mg* **Micronor** *Tab 0.35mg* **Nor-QD** *Tab 0.35mg*	**Amenorrhea, abnormal uterine bleeding:** 2.5-10mg PO qd x 5-10d during 2nd half of menstrual cycle; **endometriosis:** 5mg PO qd x 2wk, incr by 2.5mg q2wk to 15mg/d; **contraception:** (Micronor, Nor-qd)1 Tab PO qd
Progesterone, micronized	EHL 16.8-18.3h, PRC X, Lact ?
Prometrium *Cap 100mg, 200mg*	**Hormone replacement Tx to prevent endometrial hyperplasia:** 200mg PO hs 12d/mo; **secondary amenorrhea:** 400mg PO hs x 10d; **hormone replacement Tx to prevent endometrial hyperplasia:** 100mg hs continuously

17 A.1.5 Hormone Replacement Combinations

Estradiol + Norethindrone	PRC X, Lact -
Activelle *Tab 1mg + 0.5mg*	**Menopausal vasomotor symptoms, vulvar and vaginal atrophy, PRO of postmenopausal osteoporosis** →172: 1 Tab PO qd
Estradiol + Norethindrone	PRC X, Lact -
Combipatch *Film (ext.rel, TD)* *(0.05mg + 0.14mg)/24h, (0.05mg + 0.25mg)/24h*	**Menopausal vasomotor symptoms, vulvar and vaginal atrophy, female hypogonadism, castration, primary ovarian failure, PRO of postmenopausal osteoporosis** →172: 2 patch/wk
Esterified Estrogens + Methyltestosterone	PRC X, Lact -
Estratest *Tab 1.25mg + 2.5mg* **Estratest H.S.** *Tab 0.625mg + 1.25mg*	**Menopausal vasomotor symptoms:** 1 Tab PO qd
Ethinyl Estradiol + Norethindrone	PRC X, Lact -
Aygestin *Tab 0.035mg + 0.5mg* **Femhrt** *Tab 0.005mg + 1mg*	**Menopausal vasomotor symptoms, PRO of postmenopausal osteoporosis** →172: 1 Tab PO qd
Estradiol + Norgestimate	PRC X, Lact -
Ortho-Prefest *Tab (15/15) 1mg/1mg + 0.09mg*	**Menopausal vasomotor symptoms, vulvar atrophy, atrophic vaginitis, PRO of postmenopausal osteoporosis** →172: 1 pink Tab PO qd x 3d followed by 1 white Tab PO qd x 3d, cyclically and continuously

Conjugated Estrogens + Medroxyprogesterone	PRC X, Lact -
Premphase *Tab (14/14) 0.625mg/0.625mg+5mg (Premarin Tab 0.625mg + Cycrin 5mg)* **Prempro (premarin; cycrin)** *Tab (28) 0.625mg + 2.5mg (Premarin Tab 0.625mg + Cycrin 2.5mg), Tab 0.625mg + 5mg (Premarin Tab 0.625mg + Cycrin 5mg)*	**Menopausal vasomotor symptoms, vulvar/vaginal atrophy, and PRO of postmenopausal osteoporosis** →172: 1 Tab containing estrogens PO qd days 1–14, then 1 Tab containing estrogens/progestins PO qd days 15–28 (Premphase); 1 Tab PO qd (Prempro)

17 A.2 Oral Contraceptives
17 A.2.1 Monophasics

MA (monophasics): administration of the same fixed amount of an estrogen-gestagen combination qd for 21 d ⇒ antigonadotropic effects ⇒ suppression of ovulation
AE/CI (monophasic): see triphasics →444

Ethinyl Estradiol + Ethynodiol	PRC X, Lact -
Demulen *Tab (21) 0.035mg+1mg, Tab (21) 0.05mg+1mg, Tab (21/7) 0.035mg + 1mg/plac, Tab (21/7) 0.05mg+1mg/plac* **Zovia** *Tab (21) 0.035mg + 1mg, Tab (21) 0.05mg + 1mg, Tab (21/7) 0.035mg + 1mg/plac, Tab (21/7) 0.05mg + 1mg/plac*	**Contraception:** 1 Tab PO qd

Desogestrel + Ethinyl Estradiol	PRC X, Lact -
Desogen *Tab (21/7) 0.15mg + 0.03mg/plac* **Ortho-Cept** *Tab (21) 0.15mg + 0.03mg Tab (21/7) 0.15mg + 0.03mg/plac* **Generics** *Tab (21) 0.15mg + 0.03mg Tab (21/7) 0.15mg + 0.03mg/plac*	**Contraception:** 1 Tab PO qd; →361

Drospirenone + Ethinyl Estradiol	PRC X, Lact -
Yasmin *Tab (21/7) 3mg + 0.03mg/plac*	**Contraception:** 1 Tab PO qd

Mestranol + Norethindrone	PRC X, Lact -
Genora *Tab (21, 21/7) 0.05mg+1mg/plac* **Nelova** *Tab (21, 21/7) 0.05mg+1mg/plac* **Ortho-Novum** *Tab (21, 21/7) 0.05mg + 1mg/plac*	**Contraception:** 1 Tab PO qd

Ethinyl Estradiol + Levonorgestrel	PRC X, Lact -
Alesse *Tab (21, 21/7) 0.02mg + 0.1mg/plac* **Levlite** *Tab (21, 21/7) 0.02mg + 0.1mg/plac* **Levlen** *Tab (21, 21/7) 0.03mg + 0.15mg/plac* **Levora** *Tab (21, 21/7) 0.03mg + 0.15mg/plac* **Nordette** *Tab (21, 21/7) 0.03mg + 0.15mg/plac*	**Contraception:** 1 tab PO qd; **postcoital contraception:** 0.1mg ethinyl estradiol + 0.5mg levonorgestrel or 5 Tab Alesse/Levlite or 4 Tab Levlen/Levora/Nordette, rep each in 12h within 72h after sexual intercourse

Ethinyl Estradiol + Norgestrel	PRC X, Lact -
Lo/Ovral *Tab (21, 21/7) 0.03mg + 0.3mg/plac* **Low-ogestrel** *Tab (21, 21/7) 0.03mg + 0.3mg/plac* **Ogestrel 0.5/50-21** *Tab (21, 21/7) 0.05mg* *+ 0.5mg/plac* **Ovral** *Tab (21, 21/7) 0.05mg + 0.5mg/plac*	**Contraception:** 1 Tab PO qd; **postcoital contraception:** 2 Tab Ovral or 4 Tab Lo/Ovral, rep each in 12h
Ethinyl Estradiol + Norethindrone Acetate (+ Ferrous Fumarate) PRC X, Lact -	
Loestrin *Tab (21) 0.02mg + 1mg,* *Tab (21) 0.03mg + 1.5mg* **Loestrin Fe** *Tab (28) 0.02mg + 1mg, ferrous* *fumarate in plac d 22-28, Tab (28) 0.03mg + 1.5mg,* *ferrous fumarate in plac d 22-28*	**Contraception:** 1 Tab PO qd
Ethinyl Estradiol + Norethindrone	PRC X, Lact -
Brevicon *Tab (21, 28) 0.035 + 0.5mg* **Gencept** *Tab (21, 21/7) 0.035 + 0.5mg/plac,* *Tab (21, 21/7) 0.035mg + 1mg/plac* **Genora** *Tab (21, 21/7) 0.035 + 0.5mg/plac,* *Tab (21, 21/7) 0.035mg + 1mg/plac* **Modicon** *Tab (21, 21/7) 0.035 + 0.5mg/plac* **Nelova** *Tab (21) 0.035mg + 1mg, Tab (21) 0.035mg* *+ 0.5mg* **Norcept-e** *Tab (21, 21/7) 0.035 + 1mg/plac* **Norethin** *Tab (21, 21/7) 0.035 + 1mg/plac* **Norinyl** *Tab (21, 21/7) 0.035 + 1mg/plac* **Ortho-Novum** *Tab (21, 21/7) 0.035 + 1mg/plac*	**Contraception:** 1 Tab PO qd
Ethinyl Estradiol + Norethindrone	PRC X, Lact -
Ovcon-35 *Tab (21, 21/7) 0.035mg + 0.4mg/plac* **Ovcon-50** *Tab (21/7) 0.05mg + 1mg/plac* *Generics* *Tab (21, 21/7) 0.035mg + 0.5mg/plac* *Tab (21, 21/7) 0.035mg + 1mg/plac*	**Contraception:** 1 Tab PO qd; →361
Ethinyl Estradiol + Norgestimate	PRC X, Lact -
Ortho-Cyclen *Tab (21, 21/7) 0.035mg* *+ 0.25mg/plac*	**Contraception:** 1 Tab PO qd

17 A.2.2 Biphasics

MA (biphasic): first half of menstrual cycle: estrogen-only, or combination with low-dose gestagen; second half of menstrual cycle: regular estrogen-gestagen combination ⇒ inhibition of ovulation
AE/CI (biphasic): see triphasics →444

Ethinyl Estradiol + Norethindrone	PRC X, Lact -
Gencept *Tab (10/11) 0.035mg + 0.5mg/0.035mg + 1mg, Tab (10/11/7) 0.035mg + 0.5mg/0.035mg + 1mg/plac* **Ortho-Novum** *Tab (10/11) 0.035mg + 0.5mg/0.035mg + 1mg, Tab (10/11/7) 0.035mg + 0.5mg/0.035mg + 1mg/plac, Tab (7/14/7) 0.035mg + 0.5mg/0.035mg + 1mg/plac* **Generics** *Tab (7/14) 0.035mg + 0.5mg/0.035mg + 1mg, Tab (7/14/7) 0.035mg + 0.5mg/0.035mg + 1mg/plac, Tab (10/11) 0.035mg + 0.5mg/0.035mg + 1mg,* *Tab (10/11/7) 0.035mg + 0.5mg/0.035mg + 1mg/plac*	**Contraception:** 1 Tab PO qd

17 A.2.3 Triphasics

MA: 3 phases with different estrogen + gestagen combination ⇒ inhibition of ovulation
AE (estrogen-gestagen combinations): seborrhea, acne, dizziness, headache, N/V, breast tenderness, depression, vaginal candidiasis, thrombotic events
CI (estrogen-gestagen combinations): hepatic dysfunction, cholestasis, hepatic tumors, hormone-dependent malignant tumors, past or present history of thrombosis

Ethinyl Estradiol + Levonorgestrel	PRC X, Lact -
Tri Levlen, Triphasil, Trivora *Tab (6/5/10) 0.03mg + 0.05mg/0.04mg + 0.075mg/0.03mg + 0.125mg, Tab (6/5/10/7) 0.03mg + 0.05mg/0.04mg + 0.075mg/0.03mg + 0.125mg/plac*	**Contraception:** 1 tab PO qd

Ethinyl Estradiol + Norethindrone	PRC X, Lact -
Ortho-Novum *Tab (7/7/7) 0.035mg + 0.5mg/0.035mg + 0.75mg/0.035mg + 1mg, Tab (7/7/7/7) 0.035mg + 0.5mg/0.035mg + 0.75mg/0.035mg + 1mg/plac*	**Contraception:** 1 Tab PO qd

Ethinyl Estradiol + Norethindrone	PRC X, Lact -
Tri-norinyl *Tab (7/9/5) 0.035mg + 0.5mg/0.035mg + 1mg/0.035mg + 0.5mg, Tab (7/9/5/7) 0.035mg + 0.5mg/0.035mg + 1mg/0.035mg + 0.5mg/plac*	**Contraception:** 1 Tab PO qd

Ethinyl Estradiol + Norgestimate	PRC X, Lact -
Ortho tri-cyclen *Tab (7/7/7) 0.035mg + 0.18mg/0.035mg + 0.215mg/0.035mg + 0.25mg, Tab (7/7/7/7) 0.035mg + 0.18mg/0.035mg + 0.215mg/0.035mg + 0.25mg/plac*	**Contraception, adult acne** (ortho tri-cyclen): 1 Tab PO qd

17 A.2.4 Progestin Only Contraceptives (Minipill)

MA: low-dose gestagen-only administration qd for 28 d → no inhibition (suppression) of ovulation, but cervical mucus viscosity ↓
AE: irregular menstrual cycles, intracyclic menstrual bleeding!
CI: serious hepatic dysfunction

Norgestrel	PRC X, Lact -
Ovrette *Tab (28) 0.075mg*	**Contraception:** 1 Tab PO qd
Norethindrone	EHL 4-13h, PRC X, Lact -
Micronor *Tab 0.35mg* **Nor-QD** *Tab 0.35mg*	**Contraception:** (Micronor, Nor-qd)1 Tab PO qd

17 A.2.5 Other Oral Contraceptives

AE (desogestrel/ethinyl estradiol): thromboembolic disease, HTN, MI, gallbladder disease, N/V, migraine
CI (desogestrel/ethinyl estradiol): thromboembolic DO, CAD, breast/endometrial CA, estrogen-dependent neoplasia, undiagnosed abnormal vaginal bleeding, cholestatic jaundice of pregnancy, hepatic adenomas/CA

Desogestrel + Ethinyl Estradiol	PRC X, Lact -
Mircette *Tab (21/2/5) 0.15mg* *+ 0.02mg/plac/ethinyl estradiol 0.01mg*	**Contraception:** 1 Tab PO qd
Ethinyl Estradiol + Norethindrone (+ Ferrous Fumarate) PRC X, Lact -	
Estrostep 21 *Tab (5/7/9) 0.02mg + 1mg/0.03mg* *+ 1mg/Tab/0.035mg+1mg* **Estrostep FE** *Tab (5/7/9/7) 0.02mg + 1mg/0.03mg* *+ 1mg/0.035mg + 1mg/ferrous fumarate plac*	**Contraception:** 1 Tab PO qd

17 A.2.6 Other Contraceptives

AE (etonogestrel/ethinyl estradiol): thromboembolic disease, headache, edema, HTN, gallbladder disease, N/V, migraine, breakthrough bleeding, coital problems
CI (etonogestrel/ethinyl estradiol): thromboembolic DO, CAD, breast/endometrial CA, estrogen-dependent neoplasia, undiagnosed abnormal vaginal bleeding, cholestatic jaundice of pregnancy, hepatic adenomas/CA, heavy smoking (>15 cig/d) and age >35y

Etonogestrel + Ethinyl Estradiol	PRC X, Lact -
NuvaRing *Vaginal ring 0.12mg + 0.015mg/d*	**Contraception:** insert into vagina on or before the 5th d of the menstrual period; remove the ring after 3wk, insert a new ring 1wk later
Norelgestromin + Ethinyl Estradiol	PRC X, Lact -
Ortho Evra *Film (ext.rel, TD) 0.015mg + 0.02mg/d*	**Contraception:** d1-21: change 1 patch q7d; d22-28: patch free

17 A.2.7 Postcoital Contraceptives

MA: inhibition of implantation by estrogen-gestagen combination
AE: breast tenderness, N/V, menstrual irregularities, headache, abdominal pain/cramps, dizziness
CI: previous unprotected sex during the same menstrual cycle, absence of menses during preceding menstrual cycle, repeated use within one menstrual cycle, breast CA, endometrial CA, hypersensitive to any component of the product (see Prod Info for AE/CI of estrogen-gestagen combinations)

Ethinyl Estradiol + Levonorgestrel	PRC X, Lact -
Preven emergency contraceptive kit *Tab 0.05mg + 0.25mg*	**Postcoital contraception:** ini 2 Tab within 72h of unprotected intercourse, then 2 Tab 12h later (→442)

17 A.3 GnRH Agonists

MA/EF: high doses of gonadotropin releasing hormones ⇒ complete down regulation of pituitary receptors ⇒ production of sex hormones sinks to castration levels
AE (goserelin): bone pain, hot flashes, gynecomastia, impotence, breakthrough bleeding
AE (leuprolide): hot flashes, vaginal hemorrhage, bone pain, N/V, peripheral edema
AE (nafarelin): acne, hot flashes, irregular menstrual bleeding, breast enlargement
CI (goserelin): hypersensitivity to goserelin; **CI (leuprolide):** hypersensitivity to leuprolide /GnRH agonists; **CI (nafarelin):** undiagnosed vaginal bleeding, hypersensitivity to nafarelin

Ganirelix Acetate	EHL 12.8h (1x), 16.2h (multiple), PRC X, Lact -
Antagon *Inj 250µg/0.5ml*	**Infertility:** 250µg SC qd during early to mid follicular phase, continue Tx qd until day of hCG administration

Goserelin	EHL 2.3h (female), PRC X, Lact -
Zoladex *Implant System 3.6mg/syringe, 10.8mg/syringe*	**Endometriosis:** 3.6mg implant SC q28d x 6mo or 10.8mg implant SC q12wk x 6mo; **palliative Tx of breast CA →455:** 3.6mg implant SC q28d; **endometrial thinning prior to ablation for dysfunctional uterine bleeding:** 3.6mg SC 4wk preop or 3.6mg SC q4wk x 2, followed by surgery in 2–4wk

Leuprolide	EHL 3h, PRC X, Lact -
Lupron *Inj 1mg/0.2ml, Inj depot 3.75mg/vial, 7.5mg/vial, 22.5mg/vial, Inj depot 3mo 11.25mg/vial, Inj depot 4mo 30mg/vial, Inj depot ped 7.5mg/vial, 11.25mg/vial, 15mg/vial* **Viadur** *Implant System 65mg* **Generics** *Inj 1mg/0.2ml*	**Endometriosis/uterine leiomyomata (fibroids):** 3.75mg IM qmo or 11.25mg IM q3mo x 6mo (endometriosis) or x 3mo (fibroids); **central precocious puberty:** Inj: 50µg/kg/d SC, incr by 10µg/kg/d until total down regulation, Inj depot: 0.3mg/kg/4wk IM, incr by 3.75mg q4wk until adequate down regulation

Nafarelin	EHL 2.7 h, PRC X, Lact -
Synarel *Spray 0.2mg/spray*	**Endometriosis:** 200µg spray into one nostril q am, the other nostril q pm x 6mo, incr prn to 4 x 200µg/d; **central precocious puberty:** 2 sprays into each nostril q am + qpm, incr prn to 1,800µg/d

17 A.4 Fertility Drugs
17 A.4.1 Gonadotropins

AE (chorionic gonadotropin): headache, irritability, precocious puberty, gynecomastia, injection site pain;
AE (menotropins): adnexal torsion (with ovarian enlargement), ovarian cysts, flu-like symptoms,
pulmonary/vascular complications
CI (chorionic gonadotropin): precocious puberty, prostatic CA, other androgen dependent neoplasia,
hypersens. to chorionic gonadotropin; epilepsy, migraine, asthma, cardiac/renal disease; **CI** (menotropins):
vaginal/intracranial bleeding, adrenal/thyroid DO, ovarian cysts or enlargement, primary ovarian failure,
pituitary tumor, primary testicular failure

Chorionic Gonadotropins, hCG

EHL 5.6h, PRC X, Lact ?

A.P.L *Inj 5,000, 10,000, 20,000 U/vial*
Novarel *Inj 10,000 U/vial*
Pregnyl *Inj 10,000 U/vial*
Profasi *Inj 2,000, 5,000, 10,000 U/vial*
Generics *Inj 2,000, 5,000, 10,000 U/vial*

Follitropins, FSH

EHL 17-44h, PRC X, Lact ?

Bravelle *Inj 75 U/vial*
Fertinex *Inj 75 U/vial, 150 U/vial*
Follistim *Inj 75 U/vial*
Gonal-F *Inj 37.5, 75, 150 U/vial*

Menotropins, FSH/LH

EHL 2.2-2.9h, PRC X, Lact ?

Humegon *Inj 75 U/vial*
Pergonal *Inj 75 U/vial, 150 U/vial*
Repronex *Inj 75 U/vial, 150 U/vial*

Induction of ovulation and pregnancy: ini with
menotropins 75U FSH/LH IM qd x 7-12d, then
5,000-10,000 U single shot of hCG IM the day after
last menotropin dose, rep prn for 2 mor cycles, if
evidence for ovulation, incr mentropin dose prn to
max 150U FSH/LH; **induction of permatogenesis in
male hypogonadotropic hypogonadism:** 75U
FSH/LH IM tiw, prior to administration of
menotropins, hCG 5000 U IM tiw until adequate
serum testosterone levels and masculinization is
achieved, then ini 75U FSH/LH IM tiw, reduce hCG to
2000 U 2 x/wk, continue for ≥ 4mo, incr prn to 150U
FSH/LH

17 A.4.2 Ovulatory Stimulants

AE (clomiphene): blurred vision, ovarian enlargement, vasomotor flushing, abdominal pain
CI (clomiphene): uncontrolled thyroid or adrenal dysfunction, liver disease, abnormal uterine bleeding,
ovarian cysts, organic intracranial lesion

Clomiphene

Clomid *Tab 50mg*
Serophene *Tab 50mg*

EHL 5d, PRC D, Lact ?

Ovulation induction: 50mg x 5d, ini at any time if
no history of recent uterine bleeding, otherwise ini
at 5th d of cycle, prn incr to 100mg x 5d in ≥ 30d,
max 3 Tx

17 A.5 Myometrial Relaxants

AE (indomethacin): headache, GI distress
AE (magnesium): flushing, hypotension, muscle weakness
AE (nifedipine): peripheral edema, headache, dizziness, tachycardia
AE (ritodrine): N/V, restlessness, HTN, pulmonary edema, tachycardia
AE (terbutaline): tremor, tachycardia, headache, nausea, palpitations
CI (indomethacin): hypersensitivity to the drug, asthma, history of recent rectal bleeding or proctitis, allergic reactions to ASA or other anti-inflammatories
CI (magnesium): 2hr preceding delivery, heart block
CI (nifedipine): hypersensitivity to nifedipine or other CCBs, symptomatic hypotension, persistent dermatologic reactions, CHF
CI (ritodrine): hypersensitivity to ritodrine, use in medical conditions adversely affected by beta-mimetic
CI (terbutaline): hypersensitivity to terbutaline products

Indomethacin	EHL 4.5h, PRC X, Lact -
Indocin SR *Cap ext.rel 75mg* **Indocin** *Cap ext.rel 25mg, 50mg,* *Susp 25mg/5ml, Supp 50mg,* *Inj 1mg/vial* **Indo-lemmon** *Cap ext.rel 25mg, 50mg* **Indomethagan** *Supp 50mg* **Generics** *Cap ext.rel 25mg, 50mg, 75mg,* *Susp 25mg/5ml*	**Preterm labor** (2nd-3rd line): ini 50-100mg PO/PR, then 5mg PO/PR q6-12-48h; **primary dysmenorrhea:** 25mg PO tid-qid; **patent ductus arteriosus:** neonates <48h: 1st dose 0.2mg/kg, 2nd dose 0.1mg/kg, 3rd dose 0.1mg/kg, 2-7d: 1st dose 0.2mg/kg, 2nd dose 0.2mg/kg, 3rd dose 0.2mg/kg, >7d: 1st dose 0.2mg/kg, 2nd dose 0.25mg/kg, 3rd dose 0.25mg/kg

Magnesium Sulfate	EHL no data, PRC A, Lact +
Magnesium sulfate in Dextrose 5% *Inj 1g/100ml,* *2g/100ml* **Magnesium sulfate** *Inj 4g/100ml, 80mg/ml* **Generics** *Inj 500mg/ml*	**Seizure prevention in preeclampsia or eclampsia** →339: 1-4g IV x 2-4min, 5g in 250ml D5W IV inf, max 3ml/min or 4-5g of 50% sol IM q4h prn; **premature labor:** 6g IV x 20min, then 2-3g/h titrated to decrease contractions; DARF: required, monitor serum level, maint urine output 100ml/4h

Nifedipine	EHL 49-137min (pregnancy), PRC C, Lact +
Adalat *Cap 10mg, 20mg* **Adalat cc** *Tab ext.rel 30mg, 60mg, 90mg* **Procardia** *Cap 10mg, 20mg* **Procardia XL** *Tab ext.rel 30mg, 60mg, 90mg* **Generics** *Cap 10mg, 20mg, Tab ext.rel 30mg, 60mg*	**Preterm labor:** ini 10mg PO/SL q20-30min, max 40mg in 1st h of Tx, if successful, maint 10-20mg PO q4-6h or 60-160mg ext.rel PO qd; DARF: not required

Ritodrine	EHL 60-156min, PRC B/X < 20 gest. wk, Lact -
Generics *Inj 10mg/ml, 15mg/ml, 30mg/100ml* *(5% Dextrose)*	**Preterm labor:** 0.05mg/min IV inf; incr by 0.05mg/min q10min prn, usual range 0.15 -0.35mg/min x ≥ 12h until contractions cease, 150mg in 500ml D5W = 0.3mg/ml

Terbutaline	EHL 11-26 h, PRC B, Lact +
Brethine *Tab 2.5mg, 5mg, Inj 1mg/ml* **Bricanyl** *Tab 2.5mg, 5mg, Inj 1mg/ml*	**Preterm labor:** 0.25mg SC q30min up to 1mg/4h or 2.5-10µg/min IV, incr slowly to max 17.5-30µg/min or 2.5-5mg PO q4-6h

17 A.6 Labor Induction, Cervical Ripening

MA (oxytocin): contraction of uterine smooth muscle, promotion of milk ejection by stimulation of smooth muscle contraction in the mammary gland
AE (dinoprostone): GI effects, back pain, fetal HR abnormality; **AE** (misoprostol): diarrhea, abdominal pain; **AE** (oxytocin): arrhythmias, subarachnoid hemorrhage, hypotension
CI (dinoprostone): cardiac/pulmonary/renal/hepatic disease, hypersensitivity to dinoprostone products, history cesarean section/traumatic delivery, cephalopelvic disproportion, fetal distress; **CI** (misoprostol): hypersensitivity to misoprostol or prostaglandins; **CI** (oxytocin): significant cephalopelvic disproportion, unfavorable fetal positions, fetal distress, hypertonic uterus, when vaginal delivery is contraindicated, hypersensitivity to oxytocin, severe toxemia

Dinoprostone	EHL 2.5-5min, PRC X (C for cerv. ripen.), Lact ?
Cervidil *Insert ext.rel (vaginal) 10mg* **Prepidil** *Gel (endocervical) 0.5mg/syringe*	**Cervical ripening:** gel: 1 syringe via catheter placed into cervical canal below the internal os, rep prn q6h, max 3 doses. insert: 1 insert in the posterior fornix of the vagina
Misoprostol	EHL rapid, PRC X, Lact -
Cytotec *Tab 0.1mg, 0.2mg*	**Cervical ripening/labor induction:** 25–100µg oral tablet intravaginally q3-4h, max 600µg/24h or 50µg PO q4h, max 6 doses or 200µg PO q6-8h, max 2 doses
Oxytocin	EHL 3-5min, PRC X, Lact -, nasal spray +
Pitocin *Inj 10 U/ml* **Syntocinon** *Spray (nasal) 40U/ml, Inj 10 U/ml* **Generics** *Inj 10 U/ml*	**Induction/stimulation of labor:** 10U in 1000ml NS, 1-2mU/min IV as continuous inf (6-12ml/h), incr by 1-2mU/min q30min until a contraction pattern is established, max 20mU/min; **promotion of milk ejection:** 1 spray in one nostril 2min prior to nursing during 1st wk of puerperium

17 A.7 Uterotonics

AE (carboprost): emesis/diarrhea, paresthesia, fever/chills, dystonia, breast tenderness
AE (methylergonovine): HTN, N/V, dizziness, palpitations, severe headache, hallucinations
CI (carboprost): hypersensitivity to prostaglandin, acute pelvic inflammatory disease
CI (methylergonovine): hypersensitivity to methylergonovine products, HTN/toxemia

Carboprost	EHL no data, PRC C, Lact ?
Hemabate *Inj 0.25mg/ml*	**Refractory post-partum uterine bleeding:** 250µg IM, rep prn q15-90min, max 2mg
Methylergonovine	EHL 0.5-3.4h, PRC C, Lact ?
Methergine *Tab 0.2mg, Inj 0.2mg/ml*	**Increasing post-partum uterine contractions, control of post-partum bleeding:** 0.2mg IM after delivery of the placenta, delivery of the anterior shoulder, or during the puerperium, rep q2-4h prn or 0.2mg PO tid-qid during 1st wk of puerperium

see Oxytocin ↑449

17 A.8 Vaginal Preparations
17 A.8.1 Antibacterials

Clindamycin Phosphate

EHL 1.5-5h, PRC B, Lact +

Cleocin *Crm (vag) 2%,*
Supp (vaginal) 100mg

Bacterial vaginosis: 1 applicatorful (approx. 100mg clindamycin phosphate in 5g cream) intravaginally hs x 7d or one supp qhs x 3d

Metronidazole, local and systemic

EHL 6-11 h, PRC B/X (1st trimester), Lact ?

Flagyl *Tab ext.rel 750mg, Cap 375mg*
MetroCream 0.75% *Crm (vag) 0.75%*
MetroGel vaginal *Gel (vag) 0.75%*
Noritate *Crm (vag) 1%*
Protostat *Tab 250mg, 500mg*
Generics *Tab 250mg, 500mg*

Bacterial vaginosis →227 (local): 1 applicatorful (approx. 37.5mg metronidazole/5g) vag hs or bid x 5d; **bacterial vaginosis** (systemic): Flagyl ER: 750mg PO qd x 7d, other oral Tab: 500mg PO bid x 7d, in pregnancy (not 1st trimester): 250mg PO tid x 7d; **trichomoniasis:** 2g PO single dose or 250mg PO tid x 1wk or 375-500mg PO bid x 1wk, treat sex partners, too; **Giardia:** 250mg PO tid x 5-7d; **pelvic inflammatory disease:** 500mg PO bid + ofloxacin 400mg PO bid x 14d; DARF: GFR (ml/min) >10: 100%, <10: 50%

17 A.8.2 Antifungals

AE (butoconazole, clotrimazole, nystatin, terconazole, tioconazole; topical): vaginal irritation/pain
CI (butoconazole, clotrimazole, miconazole, nystatin, terconazole): hypersensitivity to product ingredients
CI (tioconazole): hypersensitivity to tioconazole or miconazole products

Butoconazole

EHL 21-24 h, PRC C, Lact ?

Femstat *Crm (vag) 2%*
Gynazole-1 *Crm (vag) 2%*
Mycelex-3 *Crm (vag) 2%*

Local Tx of vulvovaginal candidiasis (nonpregnant patients) →251: 1 applicatorful (approx. 5g) intravaginally hs x 3d,prn max 6d, in pregnant patients, 2nd and 3rd trimesters only, 1 applicatorful (approx. 5g) intravaginally hs x 6d

Clotrimazole

EHL 3.5-5h, PRC B, Lact ?

Gyne-Lotrimin *Tab (vag) 200mg, 500mg,*
Crm (vag)1%, Insert (vag)
Mycelex *Crm (vag), Solution (vag) 1%*

Local Tx of vulvovaginal candidiasis →251: 1 applicatorful 1% cream hs x 7d or 1 applicatorful 2% cream hs x 3d or 100mg Tab (vag) hs x 7d or 200mg Tab (vag) hs x 3d or 500mg Tab (vag) x 1, prn top cream for external symptoms bid x 7d

Fluconazole

EHL 30h, PRC C, Lact -

Diflucan *Tab 100mg, 150mg, 200mg, 50mg,*
Susp 40mg/ml, 10mg/ml

Vaginal candidiasis →251: 150mg PO single dose

Miconazole

EHL 24 h, PRC C, Lact ?

Monistat *Crm (vag) 2%, 4%,*
Supp (vag) 100mg, 200mg
Monistat 3 *Supp (vag) 200mg + Crm (vag) 2%*
Monistat Dual Pak *Insert (vag) 1.2g + Crm 2%*
Generics *Supp (vag) 200mg*

Vulvovaginal candidiasis: 1 applicator-ful 2% cream vag hs x 7d or 100mg supp vag hs x7d or 200mg hs x 3d or 1200mg vag insert hs x 1, top cream for external symptoms bid x 7d

Nystatin — EHL not absorbed, PRC C, Lact ?

Korostatin *Tab (vag) 100,000 U*
Nilstat *Crm 100,000 U/g, Tab (vag) 100,000 U*
Generics *Tab (vag) 100,000 U, Crm 100,000 U/g*

Local Tx of vulvovaginal candidiasis: 100,000U Tab vag hs x 2 wk, treat external lesions with cream

Terconazole — EHL 6.9 h, PRC C, Lact -

Terazol *Crm (vag) 0.4%, 0.8%, Supp (vag) 80mg*

Local Tx of vulvovaginal candidiasis: 1 applicatorful 0.4% cream vag hs x 7d or 1 applicatorful 0.8% cream vag hs x 3d or 80mg supp vag hs x 3d

Tioconazole — EHL not absorbed, PRC C, Lact -

Vagistat-1 *Oint (vag) 6.5%*

Local Tx of vulvovaginal candidiasis: 1 applicatorful (approx. 4.6 g) vag hs x 1

17 A.8.3 Postmenopausal Vaginal Preparations

Estradiol Vaginal Ring — EHL no data, PRC X, Lact -

Estring *Insert ext.rel (vaginal) 0.0075mg/24h*

Menopausal atrophic vaginitis: insert into upper 1/3 of vaginal vault, replace after 90d

Estradiol Vaginal Tablet — EHL no data, PRC X, Lact -

Vagifem *Tab (vag) 25 µg*

Menopausal atrophic vaginitis: ini 1 Tab (vag) qd x 2wk, maint 1 Tab (vag) biw

Estrogen Cream — PRC X, Lact ?

Premarin *Crm (vag, conjugated estrogens) 0.625mg/g*
Estrace *Crm (vag, estradiol) 0.01%*
Ogen *Crm (vag, estropipate) 1.5mg/g*
Ortho Dienestrol *Crm (vag, dienestrol) 0.01%*

Atrophic vaginitis/kraurosis vulvae: Premarin: 0.5-2g intravaginally qd cyclically, 3wk on and 1 wk off, Estrace: 2-4g intravaginally qd x 1-2wk, reduce slowly to maint 1g 1- 3x/wk, Ogen: 2-4g intravaginally qd cyclically, 3wk on and 1wk off, Ortho Dienestrol: 1-2 applicatorsful intravaginally qd x 1-2wk, reduce slowly to maint 1 applicatorful 1-3x/wk, apply cyclically

17 A.8.4 Other Vaginal Preparations

Progesterone Gel — EHL no data, PRC NR Lact ?

Crinone *Gel (vag) 4%, 8%*
Progestasert *Insert ext.rel (intrauterine) 38mg*

Progesterone supplementation in assisted reproduction technology: 90mg progesterone (gel 8%) vag qd; **progesterone replacement in assisted reproduction technology:** 90mg progesterone (gel 8%) vag bid; **secondary amenorrhea:** progesterone (gel 4%) vag qod x 6 doses, prn gel 8% qod x 6 doses; **contraception:** fundal insertion of progestasert IUD

17 A.9 Other Gynecologic, Obstetric Drugs

AE (clonidine): CNS depression, orthostasis, localized reactions, dry mouth; **AE** (danazol): hepatic dysfunction, weight gain, acne, menstrual disturbances; **AE** (RHO Immune Globulin): chills, headache, intravascular hemolysis; **CI** (clonidine): hypersensitivity to clonidine products, conduction defects, bleeding DO, injection site infection; **CI** (danazol): undiagnosed abnormal vaginal bleeding, hepatic/renal/cardiac dysfunction; **CI** (RHO Immune Globulin): hypersensitivity to human globulin B, Rho(D)/D(U) positive patients, Rho(D) negative patients sensitized to Rho(D)/D(U) antigens neonates, IgA deficiency

Clonidine	EHL 12 - 16 h, PRC C, Lact ?
Catapres *Tab 0.1mg, 0.2 mg, 0.3 mg* **Catapres-TTS** *Film (ext.rel, TD) 0.1mg/24h, 0.2mg/24h, 0.3mg/24h* **Generics** *Tab 0.1mg, 0.2mg, 0.3mg*	**Menopausal flushing:** 0.1-0.4mg/d PO div bid-tid or TD 0.1mg/d (1 patch qwk)

Danazol	EHL 4.5h, PRC X, Lact ?
Danocrine *Cap 50mg, 100mg, 200mg* **Generics** *Cap 50mg, 100mg, 200mg*	**Endometriosis:** ini 400mg PO bid, then decr to a dose sufficient to maintain amenorrhea x 3-6mo, max 9mo; **fibrocystic breast disease:** 100-200mg PO bid x 4-6mo; **menorrhagia:** 100-400mg PO qd x 3mo; DARF: contraind. in RF

B6, Folic Acid, B12, Calcium Carbonate	PRC A, Lact +
Premesis-Rx *Tab 75mg + 1mg + 12µg + 200mg*	**Pregnancy-induced nausea:** 1 Tab PO qd

Rho(D) Immune Globuline	PRC C, Lact ?
RhoGAM *Inj 300µg/15ml, 5%* **BayRho-D Full Dose** *Inj 300µg/15ml, 5%* **BayRho-D Mini Dose** *Inj 50µg/2.5ml* **MICRhoGAM** *Inj 50µg/2.5ml*	**PRO of isoimmunization in Rh-negative women following spontaneous or induced abortion or termination of ectopic pregnancy ≥12 wk gestation:** 50µg (Microdose) IM; **PRO of maternal sensitization ot the Rh factor in pregnancy/after childbirth:** 300µg IM if fetal packed RBC volume that entered mother's blood due to fetomaternal hemorrhage <15ml (30ml of whole blood), if >15ml, administer 600µg IM

18 B. Oncology – Therapies

Abdul–Rahman Jazieh, MD, M.P.H.
Associate Professor, Co-director, Thoracic Oncology, Barrett Cancer Center
Department of Internal Medicine, University of Cincinnati, Cincinnati, OH

18 B.1 Supportive Treatment
18 B.1.1 Depending on Symptom

	Antiemetic →125 (inhibits dopamine receptors)	**Prochlorperazine** (Compazine, Compro, Gens)	*5-10mg IM/PO q6h prn*
or	**Antiemetic** →123 (serotonine receptor antagonist = 5-HT3-receptor antagonist)	**Dolasetron** (Anzemet)	*100mg PO/IV qd*
		Granisetron (Kytril)	*1mg IV qd before chemo-Tx or 2mg PO*
		Ondansetron (Zofran)	*8mg PO/IV qd, max 8mg tid*
or	**Antiemetic** →125 (dopamine rec. antag.)	**Metoclopramide** (Reglan, Gens)	*10-20mg PO q4h prn, 10mq IV (max 2mg/kg)*
Plus	**Glucocorticoid** →148 (anti-inflammatory, immunosuppressive)	**Dexamethasone** (Decadron, Hexadrol, Mymethasone, Gens)	*10-20mg PO/IV (premed of chemo-Tx)*

Additional Options

	Antiemetic →124 (inhibits histamine rec.)	**Promethazine** (Phenergan)	*25mg IV/PO q6h*
or	**Benzodiazepine** →330 (anxiolytic)	**Lorazepam** (Ativan, Gens)	*0.5-1mg PO/IV q6h*

18 B.2 Anal Cancer

Primary Chemotherapy + Radiation

	Cytostatic antibiotic (bifunctional alkylating)	**Mitomycin C** (Muta-mycin, Mytozytrex, Gens)	*10mg/m² IV as bolus on d1, rep cyc in 6-8wk*
plus	**Pyrimidine antagonist** (inhibition of thymidine nucleotide synthesis)	**Fluorouracil** (Adrucil, Gens)	*1000mg/m² IV on d1-4, rep cyc in 6-8wk*

221. Flam 1996

Salvage Chemotherapy

	Pyrimidine antagonist (inhibition of thymidine nucleotide synthesis)	**Fluorouracil** (Adrucil, Gens)	*1000mg/m² IV on d1-4, rep cyc from d22-29*
plus	**Alkylating agent** (intrastrand cross-linking of DNA)	**Cisplatin** (Platinol, Platinol AQ, Gens)	*100mg/m² IV on d1, rep cyc from d22-29*

222. Mahjoubi et al. 1990

18 B.3 Bladder Cancer
18 B.3.1 Monotherapy

	Antimetabolite (cytidine analog, inhibits ribonucleotide reductase)	**Gemcitabine** (Gemzar)	*1200mg/m² IV over 30min on d1, d8, d15; rep cyc from d29*
or	**Spindle poison** (microtubule inhibitor, tubulin polymerization, mitosis inhibition)	**Paclitaxel** (Taxol, Gens)	*80mg/m² IV inf over 1h qwk*
Plus	**Alkylating agent** (intrastrand cross-linking of DNA)	**Carboplatin** (Paraplatin)	*AUC 6 IV over 30min on d1*

To calculate the dosage of carboplatin with the AUC-method (AUC=area under the curve of plasma concentration), use formula by A. Calvert:
Dosage of carboplatin (mg) = AUC 6 (mg/ml x min) x [GFR (ml/min) + 25]

18 B.3.2 Polychemotherapy (repeat d22)

M-VAC Methotrexate + Vinblastine + Adriamycin + Cisplatin)

	Antimetabolite →263 (folate antagonist)	**Methotrexate** (Folex, Mexate, Trexall, Gens)	*30mg/m² IV bolus on d1, d15, d22, rep cyc from d29*
plus	**Spindle poison** (inhibits microtubule formation, mitosis ↓)	**Vinblastine** (Velban, Gens)	*3mg/m² IV bolus on d2, d15, d22, rep cyc from d29*
plus	**Cytostatic antibiotic** (binds to DNA, impairs nucleic acid synthesis)	**Doxorubicin** (Adriamycin, Rubex, Gens)	*30mg/m² IV on d2, rep cyc from d29*
plus	**Alkylating agent** (intrastrand cross-linking of DNA)	**Cisplatin** (Platinol, Platinol AQ, Gens)	*70mg/m² IV on d2, rep cyc from d29*

223. Droz et al. 1998
224. Pollera et al. 1994

CISCA (Cisplatin + Cyclophosphamide + Adriamycin)

	Alkylating agent (intrastrand cross-linking of DNA)	**Cisplatin** (Platinol, Platinol AQ, Gens)	*100mg/m² IV on d1 (rep cyc from d22)*
plus	**Alkylating agent** (cross-linking of DNA)	**Cyclophosphamide** (Cytoxan, Neosar, Gens)	*650mg/m² IV on d1, rep cyc from d22*
plus	**Cytostatic antibiotic** (binds to DNA, impairs nucleic acid synthesis)	**Doxorubicin** (Adriamycin, Rubex, Gens)	*50mg/m² IV on d2 (rep cyc from d29)*

18 B.4 Brain Tumors

PCV (every 6–8 weeks)

	Alkylating agent (breakage of chromatids, inhibits mitosis)	**Procarbazine** (Matulane)	*60mg/m^2 PO on d8-21, rep cyc q6-8wk*
plus	**Alkylating agent** (inter- and intrastrand DNA crosslinks)	**Lomustine** (CCNU, CeeNU)	*160mg/m^2 PO on d1, rep cyc q6-8wk*
plus	**Spindle poison** (inhibits intracellular tubulin function/mitosis)	**Vincristine** (Oncovin, Vincasar, Gens)	*1.4mg/m^2 (max 2mg) IV on d8, d29, rep cyc q6-8wk*
or alone	**Alkylating agent** (breakage of chromatids, inhibits mitosis)	**Procarbazine** (Matulane)	*150 mg/m^2 PO qd (div tid), rep cyc q6-8wk*
or alone	**Alkylating agent** (inter-, and intrastrand DNA crosslinks)	**Carmustine** (BiCNU, BCNU)	*200mg/m^2 IV on d1, rep cyc q6-8wk*

In relapses or progression

	Alkylating agent (DNA breaks)	**Temozolomide** (Temodar)	*200mg/m^2 PO qd on d1-5, rep cyc from d28*

18 B.5 Breast Cancer

Adjuvant hormone Tx in "tumor-free" patient for relapse prophylaxis

	Antiestrogen →439 (blockade of peripheral estrogen receptors)	**Tamoxifen** (Nolvadex)	*20-40mg PO qd*
or	**Gestagen** →440 (antiestrogenic, antigonadotropic)	**Medroxyprogesterone acetate** (Amen, Provera, Gens)	*500mg PO qd*

Additive Hormone Therapy

	LH–RH–Agonist →426 (down-regulation of pituitary receptors ⇒ sex hormones ↓↓)	**Goserelin** (Zoladex)	*3.6mg SC q4wk*
	Aromatase inhibitor →439 (inhibitor of adrenal steroid and extra-adrenal estrogen synthesis)	**Aminoglutethimide** (Cytadren)	*250-500mg PO q6h*
	plus Glucocorticoid →148	**Hydrocortisone** (Gens)	*15mg PO bid*
or	**Aromatase inhibitor** →439 (inhibitor of adrenal steroid and extra-adrenal estrogen synthesis)	**Letrozole** (Femara)	*2.5mg PO qd*
or		**Anastrozole** (Arimidex)	*1mg PO qd*

225. Kaufmann et al. 1989

CMF IV

	Alkylating agent (cross-linking of DNA)	**Cyclophosphamide** (Cytoxan, Neosar, Gens)	600mg/m² IV on d1 (rep cyc from d22)
plus	**Antimetabolite** →263 (folate antagonist)	**Methotrexate** (Folex, Mexate, Trexall, Gens)	40mg/m² IV on d1 (rep cyc from d22)
plus	**Pyrimidine antagonist** (inhibition of thymidine nucleotide synthesis)	**Fluorouracil** (Adrucil, Gens)	600mg/m² IV on d1 (rep cyc from d22)

226.　Bonadonna G, et al. Adjuvant cyclophosphamide, methotrexate and fluorouracil in node-positive breast cancer: the results of 20 years of follow-up. N Engl J Med. 1995;332:901-906.

FAC

	Pyrimidine antagonist (inhibition of thymidine nucleotide synthesis)	**Fluorouracil** (Adrucil, Gens)	500mg/m² IV on d1, d8 (rep cyc from d22)
plus	**Cytostatic antibiotic** (binds to DNA, impairs nucleic acid synthesis)	**Doxorubicin** (Adriamycin, Rubex, Gens)	50mg/m² IV on d8 (rep cyc from d22)
plus	**Alkylating agent** (cross-linking of DNA)	**Cyclophosphamide** (Cytoxan, Neosar, Gens)	500mg/m² IV on d1 (rep cyc from d22)

AC (every 3 wks)

	Cytostatic antibiotic (binds to DNA, impairs nucleic acid synthesis)	**Doxorubicin** (Adriamycin, Rubex, Gens)	60mg/m² IV bolus on d1
plus	**Alkylating agent** (cross-linking of DNA)	**Cyclophosphamide** (Cytoxan, Neosar, Gens)	600mg/m² IV on d1

AC→T

	Cytostatic antibiotic (binds to DNA, impairs nucleic acid synthesis)	**Doxorubicin** (Adriamycin, Rubex, Gens)	60mg/m² IV bolus on d1 q3wk x 4 cyc
plus	**Alkylating agent** (cross-linking of DNA)	**Cyclophosphamide** (Cytoxan, Neosar, Gens)	600mg/m² IV on d1 q3wk x 4 cyc
then	**Spindle poison** (microtubule inhibitor, tubulin polymerization, mitosis inhibition)	**Paclitaxel** (Taxol, Gens)	175mg/m² IV q3wk x 4 cyc

HEC

	Cytostatic antibiotic (anthracycline derivative of doxorubicin, mitosis inhibitor)	**Epirubicin** (Ellence)	100mg/m² IV bolus on d1, rep q3wk up to 6 cyc
plus	**Alkylating agent** (cross-linking of DNA)	**Cyclophosphamide** (Cytoxan, Neosar, Gens)	830mg/m² IV bolus on d1, rep q3wk up to 6 cyc

227.　Piccart 2001

	Monoclonal antibody (anti HER-2)	**Herceptin** (Trastuzumab)	*4mg/kg loading dose, then 2mg/kg over 30min qwk*
plus	**Spindle poison** (microtubule inhibitor, tubulin polymerization, mitosis inhibition)	**Paclitaxel** (Taxol, Gens)	*175mg/m² IV inf over 3h, rep q3wk up to 6 cyc*

18 B.6 Cholangiocarcinoma, Gallbladder Carcinoma

In cholangiocarcinoma palliative Tx, indication with restraint, example:

	Pyrimidine antagonist (inhibition of thymidine nucleotide synthesis)	**Fluorouracil** (Adrucil, Gens)	*500mg/m² bolus IV on d1-5 (rep cyc from d36)*
OR	**Pyrimidine antagonist** (inhibition of thymidine nucleotide synthesis)	**Fluorouracil** (Adrucil, Gens)	*600mg/m² IV on d1, d8, d29, d36 (rep cyc from d57)*
plus	**Cytostatic antibiotic** (binds to DNA, impairs nucleic acid synthesis)	**Doxorubicin** (Adriamycin, Rubex, Gens)	*30mg/m² IV on d1, d29 (rep cyc from d57)*
plus	**Cytostatic antibiotic** (bifunctional alkylating)	**Mitomycin C** (Mutamycin, Mytozytrex, Gens)	*10mg/m² IV on d1 (rep cyc from d57)*

228. Moertel 1984

18 B.7 Choriocarcinoma

EMA-CO (Etoposide, Methotrexate + Dactinomycin +Cyclophosaphamide + Vincristine)

	Spindle poison (inhibits DNA-/protein synthesis, mitosis)	**Etoposide** (Etopophos, Toposar, Vepesid)	*100mg/m² IV on d1, d2*
plus	**Antimetabolite** →263 (folate antagonist)	**Methotrexate** (Folex, Mexate, Trexall, Gens)	*100mg/kg IV bolus, then 200mg/m² IV over 12h on d1*
plus	**Folic acid derivative** →147	**Folinic acid** (Leucovorin, Gens)	*15mg IV/PO q12h x 4,* **start 24h after MTX**
plus	**Cytostatic antibiotic** (double strand DNA breaks)	**Dactinomycin** (Cosmegen)	*0.5mg IV bolus on d1, d2*
plus	**Alkylating agent** (cross-linking of DNA)	**Cyclophosphamide** (Cytoxan, Neosar, Gens)	*600mg/m² IV on d0*
plus	**Spindle poison** (inhibits intracellular tubulin function/mitosis)	**Vincristine** (Oncovin, Vincasar, Gens)	*1mg/m² (max 2mg) on d8*

229. Lurain 1985

PEB (Cisplatin + Etoposide + Bleomycin)

	Alkylating agent (intrastrand cross-linking of DNA)	**Cisplatin** (Platinol, Platinol AQ, Gens)	*20mg/m² IV on d1-5 (rep cyc from d22)*

plus	**Spindle poison** (inhibits DNA-/protein synthesis, mitosis)	**Etoposide** (Etopophos, Toposar, Vepesid)	*100mg/m^2 IV over 1h on d1-5 (rep cyc from d22)*
plus	**Cytostatic antibiotic** (single strand breaks, DNA synthesis ↓)	**Bleomycin** (Blenoxane, Gens)	*30mg IV, on d1, d8, d15 (rep cyc from d22)*

230. Williams 1991

18 B.8 Colorectal Carcinoma
18 B.8.1 Adjuvant Therapy

Mayo Clinic Protocol

	Biomodulator (folinic acid = 5-formyl-tetrahydrofolic acid = citrovorum factor, effectiveness of 5-FU ↑)	**Folinic acid** (Leucovorin, Gens)	*20mg/m^2 IV on d1-5 (rep cyc from d29 for 6mo)*
plus	**Pyrimidine antagonist** (inhibition of thymidine nucleotide synthesis)	**Fluorouracil** (Adrucil, Gens)	*425mg/m^2 IV, on d1- d5 (rep cyc from d29 for 6mo)*
OR	**Biomodulator** →147 (folinic acid = 5-formyl-tetrahydrofolic acid = citrovorum factor, effectiveness of 5-FU ↑)	**Folinic acid** (Leucovorin, Gens)	*500mg/m^2 IV on d1, d8, d15, d22, d29 + d36 (rep cyc if effective after 2wk pause)*
plus	**Pyrimidine antagonist** (inhibition of thymidine nucleotide synthesis)	**Fluorouracil** (Adrucil, Gens)	*500mg/m^2 IV on d1, d8, d15, d22, d29, d36 (rep cyc if effective after 2wk pause)*

18 B.8.2 Metastatic Disease

Saltz Regimen (repeat cycle every 6 weeks)

	Topoisomerase I inhibitor (double strand DNA breaks)	**Irinotecan** (Camptosar)	*125mg/m^2 IV over 90min qwk x 4wk*
plus	**Biomodulator** →147 (folinic acid = 5-formyl-tetrahydrofolic acid = citrovorum factor, effectiveness of 5-FU ↑)	**Folinic acid** (Leucovorin, Gens)	*20mg/m^2 IV qwk x 4wk*
plus	**Pyrimidine antagonist** (inhibition of thymidine nucleotide synthesis)	**Fluorouracil** (Adrucil, Gens)	*500mg/m^2 IV qwk x 4wk*

231. Saltz 2000

Or Mayo Clinic Protocol

	Biomodulator →147 (folinic acid = 5-formyl-tetrahydrofolic acid = citrovorum factor, effectiveness of 5-FU↑)	**Folinic acid** (Leucovorin, Gens)	*20mg/m² IV d1-5 q4wk*
plus	**Pyrimidine antagonist** (inhibition of thymidine nucleotide synthesis)	**Fluorouracil** (Adrucil, Gens)	*425mg/m² IV d1-5 q4wk*

Or Irinotecan

	Topoisomerase I inhibitor (double strand DNA breaks)	**Irinotecan** (Camptosar)	*350mg/m² IV over 30min on d1 (rep from d22 (-d29) until progression)*

Caution: in diarrhea aggressive interaction with loperamide PO.

Or Capcitabine

	Pyrimidine antagonist (oral prodrug of 5-Fluorouracil)	**Capcitabine** (Xeloda)	*2500mg/m² PO qd (div bid) x 14d, then 1wk rest, rep cyc from d29*

18 B.9 Esophageal Carcinoma

Cisplatin+ 5 FU and Radiation

	Alkylating agent (intrastrand cross-linking of DNA)	**Cisplatin** (Platinol, Platinol AQ, Gens)	*75mg/m² IV on d1 q4wk*
plus	**Pyrimidine antagonist** (inhibition of thymidine nucleotide synthesis)	**Fluorouracil** (Adrucil, Gens)	*1000mg/m² IV over 24h x 4d q4wk*

Metastatic Disease

	Alkylating agent (intrastrand cross-linking of DNA)	**Cisplatin** (Platinol, Platinol AQ, Gens)	*100mg/m² IV on d1 q4wk*
plus	**Pyrimidine antagonist** (inhibition of thymidine nucleotide synthesis)	**Fluorouracil** (Adrucil, Gens)	*1000mg/m² IV over 24h x 4d q4wk*

18 B.10 Gastric Carcinoma

EAP (Etoposide + Adriamycin + Cisplatin)

	Spindle poison (inhibits DNA-/protein synthesis, mitosis)	**Etoposide** (Etopophos, Toposar, Vepesid)	*100-120mg/m² IV on d4-6; pat <60yr: 100mg; rep cyc from d22-29*
plus	**Cytostatic antibiotic** (binds to DNA, impairs nucleic acid synthesis)	**Doxorubicin** (Adriamycin, Rubex, Gens)	*20mg/m² IV on d1, d7, rep cyc from d22-29*

plus	**Alkylating agent** (intrastrand cross-linking of DNA)	**Cisplatin** (Platinol, Platinol AQ, Gens)	*40mg/m² IV on d2, d8, rep cyc from d22-29*

232. Preusser 1985

ELF (Etoposide + Leucovorin + Fluorouracil)

	Spindle poison (inhibits DNA-/protein synthesis, mitosis)	**Etoposide** (Etopophos, Toposar, Vepesid)	*100-120mg/m² IV on d1-3 (rep cyc from d22-29)*
plus	**Biomodulator** →147 (folinic acid = 5-formyl-tetrahydrofolic acid = citrovorum factor, effectiveness of 5-FU↑)	**Folinic acid** (Leucovorin, Gens)	*300mg/m² IV on d1-3 (rep cyc from d22-29)*
plus	**Pyrimidine antagonist** (inhibition of thymidine nucleotide synthesis)	**Fluorouracil** (Adrucil, Gens)	*500mg/m² bolus IV on d1-3 (rep cyc from d22-29)*

233. Wilke 1990

FAM

	Pyrimidine antagonist (inhibition of thymidine nucleotide synthesis)	**Fluorouracil** (Adrucil, Gens)	*600mg/m² IV on d1, d8, d29, d36 q8wk*
plus	**Cytostatic antibiotic** (binds to DNA, impairs nucleic acid synthesis)	**Doxorubicin** (Adriamycin, Rubex, Gens)	*30mg/m² on d1, d29 q8wk*
plus	**Cytostatic antibiotic** (bifunctional alkylating)	**Mitomycin C** (Mutamycin, Mytozytrex, Gens)	*10mg/m² on d1 q8wk*

FAMTX

	Pyrimidine antagonist (inhibition of thymidine nucleotide synthesis)	**Fluorouracil** (Adrucil, Gens)	*1500mg/m² IV on d1 q28d*
plus	**Biomodulator** →147 (folinic acid = 5-formyl-tetrahydrofolic acid = citrovorum factor, effectiveness of 5-FU↑)	**Folinic acid** (Leucovorin, Gens)	*15mg/m² PO q6h x 12 doses*
plus	**Cytostatic antibiotic** (binds to DNA, impairs nucleic acid synthesis)	**Doxorubicin** (Adriamycin, Rubex, Gens)	*30mg/m² on d15*
plus	**Antimetabolite** →263 (folate antagonist)	**Methotrexate** (Folex, Mexate, Trexall, Gens)	*1.5g/m² IV on d1*

18 B.11 Hepatocellular Carcinoma

	Cytostatic antibiotic (binds to DNA, impairs nucleic acid synthesis)	**Doxorubicin** (Adriamycin, Rubex, Gens)	*60mg/m² IV, bolus on d1 (rep cyc if effective after 2wk)*
OR	**Pyrimidine antagonist** (inhibition of thymidine nucleotide synthesis)	**Fluorouracil** (Adrucil, Gens)	*500mg/m² IV on d1- d5 (rep cyc from d36)*
OR	**Pyrimidine antagonist** (inhibition of thymidine nucleotide synthesis)	**Fluorouracil** (Adrucil, Gens)	*600mg/m² IV on d1, d8, d29, d36 (rep cyc from d57)*
plus	**Cytostatic antibiotic** (binds to DNA, impairs nucleic acid synthesis)	**Doxorubicin** (Adriamycin, Rubex, Gens)	*30mg/m² IV on d1, d29 (rep cyc from d57)*
plus	**Cytostatic antibiotic** (bifunctional alkylating)	**Mitomycin C** (Mutamycin, Mytozytrex, Gens)	*10mg/m² IV on d1 (rep cyc from d57)*

18 B.12 Hodgkin's Disease

See Hematology →93

18 B.13 Insulinoma

	Pyrimidine antagonist (inhibition of thymidine nucleotide synthesis)	**Fluorouracil** (Adrucil, Gens)	*400mg/m² IV on d1-5, rep cyc from d43*
plus	**Alkylating agent** (nitrosourea analog, Inhibits DNA synthesis)	**Streptozocin** (Zanosar)	*500mg/m² IV on d1-5, rep cyc from d43*
plus	**Cytostatic antibiotic** (binds to DNA, impairs nucleic acid synthesis)	**Doxorubicin** (Adriamycin, Rubex, Gens)	*50mg/m² IV on d1, d21 , rep cyc from d43*

18 B.14 Leukemia

18 B.14.1 Acute Leukemia

See Hematology →85

18 B.14.2 Chronic Myeloid Leukemia

See Hematology →84

18 B.14.3 Chronic Lymphocytic Leukemia

See Hematology →91

18 B.15 Lung Cancer
18 B.15.1 Small-cell

ACO II (extensive disease; Adriamycin + Cyclophosphamide + Oncovin)

	Cytostatic antibiotic (binds to DNA, impairs nucleic acid synthesis)	**Doxorubicin** (Adriamycin, Rubex, Gens)	*40mg/m² IV short inf on d1 (4-6 cycs q3wk)*
plus	**Alkylating agent** (cross-linking of DNA)	**Cyclophosphamide** (Cytoxan, Neosar, Gens)	*1000mg/m² IV on d1 (4-6 cycs q3wk)*
plus	**Spindle poison** (inhibits intracellular tubulin function/mitosis)	**Vincristine** (Oncovin, Vincasar, Gens)	*1mg/m² (max 2mg) IV, on d1 (4-6 cycs q3wk)*

234. ACO II Roth 1992

ACE (Adriamycin + Cyclophosphamide + Etoposide)

	Cytostatic antibiotic (binds to DNA, impairs nucleic acid synthesis)	**Doxorubicin** (Adriamycin, Rubex, Gens)	*45mg/m² IV on d1 (4-6 cycs q3wk)*
plus	**Alkylating agent** (cross-linking of DNA)	**Cyclophosphamide** (Cytoxan, Neosar, Gens)	*1000mg/m² IV on d1 (4-6 cycs q3wk)*
plus	**Spindle poison** (mitosis inhibitor, DNA-/protein synthesis inhibitor)	**Etoposide** (Etopophos, Toposar, Vepesid)	*50mg/m² IV on d1-5 (4-6 cycs q3wk)*

235. Aisner 1984

PE

	Alkylating agent (intrastrand cross-linking of DNA)	**Cisplatin** (Platinol, Platinol AQ, Gens)	*75-100mg/m² IV Inf over 2h on d1, rep q3-4wk*
plus	**Spindle poison** (mitosis inhibitor, DNA-/protein synthesis inhibitor)	**Etoposide** (Etopophos, Toposar, Vepesid)	*80-120mg/m² IV on d1-3, rep q3-4wk*

Topotecan (single-agent regimen)

	Topoisomerase I inhibitor (dsouble strand DNA breaks)	**Topotecan** (Hycamtin)	*1-1.5mg/m² IV over 30min qd on d1-5, rep cyc from d22(29) for 4-6 cyc*

Stage "limited disease" (Chemotherapy + Radiation)

	Radiation	*Concurrent chemo-Tx with radiation of 61Gy*	
plus	**Alkylating agent** (intrastrand cross-linking of DNA)	**Cisplatin** (Platinol, Platinol AQ, Gens)	*50mg/m² IV on d1, d8 (2 cycs q4wk with radiation)*
plus	**Spindle poison** (mitosis inhibitor, DNA-/protein synthesis inhibitor)	**Etoposide** (Etopophos, Toposar, Vepesid)	*50mg/m² IV on d1-5 (2 cycs q4wk with radiation)*

18 B.15.2 Non Small Cell

Combination chemotherapy Stage IV

	Spindle poison (microtubule inhibitor, tubulin polymerization, mitosis inhibition)	**Paclitaxel** (Taxol, Gens)	*175-225mg/m² IV inf over 3h on d1, rep cyc q3wk*
plus	**Alkylating agent** (intrastrand cross-linking of DNA)	**Carboplatin** (Paraplatin)	*AUC 6 IV on d1, rep q3wk*

To calculate the dosage of carboplatin with the AUC-method (AUC=area under the curve of plasma concentration), use formula by A. Calvert:
Dosage of carboplatin (mg) = AUC 6 (mg/ml x min) * [GFR (ml/min) + 25]

Or

	Spindle poison (microtubule inhibitor, tubulin polymerization, mitosis inhibition)	**Paclitaxel** (Taxol, Gens)	*135mg/m² IV over 24h on d1, rep q3wk*
plus	**Alkylating agent** (intrastrand cross-linking of DNA)	**Cisplatin** (Platinol, Platinol AQ, Gens)	*75mg/m² IV on d2, rep q3wk*

Or

	Antimetabolite (cytidine analog, inhibits ribonucleotide reductase)	**Gemcitabine** (Gemzar)	*1000mg/m² IV on d1, d8, d15, rep q4wk*
plus	**Alkylating agent** (intrastrand cross-linking of DNA)	**Cisplatin** (Platinol, Platinol AQ, Gens)	*100mg/m² IV on d1, rep q4wk*

Or

	Spindle poison (tubulin polymerization, microtubule stabilization, mitosis inhibitor)	**Docetaxel** (Taxotere)	*75mg/m² IV on d1, rep q3wk*
plus	**Alkylating agent** (intrastrand cross-linking of DNA)	**Cisplatin** (Platinol, Platinol AQ, Gens)	*75mg/m² IV on d1, rep q3wk*

236. Schiller 2002

18 B.16 Malignant Melanoma
18 B.16.1 Adjuvant Therapy

	Interferon →212 (immunostimulation, immunomodulation)	**INF alpha-2b** (Intron A)	*Ini 20 M IU/m² IV 5d/wk for 4 wk, maint 10 M IU/m² tiw for 48wk*

18 B.16.2 Advanced and Metastatic

DTIC

	Alkylating agent (depolymerization of DNA, DNA synthesis ↓)	**Dacarbazine** (DTIC-Dome, Gens)	*850-1000mg/m² IV on d1, rep cyc from d22-36*

237. Chapman PB, et al. Phase III multicenter randomized trial of the Dartmouth regimen versus dacarbazine in patients with metastatic melanoma. J Clin Oncol 1999; 17(9): 2745-2751

18 B.16.3 Combined Therapy

CVD every 21–28 days

	Alkylating agent (depolymerization of DNA, DNA synthesis ↓)	**Dacarbazine** (DTIC-Dome, Gens)	*800mg/m² IV on d1, rep cyc from d22-d29*
plus	**Alkylating agent** (intrastrand cross-linking of DNA)	**Cisplatin** (Platinol, Platinol AQ, Gens)	*20mg/m² IV on d1-5, rep cyc from d22-d29*
plus	**Spindle poison** (inhibits microtubule formation, mitosis ↓)	**Vinblastine** (Velban, Gens)	*1.6mg/m² IV on d1-5, rep cyc from d22-d29*

238. Legha SS. Current therapy for malignant melanoma. Semin Oncol. 1989;16(1 suppl 1):34-44

CDBT (Dartmouth Regimen) every 3 wks

	Alkylating agent (intrastrand cross-linking of DNA)	**Cisplatin** (Platinol, Platinol AQ, Gens)	*25mg/m² IV on d1-3, d22-24, rep cyc from d22*
plus	**Alkylating agent** (depolymerization of DNA, DNA synthesis ↓)	**Dacarbazine** (DTIC-Dome, Gens)	*220mg/m² IV on d1-3, d22-24, rep cyc from d22*
plus	**Alkylating agent** (inter-, and intrastrand DNA crosslinks)	**Carmustine** (BiCNU, BCNU)	*150mg/m² IV on d1, rep cyc from d22*
plus	**Antiestrogen** (blockade of peripheral estrogen receptors)	**Tamoxifen** (Nolvadex)	*10mg PO bid on d4, rep cyc from d22*

239. Chapman PB, et al. Phase III multicenter randomized trial of the Dartmouth regimen versus dacarbazine in patients with metastatic melanoma. J Clin Oncol 1999; 17(9): 2745-2751

Temozolomide

	Alkylating agent (DNA breaks)	**Temozolomide** (Temodar)	*150mg/m² d1-5 q28d; if well tolerated incr to 200mg/m²*

IL-2

	Interleukin 2 (IL-2) (growth factor and activator of T cells)	**Aldesleukin** (Proleukin)	*100,000 IU/kg IV qd on d1-5, d15-19, q28d*

18 B.17 Multiple Myeloma

MP (Alexanian I: Melphalan + Prednisolone)

	Alkylating agent (cross-linking DNA strands, inhibits mitosis)	**Melphalan** (Alkeran)	*9mg/m² PO on d1-4, rep cyc from d43*
plus	**Glucocorticoid** (immunosuppressive, anti-inflammatory)	**Prednisone** (Deltasone, Meticorten, Prednisone Intensol, Gens)	*60mg/m² PO on d1-4, rep cyc from d43*

VAD (Vincristine + Adriamycin + Dexamethasone)

	Spindle poison (inhibits intracellular tubulin function/mitosis)	**Vincristine** (Oncovin, Vincasar, Gens)	*0.4mg/d IV over 24h d1-4, rep cycle from d29*
plus	**Cytostatic antibiotic** (binds to DNA, impairs nucleic acid synthesis)	**Doxorubicin** (Adriamycin, Rubex, Gens)	*9mg/m² IV over 24h d1-4, rep cycle from d29*
plus	**Glucocorticoid** (anti-inflammatory, immunosuppressive)	**Dexamethasone** (Decadron, Hexadrol, Mymethasone, Gens)	*40mg PO on d1-4, d9-12, d17-20, rep cycle from d29*
Or	**Immunomodulatory** (TNF-alpha production ↓)	**Thalidomide** (Thalomid)	*100-800mg PO qd*
plus	**Glucocorticoid** (anti-inflammatory, immunosuppressive)	**Dexamethasone** (Decadron, Hexadrol, Mymethasone, Gens)	*40mg PO on d1-4, d9-12, d17-20, rep cycle from d29*

18 B.18 Non-Hodgkin Lymphoma

CHOP

	Alkylating agent (cross-linking of DNA)	**Cyclophosphamide** (Cytoxan, Neosar, Gens)	*750mg/m² IV on d1, rep cyc from d22*
plus	**Cytostatic antibiotic** (binds to DNA, impairs nucleic acid synthesis)	**Doxorubicin** (Adriamycin, Rubex, Gens)	*50mg/m² IV on d1, rep cyc from d22*
plus	**Spindle poison** (inhibits intracellular tubulin function/mitosis)	**Vincristine** (Oncovin, Vincasar, Gens)	*1.5-2mg/m² IV (not to exceed 2mg) on d1, rep cyc from d22*
plus	**Glucocorticoid** →148 (immunosuppressive, anti-inflammatory)	**Prednisone** (Deltasone, Meticorten, Prednisone Intensol, Gens)	*100mg/m² PO on d1-5, rep cyc from d22*

CHOP + Rituximab

	Alkylating agent (cross-linking of DNA)	**Cyclophosphamide** (Cytoxan, Neosar, Gens)	*750mg/m² IV on d1, rep cyc from d22*
plus	**Cytostatic antibiotic** (binds to DNA, impairs nucleic acid synthesis)	**Doxorubicin** (Adriamycin, Rubex, Gens)	*50mg/m² IV on d1, rep cyc from d22*
plus	**Spindle poison** (inhibits intracellular tubulin function/mitosis)	**Vincristine** (Oncovin, Vincasar, Gens)	*1.4mg/m² IV (not to exceed 2mg) on d1, rep cyc from d22*
plus	**Glucocorticoid** →148 (immunosuppressive, anti-inflammatory)	**Prednisone** (Deltasone, Meticorten, Prednisone Intensol, Gens)	*100mg/m² PO on d1-5, rep cyc from d22*
	Monoclonal antibody (anti CD20)	**Rituximab** (Rituxan)	*375 mg/m² on d1 (before chemo-Tx)*

ICE in relapses and primary refractory NHL

	Alkylating agent (DNA cross-linking, DNA and protein synthesis ↓)	**Ifosfamide** (Ifex, Gens)	*1000mg/m² IV over 1h on d1-2, rep cyc q28d*
plus	**Uroprotective agent** (inhibits hemorrhagic cystitis induced by ifosfamide)	**Mesna** (Mesnex, Gens)	*300mg IV before/4h + 8h after Ifosfamide, rep cyc q28d*
plus	**Alkylating agent** (intrastrand cross-linking of DNA)	**Carboplatin** (Paraplatin)	*200mg/m² on d1-2, rep cyc q28d*
plus	**Spindle poison** (mitosis inhibitor, DNA-/protein synthesis inhibitor)	**Etoposide** (Etopophos, Toposar, Vepesid)	*150mg/m² IV on d1-2, rep cyc q28d*

COP

	Alkylating agent (cross-linking of DNA)	**Cyclophosphamide** (Cytoxan, Neosar, Gens)	*800mg/m² IV on 1d, rep cyc from d22*
plus	**Spindle poison** (inhibits intracellular tubulin function/mitosis)	**Vincristine** (Oncovin, Vincasar, Gens)	*1.4mg/m² IV (not to exceed 2mg) on d1, rep cyc from d22*
plus	**Glucocorticoid** (immunosuppressive, anti-inflammatory)	**Prednisone** (Deltasone, Meticorten, Prednisone Intensol, Gens)	*60mg/m² PO on d1-5, rep cyc from d22*

CP

	Alkylating agent (mitosis inhibitor, lymphosuppression)	**Chlorambucil** (Leukeran)	*30mg/m² PO on d1, rep cyc q28d*
plus	**Glucocorticoid** →148 (immunosuppressive, anti-inflammatory)	**Prednisone** (Deltasone, Meticorten, Prednisone Intensol, Gens)	*80mg PO on d1-5, rep cyc q28d*

18 B.19 Ovarian Carcinoma

CC

	Spindle poison (microtubule inhibitor, tubulin polymerization, mitosis inhibition)	**Paclitaxel** (Taxol, Gens)	*175mg/m^2 IV on d1, rep cyc from d22*
plus	**Alkylating agent** (intrastrand cross-linking of DNA)	**Carboplatin** (Paraplatin)	*AUC 7.5 IV on d1, rep cyc from d22*

To calculate the dosage of carboplatin with the AUC-method (AUC=area under the curve of plasma concentration), use formula by A. Calvert:
Dosage of carboplatin (mg) = AUC 7.5 (mg/ml x min) x [GFR (ml/min) + 25]

Or	**Alkylating agent** (intrastrand cross-linking of DNA)	**Cisplatin** (Platinol, Platinol AQ, Gens)	*75mg/m^2 IV on d2, rep cyc from d22*
plus	**Spindle poison** (microtubule inhibitor, tubulin polymerization, mitosis inhibition)	**Paclitaxel** (Taxol, Gens)	*135mg/m^2 IV over 24h on d1, rep cyc from d22*

CAP

	Alkylating agent (cross-linking of DNA)	**Cyclophosphamide** (Cytoxan, Neosar, Gens)	*1000mg/m^2 IV on d1, rep cyc from d22*
plus	**Alkylating agent** (intrastrand cross-linking of DNA)	**Cisplatin** (Platinol, Platinol AQ, Gens)	*100mg/m^2 IV on d1, rep cyc from d22*
plus	**Cytostatic antibiotic** (binds to DNA, impairs nucleic acid synthesis)	**Doxorubicin** (Adriamycin, Rubex, Gens)	*50mg/m^2 IV on d1, rep cyc from d22*
Or	**Topoisomerase I inhibitor** (dsouble strand DNA breaks)	**Topotecan** (Hycamtin)	*1–1.5 mg/m^2 IV qd on d1-5, rep cyc from d22(29)*

18 B.20 Pancreatic Cancer

	Pyrimidine antagonist (inhibition of thymidine nucleotide synthesis)	**Fluorouracil** (Adrucil, Gens)	*600mg/m^2 IV on d1, d8, d29, d36, rep cyc from d57*
plus	**Cytostatic antibiotic** (binds to DNA, impairs nucleic acid synthesis)	**Doxorubicin** (Adriamycin, Rubex, Gens)	*30mg/m^2 IV on d1, d29, rep cyc from d57*
plus	**Cytostatic antibiotic** (bifunctional alkylating)	**Mitomycin C** (Mutamycin, Mytozytrex, Gens)	*10mg/m^2 IV on d1, rep cyc from d57*

OR	**Antimetabolite** (cytidine analog, inhibits ribonucleotide reductase)	**Gemcitabine** (Gemzar)	*1000mg/m^2 over 30min IV qwk x 7wk, then 1wk rest, then qwk x 3wk with 1wk rest*
OR	**Cytostatic antibiotic** (anthracycline derivative of doxorubicin, mitosis inhibitor)	**Epirubicin** (Ellence)	*90mg/m^2 IV on 1d, rep cyc from d29*

18 B.21 Prostate Carcinoma

Primary Therapy

	Gonadotropin-RH analog →426 (down-regulation of pituitary receptors ⇒ sex hormones ↓)	**Goserelin** (Zoladex)	*3.6mg SC q4wk or 10.8mg SC q12wk*
		Leuprolide (Eligard, Lupron, Viadur, Gens)	*7.5mg SC q4wk or 22.5mg SC q12wk*
or	**Antiandrogen** →426 (cytosol androgen receptor binding, androgen activity ↓)	**Bicalutamide** (Casodex)	*50mg PO qd*
		Cyproterone acetate (Androcur-Canada; not available in the US)	*100mg PO bid*
		Flutamide (Eulexin)	*250mg PO tid*
		Nilutamide (Nilandron)	*300mg PO qd for 30d, then 150mg PO qd*

Secondary Therapy

	Alkylating agent (cytostatic + estrogenic effects)	**Estramustine** (Emcyt)	*14mg/kg PO qd (div tid-qid)*

In Therapy Failure

	Topoisomerase II inhibitor (DNA intercalation, mitosis inhibitor)	**Mitoxantrone** (Novantrone)	*12mg/m^2 IV on d1 q3wk*
plus	**Glucocorticoid** →148 (immunosuppressive, anti-inflammatory)	**Prednisone** (Deltasone, Meticorten, Prednisone Intensol, Gens)	*5mg PO bid*
Or	**Pyrimidine antagonist** (inhibition of thymidine nucleotide synthesis)	**Fluorouracil** (Adrucil, Gens)	*500mg/m^2 IV qwk*
or	**Spindle poison** (tubulin polymerization, microtubule stabilization, mitosis inhibitor)	**Docetaxel** (Taxotere)	*75mg/m^2 IV on d1, rep q3wk*
or	**Spindle poison** (microtubule inhibitor, tubulin polymerization, mitosis inhibition)	**Paclitaxel** (Taxol, Gens)	*80mg/m^2 IV on d1, d8, d15, rep cyc from d28*

18 B.22 Renal Cell Carcinoma

IL-2 + INF Combination Therapy

	Interleukin 2 (IL-2) (growth factor and activator of T cells)	**Aldesleukin** (Proleukin)	*18 x 10^b IU/m^2 IV Cl d1-5 x 2, seperated by 6d break, then 18 x 10^6 Cl d1-5 q3wk x 4 cyc*
plus	**Interferon →212** (immunostimulating, immunomodulatory)	**INF alpha-2a** (Roferon A) **INF alpha-2b** (Intron A)	*6 M IU/m^2 SC tiw in combination with IL-2*

240. Negrier S, et al: Recombinant human interleukin-2, recombinant human interferon alfa-2a, or both in metastatic renal-cell carcinoma. Groupe Francais d'Immunotherapie. N Engl J Med 1998 Apr 30; 338(18): 1272-8

High dose IL-2 Therapy

Interleukin 2 (IL-2) (growth factor and activator of T cells)	**Aldesleukin** (Proleukin)	*600,000-720,000 IU/kg IV over 15min q8h until toxicity or 14 doses; give 2 courses separated by 5-9d, rep 2-course-cyc q6-12 wk*

18 B.23 Testicular Cancer

PEB (Cisplatin + Etoposide + Bleomycin)

	Alkylating agent (intrastrand cross-linking of DNA)	**Cisplatin** (Platinol, Platinol AQ, Gens)	*20mg/m^2 IV on d1-5 over 30min, rep cyc from d22*
plus	**Spindle poison** (mitosis ↓, DNA-/protein synthesis inhibitor)	**Etoposide** (Etopophos, Toposar, Vepesid)	*100mg/m^2 IV over 1h on d1-5, rep cyc from d22*
plus	**Cytostatic antibiotic** (single strand breaks, DNA synthesis ↓)	**Bleomycin** (Blenoxane, Gens)	*30mg IV on d1, d8, d15, rep cyc from d22*

241. Williams SD, Birch R, Einhorn LH, et al: Treatment of disseminated germ-cell tumors with cisplatin, bleomycin, and either vinblastine or etoposide. NEJM 1987; 316: 1435-14

VIP (Etoposide + Ifosfamide + Cisplatin)

	Spindle poison (mitosis inhibitor, DNA-/protein synthesis inhibitor)	**Etoposide** (Etopophos, Toposar, Vepesid)	*75mg/m^2 IV on d1-5 over 1h, rep cyc from d22*
plus	**Alkylating agent** (DNA cross-linking, DNA and protein synthesis ↓)	**Ifosfamide** (Ifex, Gens)	*1200mg/m^2 IV on d1- d5 over >1h, rep cyc from d22*
plus	**Uroprotective agent** (inhibits hemorrhagic cystitis induced by ifosfamide)	**Mesna** (Mesnex, Gens)	*400mg IV bolus, then 1200mg/m2 IV on d1-5 (rep cyc from d22)*
plus	**Alkylating agent** (DNA double str. linkage)	**Cisplatin** (Platinol AQ, CDDP)	*20mg/m^2 IV on d1-5 over 30min, rep cyc from d22*

242. Harstrick 1991

19 A. Toxicology – Drugs

19 A.1 Drugs, Antidotes

Acetylcysteine
EHL 2.27h, PRC B, Lact ?

Mucomyst, Mucosil, Generics *Sol (inhal, oral) 10%, 20%*
Acetaminophen toxicity →473: loading dose 140mg/kg PO or NG as soon as possible, then 70mg/kg q4h x 17 doses, prn mix in water; IV use: pyrogen-free IV; acetylcysteine is available only through participating poison centers; **CH** adult dose

Atropine
EHL 4h, PRC C, Lact ?

Atropine Sulfate *Inj 0.3, 0.4, 0.5, 0.6, 0.8, 1mg/ml*
Organophosphate poisoning →483: 2–5 mg IV, rep prn q10–30min; **CH** 0.05mg/kg IV, rep prn q10–30min

Charcoal
PRC B, Lact +

Actidose-Aqua *Liquid (oral) 25g/120ml*
Charcolex *Powder (oral) for Sol 15g, 30g, 40g*
Generics *Cap 260mg, Liquid (oral) 25g/120ml*
Gut decontamination →472: 25–100g (0.5–1g/kg or 10 times the amount of poison ingested) PO or NG as soon as possible, rep prn q4h; **CH** >1y: adult dose

Deferoxamine
EHL 3–6 h, PRC C, Lact ?

Desferal *Inj 500mg/vial*
Chronic iron overload →480: 500mg–1,000mg IM qd and 2g IV inf (max 15mg/kg/h) with each unit of blood or 1–2g SC qd (20–40mg/kg/d) x 8–24h via contin. inf pump; **acute iron toxicity** →480: ini 1g IM, then 500mg IM q4h x 2 doses, rep prn 500mg IM q4–12h, max 6g/24h; IV route (only in patients with CVS collapse): ini 1g slowly IV (max 15mg/kg/h), then 500mg x 4h for 2 doses at max rate of 125mg/h, prn subsequent doses of 500mg x 4–12h at max rate of 125mg/h; DARF: contraind. unless undergoing dialysis

Dimercaprol
EHL very short (no exact data), PRC N, Lact ?

BAL in oil *Inj 10%*
Arsenic/gold poisoning, mild →474: 2.5mg/kg deeply IM 4x/d x 2d, bid on 3rd day, then qd x 10d or until recovery; **arsenic/gold poisoning, severe** →474: 3mg/kg deeply IM q4h x 2d, qid on 3rd day, bid x 10d or until recovery; **mercury poisoning** →474: ini 5mg/kg, then 2.5mg/kg qd–bid x 10d; **acute lead encephalopathy** →474: 4mg/kg q4h x 2–7d, after 1st dose, combined Tx with edetate calcium disodium at separate site; **lead poisoning, mild** →474: ini 4mg/kg, then 3mg/kg q4h x 2–7d; DARF: req

Edetate Calcium Disodium
EHL 1.4–3h, PRC C, Lact -

Calcium Disodium Versenate *Inj 200mg/ml*
Lead poisoning →480: rec dosage for blood lead level >20µg/deciliter and <70µg/deciliter: $1g/m^2$/d IM x 8–12h x 5d, then interrupt Tx x 2–4d, then rep prn 5-day course of Tx, max 75mg/kg/d, mix for IM use 1ml of inj concentrate with 1ml lidocaine or procaine 1%; DARF: CrCl (mg/deciliter) 2–3: 50% q24h x 5d, rep prn qmo, 3–4: 50% q48h x 3 doses, rep prn qmo, >4: 50% qwk, rep prn qmo

Ethanol	EHL 0.232mg/(ml x h), PRC N, Lact -
Ethanol 10%	**Methanol poisoning** →480: if acidosis, visual changes, blood MeOH level >25mg/deciliter, ini loading dose 10ml/kg of 10% ethanol in D5W x 20-30min, maint 1-2ml/kg/h, maint blood ethanol level 100-150mg/ deciliter
Flumazenil	EHL 41-79min, PRC C, Lact ?
Romazicon *Inj 0.1mg/ml*	**Benzodiazepine sedation reversal** →475: 0.2mg IV x 15sec, after 30sec prn 0.2mg q1min, max 1mg total dose, usual dose 0.6-1mg; **benzodiazepine overdose reversal** →475: 0.2mg IV x 30sec, after 30sec prn 0.3mg, then prn 0.5mg q1min, max 3mg total dose; DARF: not required
Fomepizole	EHL 5h (oral), PRC C, Lact ?
Antizol *Inj 1g/ml*	**Ethylene glycol toxicity** →480: ini loading dose 15mg/kg slowly IV x 30min, then 10mg/kg slowly IV q12h x 4 doses, then 15mg/kg slowly IV q12h, then until ethylene glycol concentrations <20mg/deciliter or ini 15mg/kg PO, in 12h 5mg/kg PO, then 10mg/kg PO q12h ethylene glycol plasma levels =0; DARF: consider additional dialysis
Ipecac Syrup	PRC C, Lact ?
Generics *Syr*	**Induction of emesis** →472: 15-30ml PO, then 3-4 glasses of water, rep if vomiting does not occur within 20-30min; **CH** 1-12y: 15ml, then 1-2 glasses of water, rep if vomiting does not occur within 20-30min
Methylene Blue	PRC C, Lact ?
Generics	**Methemoglobinemia (drug induced)** →482: (1-2mg/kg IV 0.1-0.2ml/kg of 1% sol) x 5min, do not use in cyanide poisoning; DARF: use with caution in severe RF
Penicillamine	EHL 1-7.5h, PRC D, Lact -
Cuprimine *Cap 125mg, 250mg* **Depen** *Tab 250mg*	**Wilson's disease** →478: 750mg-1.5g/d resulting incupriuresis of 2mg/d, adjust dosage based on urinary copper analysis and determination of free copper in the serum; **lead poisoning** →478: 1-1.5g/d x 1-2mo given 2h before or 3h after meals; DARF: GFR (ml/ min) <50%: avoid drug
Pralidoxime	EHL 1.23h, PRC C, Lact ?
Protopam *Inj 1g/vial*	**Organophosphate toxicity (severe)** →483: 1-2g IV in 100ml saline x 15-30min or IV at max rate of 200mg/min or as a 5% sol in water IV x >5min, rep prn in 1h 1g IV, then prn continuous IV inf at rate of 500mg/h; DARF: required (no exact data available)
Sorbitol	PRC N, Lact +
Generics *Sol (oral) 70%*	**Laxative** →472: 30-150ml (70% sol) PO or 120ml (25-30% Sol) PR; **CH** 2-11y 2ml/kg (70% sol) PO or 30-60ml (25-30% sol) PR
Succimer	EHL 2h-2d, PRC C, Lact ?
Chemet *Cap 100mg*	**Lead toxicity** →481: 10-30mg/kg/d, usual dose 30mg/kg/d x 5d; **CH** ≥ 1y: if blood lead levels >45µg/deciliter, ini 10mg/kg PO or 350mg/m^2 q8h x 5d, then reduce to q12h x 2wk, interval of ≥ 4wk between edetate disodium and succimer Tx; DARF: use with caution

19 B. Toxicology – Therapies

Susan Smolinske
Managing Director
Regional Poison Control Center
Children's Hospital of Michigan
Wayne State University
Detroit, MI

19 B.1 Important Notes
19 B.1.1 General Measures

The primary removal of poisons (gastric lavage, induced vomiting etc.) is not a routine measure. Like pharmacologic therapy of poisonings, the necessity for these measures must be clearly tested and the measure must be clearly indicated. The administration of activated charcoal can replace these measures in many cases. Poison control centers can help with indications.

19 B.1.2 Pharmacologic Therapy

Drugs or antidotes can have severe adverse effects (deferoxamine, atropine, physostigmine etc.). All the same, it is often impossible to manage without their administration. Because of this, the indication for pharmacologic therapy must be carefully considered for every single case. The indication not only depends on the kind of poison, but also on the amount ingested, the time course of the poisoning, the physical condition of the patient and on other parameters. Benefits and disadvantages for the patient must be carefully considered on an individual basis.

19 B.1.3 Dosage

Absolute dosages are for adult patients. Dosages for children are specially marked. The specification mg/kg means "mg per kilogram body weight" and can usually be used for adults and children.

243.   AACT (1997) Clin Toxicol 35:699-763
244.   AACT (1999) Clin Toxicol 37:731-75

19 B.2 General Measures
19 B.2.1 Primary Gastric Decontamination

poss.	**Adsorbent** →470 (binding of poison ⇒ resorption ↓ ⇒ poison elimination ↑)	**Activated charcoal** (Actidose, CharcoAid, Insta-Char, Liqui-Char)	*0.5-1g/kg or 10 times the amount of poison ingested PO or NG*
poss.	**Emetic** →471 (induced vomiting ⇒ poison elimination)	**Syrup of ipecac** (Gens)	*Adults: 30ml;* **Ped** *6-12m: 5-10ml;* **Ped** *1-12y: 15ml, then 4-8oz H$_2$O; rep in 30min if no effect*
poss.	**Osmotic cathartic** (laxation ⇒ GI transit ↑)	**Sorbitol** (Gens)	*1-2ml/kg of 70%;* **Ped** *4.3ml/kg of 35%*

| poss. | **Gastric lavage**
(⇒ poison elimination) | **Wide bore orogastric tube**
Adults: 36–49 French
CH: 24–28 French | *200-300ml aliquots warm fluid,*
0.9% NaCl or water;
Ped *10ml/kg warm 0.9% NaCl* |
| poss. | **Whole bowel irrigation**
(⇒ poison elimination) | **PEG electrolyte solution**
(Golytely, Colyte) | *2l/h PO or NG until rectal*
effluent clear; **Ped** *35ml/kg/h* |

19 B.2.2 Secondary Poison Elimination

| poss. | **Multiple dose activated**
charcoal →470
(may disrupt entero-hepatic
circulation or adsorb drug
resorbed from the intestine;
"gut dialysis") | **Activated charcoal** (Actidose,
CharcoAid, Insta-Char, Liqui-
Char) | *0.25-0.5g/kg PO or NG every*
2-4h, sorbitol repeated only
qd-bid |
| poss. | **Extracorporeal measures**: Hemodialysis, hemoperfusion, hemodiafiltration etc. should only be undertaken after consultation with poison control centers or in special poison treatment centers. | | |

19 B.3 Specific Management
19 B.3.1 Acetaminophen

| | **Antidote** →470
(detoxification of toxic
metabolites, antioxidant) | **Acetylcysteine** (Mucomyst,
Mucosil, Gens) | *140mg/kg PO diluted to 5%,*
then 70mg/kg q4h PO for 17
doses; consider same dose IV
(investigational) if intractable
vomiting, pregnancy, ileus, or GI
bleed) |

245.   Rumack (2002) Clin Toxicol 40:3-20

10 B.3.2 Amantadine

| | **Benzodiazepine** →330
(anticonvulsant) | **Diazepam** (Valium, Gens) | *0.1-0.2mg/kg IV; may rep q1-4h*
prn |

19 B.3.3 Amphetamines

For seizures, agitation, hyperthermia

	Benzodiazepine →330 (anticonvulsant, muscle relaxant↓, hyperthermia)	**Diazepam** (Valium, Gens)	*0.1-0.2mg/kg IV;* *may rep q1-4h prn*
	Barbiturate →332 (anticonvulsant)	**Phenobarbital** (Luminal, Gens)	*10-20mg/kg slowly IV*
poss.	**Muscle relaxant** →298 (hyperthermia↓)	**Dantrolene** (Dantrium)	*2.5mg/kg IV q6h*

For tachycardia

Adenosine →37 (terminates AV nodal reentry-related dysrhythmias)	**Adenosine** (Adenocard, Adenoscan)	*3–6mg IV bolus; may rep 6–12mg q1–2min for 3 doses*
Beta- 1-selective Block. →23 (CO↓, neg. chronotropic, neg. inotropic, renin secretion↓, central sympathetic act.↓)	**Esmolol** (Brevibloc)	*50–100µg/kg/min IV inf*

For ventricular fibrillation

Antiarrhythmic →37 Class Ib	**Lidocaine** (Gens)	*Ini 100mg IV, then 2–4mg/min*

246. White (2002) Semin Resp Crit Care Med 23:27-36

19 B.3.4 Antihistamines

For QRS prolongation (diphenhydramine)

Buffer →18 (Tx of acidosis, Na$^+$ channel receptor binding↓, QRS↓)	**Sodium bicarbonate 8.4%** (50ml = 50mEq HCO$_3^-$)	*1–2mEq/kg IV (pH to 7.45–7.55)*

For seizures

Benzodiazepine →330 (anticonvulsant)	**Diazepam** (Valium, Gens)	*0.1–0.2mg/kg IV; may rep q1–4h prn*

For hypotension

Alpha- and Beta– sympathomimetic, D1 receptor agonist (pos. inotropic) →22	**Dopamine** (Intropin, Gens)	*5–15 µg/kg/min IV*

247. Clark (1992) Ann Emerg Med 21:318-321

19 B.3.5 Arsenic

Arsenic salts, arsenic acid, arsenite, and arsenate with high As urine levels, not for arsine

Chelator →471	**Succimer** (Chemet)	*10mg/kg PO tid for 5d, then 10mg/kg bid for 14d (may rep after 2wk interval, depending on arsenic excretion)*
Chelator →470 (for severe cases)	**Dimercaprol** (BAL)	*3–5mg/kg IM q4–6h*

248. Cullen (1995) Am J Emerg Med 13: 432-435

19 B.3.6 Aspirin

| | **Sodium bicarbonate** →18 (therapy of acidosis, urine alkalinization | **Sodium bicarbonate 8.4%** (50ml = 50mEq HCO$_3^-$) | *100-150mEq/l in D5W 3-4ml/kg/h with K$^+$ 20-40mEq/l (titrate to urine pH >7.5)* |
| poss. | **Benzodiazepine** →330 (anticonvulsant) | **Diazepam** (Valium, Gens) | *0.1-0.2mg/kg IV; may rep q1-4h prn* |

249. Prescott (1982) Br Med J 285:1383-1386.

19 B.3.7 Atropine

For severe anticholinergic syndrome (delirium, unstable tachycardia, coma with hypoventilation)

| poss. | **Indirect para–sympatholytic,** (cholinesterase inhibition ⇒ anticholinergic and adrenergic effectso) | **Physostigmine** (Antilirium) | *1-2mg slowly IV, may rep, although usually single dose as diagnostic;* **Ped** *0.02-0.04mg/kg slowly IV* |
| | **Benzodiazepine** →330 (anticonvulsant, antianxiety) | **Diazepam** (Valium, Gens) | *0.1-0.2mg/kg IV; may rep q1-4h prn* |

250. Burns (2000) Ann Emerg Med 35:374-381

19 B.3.8 Baclofen

| | **Dir. parasympatholytic** →37 (cholinergic effects ↓) | **Atropine** (Atropen, Gens) | *0.5-1mg IV;* **Ped** *0.02mg/kg IV* |

251. Cohen (1986) Am J Emerg Med 4: 552-553

19 B.3.9 Barbiturates

| | **Buffer** →18 (urine alkalization, poison elimination ↑) | **Sodium bicarbonate 8.4%** (50ml = 50mEq HCO$_3$-) | *100-150mEq/l in D5W 3-4ml/kg/h with K$^+$ 20-40mEq/l (titrate to urine pH >7.5; Phenobarbital only)* |

252. Frenia (1996) Clin Toxicol 34:169-175

19 B.3.10 Benzodiazepines

| | **Benzodiazepine antagonist** →471 (benzodiazepine effects ↑) | **Flumazenil** (Romazicon) | *0.2-0.6mg IV (short EHL, only in vital indication);* **Ped** *0.01-0.02mg/kg q1min to max of 1mg or 0.05mg/kg* |

253. Shalansky (1993) Clin Pharm 12:483-487

19 B.3.11 Betablockers

| | **Alpha– and Beta- sympathomimetic, D1 receptor agonist** →?? (pos. inotropic) | **Dopamine** (Intropin, Gens) | *5-20 µg/kg/min* |

	Beta- (>Alpha-) sympathomimetic →37 (pos. ino-, chrono-, bathmotropic in hypotension, bronchodilatation)	**Epinephrine** (Adrenalin, Epipen, Sus-phrine, Gens)	*0.001-0.01mg/kg IV as single dose, then depending on effects*
	Inotropic agent →154 (CO↑, HR↑ in bradycardia)	**Glucagon** (Glucagen, Gens)	*5-10mg IV bolus, then 1-5mg/h;* **Ped** *0.15mg/kg, then: 0.05mg/kg/h over 24h IV*
poss.	**Inotropic agent** →153 (BP↑)	**Insulin** (Insulin regular) **Glucose** (Gens)	*0.5 IU/kg/h with dextrose 1 g/kg/h titrate to euglycemia*
	Buffer →18 (QRS↓)	**Sodium bicarbonate 8.4%** (100ml = 100mEq HCO₃.)	*1-2mEq/kg IV (pH to 7.45-7.55)*
poss.	**Calcium** →139 (reverses myocardial depression)	**Calcium chloride 10%** (Gens)	*0.1-0.2ml/kg IV q5-10min for 3-4doses*

254. Kerns (1994) Emerg Med Clin North Am 12:365-390

19 B.3.12 Black Widow Spider Envenomation

Antivenin (complexation with venom)	**Latrodectus antivenin**	*1 vial IV, diluted to 10-50ml in saline over 30min*

19 B.3.13 Botulism

Specific antidote (poison effects↓)	**Botulinin Antitoxin (ABE)** (CDC)	*1-2 vials IV q4h for 4-5 doses, duration depends on response; not indicated in infants)*

19 B.3.14 Caffeine

For severe tachycardia or hypotension

Betablocker →23 (CO↓, neg. chronotropic, neg. inotropic, central sympathetic activity↓)	**Propranolol** (Inderal, Gens)	*1mg q2-5min up to 5mg total IV;* **Ped** *0.1mg/kg IV up to 1mg*
Betablocker →23 (CO↓, neg. chronotropic, neg. inotropic, central sympathetic activity↓)	**Esmolol** (Brevibloc)	*500µg/kg over 5min, then 50µg/kg/min for 4min; adj prn*

For ventricular fibrillation

Antiarrhythmic →37 Class Ib	**Lidocaine** (Gens)	*ini 1mg/kg IV bolus, maint 1-4mg/min*

For seizures

Benzodiazepine →330 (anticonvulsant)	**Diazepam** (Valium, Gens)	*0.1-0.2mg/kg IV; may rep q1-4h prn*

19 B.3.15 Calcium Channel Blockers

Calcium (reverses myocardial depression)	**Calcium chloride 10%** (Gens)	*0.1-0.2ml/kg IV q5-10min for 3-4 doses*
Calcium (reverses myocardial depression)	**Calcium gluconate 10%** (Gens)	*0.3-0.4ml/kg IV q5-10min for 3-4 doses*
Direct Parasympatholytic →37 (cholinergic effects↓)	**Atropine** (Atropen, Gens)	*0.5-1mg q5min to max 0.04mg/kg IV;* **Ped** *0.02mg/kg q5min; max dose 0.5mg*
Alpha- and Beta-sympathomimetic →37 (BP↑, HR↑, pos. inotropic, vasoconstriction, renal vasodilation, natriuresis)	**Epinephrine** (Adrenalin, Epipen, Sus-phrine, Gens)	*0.001-0.01mg/kg IV as single dose, then depending on effects*
Inotropic agent →154 (CO↑, HR↑ in bradycardia)	**Glucagon** (Glucagen, Gens)	*5-10mg IV bolus, then 1-5mg/h;* **Ped** *0.15mg/kg, then 0.05mg/kg/h over 24h IV*
poss. **Inotropic agent** →153 (BP↑)	**Insulin** (Insulin Regular) / **Glucose** (Gens)	*0.5 IU/kg/h with dextrose 1g/kg/h (titrate to euglycemia)*

255. Kerns (1994) Emerg Med Clin North Am 12:365-390
256. Yuan (1999) Clin Toxicol 37.463-474

19 B.3.16 Carbamate Insecticides

Direct parasympatholytic →37 (cholinergic effects↓)	**Atropine** (Atropen, Gens)	*1-5mg IV, poss. rep q5-10min until atropinized (dry pulmonary secretions, reversal bronchospasm) with 5-10mg;* **Ped** *ini 0.02mg/kg*

19 B.3.17 Cardiac Glycosides

Specific antidote →40 (glycoside effects↓)	**Digitalis Immune Fab** (Digibind, Digifab)	*vials =serum dig level (ng/ml) x body weight (kg)/100, over 30min IV. One vial binds 0.5mg dig (total dig levels after antidote falsely high)*

19 B.3.18 Chloral Hydrate

Betablocker →23 (PVCs↓)	**Propranolol** (Inderal, Gens)	*1mg q2-5min up to 5mg total IV;* **Ped** *0.1mg/kg IV up to 1mg*
Betablocker →23 (PVCs↓)	**Esmolol** (Brevibloc)	*500µg/kg over 5min, then 50µg/kg/min for 4min; adj prn*
Antiarrhythmic →37 Class Ib	**Lidocaine** (Gens)	*1mg/kg IV bolus, then 1-4mg/min*

257 Pershad (1999) Pediatr Emerg Care 15:432-435

19 B.3.19 Chloroquine

Buffer →18 (QRS↓)	**Sodium bicarbonate 8.4%** (50ml = 50mEq HCO₃-)	*1-2mEq/kg IV (pH to 7.45-7.55)*
Benzodiazepine →330 (prophylaxis of arrhythmias, seizures)	**Diazepam** (Valium, Gens)	*Ini 1-2mg/kg IV (after intubation), then 0.1-0.4mg/kg/h*
Beta- (>Alpha-) sympathomimetic →37 (pos. ino-, chrono-, bathmotropic in hypotension, bronchodilatation)	**Epinephrine** (Adrenalin, Epipen, Sus-phrine, Gens)	*0.001-0.01mg/kg IV as single dose, then depending on effects*

19 B.3.20 Clonidine

In bradycardia

Direct parasympatholytic →37 (cholinergic effects↓)	**Atropine** (Atropen, Gens)	*0.5-1mg IV,* **Ped** *0.02mg/kg IV*

For hypotension

Alpha- and Beta-sympathomimetic, D1 receptor agonist →22 (pos. inotropic)	**Dopamine** (Intropin, Gens)	*5-10µg/kg/min*

For respiratory depression

Opioid antagonist →272 (opioid effects ↓)	**Naloxone** (Narcan, Gens)	*0.4-2mg IV*

258.   Bamshad (1990) Vet Hum Toxicol 32:220-223

19 B.3.21 Cocaine

Benzodiazepine →330 (anticonvulsant)	**Diazepam** (Valium, Gens)	*0.1-0.2mg/kg IV; may rep q1-4h prn*
Barbiturate →332 (anticonvulsant)	**Phenobarbital** (Luminal, Gens)	*10-20mg/kg slowly IV (for persistent seizures relaxation)*

19 B.3.22 Copper Salts

Chelator (poison elimination↑)	**Penicillamine** (Cuprimine, Depen)	*1-1.5g PO qd, given q6-12h;* **Ped** *10-30mg/kg/d, given q8-12h*

19 B.3.23 Coral Snake Envenomation

Antivenin (complexation with venom)	**Antivenin Micrurus fulvius**	*3-5 vials IV, diluted in 50-200ml saline over 15-30min per vial; may rep for continued neurologic symptoms*

19 B.3.24 Crotalinae Envenomation

Antivenin (complexation with venom)	**Antivenin Crotalidae polyvalent** (Wyeth)	*Ini 5-10vials IV in 250-500ml saline over 60-90min; rep if progressive edema*
Antivenin (complexation with venom)	**Crotalidae antivenin immune Fab** (CroFab)	*Ini 4-6 vials IV in 250ml saline over 60-90min; maint Tx: 2 vials q6h for 3 doses after ini control; rep for recurrent edema or coagulopathy prn*

19 B.3.25 Cyanide

Met-Hb-producer (cyanide binding to Met-Hb)	**Cyanide antidote kit** (amyl nitrite) (Taylor)	*Crush 1-2 ampules and place under nose for 30sec, rep x1 (produces approx 5% Met-Hb)*
then **Met-Hb-producer** (cyanide binding to Met-Hb)	**Cyanide antidote kit** (sodium nitrite) (Taylor)	*300mg (10ml of 3%) IV over 3-5min;* **Ped** *0.15-0.33ml/kg up to 10ml; adj based on Hb conc, can rep ½ dose (→ ca. 30% Met-Hb)*
then **Cyanide binding** (form Met-Hb ⇒ change into thiocyanate ⇒ cyanide elimination)	**Cyanide antidote kit** (sodium thiosulfate) (Taylor)	*12.5g (50ml of 25%) IV at 2.5-5ml/min;* **Ped** *400mg/kg (1.6ml/kg of 25%) IV up to 50ml, can rep ½ dose*

19 B.3.26 Cyclic Antidepressants

For arrhythmias

Buffer →18 (Tx of acidosis, binding of Na channel rec.↓, QRS↓)	**Sodium bicarbonate 8.4%** (50ml = 50mEq HCO₃⁻)	*1-2mEq/kg IV (pH to 7.45-7.55)*
Antiarrhythmic →37 Class Ib	**Lidocaine** (Gens)	*1mg/kg slowly IV*

In hypotension

Alpha- and Beta-Sympathomimetic, D1 receptor agonist →22 (pos. inotropic)	**Dopamine** (Intropin, Gens)	*10-15µg/kg/min IV (do not use beta agonists)*
Alpha-Sympathomimetic →18 (periph. resist.↑, BP↑)	**Norepinephrine** (Levophed)	*Ini 0.1µg/kg/min*

259.   Mackway-Jones (1999) J Accid Emerg Med 16:139-140

19 B.3.27 Ergot Derivatives

Direct vasodilator →31 (antihypertensive therapy)	**Sodium Nitroprusside** (Nipride, Nitropress)	*0.3µg/kg/min, titrate to effect, usual range 0.5 to 10µg/kg/min IV (only in very severe cases)*

19 B.3.28 Ethylene Glycol

Alcohol Dehydrogenase blocker →471 (competitive inhibition of alcohol dehydrogenase ⇒ metabolization↓)	**Fomepizole** (Antizol)	*Ini 15mg/kg IV over 30min, then: 10mg/kg q12h for 4 doses, then incr to 15mg/kg q12h until ethylene glycol levels are <20mg/dl*
Alcohol Dehydrogenase blocker →471 (competitive inhibition of alcohol dehydrogenase ⇒ metabolization↓)	**Ethanol**	*Ini 7.5ml/kg IV of 10% in dextrose 5% or 2ml/kg PO of 50%, then: 1-2ml/kg/h IV inf. or 0.2-0.4ml/kg/h PO maint. doses (aim for ethanol conc. 100mg/dl)*
Metabolism cofactor →145 (improve glyoxylic acid elimination)	**Pyridoxine** (=Vit. B6; Gens)	*50mg IV q6h*
	Thiamine (=Vit. B1; Gens)	*100mg IV q6h*

260.   Brent. (2000) Drugs 61:979-988

19 B.3.29 Heparin

Specific antidote →72 (reversal of heparin effects)	**Protamine** (Gens)	*1-1.5mg slowly IV per 100 IU heparin if immediately after heparin dose, ½ if 30-60min, ¼ if >2h (monitor PTT)*

19 B.3.30 Iron

Chelator →470 (iron elimination↑)	**Deferoxamine** (Desferal)	*15mg/kg/h IV, max: 6g q24h (avoid inf >24h)*
Whole bowel irrigation (⇒ poison elimination)	**PEG electrolyte solution**	*Adults: 2 l/h PO or NG until rectal effluent clear* **Ped** *35ml/kg/h*

261.   Tenenbein (1996) Clin Toxicol 34:485-489
262.   Howland (1996) Clin Toxicol 34:491-497

19 B.3.31 Lead

Chelator →470 (poison elimination↑)	**Dimercaprol** (BAL)	*3-5mg/kg IM q4-6h*
Chelator (poison elimination↑)	**Ethylendiamintetra-acetic acid** (Ca-disodium EDTA)	*1000-1500mg/m^2/d, as continuous inf. of 2-4mg/ml in D5W or NS for 5d (begin 4h after BAL if combined Tx)*
Chelator →471 (poison elimination↑)	**Succimer** (Chemet)	*10mg/kg PO tid for 5d, then 10mg/kg bid for 14d*

263.   Campbell (2000) Curr Opin Pediatr 12:428-437

19 B.3.32 Levothyroxine

Betablocker →23 (CO↓, neg. chronotropic, neg. inotropic, central sympathetic activity↓)	**Propranolol** (Inderal, Gens)	*40mg PO tid*

19 B.3.33 Lithium

Saline hydration (Replace fluid/electrolyte deficits ⇒ poison elimination)	**Saline 0.45–0.9%**	*Ini 1–2l 0.9% IV; Ch 10–20ml/kg; then 0.45% at normal maintenance*
Whole bowel irrigation (⇒ poison elimination)	**PEG electrolyte solution** (Golytely, Colyte)	*Adults: 2 l/h PO or NG until rectal effluent clear;* **Ped** *35ml/kg/h*

19 B.3.34 MAO Inhibitors

	Serotonin antagonist →408	**Cyproheptadine** (Periactin, Gens)	*4mg PO q1h up to 3 doses*
poss.	**Muscle relaxant** →298 (hyperthermia ↓)	**Dantrolene** (Dantrium)	*2.5mg/kg IV q6h*
	Alphablocker →30 (BP↓)	**Phentolamine** (Regitine, Rogitine, Gens)	*1–5mg IV bolus, rep q5–10min (to diastolic <100mmHg);* **Ped** *0.02–0.2mg/kg*

19 B.3.35 Mercury

Depending on whole blood or 24 hour urine mercury concentration

Chelator →471 (poison elimination↑)	**Succimer** (Chemet)	*10mg/kg PO tid for 5d, then 10mg/kg bid for 14d*

19 B.3.36 Metformin

Insulin/Dextrose →153 (therapy of acidosis)	**Insulin** (regular) **/Dextrose 5%**	*10–20 IU IV q4h with dextrose 5–12.5g IV q4h*
Glucose (for hypoglycemia)	**Glucose 50%, then Glucose 5%**	*Depending on BS*
Buffer →18 (therapy of acidosis)	**Sodium bicarbonate 8.4%** (50ml = 50 mEq HCO$_3$⁻)	*1–2mEq/kg IV*

264. Mishin (1998) N Engl J Med 338:265-266

19 B.3.37 Methanol

Alcohol Dehydrogenase blocker →471 (competitive inhibition of alcohol dehydrogenase ⇒ inhibition of metabolization)	**Fomepizole** (Antizol)	*Ini 15mg/kg IV over 30min, then: 10mg/kg q12h for 4 doses, then incr to 15mg/kg q12 until methanol levels are <20mg/dl*

Alcohol Dehydrogenase blocker →471 (competitive inhibition of alcohol dehydrogenase ⇒ inhibition of metabolization)	**Ethanol**	*Ini 7.5ml/kg IV of 10% in dextrose 5% or 2ml/kg PO of 50%, then: 1–2ml/kg/h IV inf. or 0.2–0.4ml/kg/h PO maint. doses (aim for ethanol conc. of 100mg/dl)*
To improve formic acid elimination →147	**Folic acid** (Folicet, Folvite, Gens) **Leucovorin Calcium** (Wellcovorin, Gens)	*Leucovorin 1mg/kg (up to 50 mg) IV q4h for 2 doses, then folic acid PO 1mg/kg q4-6h*

265.   Brent (2001) N Engl J Med 344:424-429

19 B.3.38 Methaemoglobin Causing Agents

Reduction of Met–Hb →471 (poison effects ↓)	**Methylene blue** (Gens)	*1–2mg/kg IV, may rep in 30-60min for 2 doses, max 15mg/kg. Maint (if needed) 1–2mg/kg q6-8h*

19 B.3.39 Methotrexate

Specific antidote (poison effects ↓)	**Leucovorin Calcium** (Wellcovorin, Gens)	*Same dose as MTX or 75mg IV then 12mg q12h for 4 doses (give within 1h of MTX); rep doses if 24h MTX level >0.1µM to total 12 doses*

19 B.3.40 Mushrooms (Cyclopeptide)

	Adsorbent →470 (interrupt enterohepatic recirculation)	**Activated charcoal** (Actidose, CharcoAid, Insta-Char, Liqui-Char)	*0.5g/kg q4h*
poss.	**Specific antidote** →187 (inhibition of toxin uptake into liver cells)	**Penicillin G** (Penicillin, Penicillin G Potassium, Pfizerpen, Gens)	*300,000–1 M IU/kg IV qd*

266.   Floersheim (1987) Med Toxicol 2:1-9

19 B.3.41 Neuroleptics/Antipsychotics

For ventricular arrhythmias

Buffer →18 (QRS ↓)	**Sodium bicarbonate 8.4%** (50ml = 50mEq HCO$_3$-)	*1–2mEq/kg IV (pH to 7.45-7.55)*
Antiarrhythmic →37 Class Ib	**Lidocaine** (Gens)	*1mg/kg IV bolus, then 1-4mg/min*

For hypotension

Alpha– and Beta-sympathomimetic, D1 receptor agonist →22 (pos. inotropic)	**Dopamine** (Intropin, Gens)	*Dopamine (Gens)*

| Alpha-sympatho-mimetic →18 (periph. resistance ↑, BP ↑) | **Norepinephrine** (Levophed) | *Ini 0.1µg/kg/min* |
| **Dopamine agonist** →295 (adjunct in NMS) | **Bromocriptine** (Parlodel) | *2.5-10mg PO or NG 2-6 times daily* |

19 B.3.42 Opiates

| **Opioid antagonist** →272 (opioid effects↓) | **Naloxone** (Narcan) | *0.4-2mg IV q2-3min continuous inf 0.4-0.8mg/h in 0.9% Na$^+$Cl$^-$ or D5W (long-acting opioids)* |
| **Opioid antagonist** →272 (opioid effects↓) | **Nalmefene** (Revex) | *0.25-0.5mg q2-5min IV until respiration restored; may require rep doses* |

267. Clarke (2002) Emerg Med J 19:249-250

19 B.3.43 Organophosphates

| **Direct parasympatholytic** →37 (cholinergic effects ↓) | **Atropine** (Atropen, Gens) | *1-5mg IV, poss rep q5-10min until atropinized (dry pulm secretions, reversal bronchospasm) with 5-10mg;* **Ped** *ini 0.02mg/kg* |
| **Cholinesterase activator** →471 (antidote) | **Pralidoxime** (2-PAM, Protopam) | *Ini-2g IV over 5-10min;* **Ped** *25-50mg/kg; maint 200-500mg/h as 1% solution;* **Ped** *5-10mg/kg/h* |

19 B.3.44 Quinine

Membrane stabilizing effects

| **Buffer** →18 (QRS↓) | **Sodium bicarbonate 8.4%** (50ml = 50mEq HCO$_3$-) | *1-2mEq/kg IV (pH to 7.45-7.55)* |
| **Benzodiazepine** →330 (anticonvulsant, antianxiety) | **Diazepam** (Valium, Gens) | *0.1-0.2mg/kg IV; may rep q1-4h prn* |

19 B.3.45 Serotonin Reuptake Inhibitors

| **Serotonin antagonist** →408 | **Cyproheptadine** (Periactin, Gens) | *4mg PO q1h up to 3 doses* |

268. Mills (1997) Med Toxicol 13:763-783

19 B.3.46 Sulfonylureas

Antidote →128 (insulin release↓)	**Octreotide** (Sandostatin)	*50µg SC or IV q12h;* **Ped** *1-10µg*

269.　McLaughlin (2000) Ann Emerg Med 36:133-138

19 B.3.47 Theophylline

Barbiturate →332 (seizure treatment/prophylaxis)	**Phenobarbital** (Luminal, Gens)	*2mg/kg slow IV, rep q15min up to 10-20mg/kg IV*
Benzodiazepine →330 (seizure treatment/prophylaxis)	**Diazepam** (Valium, Gens)	*0.1-0.2mg/kg IV; may rep q1-4h prn*
Betablocker →23 (HR↓, BP↑)	**Propranolol** (Inderal, Gens)	*1mg q2-5 in up to 5mg total IV;* **Ped** *0.1mg/kg IV up to 1mg*
Betablocker →23 (HR↓, BP↑)	**Esmolol** (Brevibloc)	*500µg/kg over 5min, then 50µg/kg/min for 4min; adj prn*

19 B.3.48 Valproic Acid

For encephalopathy with hyperammonemia

Antidote →470 (serum ammonia↓)	**L-carnitine** (Carnitor)	*150-500mg/kg IV up to 3g/d*

270.　Raskind (2000) Ann Pharmacother 34:630-638

19 B.3.49 Warfarin/Superwarfarins

Vitamin K →146 (Vit-K antagonism↓)	**Phytonadione** (Aquamephyton, Vitamin K1, Gens)	*10-25mg PO qd (50-200mg/d may be required), 0.6mg/kg IV;* **Ped** *5-10mg PO qd (in long-acting anticoagulant rodenticides poss. over months)*

19 B.3.50 Zinc

Chelator (poison elimination↑)	**Ethylendiamintetra-acetic acid** (Ca-disodium EDTA)	*1000-1500mg/m^2/d, as cont. Inf of 2-4mg/ml in D5W or NS for 5d (ini 4h after BAL if combined Tx)*
Chelator →470 (poison elimination↑)	**Dimercaprol** (BAL)	*3-5mg/kg IM q4-6h*

Notes

Notes

Notes

Notes

Notes

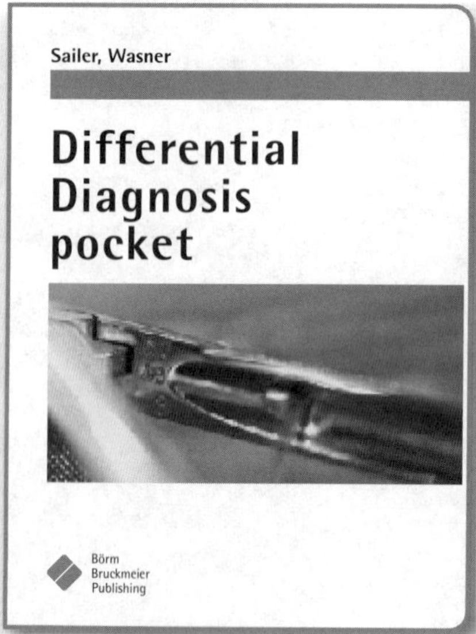

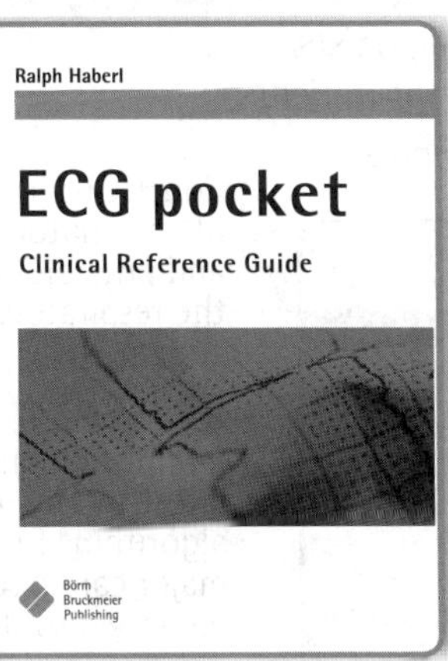

ISBN 1-59103-202-4 $12.95

- Handy reference for identifying common ECG findings

- Top-quality collection of numerous digital 12-lead ECGs

- Provides a quick reference section and a standardized ECG evaluation sheet

- For students, residents and all other health care professionals

Also available as PDA software!

ECG pocket for PDA
(670 kb, US $ 24.95)

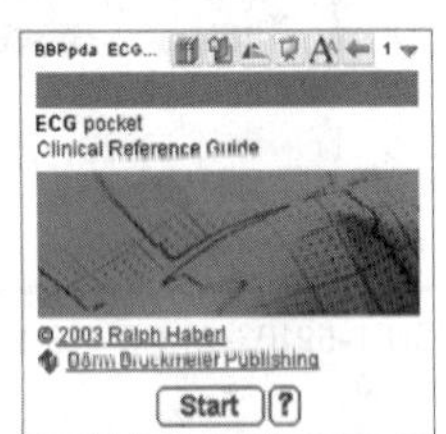

Respiratory pocket

For medical doctors, pulmonologists, respiratory therapists, medical students, and all healthcare professionals

Bajraktarević, Jakob

Respiratory pocket

Clinical Reference Guide

Börm
Bruckmeier
Publishing

ISBN 1-59103-218-0 $ 14.95

- Concise overviews of the anatomy and physiology of the respiratory system

- Assessment, monitoring and latest treatment algorithms for all major cardiopulmonary disorders

- Cites widely used guidelines and statements from major medical organizations and journals

- Superb coverage of respiratory support techniques

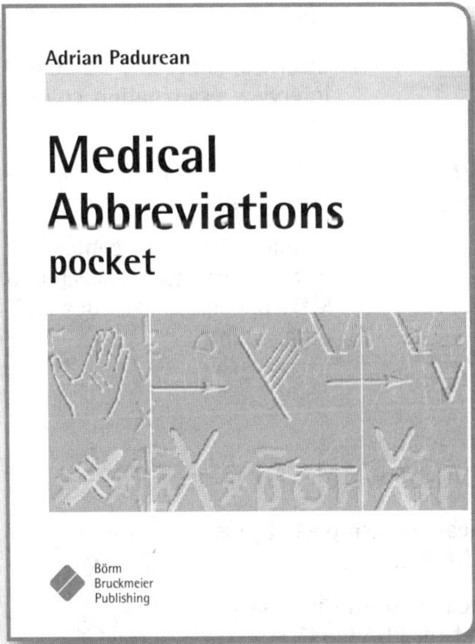

Medical Spanish pocket plus

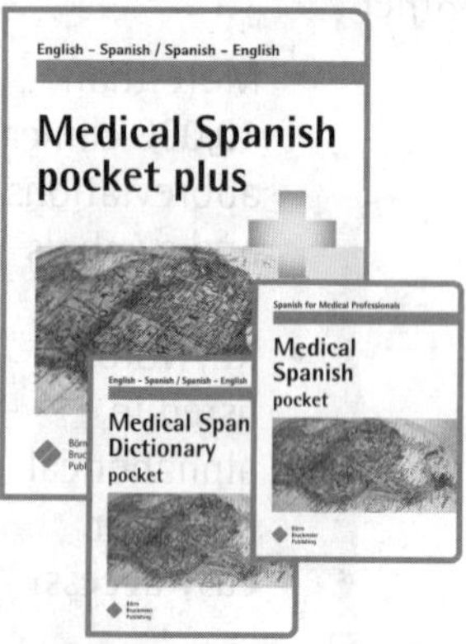

Medical Spanish pocket plus
ISBN 1-59103-213-X, US $ 22.95

- Includes contents of both
  Medical Spanish pocket and
  Medical Spanish Dictionary
  pocket

- Vital communication tool

- Clearly organized by situation:
  interview, examination, course
  of visit

- Accurate translations for almost
  every health-related term

- Bilingual dictionary contains
  medical terminology specific to
  Mexico, Puerto Rico, Cuba and
  other countries

Also available as PDA software!

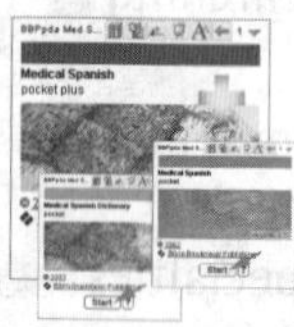

Medical Spanish pocket plus
for PDA (2487 kb)

Medical Spanish Dictionary
pocket for PDA (2343 kb)

Medical Spanish pocket
for PDA (670 kb)

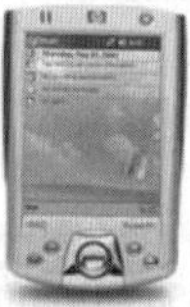

Börm Bruckmeier Publishing
PO Box 388
Ashland, OH 44805

Phone: 888-322-6657
Fax: 419-281-6883

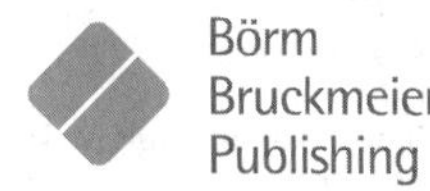

Name		E-mail	
Address			
City		State	Zip

Subtotal

Sales Tax, add only for: CA 8%; OH 6.25%

+ **Sales Tax**

Shipping & Handling for US address:
UPS Standard: 10% of subtotal with a minimum of $5.00
UPS 2nd Day Air: 20% of subtotal with a minimum of $8.00

+ **S & H**

= **Total**

Credit Card: ☐ Visa ☐ Mastercard ☐ Amex ☐ Discover
Card Number

Exp. Date   Signature

For foreign orders, quantity rebate, optional shipping and payment please inquire:
service@media4u.com

Börm Bruckmeier Products

pockets

	COPIES		PRICE/COPIES		PRICE
Anatomy pocket		X	US $ 14.95	=	
Canadian Drug pocket		X	US $ 14.95	=	
Differential Diagnosis pocket		X	US $ 14.95	=	
Drug pocket 2005		X	US $ 12.95	=	
Drug pocket plus 2004–2005		X	US $ 24.95	=	
Drug Therapy pocket 2003–2004		X	US $ 14.95	=	
ECG pocket		X	US $ 14.95	=	
EMS pocket		X	US $ 14.95	=	
Homeopathy pocket		X	US $ 14.95	=	
Medical Abbreviations pocket		X	US $ 12.95	=	
Medical Spanish pocket		X	US $ 12.95	=	
Medical Spanish Dictionary pocket		X	US $ 14.95	=	
Medical Spanish pocket plus		X	US $ 22.95	=	
Normal Values pocket		X	US $ 12.95	=	
Respiratory pocket		X	US $ 14.95	=	

pocketcards

	COPIES		PRICE/COPIES		PRICE
Antibiotics pocketcard 2005		X	US $ 3.95	=	
Antifungals pocketcard		X	US $ 3.95	=	
BLS/ALS pocketcard		X	US $ 3.95	=	
ECG pocketcard		X	US $ 3.95	=	
ECG Evaluation pocketcard		X	US $ 3.95	=	
ECG Ruler pocketcard		X	US $ 3.95	=	
ECG pocketcard Set (3)		X	US $ 9.95	=	
Emergency Drugs pocketcard		X	US $ 3.95	=	
H&P pocketcard		X	US $ 3.95	=	
Medical Abbreviations pocketcard Set (2)		X	US $ 6.95	=	
Medical Spanish pocketcard		X	US $ 3.95	=	
Neurology pocketcard (2)		X	US $ 6.95	=	
Normal Values pocketcard		X	US $ 3.95	=	
Periodic Table pocketcard		X	US $ 3.95	=	

= Subtotal